Current Trends in
Histocompatibility

VOLUME 1
IMMUNOGENETIC AND MOLECULAR PROFILES

CURRENT TRENDS IN HISTOCOMPATIBILITY

Volume 1 **Immunogenetic and Molecular Profiles**

Volume 2 **Biological and Clinical Concepts**

Current Trends in Histocompatibility

VOLUME 1
IMMUNOGENETIC AND MOLECULAR PROFILES

Edited by

Ralph A. Reisfeld
and
Soldano Ferrone

Scripps Clinic and Research Foundation
La Jolla, California

PLENUM PRESS • NEW YORK AND LONDON

Library of Congress Cataloging in Publication Data

Main entry under title:

Current trends in histocompatibility.

Includes index.
CONTENTS: v. 1. Immunogenetic and molecular profiles. – v. 2. Biological and clinical concepts.
1. Histocompatibility. 2. HLA histocompatibility antigens. I. Reisfeld, Ralph A. II. Ferrone, Soldano, 1940-
QR184.3.C87 616.07'9 80-18211

ISBN 978-1-4684-3760-7 ISBN 978-1-4684-3758-4 (eBook)
DOI 10.1007/978-1-4684-3758-4

Softcover reprint of the hardcover 1st edition 1981

A Division of Plenum Publishing Corporation
233 Spring Street, New York, N. Y. 10013

Contributors

D. Albrechtsen, The Tissue Typing Laboratory, Rikshospitalet (The National Hospital), Oslo, Norway

D.B. Amos, Division of Immunology, Department of Microbiology, Duke University Medical Center, Durham, North Carolina 27710

Peter E. Andreotti, Division of Immunology, Department of Microbiology and Immunology, Duke University Medical Center, Durham, North Carolina 27710

John R. Apgar, Division of Immunology, Department of Microbiology and Immunology, Duke University Medical Center, Durham, North Carolina 27710

Kirk W. Beisel, Department of Immunology, Mayo Clinic and Medical School, Rochester, Minnesota 55901

J. Donald Capra, Department of Microbiology, University of Texas Southwestern Medical School, Dallas, Texas 75235

John E. Coligan, Laboratory of Immunogenetics, National Institutes of Health, Bethesda, Maryland

Jacques M. Colombani, U 93 INSERM, Institute de Recherches sur les Maladies du Sang, Hôpital Saint-Louis, 75475 Paris Cedex 10, France

Richard G. Cook, Department of Microbiology, University of Texas Southwestern Medical School, Dallas, Texas 75235

Peter Cresswell, Division of Immunology, Department of Microbiology and Immunology, Duke University Medical Center, Durham, North Carolina 27710

Susan E. Cullen, Department of Microbiology and Immunology, Washington University School of Medicine, St. Louis, Missouri 63110

Hélène Dastot, U 93 ISERM, Institut de Recherches sur les Maladies du Sang, Hopital Saint-Louis, 75475 Paris Cedex 10, France

Jean Dausset, Research Unit INSERM U93, Centre Hayem, Hôpital Saint-Louis, 75475 Paris Cedex 10, France

Chella S. David, Department of Immunology, Mayo Clinic and Medical School, Rochester, Minnesota 55901

Laurent Degos, U 93 INSERM, Institut de Recherches sur les Maladies du Sang, Hôpital Saint-Louis, 75475 Paris Cedex 10, France

Victor H. Engelhard, Biological Laboratories, Harvard University, Cambridge, Massachusetts 02138

Bruce M. Ewenstein, Department of Microbiology and Immunology and Department of Cell Biology, Albert Einstein College of Medicine, Bronx, New York 10461

Soldano Ferrone, Department of Immunology, Scripps Clinic and Research Foundation, La Jolla, California 92037

Hilliard Festenstein, Department of Immunology, The London Hospital Medical College, London E1, 2AD, England

Jiří Forejt, Institute of Molecular Genetics, Czechoslovak Academy of Sciences, 142 20 Prague 4, Czechoslovakia

Braydon C. Guild, Biological Laboratories, Harvard University, Cambridge, Massachusetts 02138

R. Hartzman, Department of Pediatrics, Division of Immunologic Oncology, Georgetown University School of Medicine, Washington, D.C. 20007; and the Naval Medical Research Institute, Bethesda, Maryland 20014.

P. Ivânyi, Central Laboratory, Netherlands Red Cross Blood Transfusion Service; Laboratory of Experimental and Clinical Immunology, University of Amsterdam, Amsterdam, The Netherlands

A.H. Johnson, Department of Pediatrics, Division of Immunologic-Oncology, Georgetown University School of Medicine, Washington, D.C. 20007

Olle Kämpe, Department of Cell Research, The Wallenberg Laboratory, University of Uppsala, S-751 22 Uppsala, Sweden

Daljit Kaur, Division of Blood and Blood Products, Bureau of Biologics, Food and Drug Administration, Bethesda, Maryland 20205

Cathy S. Kindle, Department of Microbiology and Immunology, Washington University School of Medicine, St. Louis, Missouri 63110

Thomas J. Kindt, Laboratory of Immunogenetics, National Institutes of Health, Bethesda, Maryland

Jan Klein, Department of Immunogenetics, Max-Planck-Institute for Biology, Tübingen, West Germany

Thomas G. Kostyk, Biological Laboratories, Harvard University, Cambridge, Massachusetts 02138

Christopher J. Krco, Department of Immunology, Mayo Clinic and Medical School, Rochester, Minnesota 55901

William P. Lafuse, Department of Immunology, Mayo Clinic and Medical School, Rochester, Minnesota 55901

Doron Lancet, Biological Laboratories, Harvard University, Cambridge, Massachusetts 02138

Virginia Lepage, U 93 INSERM, Institute de Recherches sur les Maladies du Sang, Hôpital Saint-Louis, 75475 Paris Cedex 10, France

Pierre Lethielleux, U 93 INSERM, Institut de Recherches sur les Maladies du Sang, Hôpital Saint-Louis, 75475 Paris Cedex 10, France

José A. Lopez de Castro, Biological Laboratories, Harvard University, Cambridge, Massachusetts 02138

Dean L. Mann, Immunology Branch, National Cancer Institute, National Institutes of Health, Bethesda, Maryland 20205

M. Louise Markert, Division of Immunology, Department of Microbiology and Immunology, Duke University Medical Center, Durham, North Carolina 27710

John M. Martinko, Department of Microbiology and Immunology and Department of Cell Biology, Albert Einstein College of Medicine, Bronx, New York 10461

I.F.C. McKenzie, Department of Medicine, Austin Hospital, Heidelberg, Victoria 3084, Australia

Kamal K. Mittal, Division of Blood and Blood Products, Bureau of Biologics, Food and Drug Administration, Bethesda, Maryland 20205

Stanley G. Nathenson, Department of Microbiology and Immunology and Department of Cell Biology, Albert Einstein College of Medicine, Bronx, New York 10461

Ah-Kau Ng, Department of Immunology, Scripps Clinic and Research Foundation, La Jolla, California 92037

Harry T. Orr, Biological Laboratories, Harvard University, Cambridge, Massachusetts 02138

Peter Parham, Biological Laboratories, Harvard University, Cambridge, Massachusetts 02138

C.R. Parish, Department of Microbiology, John Curtin School of Medical Research, Australian National University, Canberra, A.C.T. 2601, Australia

Michele A. Pellegrino, Department of Molecular Immunology, Scripps Clinic and Research Foundation, La Jolla, California 92037

Per A. Peterson, Department of Cell Research, The Wallenberg Laboratory, University of Uppsala, S-751 22 Uppsala, Sweden

Hidde L. Ploegh, Biological Laboratories, Harvard University, Cambridge, Massachusetts 02138

Jordan S. Pober, Biological Laboratories, Harvard University, Cambridge, Massachusetts 02138

David Pressman, Department of Immunology Research, Roswell Park Memorial Institute, Buffalo, New York 14263

Vito Quaranta, Department of Immunology, Scripps Clinic and Research Foundation, La Jolla, California 92037

Muriel Reboul, U 93 INSERM, Institut de Recherches sur les Maladies du Sang, Hôpital Saint-Louis, 75475 Paris Cedex 10, France

Ralph A. Reisfeld, Department of Molecular Immunology, Scripps Clinic and Research Foundation, La Jolla, California 92037

Stephen M. Rose, Department of Microbiology and Immunology, Washington University School of Medicine, St. Louis, Missouri 63110

Wilhelm Schmidt, Department of Immunology, The London Hospital Medical College, London E1, 2AD, England

Jack Silver, Department of Cellular and Developmental Immunology, Scripps Clinic and Research Foundation, La Jolla, California 92037

B.G. Solheim, The Tissue Typing Laboratory, Rikshospitalet (The National Hospital), Oslo, Norway

Jack L. Strominger, Biological Laboratories, Harvard University, Cambridge, Massachusetts 02138

Nobuhiko Tada, Department of Immunology Research, Roswell Park Memorial Institute, Buffalo, New York 14263; present address: Memorial Sloan-Kettering Institute for Cancer Research, New York, New York 10021

Nobuyuki Tanigaki, Department of Immunology Research, Roswell Park Memorial Institute, Buffalo, New York 14263

Carla Testorelli, Department of Immunology, The London Hospital Medical College, London E1, 2AD, England; present address: Istituto di Farmacologia, Milan, Italy

E. Thorsby, The Tissue Typing Laboratory, Rikshospitalet (The National Hospital), Oslo, Norway

Hiroshi Uehara, Department of Microbiology and Immunology and Department of Cell Biology, Albert Einstein College of Medicine, Bronx, New York 10461

Jonathan W. Uhr, Department of Microbiology, University of Texas Southwestern Medical School, Dallas, Texas 75235

*Ellen S. Vitetta,*Department of Microbiology, University of Texas Southwestern Medical School, Dallas, Texas 75235

Edward K. Wakeland, Department of Immunogenetics, Max-Planck-Institute for Biology, Tübingen, West Germany

Leslie E. Walker, Department of Molecular Immunology, Scripps Clinic and Research Foundation, La Jolla, California 92037

Barry S. Wilson, Department of Immunology, Scripps Clinic and Research Foundation, La Jolla, California 92037

Preface

Information about histocompatibility antigens is expanding so rapidly that it is difficult to remain abreast of all advances. In these volumes, we have made an effort to bring together the most current work on topics that have generated most of the recent advances and discussions. We have asked each author to present and interpret his most current work, and we have judiciously refrained from imposing our own prejudices and viewpoints. Although there is obvious overlap in some individual topics, we have encouraged this to provide the reader with as many different and sometimes opposing viewpoints as possible. This approach will, we hope, give a broad overview of current ideas in the field.

We wish to thank all contributors for their timely and exciting manuscripts, and we sincerely hope that the reader will benefit from these volumes.

R.A. Reisfeld
S. Ferrone

La Jolla

Contents

I. Serology and Genetics

Chapter 1

Studies of HLA-DR Antigens by Complement Fixation

Jacques M. Colombani, Laurent Degos, Virginia Lepage, Hélène Dastot, Muriel Reboul, and Pierre Lethielleux

Chapter 2
Serological and Cellular Recognition of Human Histocompatibility Antigens

Peter Cresswell, Peter E. Andreotti, John R. Apgar, and M. Louise Markert

Chapter 3
Are D and DR Two Distinct Entities?

Jean Dausset

Chapter 4
Genetic Organization, Tissue Expression, and Functional Role of Murine Ia Antigens

Chella S. David, Kirk W. Beisel, Christopher J. Krco, and William P. Lafuse

Chapter 5
Expression of Syngeneic and Allogeneic H-2 Antigens on Tumor Cells

Hilliard Festenstein, Wilhelm Schmidt, and Carla Testorelli

Chapter 6

Hybrid Sterility Gene Located in the *T/t–H-2* Supergene on Chromosome 17

Jiří Forejt

Chapter 7

Interspecies MHS Relationships Studied by Serological and Cellular Cross-Reactions

P. Ivânyi

Chapter 8

The *DR* Region of *HLA:* Serological Analysis

A.H. Johnson, R. Hartzman, and D.B. Amos

Chapter 9

The Genetics of B-Cell Alloantigens

Dean L. Mann

Chapter 10

Serological Testing of the HLA Antigens: Problems and Approaches to Standardization

Kamal K. Mittal and Daljit Kaur

Chapter 11

Carbohydrate-Defined Antigens Controlled by the *I* Region

C.R. Parish and I.F.C. McKenzie

Chapter 13

The Polymorphism of *I*-Region-Encoded Antigens among Wild Mice

Edward K. Wakeland and Jan Klein

Chapter 14

HLA Polyclonal and Monoclonal Xenoantibodies: Production, Characterization, and Application to the Study of HLA Antigens

Barry S. Wilson, Ah-Kau Ng, Vito Quaranta, and Soldano Ferrone

II. Chemistry

Chapter 16

Ia Antigens: Molecular Components in Immune Regulation?

Susan E. Cullen, Stephen M. Rose, and Cathy S. Kindle

Chapter 17

Structure of H-2 Major Histocompatibility Complex Products: Recent Studies on the H-2K^b Glycoprotein and on the H-2K^b MHC Mutants

Stanley G. Nathenson, Bruce M. Ewenstein, Hiroshi Uehara, John M. Martinko, John E. Coligan, and Thomas J. Kindt

Chapter 18

Are the Classic Transplantation Antigens Primitive Cell-Surface Antibodies?

Per A. Peterson and Olle Kämpe

Chapter 19

Functional Implications of the Structural Diversity of Murine Ia and Human DR Antigens

Jack Silver

Chapter 20

Complete Primary Structure of Human Histocompatibility Antigen HLA-B7: Its Evolutionary and Functional Implications

Jack L. Strominger, Victor H. Engelhard, Braydon C. Guild, Thomas G. Kostyk, Doron Lancet, José A. Lopez de Castro, Harry T. Orr, Peter Parham, Hidde L. Ploegh, and Jordan S. Pober

Chapter 21

Antigenic Structures of HLA(A,B,C) Antigens: Chymotryptic Glycopeptides Carrying HLA(A,B,C) Determinants

Nobuyuki Tanigaki, Nobuhiko Tada, and David Pressman

Chapter 22

Structural Analysis of HLA-DR Antigens

Leslie E. Walker, Soldano Ferrone, Michele A. Pellegrino, and Ralph A. Reisfeld

I

SEROLOGY AND GENETICS

1

Studies of HLA-DR Antigens by Complement Fixation

Jacques M. Colombani, Laurent Degos, Virginia Lepage, Hélène Dastot, Muriel Reboul, and Pierre Lethielleux

1. Introduction

It was previously shown (Colombani *et al.*, 1977) that HLA-DR antigens could be detected by complement-fixation (CF) microtechnique on peripheral-blood B lymphocytes (PBBL), on peripheral-blood lymphocytes (PBL) stimulated by mitogens [phytohemagglutinin (PHA), concanavalin A (Con A), pokeweed mitogen (PWM)], and on cultured B-lymphoid lines (BLL).

We report here the results of a systematic research of complement-fixing anti-HLA-DR antibodies, showing that DR typing can be done by CF. The induction of DR antigens on PBL by mitogen stimulation and the relative DR antigenic contents of various cell types were also studied.

2. Material and Methods

The CF microtechnique was performed as previously described (Colombani *et al.*, 1971) (Table 1). PBL were obtained from whole blood by flotation on Ficoll–Isopaque (Boyum, 1974). B-enriched suspensions were prepared from PBL by elimination of lymphocytes that formed rosettes with sheep erythrocytes (Mendes *et al.*, 1973). T-enriched sus-

Jacques M. Colombani, Laurent Degos, Virginia Lepage, Hélène Dastot, Muriel Reboul, and Pierre Lethielleux • U 93 INSERM, Institut de Recherches sur les Maladies du Sang, Hôpital Saint-Louis, 75475 Paris Cedex 10, France.

TABLE 1. Complement-Fixation Microtechnique[a]

• Antibody (serum dilution or eluate)	2 μl
• Antigen preparation (cell suspension)[b]	2 μl
• Human complement diluted (2 100% hemolytic units in 2 μl)	2 μl
Mix[c] and incubate 1 hr at 37°C.	
• Sensititized sheep RBC (200,000/μ l)	2 μl
Mix[c] and incubate 30 min at 37°C.	
Centrifuge[d] and read.[e]	

[a]The test is made in microtest tissue culture plate under 6 ml viscous paraffin. Specially ordered nontreated (i.e., nonwettable) Greiner–Cooke microplates give better results than the standard (wettable) plates.

[b]Cell suspensions are made in saline supplemented with 0.1% N_3Na and 2% heat-inactivated normal human AB serum. The following cell concentrations were generally used: PBL, 15,000/μl; PHA-PBL, 5000–10,000/μl.

[c]Mixing is obtained by the vibrations produced when the plate is firmly held for 15 sec on the rotating cup of a Vortex mixer. Mixing is particularly important during the incubation with sensitized sheep RBC. It must be repeated twice during that time.

[d]Centrifugation can be done in Microtiter centrifuge carriers at 700*g* for 3 min.

[e]Reading can be done by placing the tray on a white-lighted serology reading box.

pensions were prepared from the lymphocytes not retained by a nylon wool column charged with PBL (Julius *et al.*, 1973). Cell cultures were made with RPMI 1640 or 199 medium (GIBCO) supplemented with antibiotics and 25% autologous plasma, in plastic culture vials standing upright and incubated at 37°C in a humidified 5% CO_2–air atmosphere.

3. Results and Discussion

3.1. Screening for Anti-HLA-DR Complement-Fixing Sera

This was done either from anti-HLA-A, -B hyperimmune sera or from sera containing relatively weak anti-HLA-A, -B antibodies (Table 2). A panel of 28 BLL or PHA-PBL from 9 donors were used as target cells. The results showed the high frequency (60%) of anti-DR antibodies associated with anti-HLA-A, -B in hyperimmune sera. On the other hand, 9–25% of the parous-women sera contained anti-DR antibodies with titers higher than those of anti HLA-A, -B antibodies. This was shown by screening parous-women sera by the CF technique against platelets and BLL; 25% of the sera reacted only against BLL. Their reactivity could not be absorbed on platelets, showing that it was not due to anti-HLA-A, -B antibodies. Another series of parous-women sera was screened against platelets, PBL, and PHA-PBL from a panel of 9 donors. In each case, an optimal number of cells were used: 1 × 10^6 platelets, 30,000 PBL, and 20,000 PHA-PBL; 9% of the sera reacted only with PHA-PBL. The reactivity was not abolished by absorption on platelets. These sera could thus

TABLE 2. Screening for Complement-Fixing Anti-HLA-DR Antibodies among Anti-HLA-A, -B Sera

Origin of sera	Anti-HLA-A, -B immunization[a]	Screening by CF against[b]	Frequency of anti-HLA-DR antibodies
Multitransfused patients	Strong PlCF Pos 1:5–1:500 LCT Pos 1:5–1:5000	28 BLL	68/113 (60%) positive after absorption on platelets
Parous women	Weak to mild PlCF Neg 1:5 LCT Pos 1:1–1:5	28 BLL	37/149 (25%) positive against BLL
Parous women	Same	Platelets, PBL, PHA-PBL from 9 panel donors	10/115 (9%) positive against PHA-PBL only

[a](PlCF) Platelet complement-fixation technique; (LCT) lymphocytotoxicity technique.
[b](BLL) B-lymphoid lines; (PBL) peripheral blood lymphocytes; (PHA-PBL) PHA-stimulated PBL.

be employed without the platelet absorption usually performed to remove anti-HLA-A, -B antibodies. This was true even for sera containing weak anti-HLA-A, -B antibodies detectable only with the lymphocytotoxicity (LCT) technique, which was about 5 times more sensitive than CF.

The higher percentage of positive sera found against BLL than against PHA-PBL (25 vs. 9%) could be explained by the higher reactivity of the former cells already observed with the LCT technique (Bodmer, 1978).

TABLE 3. HLA-DR Specificities Recognized by Complement Fixation on Phytohemagglutinin-Stimulated Peripheral Blood Lymphocytes[a]

Serum (dil)/antigen	++	+−	−+	−−	Total	χ^2	r
776 (1:5)/DRw5	48	5	12	131	196	122.9	0.8
BOUR (1:10)/DRw7	49	3	3	141	196	166.4	0.9
GABI (1:5)/DRw7	49	3	3	141	196	166.4	0.9
458 (1:5)/DRw2	51	8	5	132	196	138.5	0.8
ESMA (1:40)/DRw3+7	70	0	8	118	196	164.7	0.9
2298 (1:80)/DRw2+6	18	0	5	21	44	27.8	0.8
2384 (1:20)/DRw2+5+6	22	2	6	14	44	17.9	0.6
GUIM (1:10)/DRw4	7	14[b]	0	23	44	9.1	0.5
5097 (1:5)/DRw3+5	9	1	4	30	44	22.7	0.7
1079 (1:5)/DRw5	7	3	2	32	44	19.5	0.7

[a]In each test, 20,000 cultured cells were used. The BOUR, GABI, and ESMA sera were absorbed on platelets; the other sera were used unabsorbed. Comparisons are with DR specificities as defined by the LCT technique against B-enriched PBL.
[b]Ten of these cells carried a *DRw* blank allele.

Among the 115 reactive sera from the three series, 46 were extensively tested on PHA-PBL from two panels, one of 44 and the other of 196 donors, typed for HLA-DR by LCT on PBBL with 7th Histocompatibility Workshop sera (Bodmer *et al.*, 1978) and local sera. Table 3 shows the specificities recognized by the 10 best sera. The results confirmed that CF on PHA-PBL could be used for HLA-DR typing.

3.2. Expression of HLA-A, -B and -DR Antigens on Peripheral Blood Lymphocytes during Phytohemagglutinin Stimulation

The kinetics of the phenomenon are shown in Table 4. The effect of the dose of PHA is shown in Table 5. DRw7 reactivity appeared rapidly and increased during the culture in the presence of PHA, up to a peak of reactivity at days 3–4. The same evolution was observed for the control HLA-A9 antigen. A weak expression of DRw7 was apparent in the control culture without PHA. The results suggested an increase of the reactivity per cell possibly related to their increased size, as shown by the augmentation of HLA-A9. The weak DR reactivity of the cells cultured without PHA also suggested that the antigens became more accessible to their antibodies on cultured cells than on freshly prepared cells. But the high DR reactivity of the PBL cultured in the presence of PHA could be explained only by the proliferation or the selection, or both, of a cell population carrying a large number of the appropriate antigenic sites.

An attempt was made to identify this cell population. PBL and en-

TABLE 4. HLA-A9 and DRw7 Antigen Reactivity in Complement Fixation of Peripheral Blood Lymphocytes before and during Short-Term Culture with or without Phytohemagglutinin

	Days of culture					
Expt.[a]	0	1	2	3	4	5
Expt. A						
cpm[b]	0.2	5.4	18.3	20.1	9.4	10.8
A9[c]	16	4	2	1	1	2
DRw7[c]	>32	4	2	1	1	2
Expt. B						
cpm[b]	0.2	0.7	0.4	0.5	0.4	0.4
A9[c]	16	16	16	32	32	>32
DRw7[c]	>32	16	16	32	16	16

[a]PBL were cultured for the indicated periods with (Expt. A) or without (Expt. B) PHA. The cells were then assayed for their A9 (23) or DRw7 antigenic reactivity.
[b][^{3}H]Thymidine incorporation (cpm × 10^3).
[c]Minimum number of cells per test (× 10^3) giving a positive result.

TABLE 5. Expression of HLA-DR Antigen on Phytohemagglutinin-Stimulated Peripheral Blood Lymphocytes[a]: Role of the Dose of Phytohemagglutinin

	PHA dose (μl)						
	0	250	500	750	1000	2000	4000
cpm[b]	0.2	5.6	22.0	36.8	25.2	21.2	29.6
Score[c]	15	57	100	94	80	80	67

[a]Donor A26, A33, B15, B17, DRw7.
[b][^{3}H]Thymidine incorporation (cpm × 10^3).
[c]The score was calculated from the number and intensity (1–4+) of positive reactions with a battery of 31 anti-DR sera. The results are expressed as the percentage of maximum reactivity.

riched B- and T-lymphocyte populations were cultured with PHA and assayed for their HLA-DR antigenic content (Table 6). DRw5 increased significantly on PBL and B-cell populations but not on T-cell populations. The results indicated either that DR antigens could be PHA-induced only when mixed populations (B + T) were used or that the cells expressing DR were not T lymphoblasts but possibly B lymphoblasts conjointly stimulated by the T mitogen in the presence of T cells (Phillips and Roitt, 1973; Brochier *et al.*, 1976; Han and Dadey, 1978), or that both conditions obtained. The role of monocytes, which also carry HLA-DR specificities, was not clearly evaluated in these experiments.

3.3. Expression of HLA-A, -B and -DR Antigens on Peripheral Blood Lymphocytes during Concanavalin A Stimulation

The same augmentation of HLA antigen expression was observed with both Con A and PHA stimulation. But when an excess of Con A was used (Table 7), HLA-DR antigen expression decreased while that of

TABLE 6. Effect of Phytohemagglutinin or HLA-DR Expression on Various Cell Populations[a]

	Before culture			After 3 days' culture with PHA		
	PBL	B	T	PBL	B	T
cpm[b]	—	—	—	36.6	4.5	21.9
Surface Ig (%)	18.3	81.9	2.8	—	—	—
DRw5[c]	>60	20	>60	10	5	>40

[a](PBL) Peripheral blood lymphocytes; (B) B-enriched after elimination of T rosettes; (T) T-enriched after elimination of nylon-adherent cells.
[b][^{3}H]Thymidine incorporation (cpm × 10^3).
[c]Minimum number of cells per test (× 10^3) giving a positive result.

TABLE 7. Variation of HLA-DR Antigenic Reactivity on Con-A-Stimulated Peripheral Blood Lymphocytes: Role of the Dose of Con A

	PHA	Con A (μl)							
	(750 μl)	2.5	5	10	25	50	100	150	200
cpm[a]	8.35	1.7	2.35	5.15	8.4	7.2	8.15		10.35
DR score[b]	100	92	95	98	87	71	45	5	2
DRw2[b]	100	100				82			32
DRw7[b]	100	100				93			17
A3[b]	94	100				88			76
B7[b]	100	84				76			100

[a][^{3}H]Thymidine incorporation (cpm × 10^3).
[b]Results are expressed as the precentage of maximum reactivity either with a battery of 31 anti-DR sera (DR score) or with specific anti-HLA-A, -B and -DR sera.

HLA-A, -B remained stable. This phenomenon was not observed during PHA stimulation (see Table 5). These results suggested the possibility that low or high doses of Con A could stimulate different cell populations distinguished by the DR markers but all carrying the HLA-A, -B markers.

3.4. Expression of HLA-A, -B and -DR Antigens on Peripheral Blood Lymphocytes during Stimulation by a Specific Antigen

PBL from a donor sensitized to tuberculin were cultured with this antigen. This specific stimulation induced the same increase of HLA antigen expression as PHA and Con A (Table 8).

TABLE 8. Role of Cell Proliferation Induced by Specific Antigen in Culture in the Expression of HLA-A, -B and -DR Specificity

	PBL before culture[a]	PBL cultured with[a]			
		0	PPD 50	PPD 250	PHA 750
cpm[b]	—	0.36	15.55	20.57	—
A2	3.75	7	2.5	2.5	2
B5	2	5	2	2	2
DRw2	>60	20 (weak)	5	2	2.5
DR score	—	17	49	66	100

[a]PBL before culture; after 5 days' culture with 0, 50, or 250 units of tuberculin purified protein derivative (PPD); or after 3 days' culture with 750 μl PHA were assayed for their antigenic reactivity either with anti-HLA-A, -B and -DR specific antibodies [results expressed as the minimum number of cells (× 10^3) giving a positive test] or with a battery of 31 anti-DR sera (DR score: results expressed as the percentage of maximum reactivity).
[b][^{3}H]Thymidine incorporation (cpm × 10^3).

All experiments using PBL stimulated in culture showed the same striking increase of HLA-DR antigen expression. This was unexpected, since DR antigens were expressed essentially on B lymphocytes, whereas all stimulations were directed mainly at T lymphocytes. The experiment with PHA mentioned above suggested that the reactive cells were not only T lymphoblasts but also B lymphoblasts and/or B lymphocytes and/or monocytes. On the other hand, the reactivity observed was very high, suggesting that the subpopulation involved represented a substantial fraction of the total cultured-cell population. Experiments designed to isolate and identify the reactive and nonreactive cells are in progress.

3.5. Relative Reactivity of Various Cell Populations for HLA-A, -B and DR Specificities

It is possible in CF to test a single immune serum against various substrates. A direct comparison of the relative reactivities of the substrates can thus be made. Such a comparison was made for HLA-A2 specificity on three different substrates (Table 9). The results show that HLA-A2 was detected in about the same way on the three substrates when they were used at optimal doses: 1×10^6 platelets per test, 3×10^4 PBL per test, and $1–2 \times 10^4$ PHA-PBL per test. It was thus possible to screen sera against platelets and PHA-PBL simultaneously. Sera reacting against both substrates would contain anti-HLA-A, -B antibodies, and possibly anti-HLA-DR antibodies. Sera reacting only against PHA-PBL would contain anti-HLA-DR antibodies, and possibly weak anti-HLA-A, -B antibodies. Similar results were obtained when PBL or peripheral-blood T lymphocytes (PBTL) (3×10^4 cells per test) were used instead of platelets for the screening of anti HLA-A, -B antibodies.

An evaluation of the reactivity of various cell populations was made by determining the minimum reacting dose. This was done for HLA-A2 and DRw2 as shown in Tables 9 and 10. Small variations were observed

TABLE 9. Relative Reactivity of Various Cell Substrates[a] in Complement Fixation for HLA-A2 Specificity

	Platelets ($\times 10^6$)			PBL ($\times 10^4$)			PHA-PBL ($\times 10^4$)		
	2	1	0.5	6	3	1.5	4	2	1
HLA-A2 reactivity[b]	88	94	94	76	84	86	85	92	100

[a]Cell substrates were blood platelets, PBL, and PBL cultured for 3 days with PHA. Each substrate was used at three different doses per test as indicated.

[b]The degree of reactivity is shown as the percentage of maximum score calculated from the number and intensity (1–4+) of positive reactions with several dilutions of immune serum.

TABLE 10. Relative Reactivity of Various Cell Populations in Complement Fixation for HLA-A2 and DRw2 Specificities[a]

Immune serum	PBL	T[b]	B[b]	PHA-PBL[b]
Anti-HLA-A2	3	4	3	1
Anti-HLA-DRw2 (No. 458)	>30	>30	6	1
Anti-HLA-DRw2 (LER)	>30	>30	15	1

[a]Donor HLA-A2, A3, B7, B-, DRw2, DRw7. Several dilutions of immune serum were tested against several numbers of cells. The results are expressed as the minimum number of cells ($\times 10^3$) giving a positive reaction.
[b](T) T-lymphocyte suspension enriched by elimination of nylon-adherent cells; (B) B-lymphocyte suspension enriched by elimination of T rosettes; (PHA-PBL) PBL cultured 3 days with PHA.

among PBL, PBTL, and PBBL for HLA-A2, while PHA-PBL were much more reactive. For HLA-DRw2, PHA-PBL were more reactive than PBBL. PBL and PBTL were not reactive at the maximum dose used.

A comparison was made of the relative sensitivity of the CF and LCT techniques for the detection of anti-HLA-DR antibodies. As shown in Table 11, CF on PHA-PBL was about as sensitive as LCT against PBBL. A practical consequence of this observation was that CF on PHA-PBL could be efficiently used for the detection of anti-HLA-DR antibodies.

3.6. Relative Amounts per Cell of HLA-A, -B and -DR Antigens

The use in CF of anti HLA-A, -B and -DR antibodies against various substrates made possible an evaluation of their antigenic content. This was done by determining the minimum reacting dose of cells. It was based

TABLE 11. Relative Sensitivity of The Complement Fixation and Lymphocytotoxicity Techniques for the Detection of Anti-DR Antibodies

Serological test used	Dilutions of anti-DRw2 immune serum				
	1 : 10	1 : 20	1 : 40	1 : 80	1 : 160
CF on B Ly[a] (50,000 cells/test)	4	4	0	0	0
CF on PHA-PBL[a] (10,000 cells/test)	4	4	4	4	0
LCT on B Ly[b] (2,000 cells/test)	4	4	4	2	0

[a]CF was performed on enriched B-lymphocyte suspensions and on PHA-stimulated with the indicated number of cells per test. The results are shown as fixation complete (4) or absent (0).
[b]LCT was performed on enriched B-lymphocyte suspensions. The degrees of lymphocyte killing are indicated as 100% (4), 50% (2), or background level (0).

on the assumption that the smaller the number of cells needed to give a positive CF test, the higher the number of antigenic sites at the cell membrane. This is particularly true when a single immune serum is used for the comparison, since the complement-fixing ability of different sera may vary according to the classes and subclasses of the antibodies they contain. Another limitation of the method is that in excess of antibody, the degree of CF depends not only on the number but also on the concentration of the antigenic sites at the cell membrane; below a certain level, CF does not occur (Rapp and Borsos, 1970). It must be noted that the method allows only a semiquantitative evaluation of the antigenic content of a given cell population. For instance, this method was not sensitive enough to see the 1:3 ratio in HLA-A2 antigenic content on T and B lymphocytes (Pellegrino *et al.*, 1978). The results of this indirect method will thus have to be confirmed by quantitative absorption. Nevertheless, a first estimate can be made as shown in Table 12, which summarizes the results of several experiments.

For HLA-A, -B antigens, BLL and stimulated PBL were 5–10 times more reactive than resting PBL, PBBL, and PBTL. For HLA-DR antigens, BLL were 5–10 times more reactive than the resting B lymphocytes present in PBL or PBBL suspensions. The stimulated PBL suspensions, in which the number of reactive cells was unknown, were 3–5 times less reactive than the BLL. PBTL were not reactive with anti-HLA-DR antibodies, and their HLA-DR antigenic content was less than 1/20th of that of resting B lymphocytes from PBL.

4. Summary and Conclusions

A systematic search for complement-fixing anti-HLA-DR antibodies has shown that they were fairly frequent (60%) in hyper-immune sera containing high-titered anti-HLA-A, -B antibodies. In 9–25% of the sera

TABLE 12. Relative Amounts per Cell of HLA-A, -B and -DR Antigens

Substrate used in CF test	Minimum number of cells ($\times 10^3$) giving a positive test for: HLA-A, -B	HLA-DR
PBL (18% B)	5	50–100 (≈10–20 B)
B-lymphocyte-enriched PBL (≈60% B)	5–10	10 (≈6 B)
T-lymphocyte-enriched PBL (≈98% T)	5–10	Neg with 100
PHA-, Con-A-, PWM-stimulated PBL	2	2–5
Cultured BLL	1–2	1–2
Platelets	250	Neg with 2,000

containing low-titered anti-HLA-A, -B antibodies, anti-HLA-DR antibodies were observed with titers higher than those of the anti-HLA-A, -B antibodies. Such sera could be used without platelet absorption. HLA-DRw2, 3, 4, 5, 6, 7 specificities were recognized by one or several sera, on PBBL or PHA-stimulated PBL. These results showed that HLA-DR typing could be made by CF.

A study of the induction of HLA-DR specificities on PBL stimulated by PHA showed that the reactive cells were not only the T lymphoblasts but probably also the B lymphoblasts or monocytes or both. HLA-DR specificities were induced by low doses but not by high doses of Con A. Stimulation by a specific antigen (tuberculin) also induced HLA-DR specificities. Semiquantitative studies of HLA-DR antigens on various cell populations showed that the B lymphoblasts from cultured lymphoid lines contained 2–5 times more antigens than the mitogen-stimulated PBL and 5–10 times more antigens than the resting B lymphocytes from peripheral blood. HLA-DR antigenic content of PBTL was less than 1/20th of that of the PBBL.

Acknowledgments. We thank Prof. J. Dausset and his associates, who typed the panel for HLA-DR, and Mrs. F. Bayle for expert secretarial assistance. This research was supported in part by grants from INSERM, DGRST, CNRS, and the Cancer Research Institute.

References

Bodmer, J.G., 1978, Ia serology, in: *Histocompatibility Testing 1977* (W.F. Bodmer, J.R. Batchelor, J.G. Bodmer, H. Festenstein, and P.J. Morris, eds.), pp. 351–359, Munksgaard, Copenhagen.

Bodmer, W.F., Batchelor, J.R., Bodmer, J.G., Festenstein, H., and Morris, P.J. (eds.), 1978, *Histocompatibility Testing 1977*, Munksgaard, Copenhagen.

Boyum, A., 1974, Separation of blood leucocytes, granulocytes and lymphocytes, *Tissue Antigens* **4**:269–274.

Brochier, J., Samarut, C., Gueho, J.P., and Revillard, J.P., 1976, T dependence of human B lymphocyte proliferative response to mitogens, *Int. Arch. Allergy Appl. Immunol.* **51**:101–116.

Colombani, J., d'Amaro, J., Gabb, B.W., Smith, G.S., and Svejgaard, A., 1971, International agreement on a microtechnique of platelet complement fixation, *Transplant. Proc.* **3**:121–129.

Colombani, J., Dastot, H., Reboul, M., and Degos, L., 1977, Detection of human B lymphocyte alloantigens by complement fixation, *Transplantation* **24**:230–234.

Han, T., and Dadey, B., 1978, T lymphocyte dependency of B lymphocyte blastogenic response to phytomitogens, *Immunology* **34**:625–630.

Julius, M.H., Simpson, E., and Herzenberg, L.A., 1973, A rapid method for the isolation of functional thymus derived murine lymphocytes, *Eur. J. Immunol.* **3**:645–649.

Mendes, N.F., Tolnai, M.E.A., Silviera, N.P.A., Gilbertsen, R.B., and Metzgar, R.S., 1973, Technical aspects of the rosette tests used to detect human complement receptor (B) and sheep erythrocyte binding (T) lymphocytes, *J. Immunol.* **111**:860–877.

Pellegrino, M.A., Belvedere, M., Pellegrino, A.G., and Ferrone, S., 1978, B peripheral lymphocytes express more HLA antigens than T peripheral lymphocytes, *Transplantation* **25**:93–95.

Phillips, B., and Roitt, I.M., 1973, Evidence for transformation of human B lymphocytes by PHA, *Nature (London) New Biol.* **241**:254–256.

Rapp, H.J., and Borsos, T., 1970, *Molecular Basis of Complement Action*, Appleton-Century-Crofts, New York.

2

Serological and Cellular Recognition of Human Histocompatibility Antigens

Peter Cresswell, Peter E. Andreotti, John R. Apgar, and M. Louise Markert

1. Introduction

The human major histocompatibility complex (HLA) consists of a region of chromosome 6 (Smith *et al.*, 1976; Francke and Pellegrino, 1977) that contains a number of genes that code for highly polymorphic integral membrane glycoproteins. The allelic products of these genes are generally detected by their reactivity with human alloantisera from multiparous women or from individuals immunized either with lymphocytes (deliberately or by blood transfusions) or by organ grafts. Currently serologically defined are the genes *HLA-A, -B, -C,* and *-DR. HLA-A, -B,* and *-C* code for 44,000-dalton molecules that are expressed noncovalently associated with β_2-microglobulin (Springer and Strominger, 1976; Grey *et al.*, 1973), a 12,000-dalton protein coded for by a gene on chromosome 15 (Goodfellow *et al.*, 1975). HLA-DR molecules on the surface of B-lymphoid cells and monocytes consist of two noncovalently associated glycoproteins with approximate molecular weights of 35,000 and 27,000 (Cresswell and Geier, 1975; Springer *et al.*, 1977). Which of these molecules is the true product of the *HLA-DR* gene is not absolutely certain; conflicting evidence suggests that both the isolated 27,000-dalton and the 35,000-dalton molecule can bind alloantibodies to HLA-DR following denaturation and separation (Tosi *et al.*, 1978; Klareskog *et al.*, 1978).

Peter Cresswell, Peter E. Andreotti, John R. Apgar, and M. Louise Markert • Division of Immunology, Department of Microbiology and Immunology, Duke University Medical Center, Durham, North Carolina 27710.

In addition to their role as target molecules for alloantibodies, HLA antigens have been implicated in T-cell recognition. HLA-A, -B, and probably -C molecules are putative targets for cytotoxic T cells generated in the mixed-lymphocyte response (MLR) (Kristensen *et al.*, 1975; Robinson *et al.*, 1978) and are thought to participate with viral antigens in the formation of the determinants recognized by virus-specific cytotoxic T cells (McMichael *et al.*, 1977). HLA-DR has been postulated to be identical to HLA-D, the product of which is defined, not serologically, but by the ability to stimulate the blastogenic component of the MLR, which is a T-cell response (Lohrmann *et al.*, 1974; Chess *et al.*, 1974).

Most of the data that have led to the formation of these concepts are derived from statistical approaches. For example, HLA-A and -B antigens are postulated to be the targets for cytotoxic T cells because the ability of cytotoxic cells, raised in certain MLR combinations, to lyse members of a panel of target cells correlates with the presence on the targets of a particular serologically defined HLA-A or -B antigen. Similarly, HLA-DR has been postulated to be identical to HLA-D on the basis of a statistical correlation between the possession by an individual of certain HLA-DR antigens on his or her peripheral B lymphocytes, determined serologically, and the inability of his or her lymphocytes to significantly stimulate those of another person in the MLR who possesses the same serologically defined HLA-DR antigens.

Similar statistical correlations exist in the serological definition of HLA antigens. Certain *HLA-B* alleles are always found in conjunction with one member of the diallelic system known as *w4/w6* (formerly *4a/4b*), while other *HLA-B* alleles exist in conjunction with the alternate *w4/w6* allele (Bright, 1976). For example, the antigen HLA-B7 is always found together with w6, while HLA-B12 is always found together with w4.

This chapter presents recent data on molecular interpretations of some of these statistical correlations that exist in the enormous amount of data collected concerning the HLA complex since the early identification of its products as the major leukocyte determinants recognized by human alloantibodies.

2. Antibody Studies

2.1. w4 and w6 Association with HLA-A and -B Antigens

Immune precipitation of radiolabeled, solubilized membrane antigens followed by analysis of antibody-bound components in denaturing electrophoretic gel systems is a powerful tool for investigating antigen structure. We and others have used the method to establish the chain structure of HLA-A, -B and -DR antigens using both xenoantisera and alloantisera. The sequential immune precipitation technique, whereby a radiolabeled preparation is treated with antiserum A to remove antigens recognized by it, and then retested with antiserum B, can unambiguously answer the question of whether the two antisera recognize the same molecule. We have employed this technique to examine the association of the *w4/w6* diallelic system with the HLA-B series of antigens (Ayres and Cresswell, 1976).

We purified to homogeneity a papain-solubilized mixture of HLA-B7 and HLA-B12 from the cell line RPMI 4265, which is w4 and w6 positive. Throughout purification, we simultaneously monitored fractions for w4 and w6 inhibitory activity in a ^{51}Cr-release assay, and found that these activities always cochromatographed with the HLA-B specificities. The HLA-B7/B12 mixture was iodinated using the [^{125}I]Bolton–Hunter reagent and subjected to sequential immune precipitation experiments with a number of alloantisera specific for HLA-B7, B12, w4, and w6. The experiments unambiguously showed that HLA-B7 and w6 were on the same molecule, and that HLA-B12 and w4 were on the same molecule. This molecular association is precisely what would be predicted from the statistical associations, *w4* and *w6* are now referred to as *HLA-Bw4* and *Bw6*, respectively, because of this molecular association.

We have discussed the genetic implications of the association on the same molecule of a highly polymorphic series of antigens (HLA-B) with a diallelic system (*w4/w6*) (Ayres and Cresswell, 1976). The association is particularly interesting since highly cross-reactive HLA-B antigens, presumably with much structural identity, frequently differ in their Bw4 or Bw6 association. By analogy with the V region–C region dichotomy of immunoglobulins, *HLA-B* and *w4/w6* may be two separate genes, with recombination accounting for the association of cross-reactive HLA-B antigens with different *w4/w6* alleles. The effects of recombination, with the new juxtaposition of two sequences of amino acids in the recombinant molecule (one from the amino or carboxyl terminus of the HLA-B "gene product" and the other from the carboxyl or amino terminus of the w4/w6 "gene product"), could reasonably be expected to create new determinants, accounting for the fact that the recombinant product is serologically cross-reactive but not identical with the original HLA-B antigen.

We have recently examined a second interesting observed association, the reaction of individuals who are HLA-A9-positive with some sera specific for HLA-Bw4. Extensive absorption experiments have shown that subjects who are either Bw4-positive or A9-positive can remove cytotoxic activity from some Bw4 sera (Legrand and Dausset, 1975). Two explanations for the data are possible. Either there exists in tight linkage

TABLE 1. HLA-A9 and "w4-Like" Determinants Are on the Same Molecule

First precipitation[a]		Second precipitation		
Serum	cpm bound	NHS[b] (cpm bound)	Dupont (cpm bound)	L'Heritier (cpm bound)
NHS[b]	11,489 ± 113	1404 ± 22	4322 ± 147	4817 ± 76
Dupont (A9)	16,712 ± 128	1682 ± 13	1846 ± 34	2258 ± 59
L'Heritier (Bw4)	15,949 ± 80	1606 ± 63	1705 ± 16	1945 ± 18

[a]Duplicate aliquots of [^{35}S]methionine-labeled PALA DOC-soluble membranes were incubated with 30 μl sera. After 1 hr at room temperature, each mixture was added to 1.5 × 10^{10} pelleted formalin-fixed *S. aureus* and incubated for 30 min. Following centrifugation, the pellets were washed and samples comprising one third were counted. The supernatants were divided into three aliquots, which received either NHS, Dupont, or L'Heritier serum (10 μl), respectively, followed 1 hr later by *S. aureus*. These pellets were washed and counted.
[b](NHS) Normal human serum.

with HLA-A9 a gene that bears w4-like determinants or the HLA-A9 molecule itself bears such determinants. Sequential immune precipitation experiments were performed with deoxycholate (DOC)-solubilized membranes, internally labeled with [^{35}S]methionine, from the Epstein–Barr-virus-transformed cell line PALA. This is a line made from an *HLA* homozygous female, and is *HLA-A9, B8, DRw3.* The cell line also types as a Bw6. HLA-B8 is found in association with Bw6 in the general population, and based on our earlier data, HLA-B8 and Bw6 are presumably on the same molecule. Serum L'Heritier, which is a serum used to type for Bw4, also reacts with this cell. The results of an experiment employing an anti-HLA-A9 serum (Dupont) and L'Heritier are shown in Table 1. Prior precipitation of A9 with the Dupont serum and formalin-fixed *Staphylococcus aureus* removes material precipitable with the L'Heritier serum, and vice versa, indicating that HLA-A9 and "w4" are in this case on the same molecule. Both Dupont and L'Heritier precipitated the expected 44,000-dalton and 12,000-dalton peaks of HLA antigens when examined by sodium dodecyl sulfate (SDS)–gel electrophoresis and fluorography. The identity of the antibodies in L'Heritier reacting with the HLA-A9-positive cell and those antibodies reacting with HLA-B-associated w4 has been demonstrated by LeGrand and Dausset (1975) and by Kostyu (personal communication) using appropriate absorptions and testing in a microcytotoxicity assay. This would appear to be an example of cross-reactivity between an HLA-A-antigen molecule and HLA-B-antigen molecules.

As an alternative approach to studying the problem of the HLA-A9/w4 association, we have employed affinity chromatography. We previously purified HLA-DR antigens solubilized in the detergent sodium DOC by affinity chromatography using specific rabbit antibodies coupled to CNBr-activated agarose (Cresswell, 1977). The same technique has been applied in the purification of HLA-A antigens. Antisera produced in rabbits to papain-solubilized HLA-A2 can be made specific for HLA-A antigens by absorption with HLA-B antigens (Cresswell and Ayres, 1976). We absorbed 20 ml of such a rabbit antiserum (F) by repeated passage through a 3-ml-bed-volume affinity column of Biogel A15m agarose to which was bound 3 mg of a crude mixture of HLA-B7 and HLA-B12, solubilized by papain from the cell line RPMI 4265, and separated from HLA-A2 by DEAE-chromatography. Bound cross-reactive antibodies were eluted between passes with 0.1 N acetic acid. Purified IgG from this absorbed antiserum was coupled to CNBr-activated Biogel A15m.

For the HLA-A9/w4 association experiments, DOC-solubilized membranes from 5×10^9 PALA cells were applied to the column, which was equilibrated in 0.5% (wt./vol.) sodium DOC in 0.15 M NaCl, 0.01 M Tris, pH8.0 (DOCTS). Following extensive washing in this buffer, the column was eluted with 0.5% (wt./vol.) sodium DOC, 5% (vol./vol.) glycerol in 0.1 M Tris, pH 11.0, dialyzed vs. DOCTS, and concentrated by ultrafiltration using an Amicon XM-50 membrane. The starting material and the alkali-eluted material were examined for their HLA-A9, "w4," and Bw6 antigen content in an inhibition-of-complement-mediated-cytotoxicity assay using ^{51}Cr-labeled PALA cells as targets. The results are shown in Table 2. HLA-A9 activity (37.3%) and "w4" activity (34.5%) were recovered in the eluted fraction, whereas only 2.3% of the HLA-Bw6 activity was present in this fraction. This is more evidence in favor of a molecular association between a w4-like determinant and HLA-A9. The alkali-eluted material from this column shows the expected 44,000-dalton and 12,000-dalton bands when examined by SDS–gel electrophoresis, and 150–200 μg of protein can be isolated from 5×10^9 cells. We have also successfully used the column to isolate HLA-A3 from an *HLA-A3, HLA-B7* homozygous cell line, and HLA-A2 from an *HLA-A2, HLA-B7* homozygous cell line.

TABLE 2. Affinity Purification of HLA-A9 from DOC-Solubilized PALA Cell Membranes

Serum: / Specificity:	Dupont Anti-A9		L'Heritier Anti-A9,Bw4		Kavanagh Anti-Bw6	
Preparation	Pre-column	pH 11.0 eluate	Pre-column	pH 11.0 eluate	Pre-column	pH 11.0 eluate
Volume (ml)	26.0	6.0	26.0	6.0	26.0	6.0
Inhibitory titer	680	1100	495	740	345	35
Inhibitory units	17680	6600	12,870	4400	8970	210
Percent	100	37.3	100	34.5	100	2.3

HLA antigens eluted from antibody affinity columns can be used for further immunizations to produce additional xenoantibodies in rabbits or other species. We have recently, in collaboration with Drs. Michael Strong and Richard Metzgar, begun using HLA-DR antigens isolated from *HLA-DR* homozygous cell lines by affinity chromatography to produce anti-HLA-DR antisera in chimpanzees. One such serum, produced to HLA-DRw3 from the PALA cell line, proved to be an exceptionally high-titered anti-HLA-DRw3 antiserum, cross-reacting with HLA-DRw5 and HLA-DRw6. Further antisera to other specificities are currently being produced and characterized.

2.2. Two-Dimensional Electrophoretic Analysis of HLA-DR Antigens

We have recently begun studies of the electrophoretic polymorphism of the human Ia-like antigens, HLA-DR, using the two-dimensional gel technique of O'Farrell (1975).[^{35}S]Methionine-labeled membranes of *HLA-DR* homozygous cell lines are treated with neuraminidase (Parham *et al.*, 1977) to reduce electrophoretic heterogeneity caused by neuraminic acid residues, and are solubilized in the nonionic detergent octaethylene-glycol dodecyl ether [$C_{12}E_8$, 0.1% (wt./vol.) in 0.15 M NaCl, 0.01 Tris, pH 8.0.]. Immune precipitation of Ia-like antigens is effected by incubation for 1 hr at room temperature with the rabbit anti-HLA-DR serum J_{HSB} (Cresswell, 1977) followed by the addition of formalin-fixed *S. aureus* (Cowan I strain). After being washed, immune complexes are removed from the fixed bacteria by incubation in a solution containing 9.5 M urea, 2% (wt./vol.) Triton X-100, 2% (wt./vol.) ampholytes, and 5% (wt./vol.) 2-mercaptoethanol. Analysis is by isoelectric focusing in 4% (wt./vol.) acrylamide gels (pH range 5–7) in the first dimension, followed by SDS–gel electrophoresis in 11.5% (wt./vol.) acrylamide in the second. Gels are examined by fluorography.

Figure 1 shows analyses of two *HLA-DR* homozygous cell lines, TRAL (*HLA-A3, B7, DRw2*) and Sweig-1 (*HLA-A29, B40, DRw5*). Each cell type has a similar pattern, with two to four spots visible for both the 35,000-dalton and the 27,000-dalton species from each cell. We have been unable to simplify this pattern by further neuraminidase treatment of membranes either prior to or after solubilization; however, part of the complexity may possibly result from intransigent neuraminic acid residues.

Dramatic differences are apparent between the positions of the 27,000-dalton species from the two cell lines, indicating considerable heterogeneity. On superficial examination, the patterns for the 35,000-dalton species from the cell lines look identical. However, when anti-HLA-DR immune precipitates from the two cell lines are mixed and

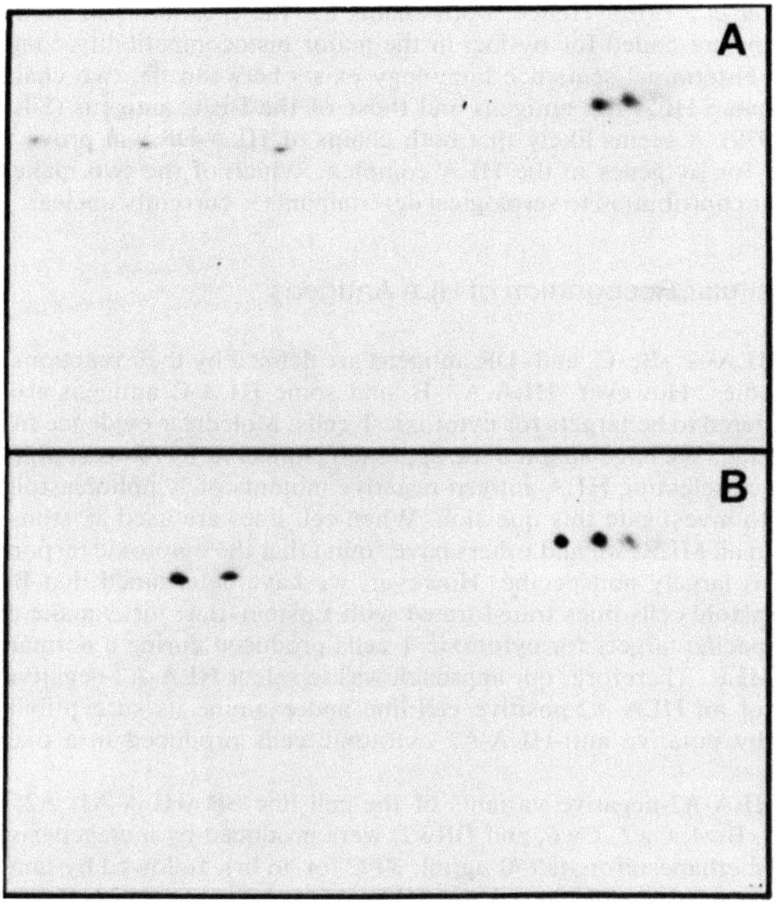

Figure 1. Two-dimensional gel analyses of [^{35}S]methionine-labeled HLA-DR antigens of homozygous cell lines precipitable by a rabbit antiserum, JHSB. The horizontal direction is the isoelectric focusing dimension, with the cathode on the left; the vertical direction, the second SDS-electrophoresis dimension. (A) Cell line TRAL (*DRw2*); (B) cell line Sweig-1 (*DRw5*). The group of spots on the right of each pattern is the 35,000-dalton species; that on the left, the 27,000-dalton species. Pronounced heterogeneity is observed for the 27,000-dalton species, more limited heterogeneity for the 35,000-dalton species.

processed together (not shown), none of the 35,000-dalton spots superimposes, indicating heterogeneity of this molecule also.

Different workers have come to different conclusions concerning which of the two molecules (the 35,000-dalton or the 27,000-dalton) is the product of *HLA-DR* (Tosi *et al.*, 1978; Klareskog *et al.*, 1978). The two chains of the *I-A* region Ia antigens of the mouse are both apparently coded for by the *I-A* region (Jones, 1977; Cook *et al.*, 1979). The two chains of the *I-E/C* region Ia antigens are coded for by the *I-A* region (27,000-dalton) and the *I-E/C* region (35,000-dalton) (Jones *et al.*, 1978;

Cook *et al.*, 1979). Hence, both chains for the two series of mouse Ia antigens are coded for by loci in the major histocompatibility complex. Since N-terminal sequence homology exists between the two chains of the human HLA-DR antigens and those of the I-E/C antigens (Silver *et al.*, 1979), it seems likely that both chains of HLA-DR will prove to be coded for by genes in the HLA complex. Which of the two makes the greater contribution to serological determinants is currently unclear.

3. Cellular Recognition of HLA Antigens

HLA-A, -B, -C, and -DR antigens are defined by their reactions with antibodies. However, HLA-A, -B, and some HLA-C antigens are also considered to be targets for cytotoxic T cells. Molecular evidence for this is lacking. We have adapted the approach pioneered by Pious *et al.* (1973, 1977) of selecting HLA-antigen-negative mutants of lymphoblastoid cell lines to investigate this question. When cell lines are used as stimulator cells in an MLR, we and others have found that the cytotoxic response to them is largely nonspecific. However, we have determined that B-lymphoblastoid cells lines transformed with Epstein–Barr virus make excellent specific targets for cytotoxic T cells produced during a normal one-way MLR. Therefore, our approach was to select HLA-A2-negative variants of an HLA-A2-positive cell line and examine its susceptibility to lysis by putative anti-HLA-A2 cytotoxic cells produced in a one-way MLR.

HLA-A2-negative variants of the cell line SB (HLA-A1, A2, B17, Bw44, Bw4, Cw2, Cw6, and DRw2) were produced by mutagenesis with ethyl methanesulfonate (50 μg/ml, 37°C for 16 hr), followed by immunoselection with a high-titered anti-HLA-A2 serum, PeC, and complement. Surviving cells were cultured for 3 weeks over a mouse fibroblast feeder layer irradiated with 2000 rads. A total of 6×10^6 cells were recovered at this stage, and these were again treated with serum PeC and complement. Surviving cells were grown up to mass culture and designated A_2m. A_2m was then cloned for 2 weeks in 0.23% (wt./vol.) soft agarose in RPMI 1640 containing 10% fetal calf serum over a human fibroblast feeder layer. Four clones were isolated and grown for further study. They were designated A_2m1, 2, 4, and 7.

3.1. Serology of the Mutant Cell Lines

The SB parent line and the four cloned variants have been extensively HLA typed by the standard NIH microcytotoxicity technique. Against a panel of 360 different antisera detecting HLA-A, -B, -C, and -DR antigens, all five cells typed identically except for five antisera. All five of these sera were anti-HLA-A2 and all killed over 95% of the parent cell while failing to lyse the mutants. No new antigens were detected on the mutant cells, and no parent cell antigen other than HLA-A2 was absent from them.

The SB parent and mutant cell lines were assayed quantitatively for HLA antigens on their surface using the [^{125}I]-*S. aureus* protein A ([^{125}I]-SpA) assay (Dorval *et al.*, 1974). PeC, the anti-HLA-A2 selection serum, and alloantisera specific for HLA-A1, HLA-Bw44, and HLA-B17, respectively, were studied. The results of these experiments on SB and the A_2m4 cell line are shown in Table 3. A_2m4 showed a 73% reduction in binding compared to SB with PeC, whereas no change was seen in binding of antibodies specific for HLA-A1, Bw44, and B17. The residual binding activity of PeC for the A_2m4 mutant could be absorbed from PeC using the uncloned A_2m cell line (Table 3). Following this absorption, the serum showed a 25% drop in lytic titer for SB, but still behaved as an anti-HLA-A2 serum, showing cross-reactivity with HLA-A28 and HLA-Aw24, when screened against a panel of normal lymphocytes. The nature of the molecules recognized by the A_2m reactive antibodies in serum PeC is currently under investigation.

We also studied the reactivity of SB and the mutant cell lines with rabbit antisera using the [^{125}I]-SpA binding assay. Table 4 shows the binding to SB and A_2m1, 2, 4, and 7 of an anti-β_2-microglobulin serum (R2), an antiserum specific for HLA-A antigens (A7/12) (Cresswell and Ayres, 1976), and an antiserum raised to a papain-solubilized mixture of HLA-B7 and B12 that predominantly recognized HLA-B antigens but that has not been absorbed to make it totally specific (Cresswell and Ayres, 1976). The four mutants show an average reduction of 26% in the

TABLE 3. Alloantibody Binding to SB and the A_2m4 Mutant Measured by the [^{125}I]-SpA Assay

Expt.	Serum[a]	Specificity	SB (cpm bound × 10^{-3})[b]	A_2m4 (cpm bound × 10^{-3})[b]
1	NHS[c]	—	9.6 ± 0.2	6.0 ± 0.1
	PeC	HLA-A2	290.5 ± 15.6	76.6 ± 0.5
	PeC/A_2m absorbed	HLA-A2	190.1 ± 6.0	7.9 ± 1.5
2	NHS[c]	—	2.7 ± 0.3	1.8 ± 0.2
	RAG	HLA-A1	36.9 ± 2.8	34.5 ± 0.2
	McGannon	HLA-Bw44	17.4 ± 0.6	15.8 ± 1.1
	Helmer	HLA-B17	12.4 ± 1.3	11.2 ± 1.4

[a]10 μl serum was used per 2 × 10^6 cells.
[b]Values are the means and ranges of duplicate determinations.
[c](NHS) Normal human serum.

TABLE 4. [^{125}I]-SpA Binding to SB Parent and A_2m Mutant Cell Lines Using Rabbit Antisera

		Cell				
		SB	A_2m1	A_2m2	A_2m4	A_2m7
Serum[a]	Specificity	(cpm bound × 10^{-3})[b]				
NRS[c]	—	7.4 ± 0.03	4.8 ± 0.15	4.8 ± 0.31	5.1 ± 0.43	4.9 ± 0.97
R2	β_2-Microglobulin	176.5 ± 1.9	135.3 ± 7.2	133.5 ± 2.8	132.6 ± 4.1	121.5 ± 7.6
A 7/12	HLA-A	103.1 ± 5.4	42.6 ± 1.0	42.1 ± 2.2	37.9 ± 1.2	38.8 ± 1.6
H	HLA-B (+ A)	146.9 ± 2.6	125.1 ± 9.7	128.9 ± 2.8	119.0 ± 8.9	115.0 ± 3.5

[a]10 μl serum was used per 2 × 10^6 cells.
[b]Values are the means and ranges of duplicate determinations.
[c](NRS) Normal rabbit serum.

expression of β_2-microglobulin, consistent with the loss of one HLA antigen assuming that HLA-C is expressed at lower levels than HLA-A and -B. All four mutants also show an average of 63% reduction in binding of the HLA-A-specific antibodies of serum A7/12. Serum H showed a minor reduction in binding of 16%, consistent with a degree of cross-reactivity of the serum with *HLA-A* locus products.

3.2. Cellular Cytotoxicity on the Mutant Cell Lines

Having demonstrated the loss of serologically detectable HLA-A2 antigen on the mutants, we investigated their susceptibility to cytotoxic cells generated in one-way MLRs. Responder peripheral blood lymphocytes (25 × 10^6) were incubated with γ-irradiated (1500 rads) stimulator lymphocytes (25 × 10^6) in 50 ml RPMI 1640 containing 10% (vol./vol.) heat-inactivated pooled human serum in round-bottomed glass centrifuge tubes at 37°C. Cells were harvested on day 7 for use as cytotoxic effector cells. Cytotoxicity assays were generally performed at a 40:1 effector target ratio using 10^4 ^{51}Cr-labeled lymphoblastoid-line target cells in V-well microtiter plates, in a volume of 110 μl RPMI 1640 with 10% fetal calf serum.

Table 5 shows the combined results of a number of experiments in which cytotoxic cells derived from a particular MLR combination were assayed for cytotoxicity on various B-lymphoblastoid cell lines. In this combination, donor PeC (A3, B7, Bw47) was sensitized to donor HaW (A2, A3, B7) to give an expected HLA-A2 cytotoxic response. It can be seen that all HLA-A2-positive cell lines tested were efficiently lysed by cytotoxic cells from this combination, while HLA-A2-negative lines were much less susceptible. Cytotoxic cells raised in this combination were

TABLE 5. PeC Anti-HaW Effectors Tested on Various B-Lymphoblastoid Cell Targets[a]

Cell line:	LTM	JY	KL	SB	HaW	Im-1	PALA	TLCL23	TRAL	PeC
HLA type:	A2,A3 B7,Bw41	A2,B7	A2, Bw35	A1,A2 Bw44,B17	A2,A3 B7	A3,A10, B12,B27	A9,B8	Aw19, Aw24,B5	A3,B7	A3,B7 Bw47
Expt. 1	—	65	61	—	—	—	7	2	—	—
Expt. 2	23	—	—	—	—	10	—	—	—	—
Expt. 3	—	—	—	—	64	—	—	—	7	—
Expt. 4	—	—	—	27	—	—	—	—	5	—
Expt. 5	—	35	—	24	—	—	—	—	1	—
Expt. 6	—	—	—	—	34	—	—	—	—	5

[a]Values are the percentage ^{51}Cr release in 4 hr at a 40: 1 effector target ratio.

also assayed on SB and A_2m1, 2, 4, and 7, along with a control cytotoxic population produced using the same responder with an HLA-A2-negative stimulator PW (HLA-A1, A10, B44, B17), who shares three antigens with SB and the mutants. In addition, a second responder PEA (HLA-A3, A26, B7, Bw39) was used with the same two stimulators to produce populations of cytotoxic cells putatively HLA-A2-specific and A1-, B44-, B17-specific populations, respectively. The results of these experiments are presented in Fig. 2.

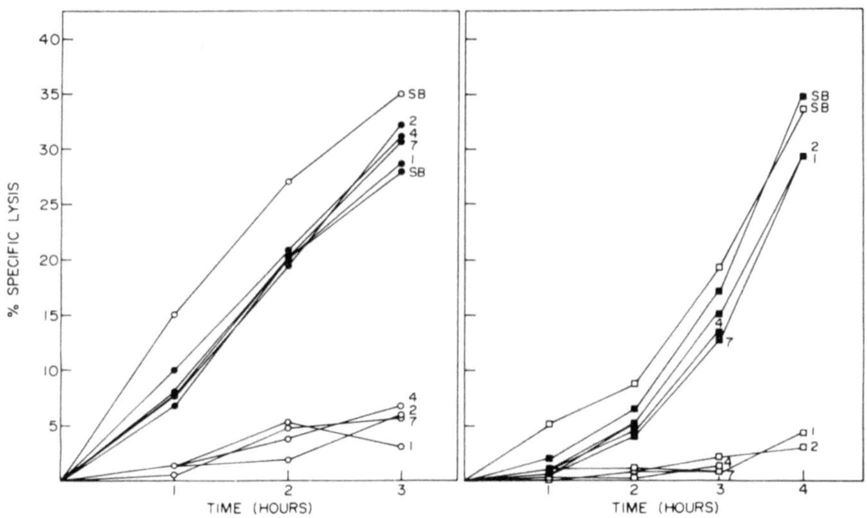

Figure 2. Cell-mediated lympholysis of ^{51}Cr-labeled SB and A_2m1, 2, 4, and 7 cell by PeC cytotoxic T cells (*left*) and PEA cytotoxic T cells (*right*). Cells sensitized to PW (A1, A10, Bw44, B17) to give control non-HLA-A2 response (●,■); cells sensitized to HaW (A2, A3, B7) to give experimental anti-HLA-A2 response (○,□). A_2m1 is indicated by 1, A_2m2 by 2, and so on.

The experiments unequivocally demonstrate that the SB cell line is susceptible to lysis by all the cytotoxic populations tested, while the four mutants have lost their susceptibility to the putatively HLA-A2-specific cells but not to the control effector cells. This experiment clearly indicates the role of the serologically detected HLA-A2 antigen as a target for cytotoxic cells, with perhaps one reservation. This is that the isolated variants could conceivably have suffered an additional mutation in a gene closely linked to the *HLA-A2* gene that rendered them resistant to lysis, or a large chromosomal deletion removed the *HLA-A2* gene along with this hypothetical second gene. This is unlikely, but cannot be discounted at present.

Preliminary biochemical evidence indicates that the A_2m4 cell synthesizes an electronegative variant of the HLA-A2 molecule, as analyzed by two-dimensional isoelectric focusing/SDS–polyacrylamide gel electrophoresis. Further studies are in progress to characterize the molecular defect conferring resistance to cytotoxicity by anti-HLA-A2 antibodies and cytotoxic cells in these mutant cell lines.

Much information has been accumulated concerning the molecular basis for antibody recognition of the many components of the major histocompatibility complex of humans and other species. However, the molecular basis of cellular recognition has proved exceptionally difficult to analyze. Selected mutants of cell lines offer an excellent approach for determining the molecular specificity of T-cell recognition of the HLA complex.

ACKNOWLEDGMENT. This research was supported by USPHS Grants AI-14016, AI-08897, and CA-14049.

References

Ayres, J., and Cresswell, P., 1976, HLA-B specificities and w4, w6 specificities are on the same polypeptide, *Eur. J. Immunol.* **6**:794.

Bright, S., 1976, Second locus HL-A antigens and 4a or 4b, *Tissue Antigens* **7**:23.

Chess, L., MacDermott, R.P., and Schlossman, S.F., 1974, Immunologic function of isolated human lymphocyte subpopulations. II. Antigen triggering of T and B cells *in vitro*, *J. Immunol.* **113**:1122.

Cook, R.G., Vitetta, E.S., Uhr, J.W., and Capra, J.D., 1979, Structural studies on the murine Ia alloantigens. V. Evidence that the structural gene for the I-E/C beta polypeptide is encoded within the I-A subregion, *J. Exp. Med.* **149**:981.

Cresswell, P., 1977, Human B cell alloantigens: Separation from other membrane molecules by affinity chromatography, *Eur. J. Immunol.* **7**:636.

Cresswell, P., and Ayres, J.L., 1976, HLA antigens: Rabbit antisera reacting with all A series or all B series specificities, *Eur. J. Immunol.* **6**:82.

Cresswell, P., and Geier, S.S., 1975, Antisera to human B-lymphocyte membrane glycoproteins block stimulation in mixed lymphocyte culture, *Nature (London)* **257**:147.

Dorval, G., Welsh, K.I., and Wigzell, H., 1974, Labeled staphylococcal protein A as an immunological probe in the analysis of cell surface markers, *Scand. J. Immunol.* **3:**405.
Francke, U., and Pellegrino, M.A., 1977, Assignment of the major histocompatibility complex to a region of the short arm of human chromosome 6, *Proc. Natl. Acad. Sci. U.S.A.* **74:**1147.
Goodfellow, P.N., Jones, E.A., van Heyningen, V., Solomon, E., Bobrow, M., Miggiano, V., and Bodmer, W.F., 1975, The β_2-microglobulin gene is on chromosome 15 and not in the HL-A region, *Nature (London)* **254:**267.
Grey, H.M., Kubo, R.T., Colon, S.M., Poulik, M.D., Cresswell, P., Springer, T., Turner, M.J., and Strominger, J.L., 1973, The small subunit of HL-A antigens is β_2-microglobulin, *J. Exp. Med.* **138:**1608.
Jones, P.P., 1977, Analysis of H-2 and Ia molecules by two-dimensional gel electrophoresis, *J. Exp. Med.* **146:**1261.
Jones, P.P., Murphy, D.B., and McDevitt, H.O., 1978, Two-gene control of the expression of a murine Ia antigen, *J. Exp. Med.* **148:**925.
Klareskog, L., Rask, L., Fohlman, J., and Peterson, P.A., 1978, Heavy HLA-DR (Ia) antigen chain is controlled by the MHC region, *Nature (London)* **275:**762.
Kristensen, T., Grunnet, N., and Kissmeyer-Nielsen, F., 1975, Cell mediated lympholysis in man: Varying strength of the HL-A (LA and Four) antigens as sensitizing or target determinants, *Tissue Antigens* **6:**221.
Legrand, L., and Dausset, J., 1975, The complexity of the HL-A gene product. II. Possible evidence for a "public" determinant common to the first and second HL-A series, *Transplantation* **19:**177.
Lohrmann, H.P., Novikovs, L., and Graw, R.G., 1974, Stimulatory capacity of human T and B lymphocytes in the mixed leukocyte culture, *Nature (London)* **250:**144.
McMichael, A.J., Ting, A., Zweerink, H.J., and Askonas, B.A., 1977, HLA restriction of cell-mediated lysis of influenza virus-infected human cells, *Nature (London)* **270:**524.
O'Farrell, P.H., 1975, High resolution two-dimensional electrophoresis of proteins, *J. Biol. Chem.* **250:**4007.
Parham, P., Albert, B.N., Orr, H.T., and Strominger, J.L., 1977, Carbohydrate moiety of HLA antigens—Antigenic properties and amino acid sequences around the site of glycosylation, *J. Biol. Chem.* **252:**7555.
Pious, D., Hawley, P., and Forrest, G., 1973, Isolation and characterization of HL-A variants in cultured human lymphoid cells, *Proc. Natl. Acad. Sci. U.S.A.* **70:**1397.
Pious, D., Soderland, C., and Gladstone, P., 1977, Induction of HLA mutations by chemical mutagens in human lymphoid cells, *Immunogenetics* **4:**437.
Robinson, M.A., Noreen, H.J., Amos, D.B., and Yunis, E.J., 1978, Target antigens of cell-mediated lympholysis: Discrimination of HLA subtypes by cytotoxic lymphocytes, *J. Immunol.* **121:**1486.
Silver, J., Walker, L.E., Reisfeld, R.A., Pellegrino, M.A., and Ferrone, S., 1979, Structural studies of murine I-E and human DR antigens, *Mol. Immunol.* **16:**37.
Smith, M., Gold, P., Shuster, J., Tanigaki, N., and Pressman, D., 1976, Chromosomal assignment of the HL-A common antigenic determinants in man–mouse somatic cell hybrids, *J. Immunogenet.* **3:**105.
Springer, T.A., and Strominger, J.L., 1976, Detergent-soluble HLA antigens contain a hydrophilic region at the COOH-terminus and a penultimate hydrophobic region, *Proc. Natl. Acad. Sci. U.S.A.* **73:**2481.
Springer, T.A., Kaufman, J.F., Terhorst, C., and Strominger, J.L., 1977, Purification and structural characterisation of human HLA-linked B cell antigens, *Nature (London)* **268:**213.
Tosi, R., Tanigaki, N., Centis, D., Ferrara, G.B., and Pressman, D., 1978, Immunological dissection of human Ia molecules, *J. Exp. Med.* **148:**1592.

3

Are D and DR Two Distinct Entities?

Jean Dausset

1. Introduction

1.1. Background

It is only recently that the human *HLA-D* locus has been recognized and analyzed. Bach and Amos (1967) and Yunis and Amos (1971) were the first to explain the "abnormal" mixed-lymphocyte reaction (MLR) between *HLA*-identical siblings by the existence of recombination between the classic *A* and *B HLA* loci and a "new" locus now called *HLA-D.*

Work on several families showing such recombinants was soon published, thus allowing the establishment of the genetic distance between *HLA-B* and *-D* as about 0.8 unit of recombination.

The VIth and VIIth Histocompatibility Workshops provided the opportunity to establish at least 11 allelic products of the *HLA-D* gene detected by homozygous typing cells.

This typing technique still has many pitfalls. It is cumbersome and needs several typing cells for each specificity, leading many research workers to search for direct serological detection of *D*-locus production. The problem has been tackled differently by several teams. The so-called "extra-reactions" so frequently observed in HLA serology were first investigated by Walford *et al.* (1975). The Merritt series described by these authors on chronic lymphocytic leukemia (CLL) lymphocytes was later found to be in the B lymphocyte. Sophisticated methods using inhibition of the MLR (Van Leeuwen *et al.*, 1973), indirect immunofluorescence (Van Rood *et al.*, 1975), or lymphocyte-dependent cytotoxicity

Jean Dausset • Research Unit INSERM U93, Centre Hayem, Hôpital Saint-Louis, 75475 Paris Cedex 10, France.

(Dossetor *et al.*, 1975) were also attempted. At the same time, the discovery of the B-lymphocyte specificities of the mouse greatly stimulated the research of similar determinants in humans. Lymphocytes from CLL or B lymphocytes in culture provided the target for detection of these anti-B lymphocyte antibodies (Winchester *et al.*, 1975; Fellous *et al.*, 1975).

Another approach was taken by our laboratory, namely, volunteer immunization between individuals differing and not differing at the *D* locus. In 1975, Legrand and Dausset (1975a) described the first B-lymphocyte antigen, Ly-Co, non-HLA-linked, by immunizing a father with his daughter's leukocytes, which were *-A*, *-B*, *-C*, and *-D* identical to those of her father, the MLR between donor and recipient remaining negative. The same year, another B-lymphocyte antigen, Ly-Li, was detected by immunization of another father with the lymphocytes of his daughter, who differed only at the *D* locus (MLR positive). This was the starting point for the definition of the public antigen Ly-Li1 and a private antigen now known as DRw5 (Legrand and Dausset, 1975b, 1976). The same approach was taken by Solheim *et al.* (1975), who found specific antibodies correlated with *D*.

It was clear at the VIIth International Workshop that the D series and the new B specificities detected by these different methods closely correlated. They were therefore called DR (D-related). However, some discrepancies remained, and a complete correlation between them could not be established. This problem is still not resolved. Clear dissociations between the D and usually corresponding DR were first observed in our laboratory (France One and Two Regional Report, 1977) and will form the basis of discussion in this chapter.

1.2. Biological Significance

The importance of these D disparities as triggers of the allogeneic immune response (at least *in vitro*) is now well established (Eijsvoogel *et al.*, 1972). A difference at the *D* locus between the responding and stimulating cells is a prerequisite not only for the proliferative response (MLR) but also for the appearance of T killer cells as detected by cell-mediated lymphocytotoxicity (CML). The specificity of these T killer cells is mainly that of HLA-A and -B antigens, but other HLA-linked targets also seem to be present.

The *HLA-D* region is the equivalent of the *H-2I* region. It is certainly as complex as the *I* region, which is already divided into five subregions: *IA*, (*IB*), *IJ*, *IE*, *IC*. Three of these subregions code for Ia (I-associated) antigens present on B lymphocytes. In humans, only one DR allelic series is well established. The existence of a second has been claimed but is not yet confirmed (Terasaki *et al.*, 1975; Mann *et al.*, 1976; Van Rood *et al.*, 1977; Walford *et al.*, 1977).

At present, it seems logical to equate human DR antigens to mouse Ia antigens, on the assumption that our knowledge of the human major histocompatibility complex (MHC) is far less complete than our knowledge of that in the mouse. However, one important difference seems to exist between the human and the mouse MHC. In the latter, no dissociation has yet been found between the products that induce proliferation *in vitro* and the products that are serologically defined. In humans, such a dissociation seems to exist, thus allowing the attribution of different characteristics to the proliferating structure (D) and the serologically defined structure (DR).

In the great majority of cases, D is associated with the corresponding DR, but occasionally this is not so. Such D/DR dissociations have been reported in caucasoids (Sasportes *et al.*, 1978a; Suciu-Foca *et al.*, 1978), as well as in Japanese (Sasazuki *et al.*, 1978) and in American Indians (Troup *et al.*, 1978). These rare haplotypes have been used to study the biological significance of these two, probably distinct, structures and their respective roles in transplantation.

2. HLA D/DR Phenotype Dissociation

2.1. Methods of Detection

Three techniques have been used to detect the products of the *D* region: (1) homozygote typing cells (HTC) used in the MLR as stimulators (MLR-I); (2) various serological methods using B lymphocytes as a target; and (3) secondary MLR (MLR-II) using responding cells twice primed *in vitro* (mostly against only one *HLA* haplotype)—this primed-lymphocyte test (PLT-I) gives an early proliferative response (2nd or 3rd day) when the specific stimulating cell is added in culture.

The relationship between the three techniques is very close, but not absolute, as can be seen in Table 1 and Fig. 1. The main observations to be drawn from these data are: (1) D stimulating products are "included"

TABLE 1. Correlations between Dw, DRw, and Specific PLT Cell Reactions

Dw/DRw	*r*	Dw/PLT	*r*	DRw/PLT	*r*
1/1	0.6				
2/2	0.7	2/2	0.8	2/2	0.8
3/3	0.8	3/3	0.5	3/3	0.9
4/4	—	4/4	—	4/4	—
5/5	0.8	5/5	0.7	5/5	0.9
6/6	0.6	6/6	0.6	6/6	0.6
7/7	0.4	7/7	0.4	7/7	0.8

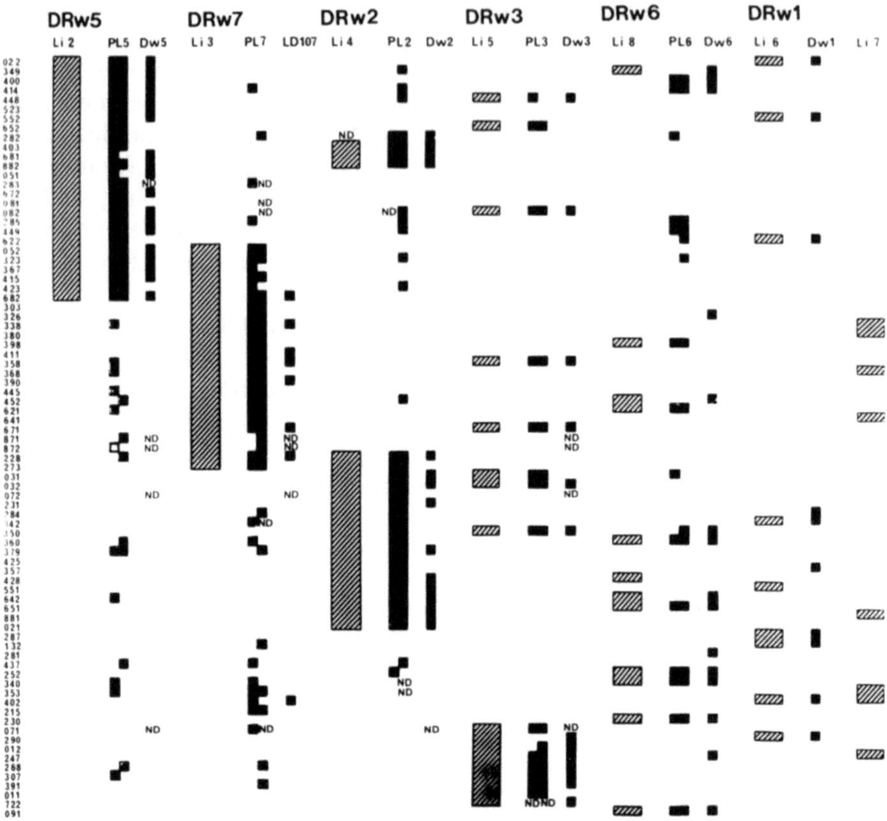

Figure 1. Panel distribution of DR, PL, and Dw specificities. The figures on the left are the individual panel members. Two PLTs were used for each specificity.

in the DR serologically detected products. That is to say many DR specificities are not accompanied by the corresponding D. (2) The PLT seems to have a better correlation with the DR than with the D series; the PLT follows the serological definition more closely than the cellular definition of D products (Sasportes *et al.*, 1978a).

2.2. Families with D/DR Dissociated Haplotypes

Studying 53 families, Dausset *et al.* (1978a) found two families in which there was a D/DR dissociation on one of the haplotypes. Family FER is depicted in Fig. 2. The dissociated haplotype was *Aw23, B8, Bw6, BfS, Dw4, DRw3.*

In family LIS (Fig. 3), the dissociated haplotype was *Aw23, Bw49, Dw4, DRw1.* In both cases, the dissociation was found to have been

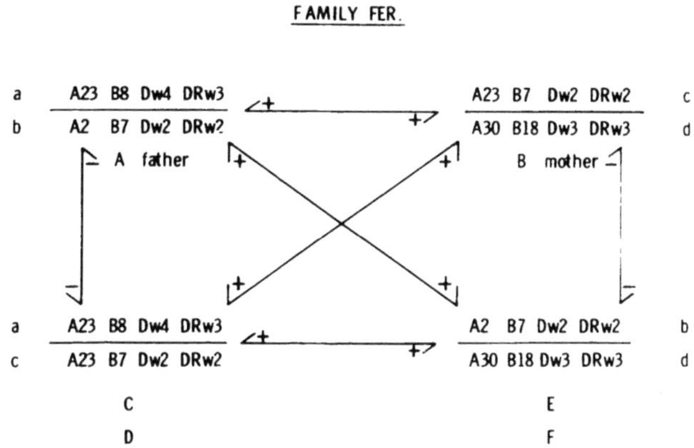

Figure 2. Schematic representation of family FER. Haplotype a bears a D/DR dissociation. (A) Father; (B) mother; (C–F) children. Results of the intrafamilial unidirectional MLR are given by + or – at the extremity of the arrow close to the stimulating cell.

transmitted from the parent to the children, and the dissociated *Dw* was *Dw4* associated with *DRw3* and *DRw1*, respectively.

It is well known that HTC determination is not an easy task and is subject to many difficulties. However, this HTC typing was done several times with local HTC or VIIth Workshop HTC from Dw1 to Dw8. For example, with cells from the FER father, typing responses were obtained with the Dw4 HTC and with Dw2 HTC (Dw2 being present in the other haplotype) (see Table 2). It was noted that HTC Dw3 gave a strong reaction with the FER dissociated haplotype, indicating that Dw3 was not present in this individual. On the other hand, no well-known cross-reactions existed between Dw3 and Dw4.

Among the 53 families studied, two others belonged to the category where an unidentified D stimulating product existed in one haplotype, together with a serologically defined DR. In these two families, the D product was not assigned; it was stimulating in MLR, but was certainly

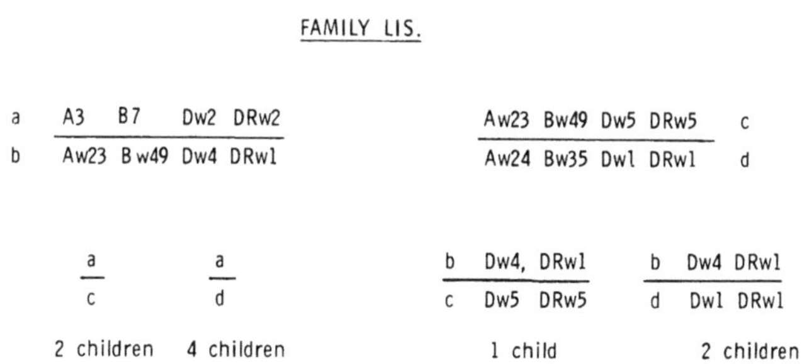

Figure 3. Family LIS. Haplotype b bears a D/DR dissociation.

TABLE 2. Typing of FER Lymphocytes on Dw2, Dw3, and Dw4 HTC[a]

Responder cells	Irradiated stimulating HTC cells[b]												
	Dw2				Dw3				Dw4				
	7w503	7w504	LERCH PARIS	DOLLE Strasbg	7w505	GOY PARIS	Mic438 Munich	7w507	7w508	7w524	7w547	Bit.Bur 180 Rennes	2.1044 Lyon
FER father	20	27	22	25	97	92	97	39	46	18	59	26	27

[a]Data are expressed as relative responses with double normalized MLR value, according to Ryder *et al.* (1975).
[b]Response against all the other HTC cells tested was positive.

not the D expected from DR typing. In family DEG, the dissociated haplotype was *A2, B12, Dw-, DRw5,* and in family CAZ, it was *A3, Cw4, Bw35, BfF, Dw-, DRw3.*

Using B-cell serology, these families were DR-typed with both local sera and VIIth Workshop sera; DRw specificities were assigned according to the criteria of the VIIth Workshop. They were also genotyped, and in no instance were two DRw specificities found on the same haplotype, and the mendelian segregation was always correct. DRw1 of family LIS was established with 5 sera, DRw3 of family FER and CAZ with 12 sera, and DRw5 of family DEG with 8 sera.

3. HLA D/DR *in Vitro* Functional Dissociation in MLR-I

3.1. Dissociation Suggested by the Intrafamilial MLR

The intrafamilial MLR was carried out for the four families quoted above. In the two families with D/DR dissociated determinants, the results were consistent with D typing. In the other families, this assay led to the deduction of the presence of a D stimulating product on the dissociated haplotype. This determinant was not as yet assigned and thus was seen to be different from the known Dw1–8 series.

Three examples are given in Table 3. In this table, for each category of *HLA*-identical sibling (a/c, a/d, b/c, or b/d), the result of only one child is shown, but the results obtained with their *HLA*-identical siblings were similar. In family FER, assuming that each DR is always accompanied by the corresponding D, the child a/c should not have stimulated the mother c/d but did. Likewise, the father a/b should not have stimulated the children b/d, but he did.

In family LIS, the father a/b should not have stimulated the children a/d, but the reactions were clearly positive [relative response (RR): 29, 32, and 23%, respectively]. Likewise, the child b/c should not have stimulated the mother c/d (RR: 18%).

In family DEG, the mother was homozygous for DRw5 but not for Dw5. She obviously gave a typing response with a Dw5 HTC. However, she possessed a haplotype *Dw5 DRw5,* since the haplotype as transmitted to three of the children (a/d and b/d) was able to react in primary MLR against five other children who had received the other haplotype *Dw-DRw5.* Likewise, the mother c/d stimulated the child a/d and the two children b/d.

Such families with an active but nonassigned D should be relatively frequent, since the DR specificities have a greater gene frequency and DR is almost always "included" in D.

TABLE 3. MLR in Three Informative Families[a]

Family	Responding cells[b]	Irradiated stimulating cells A a/b	B c/a	C a/c	C a/d	C b/c	C d/b	Haplotypes
FER	F a/b	0	34	0	—	—	24	a: Aw23, B8, *Dw4, DRw3*
	M c/d	40	0	24	—	—	8	b: A2, B7, Dw2, DRw2
	1C a/c	2	16	0	—	—	25	c: Aw23, B7, Dw2, DRw2
	1C b/d	49	9	49	—	—	0	d: Aw30, B18, Dw3, DRw3
LIS	F a/b	0	95	58	32	109	48	a: A3, B7, Dw2, DRw2
	M c/d	69	0	75	81	38	29	b: Aw23, Bw49, *Dw4, DRw1*
	2C a/c	55	144	0	132	157	161	c: Aw23, Bw49, Dw5, DRw5
	4C a/d	12	87	98	0	138	49	d: Aw24, Bw35, Dw1, DRw1
	1C b/c	47	18	79	90	0	46	
	2C b/d	67	58	117	81	110	0	
DEG	F a/b	0	97	89	62	57	100	a: A23, B12, Dw7, DRw7
	M c/d	156	0	51	46	36	45	b: A1, B8, Dw3, DRw3
	4C a/c	184	50	0	42	81	84	c: A2, B12, *Dw-, DRw5*
	1C a/d	75	27	16	0	59	45	d: Aw32, Bw35, Dw5, DRw5
	1C b/c	57	41	47	77	0	47	
	2C b/d	155	27	75	58	37	0	

[a]Results are expressed in % RR = (test − autologous cpm)/(reference cpm − autologous cpm).
[b](F) Father; (M) mother; (C) child. Only one child of each category is shown for the sake of simplicity, but the number of children is indicated (1C, 2C, etc.). Complete data are in Fradelizi *et al.* (1978).

3.2. Dissociation Suggested by the Proliferative Additive Effect of D + DR Incompatible Combinations

Data on three of the four families were studied in order to study the respective proliferative influence of D and/or DR disparity between responding and stimulating cells in MLR-I. The MLR data were classified according to four situations (Fig. 4).

1. In 35 combinations, D and DR were genetically identical when performed between *HLA*-identical siblings: the RR was almost nil (1.6).

2. In 34 combinations, D and DR were different as in the case of MLR between *HLA*-different siblings. The RR was high (86.3).

3. In the cases of MLR between *HLA*-haploidentical individuals (between parent and siblings or between two haploidentical siblings), two situations can be observed:

   a. In the case where both D and DR were incompatible between the responding and stimulating cells (88 combinations), the strength of the MLR was as expected, intermediate between the two former categories (RR: 70.4).

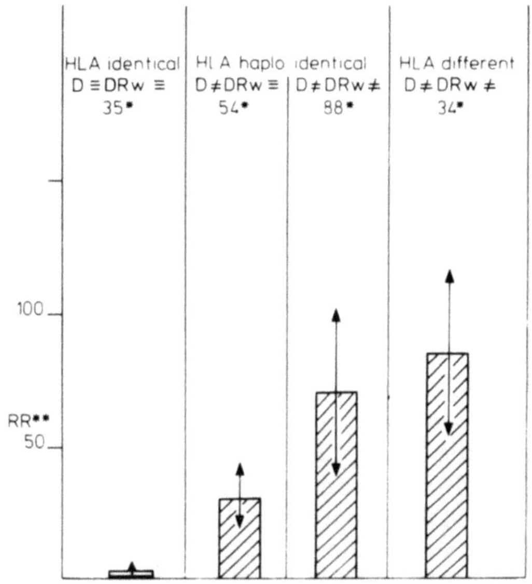

Figure 4. Influence of D or DR, or both, on the intensity of the MLR-I. *Number of MLR combinations studied (pooled results from three families); **(RR) MLR relative response.

b. However, when D was incompatible but DR was compatible (54 combinations), the MLR was weaker than in the preceding situation (RR: 28.8), showing an additive effect of D + DR disparity in MLR-I (Fradelizi *et al.*, 1978).

It was also observed that in this last category (D≠, DR≠), the strength of the reaction was not the same in the two directions. In one direction, the MLR was twice as intense as in the other (Table 4). The significance of this observation is still obscure.

A combination between HLA-haploidentical siblings with D indentical, DR different has not yet been encountered.

TABLE 4. Primary MLR between Haplotypes Bearing a Dw/DRw Dissociation

Family	MLR direction	Relative response	Mean
FER	Dw4 → Dw3	22, 24	23
	Dw3 → Dw4	9, 7	8
LIS	Dw4 → Dw1	29, 32, 23	28
	Dw1 → Dw4	11, 12, 8	10.3
DEG	Dw- → Dw5	42, 39, 37, 36	38.5
	Dw5 → Dw-	16, 10, 14, 8	12

4. HLA D/DR *in Vitro* Functional Dissociation Detected in MLR-II (PLT-I)

4.1. HTC vs. PLT in Families with D/DR Dissociation

A secondary MLR was used to ascertain the dissociation in these D/DR families. An anti-PLT directed against D/DR homozygote cells was developed between two HTC (as, for example, HTC Dw5 DRw5 → HTC Dw3, DRw3$^{=}$; this PLT cell behaves like a pure anti-DRw3). Other PLT cells were developed in intrafamilial situations between *HLA*-semiidentical individuals, i.e., against one D/DR region. Some of these cells were particularly discriminative and were used as reagents in the families.

An example of this method is illustrated in Table 5. On the assumption that PLT detects the DRw or a product of a very closely linked gene, it was shown that the dissociation between D and DR was a true one. In family FER, PLT anti-DRw3 detected this specificity in some lymphocytes, whereas Dw3 was not detected by Dw3 HTC.

4.2. Probable Existence of other DR-like Products Detected by PLT

The correlation between PLT-I and DR serology is not, however, absolute, and many "extra-reactions" were observed. Indeed, some PLT reacted with products that were not recognizable as DR (which we proposed to call the PL^{A}), but with other unknown products that we proposed provisionally to call PL^{B}.

This concept was introduced by Sasportes *et al.* (1978a,b) and by Nuñez-Roldan *et al.* (1978) and was based on the following facts.

1. The existence of apparent "extra-reactions" when PLT of a defined specificity was tested on the panel.

2. The fact that in the FER family, for example, which shared *HLA-D* between parents, it was possible to develop a PLT in the absence of primary MLR: (E, sib) Dw2, DRw2/(Dw3, DRw3) → (B$^{\neq}$ mother) Dw2, DRw2/(Dw3, DRw3). This PLT EB$^{\neq}$ tested in family FER was restimulated by all members of the family, thus indicating the presence of a stimulating product in the father (obviously *not* DRw2).

3. This conclusion was substantiated by the preparation in the same family of another PLT (FA$^{\neq}$) (F being an *HLA*-identical sibling of E): (F sib) (Dw2, DRw2)/Dw3, DRw3 → (A$^{\neq}$ father) Dw4 DRw3/(Dw2, DRw2). This PLT was also obviously not directed against DRw2 or DRw3 and behaved exactly as the PLT EB$^{\neq}$. It was restimulated by all members of the family, even including cells not possessing the Dw4 of the immunizing haplotype (for example, *Dw2, DRw2* for the mother). When this FA$^{\neq}$ PLT was tested on a panel of 33 unrelated individuals, 18

TABLE 5.

			HTC assay		PLT assay	
			HTC cell : GOY (Dw3 DRw3/ Dw3 DRw3)		PLT cell : MAI anti-GOY (Dw5 DRw5/Dw5 anti-Dw3 DRw3/Dw3 DRw3)	
Family 1	F	Dw4 DRw3/Dw2 DRw2	10.921	92%	4.225[a]	96%
	M	Dw2 DRw2/Dw3 DRw3	1.573[b]	8%	4.249	96%
	Ch1	Dw4 DRw3/Dw2 DRw2	16.208	76%	4.857	110%
	Ch2	Dw2 DRw2/Dw3 DRw3	1.310	7%	3.336	76%
HTC MAI		Dw5 DRw5/Dw5 DRw5	19.012	105%	401	9%
HTC GOY		Dw3 DRw3/Dw3 DRw3	473	2%	4.390	100%

[a]Specific DRw reactions are single-underscored.
[b]Specific Dw reactions are double-underscored.

positive reactions were observed, but no correlation with any known A, B, C, or D or DR specificity could be noted (Nuñez-Roldan *et al.*, 1978, Sasportes *et al.*, 1978a,b).

This original observation was extended to many other cases in which the D and DR were deliberately neutralized by identity for D and DR between the responding and stimulating cells. This reactivity was tested not only in the original family where these PLT cells were produced, but also in other families and in the unrelated panel. It appears that these reactions followed the HLA haplotype in each of the informative families. However, the number of families studied was still too small to provide sufficient proof that products thus detected (i.e., PL^B) are HLA products.

5. HLA D/DR *in Vitro* Functional Dissociation Detected in MLR-III (PLT-II)

The PLT cells produced by immunization *in vitro* for 10 days were stimulated a second time for a further 7 days using the same immunizing cells or cells sharing with them a DR specificity. For example, on intrafamilial PLT: Dw2 DRw2 → Dw3 DRw3 could be restimulated by the same Dw3 DRw3 cell or by another cell also bearing DRw3.

A population of hyperimmunized cells called PLT-II was thus obtained. It could be tested according to the usual MLR techniques against specific or nonspecific cells. This test is in fact an MLR-III, the responding cell being the PLT-II.

It was shown by Sasportes *et al.* (1978c) that these PLT-II cells, instead of giving an even stronger and earlier response than the PLT-I, induced on the contrary a *reduced* proliferation (Table 6), and that the reduction was specific to the DR of the immunizing cell.

This observation was extended by the use of another assay, a "third-man" test, in which irradiated PLT-II cells were added to an MLR-I. It was observed that the addition of these PLT-II cells induced a reduction of the proliferative response and that again this "suppression" is specific to the DR of the immunizing cells.

Proof that DR and not D was involved was given by using in the "third-man" test a stimulating cell bearing the D/DR dissociated haplotype *Dw4, DRw1* of family LIS. The PLT-II was specifically anti-DRw1, and reduction of the proliferation was also obtained with this D/DR dissociated cell bearing DRw1 (Table 7).

Thus, a suppressive effect was obtained after *in vitro* hyperimmunization. It was not due to the appearance of T killer cells of a DR specificity. This was shown by physical segregation (Carosella *et al.*, unpublished observation) of the two cell populations, helper and killer.

Moreover, this interpretation is unlikely, since as shown recently by Sasportes *et al.* (in prep.), the same suppressive effect can be obtained by the *supernatant* of the PLT-II culture, added in the primary MLR instead of the PLT-II cells themselves (soluble suppressor factor).

6. Miscellaneous Arguments in Favor of a Functional Dissociation between D and DR

6.1. Population Studies

In populations other than caucasoid, the same close correlation between D and DR has been observed, in most cases. However, in Japanese (Sasazuki *et al.*, 1978) and in American Indians (Troup *et al.*, 1978), different associations have been observed. For example, in Japanese, SA and HO Japanese D specificities were found strongly associated with DRw1 and DRw2 antigens, respectively.

6.2. Family Studies

Other authors have also found haplotypes with D/DR dissociated such as Suciu-Foca *et al.* (1978), who found a *Dw7, DRw2* haplotype.

TABLE 6. Decrease in the Specific Proliferative Response of Twice Primed PLTs Directed against Two DR Specificities

Responder PLT II		Restimulators		
		DR5 +	DR7 +	DR5 − DR7
LER × VDL* 2/2 5/7 10 days	→ MAI* 5/5 7 days →	<u>14,920</u>[a]	23,220[a]	17,650[a]
	→ GIL* 7/7 7 days →	23,450[a]	<u>12,170</u>[a]	14,580[a]

[a]Mean of proliferative responses (cpm). The specifically decreased reactions are underscored.

TABLE 7. PLT-II Suppresses the Response against DR Antigens Specifically[a]

[DER.F × DER.C1——10 days——→DER.C1——→7 days
DRw2/– DR2/DR1 DR2/DR1]

Responder	Third cell added (2500-rad γ-irradiated): DER.F‡ DRw2/–	Third cell added (2500-rad γ-irradiated): PLT-II	Stimulators (2500-rad γ-irradiated)		DR	Dw
DER.F	2,423	2,508 NC	DER	F a/b	2/-	2/-
DR 2/-	43,594	8,024 SC	DER	C1 a/c	2/1	2/1
	29,055	10,525	DER	C2 a/c	2/1	2/1
	44,502	12,507	LIS	F a/b	2/1	2/4
	38,018	12,911		C1 b/c	5/1	5/4
	30,355	10,170	SCH		1/1	1/1
	42,496	30,237	GIL		7/7	7/7
	30,853	28,144	VDL		5/7	5/7
	31,572	24,581	MAS		2/7	2/7
	31,674	37,555	CAM		5/-	5/-

[a]In a three-cell assay, a PLT-II anti-DRw is added to primary MLR using cells from two families (DER and LIS) and five unrelated cells. Family LIS is one of the rare families with a dissociation between DRw and Dw (the father is *Dw2,4; DRw2,1* and his child C1 is *Dw4,5; DRw1,5*). The inhibition of proliferation follows DRw1 and not Dw.

6.3. Possible Recombination between D and DR

Work on families with a possible recombination between D and DR has been published, but the data are not completely convincing and could not be taken as formal proof of the existence of two distinct genes (Festenstein *et al.*, 1977; Reinsmoen *et al.*, 1979.).

7. Discussion

The biological significance of the *HLA-D* region becomes more and more important when considered in connection with the *HLA-D* association with disease, organ transplantation, and immune response in general.

Despite numerous contributions, the subtle mechanisms controlled by this region are still unknown. It is not known whether the serological products (DR) and functions studied by *in vitro* and *in vivo* cell proliferation are under the dependence of one unique gene (*D*) or of several closely linked genes (*D* and *DR*) (see Fig. 5). Of course, many arguments can be quoted in favor of the identity D/DR, in particular: (1) the fact that anti-DR antibodies inhibit the MLR when the stimulating cells possess the

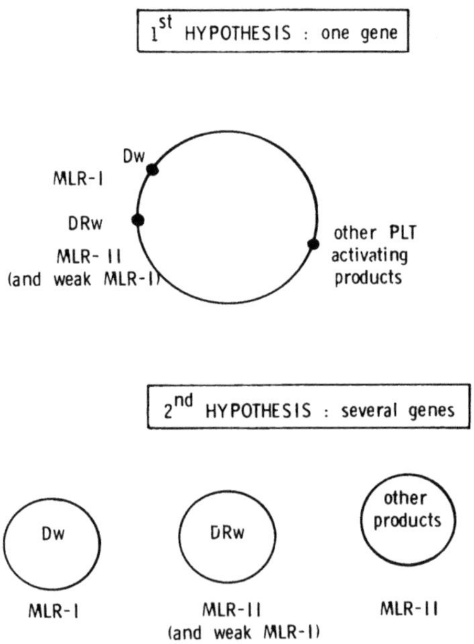

Figure 5. Schematic representation of two hypotheses, explaining the observed D/DR dissociation.

corresponding antigen; (2) the striking parallel between the D and DR specificities, which are almost always associated on the same haplotype; and (3) the same cross-reactions as detected by HTC and serology.

However, these arguments are not indisputable, since: (1) inhibition of the MLR could be due to the close proximity on the cell surface of the two determinants, thus leading to steric hindrance; (2) the parallel D/DR is not absolute—many haplotypes possess a defined DR and an undefined D; and (3) the similarity of the cross-reaction could reflect a common origin as a result of gene duplication.

We have tried to emphasize in this chapter the possibility that D and DR constitute, indeed, two discrete entities having different functions.

1. A D disparity between two lymphoid-cell populations leads spontaneously and without preimmunization to an intense proliferation of the responding cells. When one DR disparity is added to the D disparity, the primary proliferation (MLR-I) is even greater, and an additive effect is observed.

2. A DR disparity provokes a proliferation only after double sensitization (MLR-II); for this secondary MLR, a D disparity is not compulsory. The D incompatibility is not a prerequisite in the MLR-II, i.e., in the generation of reactive PLT cells. The MLR-II is not a mere booster of the MLR-I. Indeed, cells with a specificity against the DR incompatibility of the immunizing cells are produced, whatever the D of the immunizing cells and of the cells used for restimulation.

The PLT cells detect structures (PL^A) that are apparently similar to the DR specificities. The correlation between the specificity of the PLT prepared against one haplotype bearing a given DR specificity and the serological determination of the same DR is striking. It is a strong but not formal argument in favor of detection of the same determinant. When the PLT is developed between cells apparently D-different but DR-identical (thus eliminating the possibility of developing an anti-PL^A), nonetheless a reactivity remains that is directed against other determinants (PL^B), still not serologically identified, that could be coded by the HLA complex, although no correlation has been found with the HLA-A, -B, -C, -D, -DR determinants.

Thus, the PLT appears to be a very useful tool for the detection of unknown allogeneic structures on lymphoid or even nonlymphoid cell surfaces. Indeed, it constitutes a hyperimmunization carried out *in vitro*, which would be difficult to conduct *in vivo*, even in human volunteers.

The simplest hypothesis is to assign to the three categories of determinants, D, DR (PL^A), and PL^B, a decreasing proliferative power when put in contact with a homologous incompatible determinant. D possesses a spontaneous power of proliferation. It appears that each organism would thus be preimmunized against all allelic variations of its structures.

Lengthy discussion and speculation have attempted to explain the existence of so many presensitized clones of cells ready to react immediately to any alloantigen of the same species. This state of presensitization eliminates by definition all possibilities of a booster role. Another established fact is that these D structures, although different from DR, seem unable to provoke a humoral response.

On the contrary, there is *no* spontaneous sensitization against PL^A, which is probably identical to DRw. It can be assumed that the additive effect of D plus DR incompatibility during the PLT-I is due to an immunization against the incompatible DR. When a restimulation is done on the 14th day, a strong and above all early proliferative response is observed that is equivalent to a booster reaction.

The third structure, the PL^B, possessed probably the weakest proliferative power, which can be observed only when the preceding determinants are neutralized by identity. Their immunogeneity is probably weak, since no antibody directed against them has been described.

Another very important and practical question is whether or not DR is a target for cytotoxic cells. The results of skin grafts performed on human volunteers (Dausset *et al.*, 1978b) have shown clearly that DR incompatibility diminishes the survival time considerably, and this effect is cumulative and independent of the comparable effect resulting from HLA-A, -B incompatibilities. The same also seems to be true for kidney grafts.

The work of Feighery and Stastny (1979) demonstrated that the target for cytotoxic T cells was specifically the DR determinant borne by monocytes. Thus, if our hypothesis is correct, and D and DR are two discrete entities, one can visualize the detrimental effect of D + DR incompatibility as being due to the combined influence of a helper phenomenon (due to D incompatibility) and a target effect (due to DR incompatibility).

On the other hand, the demonstration that hyperimmunization leads to the appearance of DR-specific radio resistant suppressor cells (and suppressor factor) of T-cell proliferation is extremely promising. These cells are probably similar to the spontaneous suppressors described *in vivo* after pregnancy (McMichael and Sasazuki 1977; Engleman *et al.*, 1978). The suppression described here can be considered as a balanced phenomenon involving interaction between different lymphocyte populations. This phenomenon might be of great importance during pregnancy and in allograft tolerance.

8. Summary

The identity or difference between D and DR *HLA-D* region products is discussed. Despite the many arguments in favor of identity, others suggest that these could be two discrete determinants with different functions. The observation of at least two haplotypes wherein dissociation exists between defined D and DR (*Dw4, DRw3* and *Dw4, DRw1*) has allowed the study of their behavior in primary, secondary, and tertiary MLRs. MLR-I is due mainly to D disparity between responding and stimulating cells, although an additive effect is observed when a DR disparity is present. MLR-II depends mostly on the DR incompatibility. The PLT cells are DR-specific. However, they can also detect other stimulating products not yet well identified. MLR-III leads to the production of DR-specific suppressor cells and factor of the alloproliferation. Implications of these findings in transplantation are discussed.

References

Bach, F.H., and Amos, D.B., 1967, Hu-1 major histocompatibility locus in man, *Science* **153:**545.

Dausset, J., Legrand, L., Lepage V., Contu, L., Marcelli-Barge, A., Wildloecher, I., Benjamin, A., Meo, T., and Degos, L., 1978a, An haplo-type study of HLA complex with special reference to the HLA-DR series and to Bf-C2 and glyoxalase I polymorphism, *Tissue Antigens* **12**(4):297.

Dausset, J., Contu, L., Legrand, L., and Rapaport, F.T., 1978b, The influence of the HLA-DR antigens on skin allografts between haploidentical individuals, *Transplant. Proc.* **10**(4):995.

Dossetor, J.B., Kovithavongs, T., Marchk, L., Butcher, D., St. Louis, G., and Schlaut, J., 1975, A caucasoid isolate: Hutterites, correlation between ABCIL reactivity of a serum and stimulation by a typing cell, in: *Histocompatibility Testing* (F. Kissmeyer-Nielsen, ed.), pp. 620–624, Munksgaard, Copenhagen.

Eijsvoogel, V.P., Van Rood, J.J., Toit, E.D., and Schellenkens, P.T.A., 1972, Position of a locus determining mixed lymphocyte reaction distinct from the known HL-A loci, *Eur. J. Immunol.* **2:**413.

Engleman, E.G., McMichael, A.J., Batey, M.E., and McDevitt, H.O., 1978, A suppressor T cell of the mixed lymphocyte reaction in man specific for the stimulating alloantigen: Evidence that identity at HLA-D between suppressor and responder is required for suppression, *J. Exp. Med.* **147:**(1):137.

Feighery, C., and Stastny, P., 1979, HLA-D region-associated determinants serve as targets for human cell-mediated lysis, *J. Exp. Med.* **149(2)**:485.

Fellous, M., Mortchelewicz, F., Kamoun, M., and Dausset, J., 1975, The use of a lymphoid cell line to define new B lymphocyte specificities, probably controlled by the MHC region, in: *Histocompatibility Testing* (F. Kissmeyer-Nielsen, ed.), pp. 708–712, Munksgaard, Copenhagen.

Festenstein, H., 1977, Joint report: Cellular typing, in: *Histocompatibility Testing* (W.F. Bodmer, J.R. Batchelor, J.G. Bodmer, H. Festentein, and P.J. Morris, eds.), pp. 358–363, Munksgaard, Copenhagen.

Fradelizi, D., Nuñez-Roldan, A., and Sasportes, M., 1978, Human Ia-like DRw lymphocyte antigens stimulating activity in primary mixed lymphocyte reaction, *Eur. J. Immunol.* **8:**88.

France, One and Two Regional Report, 1977, in: *Histocompatibility Testing* (W.F. Bodmer, J.R. Batchelor, J.G. Bodmer, H. Festinstein, and P.J. Morris, eds.), pp. 433–448, Munksgaard, Copenhagen.

Legrand, L., and Dausset, J., 1975a, Immunogenetics of a new lymphocyte system, *Transplant. Proc.* **7**(1):5.

Legrand, L., and Dausset, J., 1975b, A second lymphocyte system (Ly-Li), in: *Histocompatibility Testing* (F. Kissmeyer-Nielsen, ed.), 665–670, Munksgaard, Copenhagen.

Legrand, L., and Dausset, J., 1976, The B lymphocyte Ly-Li system, *Transplant. Proc.* **9**(1):451.

Mann, D.L., Abelson, L., Harris, S., and Amos, D.B., 1976, Second genetic locus in the HLA region for human B-cell alloantigens, *Nature (London)* **259**(5539):145.

McMichael, A.J., and Sasazuki, T., 1977, A suppressor T cell in the human mixed lymphocyte reaction, *J. Exp. Med.* **146**(2):368.

Nuñez-Roldan, A., Sasportes, M., and Fradelizi, D., 1978, Analysis of products involved in primary and secondary allogenic proliferation in man. II. Detection of products different from Ia-like, DRw antigens, activating secondary allogenic proliferation in man, *Immunogenetics* **6**:43.

Reinsmoen, N.L., Noreen, H.J., Friend, P.S., Giblett, E.R., Greenberg, L.J., and Kersey, J.H., 1979, Anomalous mixed lymphocyte culture reactivity between HLA-A, B, C, DR identical siblings, *Tissue Antigens* **13**(1):19.

Ryder, L.P., Thomsen, M., Platz, P., and Svejgaard, H., 1975, Data reduction in LD-typing, in: *Histocompatibility Testing* (F. Kissmeyer-Nielsen, ed.), pp. 557–562, Munksgaard, Copenhagen.

Sasazuki, T., Kohno, Y., Iwamoto, I., Tanimira, M., Naito, S., Kashiwagi, N., Itakura, K., Aizawa, M., Hasegawa, T., Miyajima, T., Akiyama, N., Juji, T., Tsuji, K., Sekiguchi, S., Yoshida, T.O., Akaza, T., Matsuyama, M., and Toyoda, K., 1977, Japanese regional report: The relationship between HLA-D and WIA specificities in the Japanese population, in: *Histocompatibility Testing* (W.F. Bodmer, J.R. Batchelor, J.G. Bodmer, H. Festenstein, and P.J. Morris, eds.), pp. 489–498, Munksgaard, Copenhagen.

Sasportes, M., Fradelizi, D., Nuñez-Roldan, A., Wollman, E., Giannopoulos, Z., and Dausset, J., 1978a, Analysis of stimulating products involved in primary and secondary allogenic proliferation in man. I. Preponderant role of the Ia-like DR (Ly-Li) antigens as stimulating products in secondary allogenic response in man, *Immunogenetics* **6**:29.

Sasportes, M., Nuñez-Roldan, A., and Fradelizi, D., 1978b, Analysis of stimulating products involved in primary and secondary allogenic proliferation in man. III. Further evidence for products different from Ia-like, DRw antigens, activating secondary allogenic proliferation in man, *Immunogenetics* **6**:55.

Sasportes, M., Fradelizi, D., and Dausset, J., 1978c, HLA-DR specific human suppressor lymphocytes generated by repeated *in vitro* sensitization against allogenic cells, *Nature (London)* **276**(5687):502.

Sasportes, M., Wollman, E.E., Cohen, D., Fradelizi, D., Carosella, E., Cathely, G., and Dausset, J., 1979, Mise en évidence d'un facteur coluble capable d'inhiber la prolifération lymphocytaire allgénique chez l'Homme, *C.R. Academie Sci. Paris (Ser. D)* **289**:41.

Solheim, B.G., Bratlie, A., Winther, N., and Thorsby, E., 1975, LD antisera prepared by planned immunizations, in: *Histocompatibility Testing* (F. Kissmeyer-Nielsen, ed.), pp. 713–718, Munksgaard, Copenhagen.

Suciu-Foca, N., Rohowsky, C., Godfrey, M., Khan, R., Woodward, K., Malavet, J., and Hardy, M., 1980, Intra-HLA recombinations and mapping of DR. Communication presented at the VIIIth International Workshop of Histocompatibility, Los Angeles.

Terasaki, P.I., Opeltz, G., Park, M.S., and Mickey, M.R., 1975, Four new B lymphocyte specificities, in: *Histocompatibility Testing* (F. Kissmeyer-Nielsen, ed.), pp. 657–664, Munksgaard, Copenhagen.

Troup, G.M., Jameson, J., Thomsen, M., Svejgaard, A., and Walford, R.L., 1978, Studies of HLA alloantigens of the Navajo Indians of North America. I. Variance of association between HLA-DRW (WIA) and HLA-DW specificities, *Tissue Antigens* **12**(1):44.

Van Leeuwen, A., Schuit, R., and Van Rood, J.J., 1973, Typing for MLC (LD): The selection of non stimulator cells by MLC inhibition test using SD identical stimulator cells (MISIS) and fluorescent antibody studies, *Transplant. Proc.* **5**(2):1539.

Van Rood, J.J., Van Leeuwen, A., Keuning, J.J., and Blussé van oud Alblas, K., 1975, The serological recognition of the human MLC determinant using a modified cytotoxicity technique, *Tissue Antigens* **5**(2):73.

Van Rood, J.J., Van Leeuwen, A., and Keuning, J.J., 1977, Evidence for two series of B-cell antigens in man and their comparison with HLA-D, *Scand. J. Immunol.* **6**(5):373.

Walford, R.L., Smith, G.S., Zeller, E., and Wilkinson, J., 1975, A new alloantigenic system on human lymphocytes, *Tissue Antigens* **5**(3):196.

Walford, R.L., Ferrara, G.B., Gatti, R.A., Leibold, W., Thompson, Y.S., Mercuriali, F., Goseett, T., and Naeim, F., 1977, New groups and segregant series among B cell alloantigens of the Merrit system studies of leukemia cells, *Scand. J. Immunol.* **6**(5):393.

Winchester, R.J., Fu, S.M., Wernet, P., Kunkel, H.G., Dupont, B., and Jershild, C., 1975, Recognition by pregnancy serums of non HLA alloantigens selectively expressed on B lymphocytes, *J. Exp. Med.* **141**(5):924.

Yunis, E.J., and Amos, D.B., 1971, Three closely linked genetic systems relevant to transplantation, *Proc. Natl. Acad. Sci. U.S.A.* **68**:3031.

4

Genetic Organization, Tissue Expression, and Functional Role of Murine Ia Antigens

Chella S. David, Kirk W. Beisel, Christopher J. Krco, and William P. Lafuse

1. Introduction

The *H-2* complex, the major histocompatibility complex (MHC) of the mouse, is an extremely polymorphic and pleiotrophic group of loci located in the middle section of chromosome 17 (Fig. 1) (Klein, 1975). The genetic map of the *H-2* complex has traditionally been defined by the *H-2K* locus at the centromeric end and by the *H-2D* locus at the telomeric end. The serological markers for the *H-2K* and the *H-2D* regions are the classic *H-2* transplantation antigens with a molecular weight of 45,000 that convey genetic restriction as targets for subpopulations of cytotoxic T cells (Zinkernagel and Doherty, 1974). The *H-2D* region gene codes for two independent molecular products of the *D* and *L* loci (Neuport-Sautes *et al.*, 1978; Hansen and Sachs, 1978). The order of the *H-2L* and *H-2D* loci is not known at present and will be referred to as *D(L)*. The *H-2G* region is defined by an erythrocyte-specific antigen, H-2.7 (David *et al.*, 1975a; Klein *et al.*, 1975). Recent studies show that this antigen is also found in the serum of H-2.7-positive strains (L. Brown, personal communication) and that it could be one of the components of the complement system (Beisel, unpublished data). The *S* region codes for genes controlling the quantitative levels of the C′4 complement component (Meo *et al.*,

---

Chella S. David, Kirk W. Beisel, Christopher J. Krco, and William P. Lafuse • Department of Immunology, Mayo Clinic and Medical School, Rochester, Minnesota 55901.

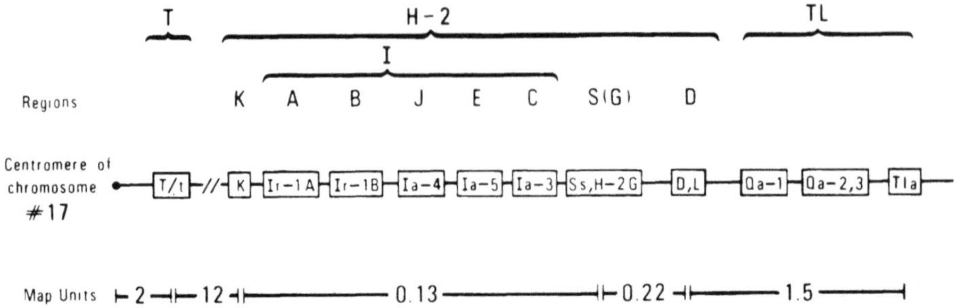

Figure 1. Genetic map of the 17th chromosome of the mouse, depicting the *I, H-2,* and *TL* complexes. Loci from left to right are as follows: (*T*) brachyury or short tail; (*K*) histocompatibility antigen; (*I*) Ia-region-associated antigen and immune response phenomena; [*S(G)*] Ss protein (4th component of complement) and H-2.7 (erythrocyte antigen); (*D*) histocompatibility antigens; (*Qa*) *Q*-region-associated antigens; (*Tla*) thymus leukemia antigen. The order of *Qa-1, Qa-2,3,* and *Tla* is not known but is arbitrarily depicted here.

1975; Shreffler, 1976) as well as a sex-limited allotypic variant (Slp) of the C′4 molecule (Passmore and Shreffler, 1970; Roos *et al.*, 1978). Since the *S* and *G* regions are separated by only one "questionable" recombinant, it is possible that the H-2.7 antigen actually maps in the *S* region.

The *TL* region, which maps to the right of the *H-2D(L)* region, was first identified by a polymorphic locus *(Tla)* that controls the expression of antigens on leukemia cells, normal cells, and subpopulations of lymphocytes (Old and Stockert, 1977). Present data suggest that there are six loci within the *TL* region, the two *Qa* loci (*Qa-1* and Qa-2,3), *H-2T, H-31, H-32,* and the *Tla* loci. This region has recently been referred to as the *H-2T* region (Klein *et al.*, 1978). We will refer to this region as the *H-2TL* region, since it was first defined by Tl antigens. Further, it would be best to reserve the term "*T* region" or "*T* complex" to denote the chromosomal segment coding for *T/t* loci (Bennett, 1975). It is becoming increasingly apparent that the *TL* region should be included in the MHC of the mouse, since its immunologically related properties are similar to those of *H-2. Qa-1* and *Qa-2,3* control serologically detectable determinants found on subpopulations of T lymphocytes (Flaherty, 1976; Stanton and Boyse, 1976; Flaherty *et al.*, 1978). Structurally, the *Qa*-loci antigens bear a remarkable similarity to the transplantation antigens of the *K* and *D* regions (Uhr *et al.*, 1976; Michaelson *et al.*, 1977). The *TL* region also maps two histocompatibility loci, *H-31* and *H-32* (Flaherty and Wachtel, 1975), as well as a cell-mediated lymphocytotoxicity (CML) locus, *H-2T* (Klein and Chiang, 1978). It is possible that the histocompatibility and cytotoxic effects of these three loci are a result of the Qa antigens.

2. Identification of Ia Antigens

The *H-2I* region mapping between the *H-2K* and*S* regions was first defined by immune response *(Ir)* genes to the synthetic amino acid polymer (H,G)-A–L (McDevitt *et al.*, 1972). Since the *Ir* genes were hypothesized to code for antigen receptors on T cells (Benacerraf and McDevitt, 1972), several laboratories attempted to produce antisera against these putative receptors. It was hoped that the resulting antisera would enable the further characterization of the *Ir* gene products. At that time, two sets of recombinant strains of mice were available that were identical at *H-2K* and *H-2D* but differed for the *S* region as well as the *Ir* genes (Fig. 2). They were A.TH ($K^sI^sS^sD^d$), A.TL ($K^sI^kS^kD^d$) (David and Shreffler, 1972) and B10.AQR ($K^qI^kS^dD^d$), B10.T(6R) ($K^qI^qS^qD^d$) (Klein *et al.*, 1970). Reciprocal immunizations with these strains of mice yielded antisera that were shown to react with a subpopulation of lymphocytes (David *et al.*, 1973; Hauptfeld *et al.*, 1973a). Later studies suggested predominant reactivity of these antisera with B lymphocytes (Sachs and Cone, 1973; Götze *et al.*, 1973; Hämmerling *et al.*, 1974). Since there was no direct proof that these antisera were reacting with the *Ir* gene product, the antigens were designated as immune-response-associated (Ia) antigens (Shreffler *et al.*, 1974). Later studies showed that most anti-H-2 sera contained antibodies to the Ia antigens (David and Shreffler, 1974a,b). Immunochemical analysis using anti-la sera demonstrated that the Ia determinants are found on the protein component of a glycoprotein containing two peptide chains of 28,000 and 33,000 daltons (Cullen *et al.*, 1974). This is contrasted with the transplantation antigens of the MHC, which are expressed on 45,000-dalton glycoproteins.

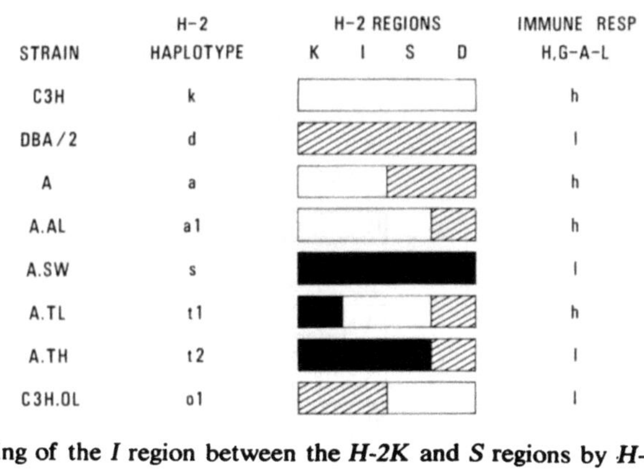

Figure 2. Mapping of the *I* region between the *H-2K* and *S* regions by *H-2* recombinant strains.

3. Genetic Fine Structure of the *I* Region

After the initial identification of the *Ir-1* locus by McDevitt *et al.* (1972), studies in several laboratories showed that control of immune responses to most antigens could also be influenced by the *Ir-1* locus or genes closely linked to the *Ir-1* locus. Lieberman *et al.* (1972) showed that responses to defined immunoglobulin G (IgG) and IgA allotypes were controlled by two adjacent loci. Immune response to the IgA allotype was associated with the *Ir-1* locus, while the *Ir* gene determining the IgG-allotype response was designated *Ir-IgG* and mapped to the new *I* subregion, *Ir-1B*. Strain B10.A(5R), a recombinant derived from crossing over between haplotypes $H\text{-}2^a$ and $H\text{-}2^b$, showed immune responses characteristic of $H\text{-}2^b$ at the *Ir-1A* and *Ir-1B* loci, but still expressed the Ia specificity (Ia.7) characteristic of the $H\text{-}2^a$ haplotype. This new *I* subregion (David *et al.*, 1975b) (Fig. 3) was designated *I-C*, and *Ir-1A* and *Ir-1B* were changed to *I-A* and I-B.

The recombinant B10.A(5R) was also involved in the identification and definition of another *I* subregion, *I-E*. The genetic material of B10.A(5R) was thought to consist primarily of the $H\text{-}2^b$ and the $H\text{-}2^d$ derived loci. However, $(b \times d)F_1$ anti-I^k antisera were found to react with B10.A(5R) lymphocytes (Colombani *et al.*, 1976; Shreffler *et al.*, 1977). This suggested a functional segment of chromosome in B10.A(5R) between the *I-B* and *I-C* regions derived from $H\text{-}2^a$ that was presumably of $H\text{-}2^k$ origin (Fig. 4). The crossing over in B10.A(5R) occurred between *I-B* and the new subregion, designated as *I-E*. The Ia specificity mapping in the *I-E* subregion was designated Ia.22.

Two laboratories identified antigen-specific suppression controlled by genes within a new region, *I-J* (Tada *et al.*, 1976a; Murphy *et al.*, 1976). A keyhole limpet hemocyanin (KLH)-specific suppressor factor derived from the $H\text{-}2^k$ haplotype was able to suppress the response of B10.A (5R),

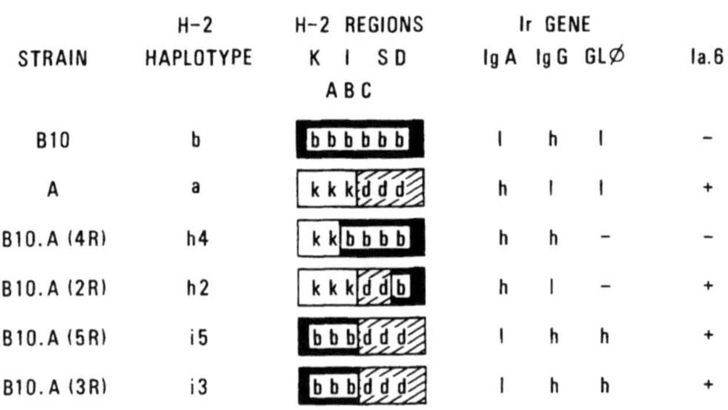

Figure 3. Mapping of the *I-A*, *I-B*, and *I-C* subregions within the *H-21* region.

STRAIN	H-2 HAPLOTYPE	H-2 REGIONS K I S D (A B J E C)	Ia 7	Ia 22 (I-E)	Ia 23	MLR SuPPR H-2^d FACTOR	KLH SuPPR H-2^k FACTOR
B10	b	b b b b b b b b	-	-	-	-	-
B10.BR	k	k k k k k k k k	+	+	-	-	+
B10.D2	d	d d d d d d d d	-	+	+	+	-
B10.A	a	k k k k k d d d	+	+	-	+	+
B10.A (5R)	i5	b b b k k d d d	+	+	-	+	+
B10.A (3R)	i3	b b b b k d d d	+	+	-	+	-

Figure 4. Further division of the *I* region by the description and mapping of the *I-E* and I-J subregions.

but not that of B10.A(3R). These two recombinants derived from H-2^a and H-2^b were thought to be identical. A B10.A (3R) anti-B10.A(5R) serum could absorb the suppressor factor from H-2^k, but not that from H-2^b. On the other hand, B10.A(5R) anti-B10.A(3R) serum could absorb suppressor factors from H-2^b, but not those from H-2^k. B10.A(5R) was $A^bB^bJ^kE^kC^d$ and B10.A(3R) was $A^bB^bJ^bE^kC^d$. mapping *I-J* between the *I-B* and the *I-E* subregion (Fig. 4). These results were confirmed using another set of recombinants, B10.S(9R) and B10.HTT, which were also identical at *I-A* and the *I-E* subregion, but differed at the *I-J* subregion.

Haplotype H-2^a became the only recombinant separating *I-E* and I-C. Sequential immunoprecipitation studies showed that Ia.7, previously mapping to the I-C subregion, coprecipitated with a Ia.22 in H-2^k strains and with Ia.23 in H-2^d strains, thereby mapping Ia.7, 22, and 23 in the *I-E* subregion (David and Cullen, 1978). The existence of *I-C* as a distinct subregion was confirmed by the finding of Rich *et al.* (1979) that alloantigen-activated-mixed-lymphocyte reaction (MLR) suppressor factor induced in and specific for H-2^d haplotype could suppress B10.A and C3H.OL but not B10.BR, thereby mapping it in *I-C* between the *I-E* and *S* regions (Fig. 4).

The current map of *H-21* regions consists of five subregions, *I-A, I-B, I-J, I-E,* and *I-C.* In the rest of this section, we will review the different traits associated with each of these subregions and the possible number of genes mapping within them. Table 1 shows the *H-2* gene complex composition of recombinant strains with crossing over between *H-2K* and the *S* regions.

3.1. *I-A* Subregion

The *I-A* subregion is currently defined by the recombinants A.TL (K^sA^k) and AQR (K^qA^k) on the left side and B10.A(4R) (A^kB^b) on the

TABLE 1. List of *I*-Region Recombinants

Strain	*H-2* haplotype	Parental *H-2* haplotypes	Origin of regions[a] *K A B J E C S*	Ia specifications *A*	*E*
A,B10.A	*a*	*k/d*	*k k k k k/d d*	1,2,3,15,17,18,19	7,22
AIR-1[b]	*a2*	*a1/i8*	*k k k k k · b*	1,2,3,15,17,18,19	7,22
A.TFR-3	*ap3*	*f/t2*	*f f· · · · s*	1,5,9,14,16,17,18	—
A.TFR-4	*ap4*	*lf/t2*	*f f· · · · s*	1,5,9,14,16,17,18	—
A.TFR-5	*ap5*	*lf/t1*	*f· · · k k k*	1,5,9,14,16,17,18	7, (22?)
B10.LG	*dx*	*d/?*	*d/f fff ff*	1,5,9,14,16,17,18	—
B10.S(8R)	*as1*	*a/s*	*k k · · s s s*	1,2,3,15,17,18,19	7,22
TBR2	*at2*	*t1/b*	*s k/b b b b b*	1,2,3,15,17,18,19	—
TBR3	*at3*	*t1/b*	*s k/b b b b b*	1,2,3,15,17,18,19	—
B10.F(13R)	*av1*	*p/b*	*p p p p p p/b*	3,5,13	7,21
D2.GD	*g2*	*d/b*	*d d d/b b b b*	8,11,15,16	—
B10.A(4R)	*h4*	*a/b*	*k k/b b b b b*	1,2,3,15,17,18,19	—
B10.BAR4	*h6*	*k/b*	*k k/b b b b b*	1,2,3,15,17,18,19	—
B10.A(3R)	*i3*	*b/a*	*b b b b k/d d*	3,8,9,15,20	7,22
B10.A(5R)	*i5*	*b/a*	*b b b/k k d d*	3,8,9,15,20	7,22
B10.QAR	*m1*	*a/q*	*k k k k k · q*	1,2,3,15,17,18,19	7,22
C3H.OL	*o1*	*d/k*	*d d d d d d/k*	8,11,15,16	7,23
B10.F(14R)	*bp*	*b/p*	*b b b b b b/p*	3,8,9,15,20	—
B10.QSR-2	*sq2*	*s/q*	*s s · · · · q*	4,5,9,12,17,18	—
A.TL,B10.TL	*t1*	*s/a1*	*s/k k k k k k*	1,2,3,15,17,18,19	7,22
B10.HTT	*t3*	*s/t1*	*s s s s/k k k*	4,5,9,12,17,18	7,22
B10.S(9R)	*t4*	*s/a*	*s s · k k d d*	4,5,9,12,17,18	7,22
BSVS	*t5*	*s/d*	*s s s s s s/d*	4,5,9,12,17,18	—
B10.AQR	*y1*	*q/a*	*q/k k k k d d*	1,2,3,15,17,18,19	7,22

[a](·) Unknown. [b]Tentative.

right side. Immune responses to most of the antigens studied so far are controlled by *Ir* genes in the *A* subregion, and the majority of the Ia specificities map primarily in the *A* subregion. Studies by Schmitt-Verhulst and Shearer (1978) have suggested an *Ir* gene mapping to the left of the crossover in A.TL strain that codes for response to trinitrophenyl-modified *H-2D*^{d} antigen. Zaleski and Klein (1977) have also shown that a complementing *Ir* gene to Thy-1.1 antigen maps within the *K* region on the basis of studies utilizing *H-2K* mutants. These investigations suggest that the *I* region may not be unique in coding for genes involved in human response.

The loci mapping in the *A* subregion are the most polymorphic among the *I* regions. Benacerraf and Dorf (1976) have mapped a complementing immune suppression gene also to the *A* subregion. It is still not clear whether the same locus (*Ir-1*) controls the immune response to all the different antigens or two or more closely linked genes within the *A* subregion control these responses. Every haplotype studied has a unique private Ia specificity mapping in the *I-A* subregion. The data on the Ia antigens suggest that one locus controls the Ia molecule carrying multiple specificities (Cullen *et al.*, 1976a). Whether the same locus also controls immune response is still an open question. Expression of Ia antigens on B cells, T cells, and macrophages seems to be controlled by the same loci. Tada *et al.* (1976b) have shown that an *A*-region gene product is expressed on the enhancing helper factor. Further, an acceptor site found in a subpopulation of T cells that receive this helper signal seems to be controlled by a different gene within the *A* region. Certain strains are able to generate the enhancing helper factor, but are unable to receive the helper signal. Taussig *et al.* (1975) demonstrated that an *A*- region gene product was expressed on a helper-T-cell replacing factor for the response to (T,G)-A—L. The acceptor molecule, which receives this helper signal and is expressed on B cells, is presumably controlled by a different gene within the *A* region (Ia?). The *I-A* subregion also contains a histocompatibility (*H*) locus (Klein *et al.*, 1974) and an *Lad* locus (Meo *et al.*, 1973), and can serve as a CML target (Nabholtz *et al.*, 1975).

At this time, we can postulate that there are a minimum of five genes mapping within the *A* subregion. Three (A_α, A_β, A_e) control Ia antigens expressed on B cells, T cells, and macrophages. A fourth gene has the capability of antigen recognition and/or generation of helper factors, while the fifth gene controls "receptors" on a subpopulation of T cells and/or B cells that are triggered by these *A*-subregion helper factors. This is a minimum estimate, and most probably several more genes may map within the *A* subregion. So far, no recombinants have been produced to separate the different phenomena associated with the *A* subregion. There could be crossover inhibition functioning to prevent recombination or separation of the *A* region genes, since linkage among these gene products may be critical for optimal interaction. One cannot assume that the cross over points in A.TL and AQR are identical, and further studies involving these two recombinants could suggest possible differences. A new recombinant, B10.LG (K^d I^f), should also aid in these fine-structure studies.

3.2. *I-B* Subregion

The *I-B* subregion was originally defined by the immune response to the IgG allotype. The region is defined by recombinant B10.A(4R) (K^k A^k B^b) on the left side and by B10.A(5R) (A^b B^b J^k) on the right. So far, neither Ia antigens nor MLRs can be attributed to the *I-B* subregion. The detection of complementing genes for certain antigens (Dorf and Benacerraf, 1975; Melchers and Rajewsky, 1975; Zaleski and Klein, 1976) raised the question of whether the Ir-IgG response described by Lieberman *et al.*, (1972) could be accounted for by complementing *Ir* genes mapping in the *A* and *E/C* subregions. But recently, new phenomena have been mapped to this subregion. Studies by Urba and Hildemann (1978) mapped a recessive *Ir* gene to trinitrophenylated mouse serum albumin in this region. Also, an "immune-response"-type gene controlling skin graft acceptance or rejection for H-Y incompatibility maps in this region (Hurme *et al.*, 1978). Hence, the *I-B* region is defined by a functional phenotypic marker but lacks Ia, MLR, and H determinants, suggesting that it is not synonymous to the *A* subregion. Possibly, crossing over has separated some of the *Ir* genes from the *A* region. This would give credence to the postulation that immune responses are controlled by more than one closely linked gene mapping in the *A* subregion. Recently, a few more recombinants have been identified that seem to have crossing over in this segment of the chromosome (AIR1, TBR2, and TBR3) (Beisel *et al.*, 1980). Further analysis of these recombinants along with B10.A(4R) and D2.GD for immune responses to all *H-2*-associated antigens might provide further information on this aspect. So far, neither does this region express any products on B cells or macrophages nor have T-cell factors been associated with this region. Without the availability of an antiserum detecting a gene product in this region, further serological, biochemical, and functional analyses have not been possible.

3.3. *I-J* Subregion

The *I-J* subregion was originally defined by the identification of the genes controlling the antigen-specific suppressor factors to KLH antigen and by antigens expressed on allotype suppressor cells (Tada *et al.*, 1976a; Murphy *et al.*, 1976). The region is defined by recombinant B10.A(5R) ($B^b J^k$) on the left side and by recombinant B10.A(3R) ($B^b J^b E^k$) on the right side. Most of the studies suggest that the *J* subregion codes for genes primarily involved in the suppressive mechanisms. The gene products seem to be expressed primarily on suppressor T lymphocytes, but there is controversy as to their expression on macrophages (Cowing *et al.*, 1978; Neiderhuber, 1978). Studies by Tada (1977) with the KLH antigens suggest that one gene within the *J* subregion controls the generation of the antigen-specific suppressor factor. A second *I-J* gene, expressed on a subpopulation of suppressor T cells, controls the site or receptor that receives the *I-J* suppressor factor. Strain A/J, for example, cannot produce or generate the suppressor factor even though they can accept a suppressive signal. These studies would suggest that there are at least two loci within the *J* subregion. These two genes are probably very closely linked, and selection might discourage crossing over. Recently, Howie *et al.* (1979) have shown that *I-J* determinants may be expressed on a GAT helper factor. Tada *et al.* (1978) have described carrier-specific helper T cells that act to augment B-cell response to hapten. This subpopulation of T cells carries an Ia antigen controlled by the *I-J* subregion. This would mean that the *I-J* region could also include helper-type genes even though it controls predominantly suppressor functions. Studies in our laboratory (Okuda *et al.*, 1977) showed that *I-J* determinants expressed on T cells are capable of stimulating in the MLR and that this reaction can be inhibited by anti-I-J sera. No *H* loci have been demonstrated for this region.

3.4. *I-E* Subregion

The *I-E* subregion was defined by the identification of Ia.22, which is a private specificity of I^k strains (Shreffler *et al.*, 1977). The region is defined on the left side by recombinant B10.A(3R) (J^b E^k) and B10.HTT (J^s E^k) and on the right side by haplotype $H\text{-}2^a$ (E^k C^d). Specificity Ia.7, which was previously mapped to the *I-C* subregion, is mapped to the *I-E* subregion (David and Cullen, 1978). A private *I-E* subregion specificity for the $H\text{-}2^d$ haplotype has also recently been mapped (Ia.23). The *I-E* product is also expressed on haplotypes $H\text{-}2^p$ and $H\text{-}2^r$ (Ia.7). Gene products associated with haplotypes $H\text{-}2^b$, $H\text{-}2^s$, $H\text{-}2^f$, and $H\text{-}2^q$ have not been identified using alloantisera. Studies utilizing xenoantisera to identify the gene products in these haplotypes are currently under way in our laboratory and will be described in a later section. The *I-E* gene products are expressed predominantly on B cells and also on a subpopulation of T cell. MLR studies with the *I-J* subregion suggested that at least some of the *I-J*-bearing T cells might express an *E* product (Okuda *et al.*, 1977). Weak expression of the *I-E/I-C* gene product has also been shown for macrophages (Cowing *et al.*, 1978).

The polymorphism of the *I-E* gene products seems to be far less than that of the *I-A* subregion. Serological cross-reactions between Ia antigens of the *A* and *E* loci suggest that these two loci might have resulted from gene duplication (Murphy and Shreffler, 1975; David *et al.*, 1978). Further, recent studies by Jones *et al.* (1978) suggest that expression of an *I-A*-region gene product might depend on a genetic complementation with the *I-E*-region gene. Preliminary amino acid sequence analyses of McMillan *et al.* (1977) and Silver *et al.* (1978) show that the human B-cell Ia molecule has a high homology with the *I-E*-region mouse Ia molecule but not with the mouse *I-A*-region molecule. These results suggest that the *I-E* subregion might constitute the ancestral locus, while the *I-A* subre-

TABLE 2. Traits Associated with *I*-Subregions

Trait	Subregion *A*	*B*	*J*	*E*	*C*
Tissue expression					
B cells	+	−	−	+	−
T cells	+	−	+	+	+
Macrophages	+	−	−	+	−
Epidermal (Langerhans)	+	−	−	+	−
Neutrophils	+	−	−	+	−
Eosinophils	+	−	−	+	−
Peyer's patch	+	−	−	+	?
Tumor cells	+	−	?	+	−
Serum	+	−	−	+	−
Ir genes	+	+	−	−	+
Is genes	+	−	−	−	+
Helper factors					
T cell	+	−	+	−	−
Macrophage	+	−	−	−	−
Suppressive factors					
Antigen-specific	−	−	+	−	−
Alloantigen (MLR)	−	−	−	−	+
Contact sensitivity	−	−	−	−	+
Receptors on T cells	+	?	+	−	+
Receptors on B cells	+	−	−	−	−
Antigen presentation (?)	+	−	−	+	−
Antigen recognition (?)	+	+	+	−	+
Minimum number of genes	3	1	3	1	2

gion evolved after duplication of the ancestral gene to code for unique gene products mediating immune phenomena. The *I-E* subregion also maps histocompatibility loci and MLR loci.

3.5. *I-C* Subregion

The *I-C* subregion was originally identified on the basis of an Ia specificity, Ia.7 (David *et al.*, 1974). Recent studies have moved all Ia specificities expressed on B cells to the *I-E* subregion, leaving the *I-C* subregion coding primarily for antigens or products on T cells (David and Cullen, 1978). One Ia specificity, Ia.6, expressed on T cells and capable of stimulating MLR, is mapped in the $I\text{-}C^d$ subregion (Okuda and David, 1978). The region is defined by the $H\text{-}2^a$ haplotype ($E^k\ C^d\ S^d$) on the left side and by C3H.OL ($C^d\ S^k$) on the right side. This region is characterized primarily on the basis of MLR and functional tests. A gene product for *I-C* has not been biochemically identified. There is some indication that this antigen may be expressed on macrophages, but the results are inconclusive. An MLR-suppressor factor generated by alloantigens has clearly been shown to be generated by genes within the *I-C* subregion (Rich *et al.*, 1979). These studies show that one gene may be responsible for generation of suppressor factor, whereas a second gene mapping within the same region may be involved in the acceptance of the suppressive signal. Preliminary studies by Moorhead (personal communication) suggest that the suppressor factor involved in dinitrofluorobenzene (DNFB) contact sensitivity expresses *I-C*-region gene products. Benacerraf and Dorf (1977) have mapped the complementing immune suppression and immune response genes to this region. Hence, this region may map both immune-response- and immune-suppression-type phenomena. This could be the ancestral *Ir* locus, and duplication could have given rise to diverse *Ir* genes in the *I-A* subregion.

Table 2 lists the major traits associated with the five *I* subregions. Figure 5 shows the crossing-over frequencies and the number of recombinants defining the crossover points.

4. Polymorphism of Ia Antigens

One of the early antisera produced, A.TH anti-A.TL (anti-I^k), suggested the complexity of the Ia antigens by their extensive cross-reactivity (David *et al.*, 1973). This antiserum reacted with independent haplotypes H-2^b, H-2^d, H-2^f, H-2^k, H-2^p, H-2^q, H-2^r, H-2^u, and H-2^v. Absorption studies suggested more than one antibody population in this serum. By producing restricted antisera, individual antigenic specificities were identified. Detailed definitions of each of the Ia specificities have

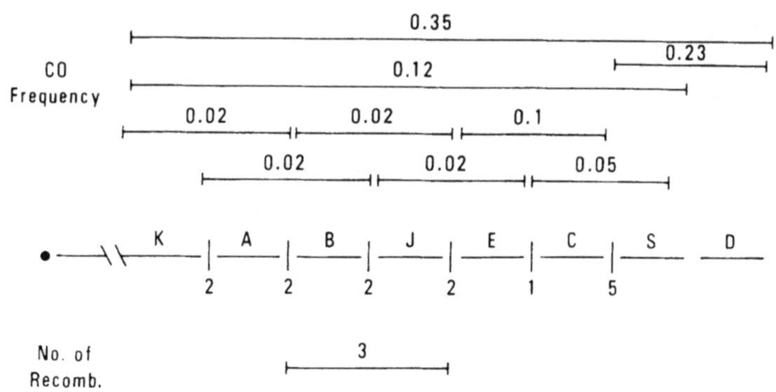

Figure 5. Recombination frequencies among the different regions and subregions of the *H-2* complex.

been covered in earlier reviews (Shreffler and David, 1975; David, 1976, 1977). In this section, we will briefly review the definitions of the currently known Ia specificities, define five new specificities, and include any changes in the distribution of Ia antigens that have occurred since the last review.

Ia specificities 1, 2, 3, 4, 5, and 7 were identified by the first two anti-Ia sera produced, A.TL anti-A.TH (I^k anti-I^s) and A.TH anti-A.TL (I^s anti-I^k) (David and Shreffler, 1974a). Specificity Ia.1 was defined as a cross-reaction of antiserum A.TH anti-A.TL with $H\text{-}2^f$ haplotypes (anti-I^k with I^f). Later studies showed that haplotypes $H\text{-}2^r$ and $H\text{-}2^u$ also expressed specificity Ia.1. Specificity Ia.2 was defined as the private specificity of haplotype $H\text{-}2^k$, antibodies against which are present in most anti-I^k sera. Specificity Ia.3 was first identified by a cross-reaction of A.TH anti-A.TL with the $H\text{-}2^b$ haplotypes (anti-I^k with I^b). Ia.3 was also found to be expressed in haplotypes $H\text{-}2^j$, $H\text{-}2^q$, $H\text{-}2^r$, and $H\text{-}2^v$. Recent studies by Guimezanes *et al.* (1979) strongly suggest that the $H\text{-}2^p$ haplotype also expresses the Ia.3 specificity. They showed that after A.TH anti-A.TL serum was bound to the B10 ($H\text{-}2^b$) lymphocytes (Ia.3), the eluted antibodies reacted with B10.P ($H\text{-}2^p$). B10.P could absorb anti-Ia.3 activity for B10 target cells. The reaction of the A.TH anti-A.TL serum with B10.D2 strains (anti-I^k with I^d) was defined as specificity Ia.7. Ia.7 is also expressed on haplotypes $H\text{-}2^j$, $H\text{-}2^p$, $H\text{-}2^r$, $H\text{-}2^u$, and $H\text{-}2^v$. The Ia typing on haplotypes $H\text{-}2^u$ and $H\text{-}2^v$ was recently reported by Klein *et al.* (1978).

The reciprocal antiserum A.TL anti-A.TH reacted with $H\text{-}2^f$, $H\text{-}2^j$, $H\text{-}2^p$, $H\text{-}2^q$, $H\text{-}2^r$, $H\text{-}2^s$, and, more recently, $H\text{-}2^u$ and $H\text{-}2^v$. Most of the absorption studies showed that any one of the cross-reacting haplotypes could remove the activity for all the other haplotypes, suggesting two antibody populations in this antiserum. Specificity Ia.4 was defined as the private specificity of $H\text{-}2^s$ haplotypes and Ia.5 was defined as a cross-reaction of A.TH anti-A.TH with B10.M (anti-I^s with I^f). Ia.5 was found to be expressed on all the other haplotypes that cross-reacted with this antiserum. All these cross-reactions have not been confirmed by immunoprecipitation analysis. There is some question as to whether some of the cross-reaction could be due to a Qa antigen, since A.TL anti-A.TH antiserum is known to contain anti-Qa antibodies (Flaherty *et al.*, 1975).

In an attempt to produce Ia antigens associated with the *Ir-IgG* loci, reciprocal immunizations were carried out between recombinants B10.A(4R) and B10.A(2R), which differed primarily for this region along with the *S* and *G* regions (David and Shreffler, 1974b). The antiserum B10.A(2R) anti-B10.A(4R) did not have detectable antibodies, whereas B10.A(4–R) anti-B10.A(2R) gave very weak cytotoxic reactivity. The reaction with the $H\text{-}2^d$ haplotypes was stronger than with the $H\text{-}2^k$

haplotypes. Absorption of this antiserum with $H\text{-}2^k$ strains left weak residual activity for $H\text{-}2^d$ strains. The antigen expressed on the $H\text{-}2^d$ haplotypes reacting with B10.A(4R) anti-B10.A(2R) serum was defined as specificity Ia.6. This specificity first suggested the existence of the *I-C* subregion. Recently, it has been very difficult to produce antisera against the Ia.6 specificity.

Specificities Ia.8 and Ia.9 were defined on the basis of cross-reactions (Sachs *et al.*, 1975). Ia.8 was defined by a cross-reaction of B10.A anti-B10 serum (anti-$H\text{-}2^b$) with B10.D2 ($H\text{-}2^d$) (anti-I^b with I^d). The reactivity of the same antiserum with B10.S ($H\text{-}2^s$) and B10.G ($H\text{-}2^q$) was defined as Ia.9 (anti-I^b with I^s). Specificity Ia.9 was also found to be expressed on $H\text{-}2^u$ and $H\text{-}2^v$ haplotypes. Originally, the cross-reaction of the antiserum B10.A anti-B10 with B10.M ($H\text{-}2^f$) was ascribed to an *H-2* specificity, H-2.39. Immunoprecipitation studies by Cullen (personal communication) suggest that this cross-reaction involves both *H-2* (H2.39) and an Ia specificity (Ia.9). Specificity Ia.10 was defined by the antiserum B10.AQR anti-B10.T(6R) (anti-I^q) as a private specificity of haplotype $H\text{-}2^q$ (Hauptfeld *et al.*, 1973b). Recent studies suggest that specificity Ia.10 is also expressed on the $H\text{-}2^j$ haplotype.

Specificity Ia.11 was defined as a private specificity of haplotype $H\text{-}2^d$ by absorption of antiserum (B10 × A)F_1 anti-B10.D2 (anti-K^d I^d) with B10.D2 erythrocytes (to remove anti-H-2) and B10.Q lymphocytes (to remove anti-Ia.16) and showing specific Ia activity only with the $H\text{-}2^d$ haplotypes (Davies and Hess, 1974). The cross-reaction of the unabsorbed antiserum with B10.Q ($H\text{-}2^q$) was defined as Ia.16 (Staines *et al.*, 1974). Cross-reactions on the basis of secondary MLR suggest that Ia.16 may also be expressed on the $H\text{-}2^f$ haplotype (Fathman *et al.*, 1977). Specificities Ia.12, 13, and 14 were defined by cross-reactions of anti-$H\text{-}2^r$, anti-$H\text{-}2^p$, and anti-$H\text{-}2^f$ sera (David *et al.*, 1976b). Reaction of antiserum [B10.A(2R) × C3H.NB]F_1 anti-B10.RIII with B10.S strains defined Ia.12 (anti-I^r with I^s). A new antiserum [(B10.RIII (20R) × A]F_1 anti-B10.RIII identifies a private Ia specificity of the $H\text{-}2^r$ haplotype that has been given the workshop designation IaW34 (Lafuse, Beisel, and David, unpublished data). Specificity Ia.13 was defined by the cross-reaction of the antiserum (B6 × A)F_1 anti-B10.P with B10.Q (anti-I^p with I^q). When this antiserum was absorbed with B10.P platelets (to remove anti-H-2) and B10.Q lymphocytes (to remove anti-Ia.13), a private Ia specificity (Ia.21) of haplotype $H\text{-}2^p$ was detected (Cullen *et al.*, 1976b). Recently, an antiserum produced in the combination (B10 × BZ.H)F_1 anti-B10.A(13R) identified a private specificity of haplotype $H\text{-}2^p$ different from Ia.21. This specificity has been tentatively designated IaW35 (David, unpublished data). Ia.14 was defined by the antiserum A.TFR-1 anti-A.CA after absorption with A.CA platelets leaving a private specificity for $H\text{-}2^f$ haplotype.

Specificity Ia.15 was defined by the antiserum (A.TH × B10.HTT)F_1 anti-A.TL reacting with B10.D2 (anti-I^k with I^d). Strains carrying *H-2*^{d}, *H-2*^{d}, and *H-2*^{k} shared the Ia.15 specificity. Specificities Ia.17, 18, and 19 were defined by antiserum (C3H.Q × B10.D2)F_1 anti-AQR by cross-reactions (Colombani *et al.*, 1976). Specificities Ia.17 and 18 were defined as a cross-reaction of this antiserum with B10.S (I^k with I^s). Specificity Ia.17 was also expressed in haplotypes *H-2*^{f}, *H-2*^{j}, and *H-2*^{r}, while Ia.18 was also present in *H-2*^{f}. Specificity 19 was defined by cross-reaction of this antiserum with B10.RIII after absorption with B10.S (I^k with I^r). Specificity Ia.22 was mapped on the basis of the reaction of this antiserum with B10.A(5R) (Shreffler *et al.*, 1977). In this case, Ia.22 is not a cross-reactive specificity but a private specificity of the *H-2*^{k} haplotype mapping to the *I-e* subregion, which will be discussed later. Specificity Ia.23 was identified as a private specificity of the *H-2*^{d} haplotype, mapping in the *I-E* subregion by absorbing antiserum (B10 × A)F_1 anti-B10.D2 with D2.GD lymphocytes. The D2.GD lymphocytes removed antibodies reacting against antigens mapping in the *K* and the *A* subregion (David and Cullen, 1978).

Specificities Ia.24, 31, 32, and 33 were recently reported (Klein *et al.*, 1978). Specificities W25, W26, W27, W28, W29, and W30 were identified by Gotze (1976) using lymphoblasts for immunization. Such immunizations could produce antibodies against components of the lymphoblasts not present in normal cells, and against other cell-surface components. We have recently identified private Ia specificities, IaW36, IaW37, and IaW38, belonging to haplotypes *H-2*^{u}, *H-2*^{j}, and *H-2*^{v}, respectively (David *et al.*, unpublished data). W36 was identified by absorbing antiserum (A × B10.S)F_1 anti-B10.PL with B10.PL platelets, W37 was identified by absorbing antiserum (B10 × A)F_1 anti-B10.WB with B10.WB platelets and W38 was identified by absorbing antiserum [A × B10.SM(22R)]F_1 anti-B10.SM with B10.SM platelets. All the identifications discussed above were confirmed by immunoprecipitation studies. Table 3 shows the distribution of Ia specificities of independent haplotypes. Table 4 shows the current recipient–donor combinations to provide anti-Ia sera.

4.1. Mapping of Ia Specificities

The majority of the Ia specificities identified so far are associated with the *I-A* subregion, which also controls most of the immune responses (Cullen *et al.*, 1976a). Hence, the *I-A* subregion is the most polymorphic Ia locus. Every independent haplotype expresses at least one private specificity associated with the *I-A* subregion and several public specificities. Specificities Ia.1, 2, 3, 8, 9, 11, 15, 17, 18, 19, and 20 were

TABLE 3. Distribution of Ia Specificities in the Independent Halpotypes

H-2 haplo-type	Type strain	Specificity[a]																											
		1	2	3	4	5	6	7	8	9	10	11	12	13	14	15	16	17	18	19	20	21	22	23	W34	W35	W36	W37	W38
b	B10	–	–	3	–	–	–	–	8	9	–	–	–	–	–	15	–	–	–	–	20	–	–	–	–	–	–	–	–
d	B10.D2	–	–	–	–	–	6	7	8	–	–	11	–	–	–	15	16	–	–	–	–	–	–	23	–	–	–	–	–
f	B10.M	1	–	–	–	5	–	–	–	9	–	–	–	–	14	–	16	17	18	–	–	–	–	–	–	–	–	–	–
j	B10.WB	–	–	3	–	–	·	7	–	9	10	–	–	–	–	·	–	17	–	–	–	–	–	–	–	–	–	W37	–
k	B10.K	1	2	3	–	–	–	7	–	–	–	–	–	–	–	15	–	17	18	19	–	–	22	–	–	–	–	–	–
p	B10.P	–	–	3	–	5	6	7	–	–	–	–	–	13	–	–	–	–	–	–	–	21	–	–	–	W35	–	–	–
q	B10.Q	–	–	3	–	5	–	–	–	9	10	–	–	13	–	–	16	–	–	–	–	–	–	–	–	–	–	–	–
r	B10.RIII	1	–	3	–	6	–	7	–	–	–	–	12	–	–	–	–	17	–	19	–	–	–	–	W34	–	–	–	–
s	B10.S	–	–	–	4	5	–	–	–	9	–	–	12	–	–	–	–	17	18	–	–	–	–	–	–	–	–	–	–
u	B10.PL	1	–	·	–	5	·	7	8	9	–	–	–	–	·	·	–	?	?	?	–	–	–	–	–	–	W36	–	–
v	B10.SM	–	–	3	–	5	·	7	–	9	–	–	–	–	·	·	–	?	?	?	–	–	–	–	–	–	–	–	W38

[a](–) Absence of a specificity; (·) unknown; (?) uncertain presence or absence of specificity.

TABLE 4. Donor–Recipient Combinations for Production of Anti-Ia Sera

Specificity	Recipient	Donor	Target strain	Absorbed in	Other antibodies	Region detected
1	$(A.BY\times B10.HTT)F_1$	A.TL	A.CA	—	Ia.2	$(A,B,J)^k$
2	$[B10.S(9R)\times A.TFR\text{-}5]F_1$	A.TL	A.TL	—	Ia.3	A^k
3	$(A.TH\times B10.HTT)F_1$	A.TL	B10	—	Ia.1,2,15	$(A,B,J)^k$
4	$[A.TL\times B10.A(1R)]F_1$	B10.S(9R)	B10.S(9R)	—	Ia.5	A^s
5	$(A.TL\times A)F_1$	A.TH	A.CA	—	Ia.4	I^s
6	B10.A(4R)	B10.A(2R)	B10.D2	—	Ia.7?,22?	$(B,J,E)^k\ C^d$
7	$(B10\times HTI)F_1$	B10.A(5R)	B10.D2	—	Ia.22	E^k,C^d
8	$(B10.A\times A)F_1$	B10.A(5R)	B10.D2	—	Ia.20,H-2.33	$(K,A,B)^b$
9	$(B10.A\times D2.GD)F_1$	B10.A(5R)	B10.S	—	Ia.20,H-2.33	$(K,A,B)^b$
10	$(B10.AQR\times A)F_1$	B10.T(6R)	B10.Q	—	?	I^q
11	$(B10.LG\times C3H)F_1$	C3H.OL	D2.GD	—	—	I^d
12	$(B10.A\times C3H.NB)F_1$	B10.RIII	B10.S	—	Ia.W34	$H\text{-}2^r$
13	$(B10\times A)F_1$	B10.P	B10.Q	—	Ia.21,W35	$H\text{-}2^p$
14	$(A.TL\times B10.Q)F_1$	A.TFR-5	B10.LG	B10.M (platelets)	—	$(K,A,B,J)^f$
15	$(A.TH\times B10.HTT)F_1$	A.TL	B10.D2	—	Ia.1,2,3	$(A,B,J)^k$
16	$(B10\times A)F_1$	B10.GD	B10.Q	—	Ia.11	$(K,A,B)^d$
17	$(C3H.Q\times B10.D2)F_1$	B10.AQR	B10.WB	—	Ia.2,18,19,22	I^k
18	$(C3H.Q\times B10.D2)F_1$	B10.AQR	B10.S	B10.RIII	Ia.2,17,19,22	I^k
19	$(C3H.Q\times B10.D2)F_1$	B10.AQR	B10.RIII	B10.S	Ia.2,17,18,22	I^k
20	$(B10.GD\times C3H.Q)F_1$	B10	B10	B10 (platelets)	—	$(K,A,B)^b$
21	$(B10\times A)F_1$	B10.F(13R)	B10.P	B10.P (platelets)	Ia.13,W35	$(K,I)^p$
22	$[129\times B10.A(4R)]F_1$	B10.A(2R)	B10.K	B10.D2	Ia.7	$E^k\ C^d$
23	$(D2.GD\times B10.A)F_1$	B10.D2	B10.HTG	—	—	$(J,E)^d$
W34	$[B10.RIII(20R)\times A]F_1$	B10.RIII	B10.RIII	B10.RIII (platelets)	—	I^r
W35	$(B10\times A)F_1$	B10.F(13R)	B10.P	B10.P (platelets)	Ia.13,21	I^p
W36	$(A\times B10.S)F_1$	B10.D2	B10.D2	B10.PL (platelets)	—	I^u
W37	$(B10\times A)F_1$	B10.WB	B10.WB	B10.WB (platelets)	—	I^j
W38	$[B10\times B10.SM(22R)]F_1$	B10.SM	B10.SM	B10.SM (platelets)	—	I^v

assigned to the *I-A* subregion on the basis of specific recombinants. Specificities Ia.22 and 23 were mapped to the *I-E* subregion also on the basis of specific recombinants. Specificities Ia.7 and 21 were mapped to the *I-E* subregion on the basis of sequential immunoprecipitation. Specificities Ia.4, 5, 12, and 13 could map in either the *A* or the *B* subregion, but since no Ia specificity has been identified so far in the *I-B* subregion, they most probably map at the *I-A* subregion. Specificities Ia.14 and Ia.16 could map in either the *I-A*, *I-B*, or *I-J* subregion. No precipitable Ia gene products have been associated with the *I-B* and *I-J* subregions, so Ia.14 and Ia.16 probably map in the *I-A* subregion. Specificity Ia.10 could map anywhere in the *I* region. Studies are under way to definitively map specificities Ia.4, 5, 10, 12, 13, 14, and 16 by sequential immunoprecipitation. The new Ia specificities have not yet been mapped. Specificity Ia.6, which is expressed on a subpopulation of T cells, is tentatively mapped to the *I-C* subregion. Since immunoprecipitation studies have been impossible with this specificity, conclusive mapping cannot be made.

4.2. *I-E*-Subregion Gene Products in "Silent" Haplotypes

The *I-E* subregion was first serologically and biochemically defined in haplotype $H\text{-}2^k$ (Ia.7,22) and more recently in haplotype $H\text{-}2^d$ (Ia.7,23) (Shreffler *et al.*, 1977; David and Cullen, 1978). Since the antisera directed against specificity Ia.7 also react with haplotypes *j*, *p*, *r*, *u*, and *v*, we can assume that these haplotypes also express a product in the *I-E* subregion. Alloimmunizations to detect the *I-E*-subregion products in the $H\text{-}2^b$ and $H\text{-}2^s$ haplotypes have so far been unsuccessful (David, unpublished data). Immunizations, B10.A(2R) anti-B10.A(4R), B10.A(5R) anti-B10.A(18R), B10.HTG anti-B10.GD, and several other combinations failed to yield antibodies against the $I\text{-}E^b$ product. Immunizations B10.S(9R) anti-B10.S(7R), B10.HTT anti-B10.S(7R), and several other combinations also failed to produce antibodies against the $I\text{-}E^s$ product. All immunizations involving the $H\text{-}2^f$ and $H\text{-}2^q$ have so far primarily yielded antibodies reacting with *I-A* products. The serological studies have been confirmed by MLR tests (Meo, unpublished data).

We can postulate several reasons that antibodies against the *I-E*-subregion gene products in these haplotypes are not generated (we will refer to these haplotypes as "*I-E* silent" haplotypes): (1) Antigens coded by the *I-E* subregion genes in *b*, *f*, *q*, and *s* haplotypes are probably not very immunogenic and fail to initiate the production of antibodies. This explanation seems unlikely, since every possible method to enhance the immunogenicity has failed. Sensitive detection assays have also been tried to detect very low titer or nonbinding antibodies. (2) Recipients used for immunizations may be low responders to these particular Ia antigens.

This is also unlikely, since so many different donor–recipient combinations have been tried. (3) In haplotypes *b*, *f*, *q*, and *s*, there may be a deletion for this chromosomal segment resulting in the lack of any gene products associated with this region. Since the *I-J* subregion and the *S* region have been identified in all these haplotypes, the possibility of deletion involving just the *I-E* subregion (and *I-C*) seems unlikely. Studies are under way to detect the *I-C* subregion in these haplotypes. (4) The *I-E*-subregion locus apparently codes for nonpolymorphic gene products. Haplotypes in which the *I-E* gene product has been identified could possibly represent recent mutation events. These gain-type mutations were identified by alloimmunizations utilizing recipient strains that lacked the antigens and are designated Ia.7, 21, 22, 23, and so on. The reciprocal immunization does not imply any incompatibility, and hence, no antibodies are produced. If this is true, xenoimmunizations, but not alloimmunizations, will lead to production of antibodies to detect this gene

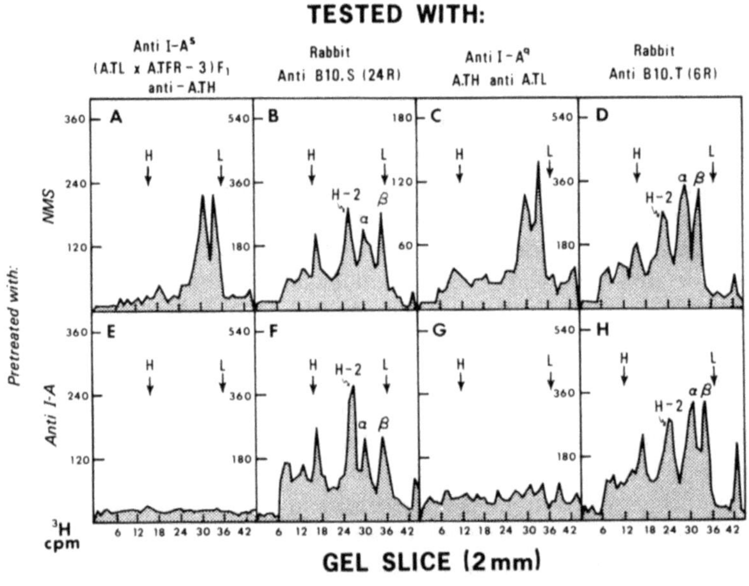

Figure 6. Electrophoretic patterns of Ia antigens sequentially precipitated from B10.S (panels A, B, E, and F) and B10.Q (panels C, D, G, and H) strains. NP-40 extracts labeled with [^{3}H]leucine were first treated with an excessive amount of normal mouse serum or anti-I-A serum as indicated on the left side of the panels. The immune complexes were removed with protein-A-bearing staphylococci. The supernatants were aliquoted and subjected to a second precipitation using the sera indicated at the top of the figure. The immune complexes were removed with protein-A-bearing staphylococci, solubilized, reduced, and electrophoresed. (H, L) Positions of ^{14}C-labeled heavy and light chains of a human IgM electrophoresed on a parallel gel.

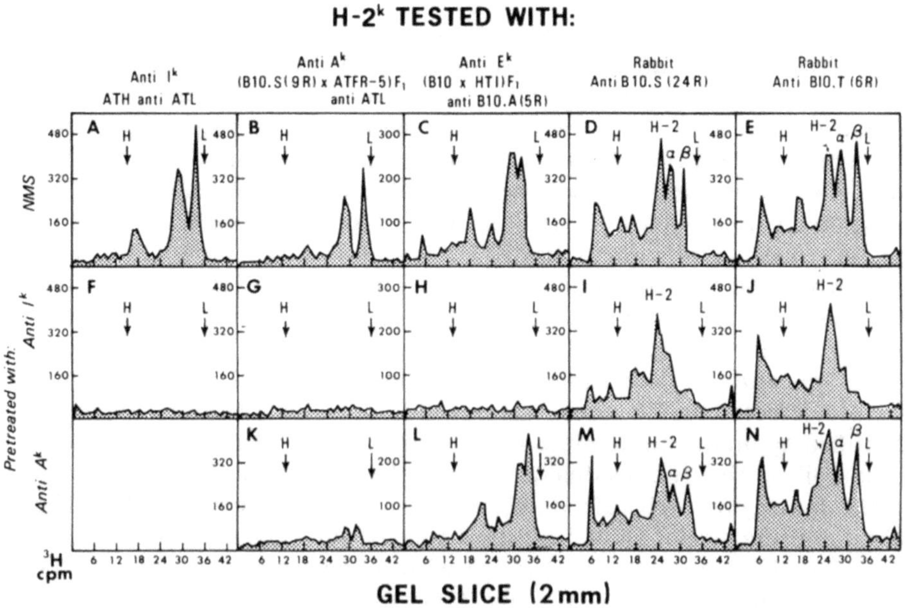

Figure 7. Sequential immunoprecipitation analysis of Ia antigens of B10.AM mice. Pretreatment with normal mouse serum (top row) left molecules reactive with anti-*I*k, anti-*A*k, anti-*E*k, rabbit anti-B10.S(24R), and rabbit anti-B10.T(6R) sera. Pretreatment with A.TH anti-A.TL (anti-*I*k) sera (middle row) removed molecules reactive with both the rabbit antisera. Pretreatment with anti-*I-A*k sera (bottom row) failed to remove all the I-A antigens reactive with rabbit anti-B10.S(24R) and B10.T(6R) sera.

product. In the rest of this section, we will describe our preliminary results with xenoantisera.

Cells from the spleen, lymph node, and thymus of mice carrying the *I* region of *b, f, q,* and *s* haplotypes were solubilized with 0.5% Triton X-100 in Tris-buffered saline. The lysates were ultracentrifuged and the supernatants mixed with equal volumes of complete Freund's adjuvant for immunization with rabbits. First, antisera were tested to determine whether they had activity against Ia molecules. Potentially, the antisera could also contain antibodies to mouse immunoglobulins, H-2 molecules, and other cell-surface glycoproteins. ^3H-labeled spleen cells were lysed with Triton X-100 and purified by lentil lectin affinity chromatography. The lysates were pretreated with a rabbit anti-mouse Ig and protein-A-bearing *Staphylococcus aureus* to remove immunoglobulins before immunoprecipitation with rabbit antisera. After overnight incubation of lysates with rabbit antisera, immune complexes were then removed with *S. aureus* and run on sodium dodecyl sulfate (SDS)–polyacrylamide gels. All four of the anti-sera gave substantial Ia peaks on SDS gels.

Sequential precipitations were done to remove the molecules associated with the *I-A* subregion. After removal of the *I-A*-subregion molecules, Ia peaks were seen with rabbit antisera as shown in Fig. 6. This of course does not prove that the residual Ia molecule is associated with the *I-E* subregion. All this shows is that molecules associated with the *I-A* subregion were removed, but the residual activity remaining could be associated with any part of the *I* region. Two of the antisera were examined in sequential precipitations of $H\text{-}2^k$ lysates in which products of both the *I-A* and the *I-E* subregion are removed with A.TH anti-A.TL serum. As shown in Fig. 7, after removal of both *I-A* and *I-E* molecules, there are no residual Ia peaks detected by the rabbit antisera. This suggests that the rabbit xenoantisera detect the same *I*-region-associated Ia molecules that are also detected by the mouse alloantisera. Since Ia molecules have been identified by immunoprecipitation only for the *I-A* and *I-E* subregions, it is most likely that the residual activity of the xenoantisera after removal of the *I-A* region molecule is against the *I-E*-subregion molecules. The rabbit antisera do not show haplotype specificity, suggesting that at least part of their reactivity is associated with a species-specific site on the molecule. The heterogeneity of the Ia molecule associated with the *I-E* silent haplotypes can be checked only by peptide mapping and amino acid sequencing. Studies are under way to detect whether the xenoantisera preferentially react with either the α or the β polypeptide chains.

5. Tissue Distribution

Early studies on Ia antigens suggested predominant expression on B lymphocytes (David *et al.*, 1973; Hauptfeld *et al.*, 1973a,b; Sachs and Cone, 1973; Götze *et al.*, 1973; Hämmerling *et al.*, 1974). Studies by Frelinger *et al.* (1974) demonstrated Ia antigen expression on a subpopulation of T lymphocytes. Later studies by David *et al.* (1976b) utilizing concanavalin-A-stimulated thymocyte blast cells unequivocally demonstrated strong reactions of anti-Ia sera with T cells by cytotoxicity and absorption analyses. Subsequently, several studies have demonstrated Ia antigen expression on subpopulations of T lymphocytes by a variety of methods including autoradiography and fluorescence-activated cell sorting (Goding *et al.*, 1975; Fathman *et al.*, 1975; B. D. Schwartz *et al.*, 1977). Macrophages were also shown to be Ia-positive by immunofluorescence (Unanue *et al.*, 1974) and by immunoprecipitation studies (R. H. Schwartz *et al.*, 1976). Recent studies by Cowing *et al.* (1978) suggest that Ia expression on macrophages is associated with *I-A* and *I-E/I-C* subregions, similar to B cells.

Recent investigations in the past few years, in our laboratory as well as in other laboratories, have demonstrated the presence of Ia antigens on cells other than those of the classic T- and B-lymphocyte lineage. The rest of this section will outline some of these findings as well as ongoing research in our laboratory.

5.1. Epidermal Cells

Hämmerling *et al.* (1975) originally reported that mouse epidermal cells express Ia antigens. Subsequent studies by Klein *et al.* (1976) and Frelinger *et al.* (1978) have confirmed those findings. More recently, work in the human and guinea pig systems (Stingl *et al.*, 1977, 1978) has led to the suggestion that a subpopulation of epidermal cells, the Langerhans cells, may express the human and guinea pig equivalent of murine Ia antigens. In view of the postulated role of Langerhans cells in antigen trapping and contact hypersensitivity, we have investigated whether specific *I*-region gene products can be detected on mouse tail epidermal cells (Krco *et al.*, 1979).

Using an anti-A^k serum, approximately 35% specific lysis of B10.A epidermal cells was observed in the presence of guinea pig complement (Fig. 8). Comparable reactions were observed using an anti-(J^k E^k C^d) serum. The marginal reactions observed using anti-C^d serum suggest that *I-C* gene products may be also expressed on epidermal cells. Based on work in the guinea pig, the Langerhans cells comprise 4–5% of an epidermal cell population and are the cells that express Ia antigens. In contrast, our results suggest that the mouse has a far greater percentage of the cells expressing Ia antigens. The obvious question is whether all the Ia-positive

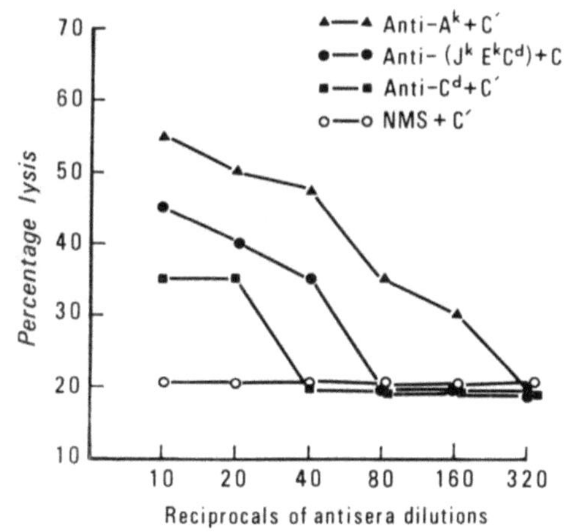

Figure 8. Detection of Ia antigens on B10.A epidermal cells.

cells are also Langerhans cells. This problem is currently being approached through combined histochemical and serological techniques.

The possibility that epidermal cells may possess characteristics of reticuloendothelial cells, namely, the presence of constant-fragment (Fc) receptors and the ability to phagocytize particulate matter, was examined. These studies show that 10% of mouse epidermal cells express IgG Fc receptors, and 15% of cells can ingest latex particles. These studies suggest that not all the Ia+ cells in the mouse are Langerhans cells. The importance of this finding is not yet understood.

5.2. Peritoneal Neutrophils

Neutrophils comprise nearly half the peritoneal leukocyte population. In view of the similar morphology and phagocytic capabilities of neutrophils and macrophages, the possibility of Ia antigen expression on these cells was investigated (Okuda *et al.*, 1979). Neutrophils were isolated using a modified procedure of Cohn and Morse (1959). Briefly, 10 ml of a 0.1% glycogen solution prepared in saline is injected into the peritoneal cavities of mice. After 5 hr, the cells obtained from the peritoneal cavities are collected and washed. The cell population at this stage comprises 95% neutrophils, 5% monocytes, and 1% eosinophils. The cells are then centrifuged over a Ficoll–Hypaque density gradient, which results in a 99% pure neutrophil population. These cells are then tested in cytotoxicity assays.

Under conditions in which 70–80% of the neutrophils are killed in the presence of anti-D^k or anti-K^k serum and rabbit complement, approximately 75% of the neutrophils are killed by an anti-I^k serum. Antisera specific for *I-C* or *I-J* determinants do not result in significant cell death. However, strong cytotoxicity (60% cell death) is observed using antisera specific for either $I\text{-}E^k$ or $I\text{-}A^k$ Ia antigens. The results of absorption analyses indicate that the density of Ia antigens on neutrophils is much less than on B lymphocytes. Immunoprecipitation analyses using A.TH anti-A.TL serum on B10.BR neutrophils yielded Ia products of conventional molecular weight like those obtained from spleen cells, namely, glycoproteins of molecular weights 31,000 and 27,000. The presence of Ia antigens on neutrophils has also been demonstrated by the ability of A.TL neutrophils to stimulate A.TH lymphocytes in a mixed-lymphocyte culture.

5.3. Eosinophils

Eosinophils have been implicated in several immunological phenomena including allergic, inflammatory, parasitic, and neoplastic immune responses. Thus, one might expect to observe Ia antigen expression by these immunocompetent cells. Eosinophils were obtained from the peritoneal washes of mice that had been injected with paraffin oil (Neely and Yokota, in prep.). The cells thus obtained were passed through nylon wool columns. The column eluate was then fractionated on a metrizamide gradient that was centrifuged at 12 *g* for 40 min at 5°C. Approximately 90–97% pure eosinophil cell suspension was obtained by this technique. These cells were then subjected to cytotoxicity, immunoprecipitation, mixed-lymphocyte cultures, and antigen-presentation assays. Using an A.TH anti-A.TL serum and rabbit complement, approximately 60% cell death was observed. Antisera specific for *I-A* and *I-E* subregions kill about 40% of the cells, while no killing was observed using antisera specific for the *I-B*, *I-J*, or *I-C* subregion. Investigations of other parameters of Ia antigen expression on eosinophils are currently being done.

5.4. Peyer's Patch Cells

Peyer's patch cells are lymphoid tissue islands that are abundant in intestinal tissue of mammals. Peyer's patch cells contain both T and B cells. The B cells are thought to be predominantly precursors of IgA-producing cells. It is quite easy to demonstrate that B cells within the Peyer's patches can mature into antibody-secreting cells. However, there has been controversy concerning the immunocompetence of T cells within the Peyer's patches. Characterization of Ia antigen expression by B cells, T cells, and phagocytic cells within Peyer's patches was attempted (Krco *et al.*, 1980).

Table 5 summarizes the results concerning the characterization of the cell profile of Peyer's patch cells compared with standard lymphoid tissues. Peyer's patch cells were found to be composed of approximately 50% B cells, 37% T cells, 6% phagocytic cells, and less than 5% adherent cells. Due to the large number of B cells, strong cytotoxicity reactions were observed using anti-I^k sera as tested on CBA Peyer's patch cells.

TABLE 5. Cellular Characteristics of Peyer's Patch Cells from CBA/J Mice Compared with Other Lymphoid Tissues (Mean ± S.D.)

Cell type	Criterion	Peyer's patch	Spleen	Lymph node
B cell	Anti-kappa-positive	49 ± 3	44 ± 7	17 ± 5
T cell	Anti-Thy-1,2-positive	37 ± 5	41 ± 9	68 ± 9
Phagocytic	Latex ingestion	5.2 ± 1.1	11.1 ± 2.5	5.7 ± 1.8
Adherent	Glass-adherent	3.8 ± 2.6	13.1 ± 2.8	6.4 ± 1.9
	TOTAL:	95	109.2	97.1

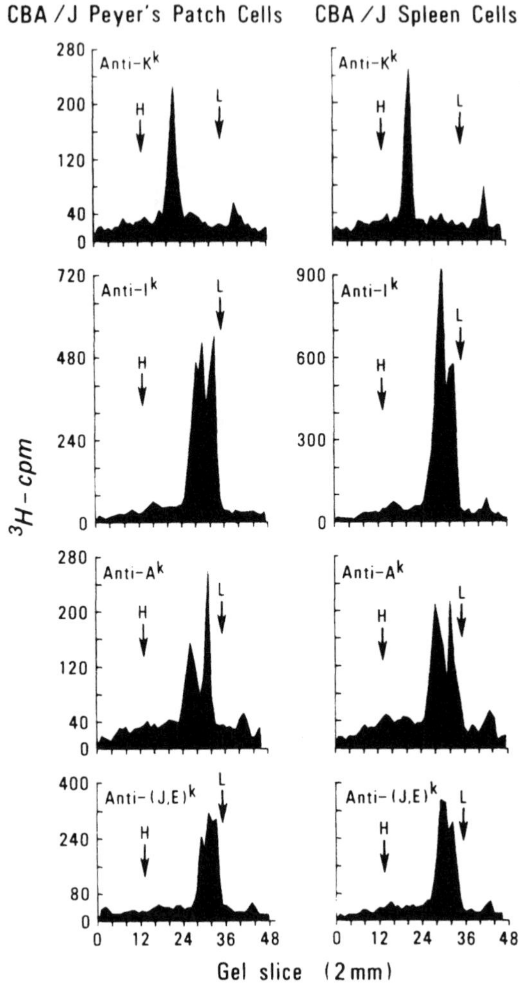

Figure 9. Detection of Ia antigens on Peyer's patch cells from CBA/J mice by immunoprecipitation.

About 70% of Peyer's patch cells were killed by anti-I^k serum, while 65% killing was seen with anti-IA^k and anti-I-E^k/C^k sera in complement-dependent cytotoxicity assays. In addition, Ia antigen expression was not limited to B cells, in that cell death was observed using the same anti-I sera when testing against nylon-wool-purified T cells or adherent cells (macrophage-enriched). Immunoprecipitation studies with Peyer's patch cells showed typical H-2 and Ia peaks (Fig. 9).

However, despite the large amount of Ia antigen expression by Peyer's patch adherent cells, these cells fail to present antigen. The adherent cells, after pulsing with ovalbumin, fail to present antigen to ovalbumin-sensitized lymph node cells. Under identical conditions, spleen and lymph node adherent cells present antigen effectively. Preliminary evidence suggests that the failure to present antigen was not due to the presence of a suppressor-cell population. Characterization of the adherent cells from Peyer's patches demonstrated that a large proportion of the adherent cells from Peyer's patch are not phagocytic. There appears to exist a glass-adherent, Ia+, nonphagocytic, non-antigen-presenting cell within the Peyer's patch. Investigations are in progress to determine the function of this cell type.

5.5. T-Cell Lymphomas

The Ia antigen expression by primary T-cell lymphomas induced in C3H-Bi mice by Gross murine leukemia virus is being studied at present (Peterson and David, in prep.). Several T-cell lymphoma lines have been established from such primary tumors by subcutaneous transplantation. Each of the lymphoma lines has been characterized with respect to Ia antigen expression. Tumor lines 1, 2, 5, and 11 can absorb substantial amounts of anti-Ia antibodies. Lines 2, 4, 12, and 13 do not absorb anti-Ia activities. Lymphoma line number 14 shows partial absorption. These tumors are monoclonal. The expression of individual *I* subregions in these tumor lines is also being determined.

6. Functional Role

6.1. MHC Genes in Immune Surveillance

The 17th chromosome of mice codes for several genes that are involved in immune mechanisms. The *T* complex codes for a series of genes that are expressed on certain embryonic cells, teratoma cells, and sperm and seem to be involved in morphogenesis and cellular differentiation (cell–cell interaction and recognition) during embryogenesis (Martecorena *et al.*, 1978). These genes function sequentially, and any defects along the pathway result in abnormal development. Serological studies have shown that antibodies can be generated to cell-surface structures controlled by these genes. The gene products so far identified seem to be a 45,000-molecular-weight molecule (Vitetta *et al.*, 1974, 1975). On the right-hand side of the *H-2* gene complex, the *TL* region previously was thought to code primarily for antigens expressed on thymus leukemia cells and certain normal cells (Old and Stockert, 1977). Recently, there have been found to map in that region several closely linked loci designated *Qa-1, 2,* and *3* that discriminate functionally distinct T-cell subclasses (Flaherty, 1976; Stanton and Boyse, 1976; Flaherty *et al.*, 1978). The gene products of several of these genes are molecules of 44,000–45,000 molecular weight (Michaelson *et al.*, 1977; Uhr *et al.*, 1976).

The *H-2* gene complex consists of at least three loci coding for 45,000-molecular-weight gene products, one in the *K* region and two in the *D* region (*D* and *L*) (Hansen *et al.*, 1977). The *K*- and the *D*-region antigens serve as targets for cytotoxic T lymphocytes generated against viral-infected and chemically modified self cells (Blandon *et al.*, 1975; Shearer *et al.*, 1975). *H-2K* and *H-2D* also mediate *H-2* restriction in cell-mediated lympholysis of minor and Y-chromosome-associated histocompatibility antigens (Bevan, 1975; Gordon *et al.*, 1975). Recent studies indicate that cell-mediated lympholysis directed against tissue-specific antigens on epidermis cells requires identity at the *H-2K* locus (Steinmuller *et al.*, in prep.). The immune response to Thy-1.1 antigen also seems to be associated with the *H-2K* locus (Zaleski and Klein, 1977). The *H-21* region is unique in the sense that the genes code for 28,000- and 33,000-molecular-weight products (Cullen *et al.*, 1974). Within the *I* region, two loci, *I-A* and *I-E*, code for Ia gene products (David and Cullen, 1978).

The MHC-associated regions defined in the 17th chromosome have several similar properites. For example, a histocompatibility locus has been associated with most of these regions. Most of these regions have associated *Lad* loci, i.e., antigens that can stimulate in an MLR. In general, most of these antigens can serve as targets for cytotoxic T cells. When cytotoxic T cells are generated by incompatibility at one of the regions in the 17th chromosome, no MHC restriction is seen. This suggests that each of the MHC loci can serve as targets without being restricted by another locus within the complex. With the exception of the *T* locus, the products are expressed on lymphocytes, even though the proportions and subpopulations vary.

For a long time, immune-response-type phenomena were associated primarily with the *I* region. Recent studies show that the capacity to generate cytotoxic T cells may be controlled by *Ir*-type genes mapping in the *K* region (Schmitt-Verhulst and Shearer, 1978; Zinkernagel *et al.*, 1978). Zinkernagel (personal communication) postulates that the *H-2K* restricting element and the *Ir* gene product may be identical. We postulate that the two functions are mediated by closely linked genes mapping within the *H-2K* region. One gene codes for the 45,000-molecular-weight product involved in both presentation of the viral antigens and the target of cytotoxic T cells, while a second gene codes for the "recognizer molecule" involved in generation of the cytotoxic "killer" cells.

Besides the restrictions associated with the *H-2D* molecule, the *D* end seems to map numerous other traits: recovery from Friend virus infection (Chesebro and Wehrly, 1978), resistance to radiation-induced leukemia (Meruelo *et al.*, 1978), hybrid histocompatibility (Cudkowicz and Lotzová, 1973), suppression of contact sensitivity associated with DNFB (Moorhead, 1977), and, more recently, suppression to autoimmune thyrodiditis (Kong *et al.*, 1979). We would postulate that the *H-2D* molecule is also involved in presenting antigens and triggering a "recognizer molecule" controlled by a closely linked gene. The "recognizer molecule" invokes the generation of cytotoxic "killer" cells directed against either the helper cell (autoimmune diseases, delayed-type hypersensitivity) or a suppressor cell (neoplasia).

In conclusion, the *T* complex could be involved in immune surveillance and cell–cell interaction during the embryonic and developmental stages. The *K* region mediates immune surveillance to viral antigens, tissue-specific antigens, chemically modified, and minor histocompatibility antigens. The *I-A* subregion functions in surveillance for most foreign antigens, while the *I-E* subregion may function in triggering "recognizers" that could generate the production of suppressor factor, either antigen-specific (*I-J*) or alloantigen-mediated *(I-C)* or both. The *D* region has been implicated in response or suppression to self antigens or altered-self antigens. Hence, several molecules controlled by genes mapping in the 17th chromosome (MHC) could be capable of immune surveillance and antigen presentation even though to different classes of antigens. Since most normal individuals in a population are heterozygous, the number of molecules that may function in immune surveillance would be doubled. Further, there are examples where complementation of two MHC genes would produce a unique product (Jones *et al.*, 1978) and complementation of genes expressed in two haplotypes in an F_1 would also produce unique (hybrid) products (Fathman *et al.*, 1977). Thus, the number of molecules in an individual that could function in immune surveillance (processing and presentation of antigens) could be numerous. By taking the Ia antigens as a model, we will propose a scheme by which they could present antigen. The same hypothesis could be applied to the other MHC gene products.

6.2. Ia Antigens in Antigen Presentation

In the past few years, several hypotheses have been suggested implying a role for Ia antigens in antigen presentation (Rosenthal and Shevach, 1973; R. H. Schwartz, 1978; Benacerraf, 1978). We will include several of the ideas from these authors in our speculation suggesting how Ia antigens may be involved in immune response. We will focus attention primarily on the "classic Ia antigens," the gene products of molecular weight 28,000–33,000.

During the process of phagocytosis, engulfment, and digestion of the foreign molecule, a subpopulation of macrophages would process the different antigens. The antigenic sites are those segments in the molecule that are most antigenic and are released as fragments (Fig. 10). A second population of macrophages, the antigen-presenting cells (APC), express the classic Ia molecules. The antigenic fragments are attracted to the APC and come in contact with the Ia molecules. If there is complementarity between the Ia molecule and the antigenic fragment, then binding takes place. Ia molecules bound to the antigen fragment are released into circulation. The "T-cell-recognizer" molecule sees this (Ia molecule + antigen) complex, possibly through actual contact via the Ia molecule on the T cell. This could either convert this T cell into a helper or suppressor T cell (or in turn stimulate a particulate subset of T helper or T suppressor cells). These converted T lymphocytes in turn would generate either the helper factor or the suppressor factor. Studies have shown that these factors actually contain the antigenic fragment (Erb *et al.*, 1976). The events that lead to the generation of helper or the suppressor factor are still very unclear. These factors then either stimulate or suppress the generation of cytotoxic T cells. Possibly, these factors could also turn the B cells on or off when the humoral immunity is involved. The classic Ia antigens on the B cells could also serve a role in the binding of the (Ia molecule + antigen) complex to the B cell in certain cases. The primary function of Ia molecules may be the presentation of antigens that occurs at the level of the macrophages. The secondary function may be the binding or recognition of the (Ia molecule + antigen) complex by the T cells or B cells or both.

There may be circumstances in which Ia antigens on T cells or B cells

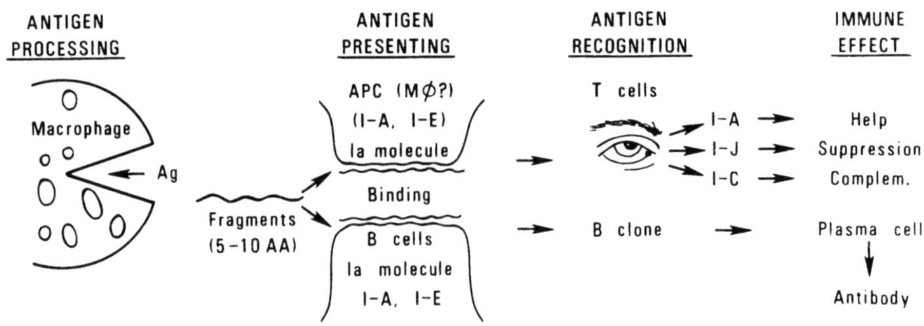

Figure 10. Diagram depicting the role of *I*-region gene products in antigen presentation and recognization for immune functions of help, suppression, complementation, and antibody formation.

can directly present the antigen, thus bypassing the role of macrophages. With a low-responder haplotype for any particular antigen, the defect could be at any one of several steps. The defect could be at the level of antigen processing by the macrophages. A lack of complementarity between the Ia molecule on the APC and the antigenic fragment would lead to nonbinding and thereby nonpresentation. The T cell "recognizers" could either fail to respond to the (Ia + antigen) complex or trigger the suppressor T cells. There could be a defect in the helper T cell in the generation of helper factor or a defect in the helper factor in triggering the cytotoxic T cells. Defects in humoral antibody production could result, if the helper factors cannot signal the B cells or if the plasma cells cannot secrete antibody.

6.3. Ia Function—A Molecular Approach

In collaboration with Dr. Zouhair Atassi and his associates, we have initiated experiments to test our hypothesis. Sperm whale myoglobin was selected for these studies. Atassi and his associates (reviewed in Atassi and Kazim, 1977) have determined the antigenic sites on the sperm whale myoglobin molecule. The amino acid sequence and the helical structure of sperm whale myoglobin have already been determined (Kendrew *et al.*, 1961; Edmundson, 1965). Sperm whale myoglobin has a molecular weight of 17,000 consisting of 153 amino acids. Five antigenic sites have been demonstrated on the molecule. The amino acid sequences involving those five sites are: site 1, 15–22; site 2, 56–62; site 3, 94–99; site 4, 113–119; site 5, 145–151. Synthetic peptides of each of these antigenic determinants have been prepared by Dr. Atassi and his colleagues. All these studies were performed using rabbit antibody. The sperm whale myoglobin was demonstrated to be under *H-2*-linked *Ir* gene control in mice (Okuda *et al.*, 1978). T-cell-proliferation experiments were carried out in independent and recombinant haplotypes of mice with whole sperm whale myoglobin. The T-cell-proliferation assays showed that haplotypes $H\text{-}2^d$, $H\text{-}2^s$, and $H\text{-}2^f$ are high responders to the sperm whale myoglobin, whereas haplotypes $H\text{-}2^b$, $H\text{-}2^k$, $H\text{-}2^q$, $H\text{-}2^j$, $H\text{-}2^r$, and $H\text{-}2^p$ are low responders. Studies with recombinant haplotypes demonstrated that most of the responses were associated with the *I-A* subregion, even though a possible second *Ir* gene could also be mapped in the *I-C* subregion. Studies by Berzofsky (1978) have also shown that antibody responses to the sperm whale myoglobin are under *H-2*-linked *Ir* gene control.

Subsequent studies involved the immune response to the synthetic peptides (Okuda *et al.*, 1979). In these studies, mice of independent haplotypes and recombinant haplotypes were primed with whole sperm whale myoglobin and then challenged by the PETLES (peritoneal exudate T-lymphocyte-enriched cells) assay with each of the synthetic peptides involving the five antigenic sites. In addition, two peptides, which are not recognized as antigenic determinants by the rabbit anti-myoglobin serum, were also used as a control. Further, a nonsense peptide that did not resemble the sperm whale myoglobin in its sequence was also used. These studies showed that among the high responders, haplotype $H\text{-}2^d$ responded to sites 1, 2, and 5; haplotype $H\text{-}2^s$ responded to sites 1, 2, 3, and 5; and haplotype $H\text{-}2^f$ responded to sites 1, 2, and 3. Among the nonresponders, surprisingly, haplotypes $H\text{-}2^b$ and $H\text{-}2^k$ responded to site 4. The other nonresponder haplotypes (i.e., *q, j, r, p*) did not respond to any of the sites. The response to sites 1, 2, 4, and 5 was mapped specifically to the *I-A* subregion, while the response to site 3 could not be positively mapped within the *H-2* gene complex. Response to sites 1 and 2 was also controlled by a second *Ir* gene, mapping in the *I-C* subregion. On the basis of these preliminary findings, the following conclusions could be made: (1) immune response, as far as myoglobin is concerned, is at the level of individual determinants based on primary sequence; (2) different haplotypes may respond to different sites on the same molecule; (3) besides gene complementation, there could also be additive gene effects involving two different antigenic determinants that in the F_1 animal might resemble complementation; and (4) certain sites on the molecule could trigger a suppressive effect in certain haplotypes.

In collaboration with Dr. Atassi, similar studies are being done using a second native protein, lysozyme, the antigenic determinants of which are determined by spatially adjacent surface residues that are mostly distant in sequence (Atassi, 1978). It will be interesting to see whether T cells can also recognize the "discontinuous sites" of a lysozyme as they did with the "continuous sites" of myoglobin. Recently, Kazim and Atassi (1977) have synthesized two antigenic regions of human hemoglobin (one each on the α and β chains) by extrapolation of the three-dimensional location of an antigenic site of sperm whale myoglobin. We have also included hemoglobin, a larger and complex molecule, in our studies on the molecular probe of *Ir* gene function. In collaboration with Dr. Atassi, we have also initiated studies on the more commonly used native protein, albumin. The present immunochemical studies on bovine serum albumin reveal a novel feature, namely, that it contains repeating identical or very similar antigenic determinants (Habeeb, 1978). Studies with these four unique native proteins and their antigenic sites should reveal the gene action involved in immune recognition.

Studies have just begun to check the hypothesis of antigen presentation by Ia molecules. The experimental protocol calls for purification of Ia molecules from high-responder and low-responder primed and nonprimed mice to determine whether these molecules bind to specific synthetic peptides. If the data demonstrate that there is binding, then the [Ia molecule–antigen peptide complex] could be used as a probe in studies to delineate antigen recognition by T cells. This work is in a very preliminary stage.

ACKNOWLEDGMENTS. The authors are greatly indebted to Sharon Ames for patient and skillful preparation of the manuscript. We also thank Rosemary Johnson for the illustrative material in this manuscript. The studies done in our laboratory were supported by grants from the National Institute of Allergies and Infectious Diseases (AI-14764), the National Cancer Institute (CA-24473), and the Mayo Foundation. K.W.B. was supported by American Cancer Society Postdoctoral Fellowship PF-1545. C.J.K. was supported by NIH Research Service Award AI-05584. W.P.L. was supported by NCI Postdoctoral Training Grant CA-18900.

References

Atassi, M.Z., 1978, Precise determination of the entire antigenic structure of lysozyme, *Immunochemistry* **15:**909.

Atassi, M.Z., and Kazim, A.L., 1977, First consequences of the determination of the entire antigenic structure of sperm whale myoglobin, in: *Immunobiology of Proteins and Peptides* (M.Z. Atassi and A.B. Stavitsky, eds.), pp. 19–40, Plenum Press, New York.

Beisel, K.W., Passmore, H.C., and David, C.S., 1980, Intra-*H-2* recombination in the mouse. III. I region Characterization of haplotypes $H\text{-}2^{at2}$, $H\text{-}2^{at3}$ and $H\text{-}2^{a2}$, *Immunogenetics* **11:**123.

Benacerraf, B., 1978, Opinion: A hypothesis to relate the specificity of T lymphocytes and the activity of *I* region-specific *Ir* genes in macrophages and B lymphocytes, *J. Immunol.* **120:**1809.

Benacerraf, B., and Dorf, M.E., 1977, Genetic control of specific immune responses and immune suppressions by *I*-region genes, *Cold Spring Harbor Symp. Quant. Biol.* **41:**465.

Benacerraf, B., and McDevitt, H.O., 1972, Histocompatibility-linked immune response genes, *Science* **175:**273.

Bennett, D., 1975, The *T* locus of the mouse: A review, *Cell* **6:**441.

Berzofsky, J.A., 1978, Genetic control of the immune response to mammalian myoglobins in mice. I. More than one *I*-region gene in *H-2* controls the antibody response, *J. Immunol.* **120:**360.

Bevan, M.J., 1975, Interaction antigens detected by cytotoxic T cells with the major histocompatibility complex as modifier, *Nature (London)* **256:**419.

Blandon, R.V., Doherty, P.C., Dunlop, M.B.C., Gardner, I.D., Zinkernagel, R.M., and David, C.S., 1975, Genes required for T cell-mediated cytotoxicity against virus-infected target cells are in the *K* and *D* regions of the *H-2* complex, *Nature (London)* **254:**269.

Chesebro, B., and Wehrly, K., 1978, *Rfv-1* and *Rfv-2*, two *H-2*-associated genes that influence recovery from Friend leukemia virus-induced splenomegaly, *J. Immunol.* **120:**1081.

Cohn, Z.A., and Morse, S.I., 1959, Interaction between rabbit polymorphonuclear leucocytes and staphylococci, *J. Exp. Med.* **110:**419.

Colombani, J., Colombani, M., Shreffler, D.C., and David, C., 1975, Separation of anti-Ia (*I* region associated antigens) from anti-*H-2* in complex sera by absorption on blood platelets: Description of three new Ia specificities, *Tissue Antigens* **7**:74.

Cowing, C., Pincus, S.H., Sachs, D.H., and Dickler, H.B., 1978, A subpopulation of adherent accessory cells bearing both *I-A* and *I-E* or *C* subregion antigens is required for antigen-specific murine T lymphocyte proliferation, *J. Immunol.* **121:**1680.

Cudkowicz, G., and Lotzová, E., 1973, Hemopoietic cell-defined components of the major histocompatibility complex of mice: Identification of responsive recipients for bone marrow transplants, *Transplant. Proc.* **5:**1399.

Cullen, S.E., David, C.S., Shreffler, D.C., and Nathenson, S.G., 1974, Membrane molecules determined by the *H-2*-associated immune response region: Isolation and some properties, *Proc. Natl. Acad. Sci. U.S.A.* **71:**648.

Cullen, S.E., David, C.S., Cone, J.L., and Sachs, D.H., 1976a, Evidence for more than one Ia antigenic specificity on molecules determined by the *I-A* subregion of the mouse major histocompatibility complex, *J. Immunol.* **116:**549.

Cullen, S.E., Sachs, D.H., and David, C.S., 1976b, Use of immune precipitation to identify and suggest mapping position for new Ia specificities, in: *Leukocyte Membrane Determinants Regulating Immune Activity* (V.P. Eijsvoogel, D. Roos, and W.P. Zeijimaker, eds.), pp. 507–508, Academic Press, New York.

David, C.S., 1976, Serological and genetic aspects of murine Ia antigens, *Transplant. Rev.* **30:**299.

David, C.S., 1977, The major histocompatibility system of the mouse, in: *The Major Histocompatibility System in Man and Animals* (D. Götze, ed.), pp. 255–290, Springer-Verlag, New York.

David, C.S., and Schreffler, D.C., 1972, Studies on recombination within the mouse *H-2* complex. II. Serological analyses of four recombinants $H\text{-}2^{al}$, $H\text{-}2^{ol}$, $H\text{-}2^{tl}$, $H\text{-}2^{th}$, *Tissue Antigens.* **2:**241.

David, C.S., and Cullen, S.E., 1978, Murine Ia antigens: Identification and mapping of Ia.23 and further definition of the *I-E* subregion, *J. Immunol.* **120:**1659.

David, C.S., and Shreffler, D.C., 1974a, Lymphocyte antigens controlled by the *Ir* region of the mouse *H-2* complex: Detection of new specificities with anti-H-2 reagents, *Transplantation* **17:**462.

David, C.S., and Shreffler, D.C., 1974b, *I*-region associated antigen system (Ia) of the mouse *H-2* gene complex, *Transplantation* **18:**313.

David, C.S., Shreffler, D.C., and Frelinger, J.A., 1973, New lymphocyte antigen system (Lna) controlled by the *Ir* region at the mouse *H-2* complex, *Proc. Natl. Acad. Sci. U.S.A.* **70:**2509.

David, C.S., Frelinger, J.A., and Shreffler, D.C., 1974, New lymphocyte antigens controlled by the *Ir-IgG* region of the *H-2* gene complex, *Transplantation* **7:**122.

David, C.S., Stimpfling, J.H., and Shreffler, D.C., 1975a, Identification of specificity H-2.7 as an erythrocyte antigen: Control by an independent locus, *H-2G* between the *S* and *D* regions, *Immunogenetics* **2:**131.

David, C.S., Cullen, S.E., and Murphy, D.B., 1975b, Serological and biochemical studies with the *H-2* gene complex of mice: Further evidence for the *I-C* subregion, *J. Immunol.* **114:**1205.

David, C.S., Colombani, J., Colombani, M., and Cullen, S.E., 1976a Murine *I* region-associated antigen (Ia) system: Identification and chemical characterization of specificities Ia.12, 13 and 14, *Transplantation* **21:**520.

David, C., Meo, T., McCormick, J., and Shreffler, D.C., 1976b, Expression of individual Ia specificities on T and B cells. I. Studies with mitogen induced blast cells, *J. Exp. Med.* **143:**218.

David, C.S., McCormick, J.F., and Stimpfling, J.H., 1978, Further serological and genetic characterization of *I-E* and *I-C* subregions, in: *Ir Genes and Ia Antigens* (H.O. McDevitt, ed.), pp. 9–20, Academic Press, New York.

Davies, D.A.L., and Hess, M., 1974, New alloantigen genetically linked to the major histocompatibility locus of the mouse, *Nature (London)* **250:**228.

Dorf, M., and Benacerraf, B., 1975, Complementation of *H-2*-linked *Ir* genes in the mouse, *Proc. Natl. Acad. Sci. U.S.A* **72:**3671.

Edmundson, A.B., 1965, Amino-acid sequence of sperm whale myoglobin, *Nature (London)* **205:**883.

Erb, P., Feldmann, M., and Hogg, N., 1976, Role of macrophages in the generation of T helper cells. IV. Nature of genetically related factor derived from macrophages incubated with soluble antigen, *Eur. J. Immunol.* **6:**365.

Fathman, C.G., Cone, J.L., Sharrow, S.O., Tyrer, H., and Sachs, D.H., 1975, Ia alloantigen(s) detected on thymocytes by use of a fluorescence-activated cell sorter, *J. Immunol.* **115:**584.

Fathman, C.G., Callavo, D., Davies, S., and Nabholz, M., 1977, *In vitro* secondary MLR. I. Kinetics of proliferation and specificity in *in vitro* primed responder cells, *J. Immunol.* **118:**1232.

Flaherty, L., 1976, The *Tla* region of the mouse: Identification of a new serologically defined locus, *Qa-2*, *Immunogenetics* **3:**533.

Flaherty, L., and Wachtel, S.S., 1975, H (Tla) system: Identification of two new loci, *H-31* and *H-32*, and alleles, *Immunogenetics* **2:**81.

Flaherty, L., Stanton, T.H., and Boyse, E.A., 1975, Contamination of Ia antiserum A.TL anti-A.TH with antibodies related to the *Tla* region, *Immunogenetics* **4:**101.

Flaherty, L., Zimmerman, D., and Hansen, T.H., 1978, Further serological analysis of the Qa antigens: Analysis of an anti-H-2.28 serum, *Immunogenetics* **6:**245.

Frelinger, J.A., Niederhuber, J.E., David, C.S., and Shreffler, D.C., 1974, Evidence for the expression of Ia (*H-2*-associated) antigens on thymus-derived lymphocytes, *J. Exp. Med.* **140:**1273.

Frelinger, J.G., Wettstein, P.J., Frelinger, J.A., and Hood, L., 1978, Epidermal Ia molecules from the *I-A* and *I-E/C* subregions of the mouse *H-2* complex, *Immunogenetics* **6:**125.

Goding, J.W., Nossal, G.J.V., Shreffler, D.C., and Marchalonis, J.J., 1975, Cellular localization of an I-associated (Ia) antigen, *J. Immunogenet.* **2:**41.

Gordon, R.D., Simpson, E., and Samelson, L.E., 1975, *In vitro* cell-mediated immune responses to the male specific (H-Y) antigen in mice, *J. Exp. Med.* **142:**1108.

Götze, D., 1976, Serological characterization of Ia antigens of the $H\text{-}2^k$, $H\text{-}2^s$, and $H\text{-}2^q$ haplotypes by antisera produced against skin, lymphocytes, and lymphoblasts: Strain distribution pattern of Ia antigens and their relationship to *Ir* genes, *Immunogenetics* **3:**139.

Götze, D., Reisfeld, R.A., and Klein, J., 1973, Serological evidence for antigens controlled by the *Ir* region in mice, *J. Exp. Med.* **138:**1003.

Guimezanes, A., Colombani, M., and Colombani, J., 1979, Secondary mouse mixed lymphocyte reaction (MLR) *in vitro:* Correlation between primed cells reactivity and serological typing for Ia specificities, *Immunogenetics* **8:**127.

Habeeb, A.F.S.A., 1978, Immunochemistry of bovine serum albumin, in: *Immunobiology of Proteins and Peptides* (M.Z. Atassi and A.B. Stavitsky, eds.), pp. 101–118, Plenum Press, New York.

Hämmerling, G.J., Deak, B.D., Mauve, G., Hämmerling, U., and McDevitt, H.O., 1974, B lymphocyte alloantigens controlled by the *I* region of the major histocompatibility complex in mice, *Immunogenetics* **1:**68.

Hämmerling, G.J., Mauve, G., Goldberg, E., and McDevitt, H.O., 1975, Tissue distribution of Ia antigens: Ia on spermatozoa, macrophages, and epidermal cells, *Immunogenetics* **1:**428.

Hansen, T.H., Sachs, D.H., 1978, Isolation and antigenic characterization of the product of a third polymorphic *H-2* locus, *H-2L*, *J. Immunol.* **121:**1469.

Hansen, T.H., Cullen, S.E., and Sachs, D.H., 1977, Immunochemical evidence for an additional *H-2* region closely linked to *H-2D*, *J. Exp. Med.* **145:**438.

Hauptfeld, V., Klein, D., and Klein, J., 1973a, Serologic detection of antigens controlled by the *Ir* region of the *H-2* complex in the mouse, *Transplant. Proc.* **4:**1811.

Hauptfeld, V., Klein, D., and Klein, J., 1973b, Serological identification of an *Ir*-region product, *Science* **181:**167.

Howie, S., Parish, C., David, C.S., McKenzie, I.F.C., Maurer, P.H., Moses, E., and Feldman, M., 1979, Serological analysis of antigen specific helper factors for (T,G)-A—L and GAT, *Eur. J. Immunol.* **9:**501.

Hurme, M., Chandler, P.R., Hetherington, C.M., and Simpson, E., 1978, Cytotoxic T-cell responses to H-Y: Correlation with the rejection of syngeneic male skin grafts, *J. Exp. Med.* **147:**768.

Jones, P.P., Murphy, D.B., and McDevitt, H.O., 1978, Two gene control of the expression of a murine Ia antigen, *J. Exp. Med.* **148:**925.

Kazim, A.L., and Atassi, M.Z., 1977, Prediction and confirmation by synthesis of two antigenic sites in human haemoglobin by extrapolation from known antigenic structure of sperm-whale myoglobin, *Biochem. J.* **167:**275.

Kendrew, J.C., Watson, H.C., Stadberg, B.E., Dickerson, R.E., Phillips, D.C., and Shore, V.C., 1961, A partial determination of X-ray methods and its correlation with chemical data, *Nature (London)* **190:**666.

Klein, J., 1975, *Biology of the Mouse Histocompatibility Complex*, p. 620, Springer-Verlag, New York.

Klein, J., and Chiang, C.L., 1978, A new locus *(H-2T)* at the *D* end of the *H-2* complex, *Immunogenetics* **6:**235.

Klein, J., Klein, D., and Shreffler, D.C., 1970, *H-2* types of translocation stocks T (2;9) 138Ca, T (9;13) 190 Ca and an *H-2* recombinant, *Transplantation* **10:**309.

Klein, J., Hauptfeld, M., and Hauptfeld, V., 1974, Evidence for a third, *Ir*-associated histocompatibility region in the *H-2* complex of the mouse, *Immunogenetics* **1:**45.

Klein, J., Hauptfeld, V., and Hauptfeld, M., 1975, Evidence for a fifth *(G)* region in the *H-2* complex of the mouse, *Immunogenetics* **2:**141.

Klein, J., Geib, R., Chiang, C., and Hauptfeld, V., 1976, Histocompatibility antigens controlled by the *I* region of the murine *H-2* complex. I. Mapping of *H-2A* and *H-2C* loci, *J. Exp. Med.* **143:**1439.

Klein, J., Flaherty, L., VandeBerg, J.L., and Shreffler, D.C., 1978, *H-2* haplotypes, genes, regions, and antigens: First listing, *Immunogenetics* **6:**489.

Kong, Y.M., David, C.S., Giraldo, A.A., Elrehewy, M., and Rose, N.R., 1979, Regulation of autoimmune response to mouse thyroglobulin: Suppressive effect of *H-2D*-end genes, *J. Immunol.* **123:**15.

Krco, C.J., Steinmuller, D., and David, C.S., 1979, Expression of *I* region gene products on mouse tail epidermis cells, *Cell. Immunol.* **46:**239.

Krco, C.J., Challacombe, S.J., LaFuse, W.P., David, C.S., and Tomasi, T.B., 1980, Expression of Ia antigens by mouse Peyer's patch cells, *Cell. Immunol.*

Lieberman, R., Paul, W.E., Humphrey, W., Jr., and Stimpfling, J.H., 1972, *H-2*-linked immune response *(Ir)* genes: Independent loci for *Ir-IgG* and *Ir-IgA* genes, *J. Exp. Med.* **136:**1231.

Martecorena, P., Artzt, K., and Bennett, D., 1978, Relationship of F9 antigen and genes of the T/t complex, *Immunogenetics* **7**:337.

McDevitt, H.O., Deak, B.D., Shreffler, D.C., Klein, J., Stimpfling, J.H., and Snell, G.D., 1972, Genetic control of the immune response: Mapping of the *Ir-1* locus, *J. Exp. Med.* **135**:1259.

McMillan, M., Cecka, J.M., Murphy, D.B., McDevitt, H.O., and Hood, L., 1977, Structure of murine Ia antigens: Partial NH_2-terminal amino acid sequences of products of the *I-E* or *I-C* subregion, *Proc. Natl. Acad. Sci. U.S.A.* **74**:5135.

Melchers, I., and Rajewsky, K., 1975, Specific control of responsiveness by two complementing *Ir* loci in the *H-2* complex, *Eur. J. Immunol.* **5**:753.

Meo, T., Vives, J., Miggiano, V., and Shreffler, D.C., 1973, A major role for the *Ir-1* region of the mouse *H-2* complex in the mixed lymphocyte reaction, *Transplant. Proc.* **5**:1507.

Meo, T., Krasteff, T., and Shreffler, D.C., 1975, Immunochemical characterization of murine *H-2* controlled Ss (serum substance) protein through identification of its human homologue as the fourth component of complement, *Proc. Natl. Acad. Sci. U.S.A.* **72**:4536.

Meruelo, D., Nimelstein, S.H., Jones, P.P., Lieberman, M., and McDevitt, H.O., 1978, Increased synthesis and expression of H-2 antigens on thymocytes as a result of radiation leukemia virus infection: A possible mechanism for *H-2*-linked control of virus-induced neoplasia, *J. Exp. Med.* **147**:470.

Michaelson, J., Flaherty, L., Vitetta, E., and Poulik, M.D., 1977, Molecular similarities between the Qa.2 alloantigen and other gene products of the 17th chromosome of the mouse, *J. Exp. Med.* **145**:1066.

Moorhead, J.W., 1977, Soluble factors in tolerance and hypersensitivity to DNFB in mice, *J. Immunol.* **119**:1773.

Murphy, D.B., and Shreffler, D.C., 1975, Cross-reactivity between *H-2K* and *H-2D* products. I. Evidence for extensive and reciprocal serological cross-reactivity, *J. Exp. Med.* **141**:374.

Murphy, D.B., Herzenberg, L.A., Okumura, K., Herzenberg, L.A., and McDevitt, H.O., 1976, A new *I* subregion (*I-J*) marked by a locus (*Ia.4*) controlling surface determinants on suppressor T lymphocytes, *J. Exp. Med.* **144**:699.

Nabholtz, M., Vives, J., Young, H.M., Meo, T., Miggiano, V., Rijnbeck, A., and Shreffler, D.C., 1975, *I*-region associated determinants: Expression on mitogen stimulated lymphocytes and detection by cytotoxic T cells, *Eur. J. Immunol.* **5**:594.

Neauport-Sautes, C., Joskowicz, M., and Demant, P., 1978, Further evidence for two separate loci (*H-2D* and *H-2L*) in the *D* region of the *H-2* complex, *Immunogenetics* **6**:513.

Niederhuber, J.E., 1978, The role of *I* region gene products in macrophage–T lymphocyte interaction, *Immunol. Rev.* **40**:28.

Okuda, K., and David, C.S., 1978, A new lymphocyte-activating determinant locus expressed on T cells, and mapping in *I-C* subregion, *J. Exp. Med.* **147**:1028.

Okuda, K., David, C.S., and Shreffler, D.C., 1977, The role of gene products of the *I-J* subregion in mixed lymphocyte reactions, *J. Exp. Med.* **146**:1561.

Okuda, K., Christadoss, P., Twining, S., Atassi, M.Z., and David, C.S., 1978, Genetic control of immune response to sperm whale myoglobin in mice. I. T lymphocyte proliferative response under *H-2*-linked *Ir* gene control, *J. Immunol.* **121**:866.

Okuda, K., Neely, B., and David, C.S., 1979, Expression of H-2 and Ia antigens on mouse peritoneal neutrophils, *Transplantation* **28**:354.

Okuda, K., Twining, S.J., David, C.S., and Atassi, M.Z., 1979, Genetic control of immune response to sperm whale myoglobin in mice. II. T-lymphocyte proliferative response to the synthetic antigenic sites, *J. Immunol.* **123**:182.

Old, L.J., and Stockert, E., 1977, Immunogenetics of cell surface antigens of mouse leukemia, *Annu. Rev. Genet.* **17:**127.

Passmore, H.C., and Shreffler, D.C., 1970, A sex-limited serum protein variant in the mouse: Inheritance and association with the *H-2* region, *Biochem. Genet.* **4:**351.

Rich, S.S., David, C.S., and Rich, R.R., 1979, Regulatory mechanisms in cell-mediated immune responses. VII. Presence of *I-C* subregion determinants on mixed leukocyte reaction suppressor factor, *J. Exp. Med.* **149:**114.

Roos, M.H., Atkinson, J.P., and Shreffler, D.C., 1978, Molecular characterization of the Ss and Slp (C4) proteins of the mouse *H-2* complex: Subunit composition, chain size, polymorphism, and an intracellular (pro-Ss) precursor, *J. Immunol.* **121:**1106.

Rosenthal, A.S., and Shevach, E.M., 1973, Function of macrophages in antigen recognition by guinea pig T lymphocytes. I. Requirement for histocompatible macrophages and lymphocytes, *J. Exp. Med.* **138:**1194.

Sachs, D.H., and Cone, J.L., 1973, A mouse B-cell antigen determined by gene(s) linked to the major histocompatibility complex, *J. Exp. Med.* **138:**1289.

Sachs, D. H., Cullen, S. E., and David, C. S., 1975, Immune response associated lymphocyte antigen system (Ia): Definition of specificities Ia.8 and Ia.9 controlled by the I^b region, *Transplantation* **19:**388.

Schmitt-Verhulst, A., and Shearer, G.M., 1978, Involvement of *I* region product in T-cell immunity against TNP-modified autologous cells, in: *Ir Genes and Ia Antigens* (H.O. McDevitt, ed.), pp. 379–385, Academic Press, New York.

Schwartz, B.D., Kask, A. M., Sharrow, S.O., David, C.S., and Schwartz, R.H., 1977, Partial chemical characterization of Ia antigens derived from murine thymocytes, *Proc. Natl. Acad. Sci U.S.A.* **74:**1195.

Schwartz, R.H., 1978, A clonal model for *Ir* gene control of the immune response, *Scand. J. Immunol.* **7:**3.

Schwartz, R.H., Dickler, H.B., Sachs, D. H., and Schwartz, B.D., 1976, Studies of Ia antigens on murine peritoneal macrophages, *Scand. J. Immunol.* **5:**731.

Shearer, G.M., Rehn, T.G., and Garbarino, C.A., 1975, Cell-mediated lympholysis of trinitrophenyl-modified autologous lymphocytes: Effector cell specificity to modified cell surface components controlled by H-2K and H-2D serological regions of the murine major histocompatibility complex, *J. Exp. Med.* **141:**1364.

Shreffler, D.C., 1976, The *S* region of the mouse major histocompatibility complex (*H-2*): Genetic variation and functional role in complement system, *Transplant. Rev.* **32:**140.

Shreffler, D.C., and David, C.S., 1975, The *H-2* major histocompatibility complex and the *I* immune response region: Genetic variation, function and organization, *Adv. Immunol.* **20:**125.

Shreffler, D., David, C., Götze, D., Klein, J., McDevitt, H., and Sachs, D., 1974, Genetic nonmenclature for new lymphocyte antigens controlled by the *I* region of the *H-2* complex, *Immunogenetics* **1:**189.

Shreffler, D.C., David, C.S., Cullen, S.E., Frelinger, J.A., and Niederhuber, J.E., 1977, Serological and functional evidence for further subdivision of the *I* regions of the *H-2* gene complex, *Cold Spring Harbor Symp. Quant. Biol.* **41:**477.

Silver, J., Russell, W.A., Reis, B.L., and Frelinger, J.A., 1978, Chemical characterization of murine Ia alloantigens determined by the *I-E/I-C* subregions of the *H-2* complex, *Proc. Natl. Acad. Sci. U.S.A.* **74:**5131.

Staines, N.A., Guy, K., and Davies, D.A.L., 1974, Passive enhancement of mouse skin allografts: Specificity of the antiserum for major histocompatibility complex antigens, *Transplantation* **18:**192.

Stanton, T.H., and Boyse, E.A., 1976, A new serologically defined locus, *Qa-1*, in the *Tla* region of the mouse, *Immunogenetics* **3:**525.

Stingl, G., Wolff-Schreiner, E.C., Pichler, W.J., Gochnait, F., Knepp, W., and Wolff, K., 1977, Epidermal Langerhans cells Fc and C3 receptors, *Nature (London)* **268:**245.

Stingl, G., Katz, S.I., Clement, L., Green, I., and Shevach, E.M., 1978, Immunologic functions of Ia-bearing epidermal Langerhans cells, *J. Immunol.* **121:**2005.

Tada, T., 1977, Regulation of the antibody response by T cell products determined by different *I* subregions, in: *Immune Systems: Genetics and Regulation* (E.E. Sercarz, L.A. Herzenberg, and C.F. Fox, eds.), pp. 345–362, Academic Press, New York.

Tada, T., Taniguchi, M., and David, C.S., 1976a, Properties of the antigen-specific suppressive T-cell factor in the regulation of antibody response of the mouse. IV. Special subregion assignment of the gene(s) that codes for the suppressive T-cell factor in the *H-2* histocompatibility complex, *J. Exp. Med.* **144:**713.

Tada, T., Taniguchi, M., and David, C.S., 1976b, Suppressive and enhancing T-cell factors as *I*-region gene products: Properties and the subregion assignment, *Cold Spring Harbor Symp. Quant. Biol.* **41:**119.

Tada, T., Takemori, T., Okumura, K., Nonaka, M., and Tokuhisa, T., 1978, Two distinct types of helper T cells involved in the secondary antibody response: Independent and synergistic effects of Ia− and Ia+ helper T cells, *J. Exp. Med.* **147:**446.

Taussig, M.J., Munro, A.J., Campbell, R., David, C.S., and Staines, N.A., 1975, Antigen-specific T-cell factor in cell cooperation: Mapping within the *I* region of the *H-2* complex and ability to cooperate across allogenic barriers, *J. Exp. Med.* **142:**694.

Uhr, J.W., Vitetta, E.S., Klein, J., Poulik, M.D., Klapper, D.G., and Capra, J.D., 1976, Structural studies of H-2 and TL alloantigens, *Cold Spring Harbor Symp. Quant. Biol.* **41:**363.

Unanue, E.R., Dorf, M.E., David, C.S., and Benacerraf, B., 1974, The presence of *I*-region-associated antigens on B cells in molecules distinct from immunoglobulins and *H-2K* and *H-2D*, *Proc. Natl. Acad. Sci. U.S.A.* **71:**5014.

Urba, W.J., and Hildemann, W.M., 1978, *H-2*-linked recessive *Ir* gene regulation of high antibody responsiveness to TNP hapten conjugated to autogenous albumin, *Immunogenetics* **6:**433.

Vitetta, E., Artzt, K., Bennett, D., Boyse, E.A., and Jacob, F. 1975, Structural similarities between product of the *T/t* locus isolated from sperm and teratocarcinoma cells and H-2 alloantigen isolated from splenocytes, *Proc. Natl. Acad. Sci. U.S.A.* **72:**3215.

Zaleski, M.B., and Klein, J., 1976, Immune response of mice to the Thy-1.1 antigen: Intra-*H-2* mapping of the complementary *Ir-Thy-1* loci, *J. Immunol.* **117:**814.

Zaleski, M., and Klein, J., 1977, *H-2* mutation affecting immune response to Thy-1.1 antigen, *J. Exp. Med.* **145:**1602.

Zinkernagel, R.M., and Doherty, P.C., 1974, Immunological surveillance against altered self components by sensitized T lymphocytes in lymphocytic choriomeningitis, *Nature (London)* **251:**547.

Zinkernagel, R.M., Althage, A., Cooper, S., Kreeb, G., Klein, P.A., Sefton, B., Flaherty, L., Stimpfling, J., Shreffler, D., and Klein, J., 1978, *Ir*-genes in *H-2* regulate generation of anti-viral cytotoxic T cells: Mapping to *K* or *D* and dominance of unresponsiveness, *J. Exp. Med.* **148:**592.

5

Expression of Syngeneic and Allogeneic H-2 Antigens on Tumor Cells

Hilliard Festenstein, Wilhelm Schmidt, and Carla Testorelli

1. Introduction

It is now well established that the major histocompatibility system (MHS), Ly, and other alloantigenic systems play important roles in cell–cell interactions, which are particularly relevant in immune reactivity. For example, *I*-region gene products are involved in the presentation of antigen by macrophages and may be part of antigen-specific and -nonspecific factors that are released by helper and suppressor cells, respectively. In contrast, T-cell *in vitro* cytotoxicity appears to be dependent on the sharing of *H-2K/D*-like gene products between target and effector cells in specific instances. This appears to be true for virally infected and chemically modified cells and for effector cells sensitized against the H-Y antigen and a variety of non-H-2 antigens including certain tumor-associated antigens. Any modification of the antigenic profile of effector or target cells, or both, may thus substantially influence the outcome of immune reactivity (for references, see Snell, 1979).

The antigenic profile of tumor cells may be modified by a variety of factors and mechanisms and the consequences, e.g., loss of determinants, may result in less efficient surveillance of the tumor and hence

Hilliard Festenstein, Wilhelm Schmidt, and Carla Testorelli • Department of Immunology, The London Hospital Medical College, London E1, 2AD, England. Dr. Testorelli's present address is Istituto di Farmacologia, Milan, Italy.

more rapid growth. In contrast, the unexpected gain of H-2 and non-H-2 alloantigens on syngeneic tumors may provide the means by which the immune system can bring them under control. However, some of these may stimulate the production of suppressor cells or introduce new restricting elements for the efficient killing of the targets, e.g., if they require K/D identity or induce less efficient *I*-region-independent cooperation and hence unimpeded growth of tumor(s).

One of the simplest reasons for the quantitative alteration of the antigenic profile of a tumor cell is the increased rate of turnover of the cell membrane that is often associated with rapidly dividing cells (Cikes and Friberg, 1971). Variations in the antigenic profile of tumor cells may also be due to endogenous virus encoding cell-membrane products of viral origin. Mutations may readily alter the profile with gain or loss, or both, of determinants. Variations in genetic regulatory function may also be responsible for the quantitative changes in the expression of H-2, differentiation, and other alloantigens. In addition, epigenetic mechanisms, e.g., defective glycosylation, may also result in failure of expression of these antigens, but would be unlikely to influence selectively, say, the K-end and not the D-end antigens.

Disturbances in the genetic regulatory mechanism could result in the repression of genes with failure of expression of normal syngeneic antigens and the derepression of silent structural genes. The latter hypothesis would imply that there is an alternative mechanism for the generally accepted explanation of allelism for H-2 antigens; such a hypothesis involving regulatory genes has already been invoked to explain the modulation of TL antigens in leukemia and other systems because, for example, in Gross virus leukemia, there is expression of TL antigens, not only of the relevant syngeneic strain but also of those strains belonging to foreign haplotypes. The *Tla* structural genes of all strains of the species must thus be inherited by all mice, but only one kind of TL antigen is expressed at a time. Control is through regulatory genes that determine which haplotype is normally expressed. In Gross virus leukemia, this mechanism is disturbed. The genes become derepressed and TL antigens of all the different haplotypes of inbred mice are found on the leukemic cells (for references, see the review by Old and Stockert, 1977). Amos (1971) proposed that a similar mechanism may control the polymorphism of the HLA system. However, firm experimental data showing that the MHS probably operates in this way have only recently been published (see Abstracts, 1979; Workshop Issue, 1980). In our own experiments, we found alterations in the MHS antigenic profile of tumors that could not readily be explained by classic Mendelian interpretations. The results were obtained using a variety of serological and immunochemical techniques and assays of cell-mediated immunity, including mixed-lymphocyte culture tests and tests of cell-mediated cytotoxicity (CMC), cytostasis, and transplantation (Festenstein, 1978; Festenstein *et al.*, 1979a). By serological testing, we found *H-2D*^{k}-like specificities on *H-2*^{d} tumors, while *H-2K*^{k} specificities were absent from a tumor that arose in a C3H (*H-2*^{k}) mouse (Garrido *et al.*, 1976a,b). For these serological assays, we used a specifically devised "postlabeling" assay. The capacity of tumor cells to incorporate anti-H-2 radiolabeled [^{14}C]-uridine or -thymidine was measured after treatment with antibody and complement (Garrido *et al.*, 1977a). Sera were absorbed with normal cells and tumor cells (Garrido *et al.*, 1977b) carrying the extra specificities and then retested on the tumor cells and normal cells, respectively. By these criteria, we could not distinguish between the putative extra H-2 allospecificities of foreign haplotypes on syngeneic tumours and the normal H-2 specificity or specificities on cells of the relevant haplotype. However, we had to be sure that these reactions were not unexpectedly directed against H-2 products, or normal differentiation antigens, because contaminating or cross-reacting antibodies in the sera could disclose the existence of hitherto undetected H-2 public specificities or differentiation antigens better represented on the tumor cells than on normal cells. However, even though we considered this theoretical possibility unlikely, we employed F_1 hybrid cells incorporating the strain of origin of the tumor as responding cells to rule it out (Festenstein *et al.*, 1979a). When H-2 congeneic sensitizations were made using responder cells syngeneic with the strain of origin of the tumor, and the CMC tests were carried out with them, they were still positive against the syngeneic tumor targets. We concluded that the tumor(s) had H-2-like determinants, in common with the haplotype of the H-2 congeneic stimulating strain, that were absent from the responder strain. To explain these results, we favor the repression–derepression hypothesis outlined above. According to this theory, the targets could be the products of derepressed silent *H-2* structural genes normally belonging only to mouse strains of allogeneic types. During tumorigenesis, these products become expressed following disturbance of the normal regulatory mechanism.

2. Studies with the K36 Spontaneous Leukemia

To investigate the mechanism further, we extended the studies on the K36 tumor—the spontaneous AKR (*H-2*^{k}) leukemia (Table 1). It was originally isolated at the Sloan-Kettering Institute for Cancer Research, New York (Old *et al.*, 1965). Since then, it has been distributed to many laboratories throughout the world and has been propagated both *in vivo* and *in vitro*. The first subline of this tumor was obtained from J.P. Levy (Paris) and was propagated *in vitro*. Twenty clones were isolated. Later,

TABLE 1. Characterization of the K36 Tumor

Origin		
AKR (*H-2*^{k}, *Tla*^{b}, *Qa1*^{b}, *Qa2*^{b}, *Qa3*^{b})		
Induction		
Spontaneous leukemia		
Cell-surface markers		
H-2K^k (specificities *23,3,8,11,25*) −		
H-2D^k (specificities *32,1,5,*) +		
H-2D^d (specificities *4,28*) +		
S-Igl −	Thy 1.1 +	gp70 +
Ia^k −	GIX +	p30 +
TL1,2,3,4 −	GCSA +	p15 +

we obtained the original strain from Elizabeth Stockert of the Sloan-Kettering Institute. Several of these strains were tested, and all (including the clones) behaved concordantly. The anomalous atypical, as well as the typical, expected reactions were consistently reproduced. Representative results of CMC and serology, including absorptions, are shown in Table 2. Certain gene products, e.g., those of the *H-2K*^{k} gene, were absent even though the K36 tumor had spontaneously arisen in an AKR (*H-2*^{k}) mouse (Schmidt *et al.*, 1979), while certain allospecificities of *H-2*^{d} were unexpectedly present (Schmidt and Festenstein, 1980). The expected *H-2D*^{k} gene products were unaltered. It can also be seen from Table 2 that the results of direct serological cytotoxic tests on the tumor with for example, serum 8, were sometimes discordant with the results of tests on normal cells after the sera were first absorbed with the tumor cells (a cytotoxicity-positive/absorption-negative result).

2.1. Absence of the *H-2K*^{k} Gene Product(s)

2.1.1. Serology

K36 was negative with anti-H-2.23 sera detecting the *K*^{k} private specificity as well as with anti-11 and anti-25 sera, the public specificities of the *K*^{k} haplotype. Furthermore, K36 was unable to absorb out anti-K^k-H-2.23, 8 11, or 25 activity from the relevant sera when tested on B10.A (*K*^{k}*D*^{d}) test cells, while normal AKR (*K*^{k}-positive) cells removed activity from all these sera and the *K*^{k}-negative cell BALB/c (*H-2*^{d}) failed to remove any activity as expected (Table 2).

In contrast, the K36 tumor cell line behaved like its AKR strain of origin with respect to its *D*^{k} product(s) when tested with the relevant antisera (32, 1, and 5). In addition, the K36 tumor cell as well as lymph node cells of the B10.A, AKR, and C3H.OH strains were tested with monoclonal anti-K^k sera (Table 3). There was no reactivity against the K36 tumor cell or the C3H.OH cell line with the anti-H-2.11 antibody, but positive cytotoxic reactions were obtained against B10.A and AKR lymphoid cells. This is regarded as further proof for the absence of the K^k product on K36.

To confirm further the absence of the K^k product, extensive immunization of C57BL/10 (H-2^b) and B10.D2 (H-2^d), BALB.B (H-2^b) and BALB.K (H-2^k) mice with K36 tumor cells was carried out. The resulting antisera reacted with B10.A (K^k D^d) as well as with the complete *H-2* haplotype (*AKR*, K^k D^k, cells) and on the basis of this result, one might expect the reaction to be directed against the K^k gene product(s). However, this cannot be so because absorption with C3H.OH (dddd*dk*) spleen cells completely removed the activity from the sera when tested against B10.A lymphoid cells (Table 4). These results confirm the absence of K^k from K36 because the reactivity against B10.A was due to a biregional public specificity of the H-2^k haplotype.

2.1.2. Cell-Mediated Cytotoxicity Tests

The CMC assays were done following *in vitro* sensitization or *in vivo* priming of the B10 H-2 congeneic mice and stimulated by various H-2 congeneic allogeneic lymphoid cells and PHA blasts.

TABLE 2. Reactivity of K36.16 with H-2 Antisera

Antiserum	H-2 antigen detected	C′-dependent cytotoxicity[a]		Absorption[b]			Test cells
		AKR	K36.16	AKR	BALB/c	K36.16	
23	K^k	+	−	Abs	N	N	B10.A
8	Public	+	+	Abs	Abs	N	B10.A
11	Public	+	−	Abs	N	N	B10.A
25	Public	+	−	Abs	N	N	B10.A
32	D^k	+	+	Abs	N	Abs	B10.BR
1	Public	+	+	Abs	N	Abs	B10.BR
3	Public	+	−	Abs	Abs	N	B10.BR
5	Public	+	+	Abs	N	Abs	B10.BR
4	D^d	−	(±)	N	Abs	Abs	B10.D2
28	Public	−	(±)	N	Abs	Abs	B10.D2
2	D^b	−	−	N	N	N	B10
31	K^d	−	−	N	Abs	N	B10.D2
33	K^b	−	(±)	N	N	N	B10

[a](+) Antiserum is cytotoxic for the test cell; (−) negative reaction.
[b](Abs) Absorption of alloantibody from the antiserum, when tested against the indicated test cells; (N) no absorption.

TABLE 3. Reactivity of Monoclonal Antibodies with K36.16 Tumor and Control Lymphoid Cells

Monoclonal antibody[a]:			R100/5	R100/27	R100/30
Suggested specificity[b]:			H-2.11	H-2.25	H-2.5
Target cell[c]	*H-2*		Cytotoxicity[d] (%) (titer[e])		
K36.16	—	D^k	0	66 (1:12,500)	68 (1:4000)
AKR	K^k	D^k	73 (1:8,000)	84 (1:32,000)	N.D.
B10.A	K^k	D^d	74 (1:16,000)	N.D.	73 (1:8000)
C3H.OH	K^d	D^k	56 (1:100)	28 (1:16,000)[f]	22 (1:<100)

[a]Kindly provided by Dr. H. Lemke, Cologne.
[b]From Hämmerling *et al.* (1978).
[c]Target cells were ^{51}Cr-labeled. K36.16 tumor cells were grown *in vitro*, and AKR, B10.A, and C3H.OH were mesenteric lymph node cells.
[d](N.D.) Not determined.
[e]50% titer.
[f]Based on 28% endpoint.

The cytotoxicity studies showed in two ways that the K^k product was missing: (1) when B10.D2 cells were immunized with B10.A lymphoid cells and these effector cells were then tested against the K36 tumor cells, there was no significant killing, while the effector cells readily killed B10.A PHA blasts (Testorelli *et al.*, 1980) (Table 5); (2) K36 itself was able to generate anti-D^k killers in B10.D2 responders, but failed to generate killers against the K^k haplotype (Table 6).

In addition to these direct cytotoxicity experiments, cold target-cell-inhibition experiments were also performed. Specific blocking of cyto-

TABLE 4. Lack of Anti-H-2.23 Appearance after Immunization with K36

Antiserum[a]	Treatment	Cytotoxic activity against ^{51}Cr-labeled B10.A lymphoid cells (titer)
BALB/c anti-K36	Unabsorbed	63 (1:8000)
	C3H.OH abs.[b]	27 (1:<20)
Balb.B anti-K36	Unabsorbed	47 (1:400)
	C3H.OH abs.[b]	0

[a]Hyperimmune sera were produced by repeated injections of 10^7 tumor cells.
[b]Antisera were absorbed with 5×10^8 lymphoid cells from C3H.OH (K^d D^k) per microliter of antiserum.

TABLE 5. Absence of killing of K36 (*H-2*^{k}) by Effector Cells Sensitized against *H-2K*^{k} Gene Products

Responding cells	Stimulating cells	Targets[a]	^{51}Cr release (%) E/T ratio 40	20	10
B10.D2 (dddddd)	B10.BR (*kkkkkk*)	B10.BR	31	24	20
		AKR	29	24	15
		K36	35	31	16
B10.D2 (dddddd)	B10.A (*kkk*ddd)	B10.A	32	26	18
		AKR	31	25	16
		K36	13	11	6
C3H.OH (ddddd*k*)	C3H (*kkkkkk*)	C3H	52	40	nd
		AKR	33	26	nd
		K36	9.5	9	nd

[a]K36.16 tumor cells grown in tissue culture and PHA blasts.

toxicity was obtained with the appropriate normal *H-2K*^{k} (B10.A) *H-2*^{k} (AKR) (Table 7) (Testorelli *et al.*, 1980). K36 tumor cells, however, failed to block anti-K^{k} sensitization—probably due to the absence of *K*^{k} gene product(s).

TABLE 6. Inability of K36 to Stimulate Effectors in B10.D2 Responder Cells against *H-2K*^{k} Gene Products

Responder	Stimulator	Target[a]	^{51}Cr release (%) E/T ratio 40	20	10
B10.D2 (dddddd)	K36	B10.A (*kkk*ddd)	3	1	0.4
		C3H.OH (ddddd*k*)	20	14	7
		AKR (*kkkkkk*)	19	15	7
		K36	12	9	5

[a]PHA blasts or K36.16 tumor cells grown in tissue culture.

TABLE 7. Failure of K36 to Inhibit Anti-H-2K^k Cytotoxic Lymphocytes (B10.D2 Anti-B10.A)

Responding cells	Stimulating cells	Targets	Inhibitors[a]	^{51}Cr release (%)[b] 10^5	^{51}Cr release (%)[b] 10^4	Inhibition (%) 10^5	Inhibition (%) 10^4
B10.D2	B10.A	B10.A	—	35		—	
(dddddd)	(*kkk*ddd)	(*kkk*ddd)	B10.A (K^k-pos)	9.8	18.2	72	48
			AKR (K^k-pos)	12.3	19.2	65	45
			K36 (K^k-neg)	31.1	33.9	11	3
			LSTRA (K^k-neg)	28.0	33.6	20	6

[a]B10.A and AKR PHA blasts; K36.16 of AKR origin, grown in tissue culture; LSTRA tumor cells grown in ascites form in BALB/c mice (*H-2*^{d}).
[b]Effector/target cell ratio was 40:1. ^{51}Cr release is given for 10^5 and 10^4 inhibitors.

2.1.3. *Immunochemical Analysis*

The absence of the *H-2K*^{k} product from K36 was also investigated by immunoprecipitating [^{3}H]arginine-labeled glycoprotein of the K36 membrane with anti-H-2.23 sera and comparing the results with control reactions of [^{14}C]arginine-labeled glycoprotein from B10.BR cells with anti-H-2.23 sera. The 45D peak was analyzed. The anti-H-2.23 sera reactdd with K36 as well as the control B10.BR glycoprotein, but activity against K36 as well as B10.BR glycoprotein was eliminated by prior absorption of the sera with B10.A while absorption with Eo2G (*H-2*^{b} GCSA positive) and C57BL/6 removed anti-K36 activity without affecting anti-B10.BR glycoprotein activity. These results can best be explained by the presence of contaminating antibody precipitating viral gp45. The conclusion from these results is that the K^k product is indeed absent from K36 (Schmidt *et al.*, 1979).

2.2. *H-2*^{d} Products on K36 of AKR (*H-2*^{k}) Origin

One would not normally expect to find *H-2*^{d} gene products on a cell of AKR (*H-2*^{k}) origin, yet by several different criteria, these reactions were present.

1. By conventional serological cytotoxicity and absorption studies (see Table 1), both H-2.4 (the private) and H-2.28 (one of the public specificities of *H-2D*^{d}) were present. These "anomalous" reactions were present in the cloned as well as the original tumors (see Tables 1 and 2, Schmidt and Festenstein, 1980).
2. The extra reactions of the D^d haplotype were also investigated by

immune precipitation techniques. Using [^{3}H]arginine glycoprotein of LSTRA (*H-2*^{d}) and anti-H-2.4 (the private specificity of *D*^{d}) sera without anti-gp70 activity, various absorptions were done prior to testing. Meth.A and BALB/c, all *H-2*^{d}, as well as K36 carrying the putative extra H-2.4, were effective in removing this activity, while AKR and E♂G2 (*H-2*^{k} and *H-2*^{b}, respectively) failed to do so (Figs. 1 and 2).

3. CMC testing was then done. B10.A (K^k and D^d) lymphoid cells were used to stimulate (AKR × B10)F_1 (K^k/K^b-D^k/D^d) responder cells. The cytotoxic effectors killed not only B10.D2 (K^d D^d) and B10.A (K^k

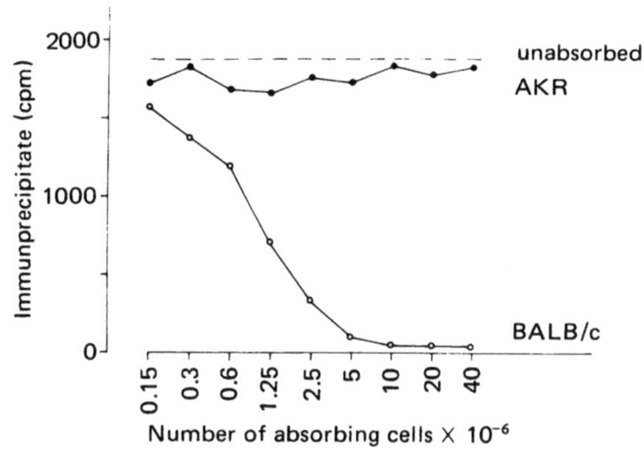

Figure 1. Immunoprecipitation of 45,000-dalton H-2D^d from purified LSTRA (*H-2*^{d}) glycoprotein by anti-H-2.4 sera after absorption with BALB/c (H-2.4-positive) (○) or AKR (H-2.4-negative) (●) lymphoid cells. (----) Unabsorbed H-2.4 serum.

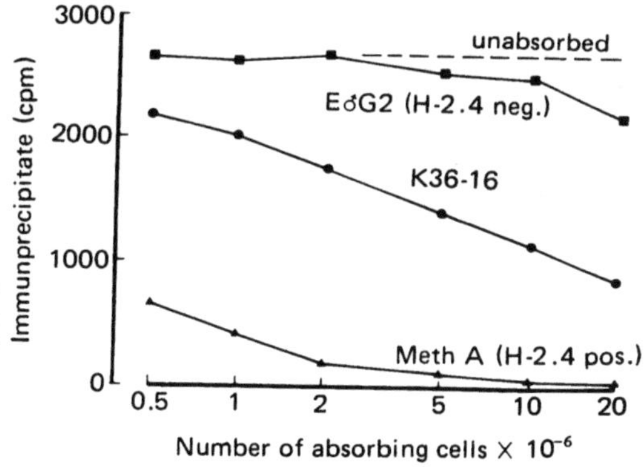

Figure 2. Absorption of anti-H-2.3 sera by K36.16 (16th clone of K36), Meth.A (H-2.4-positive), and all E♂G2 (H-2.4-negative) tumor cells and testing by immunoprecipitation of the 45,000-dalton H-2D^d from purified LSTRA glycoprotein. From Festenstein *et al.*, (1979b).

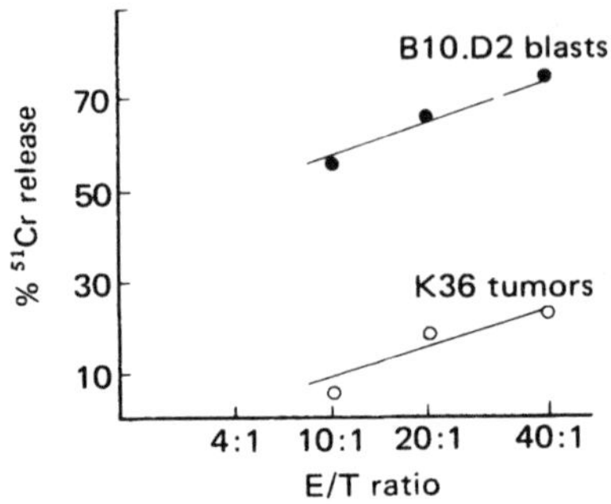

Figure 3. Killing of K36 (H-2^k-derived) by (AKR × B10)F_1 effectors sensitized against B10.D2 (H-$2D^d$).

D^d), but also K36 (K^-D^k). The K36 tumor was killed as though it carried, in addition to its normal D^k antigenic specificities, D^d (Fig. 3) determinants. Their presence on K36 cells was confirmed by experiments in which K36 tumor cells were used to inhibit the killing of B10.A (K^kD^d) PHA target cells by (AKR × B10)F_1 lymphoid cytotoxic effectors (Fig. 4).

4. Immunochemical studies were then performed. Sodium dodecyl

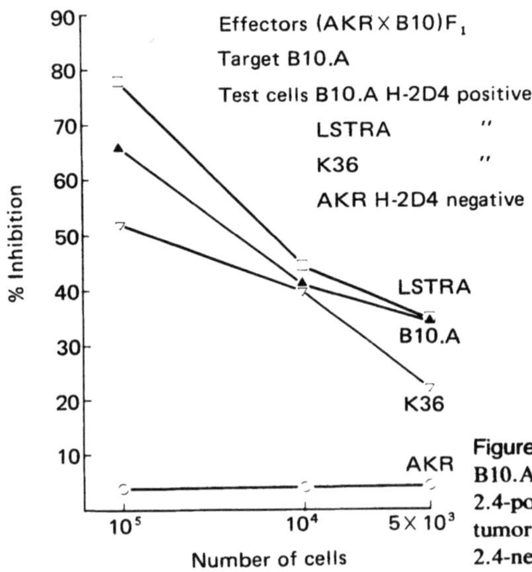

Figure 4. Inhibition of AKR × B10 anti-B10.A cytotoxicity by K36 and H-2.4-positive (B10.A, LSTRA) normal and tumor cells with no inhibition by H-2.4-negative (AKR) control.

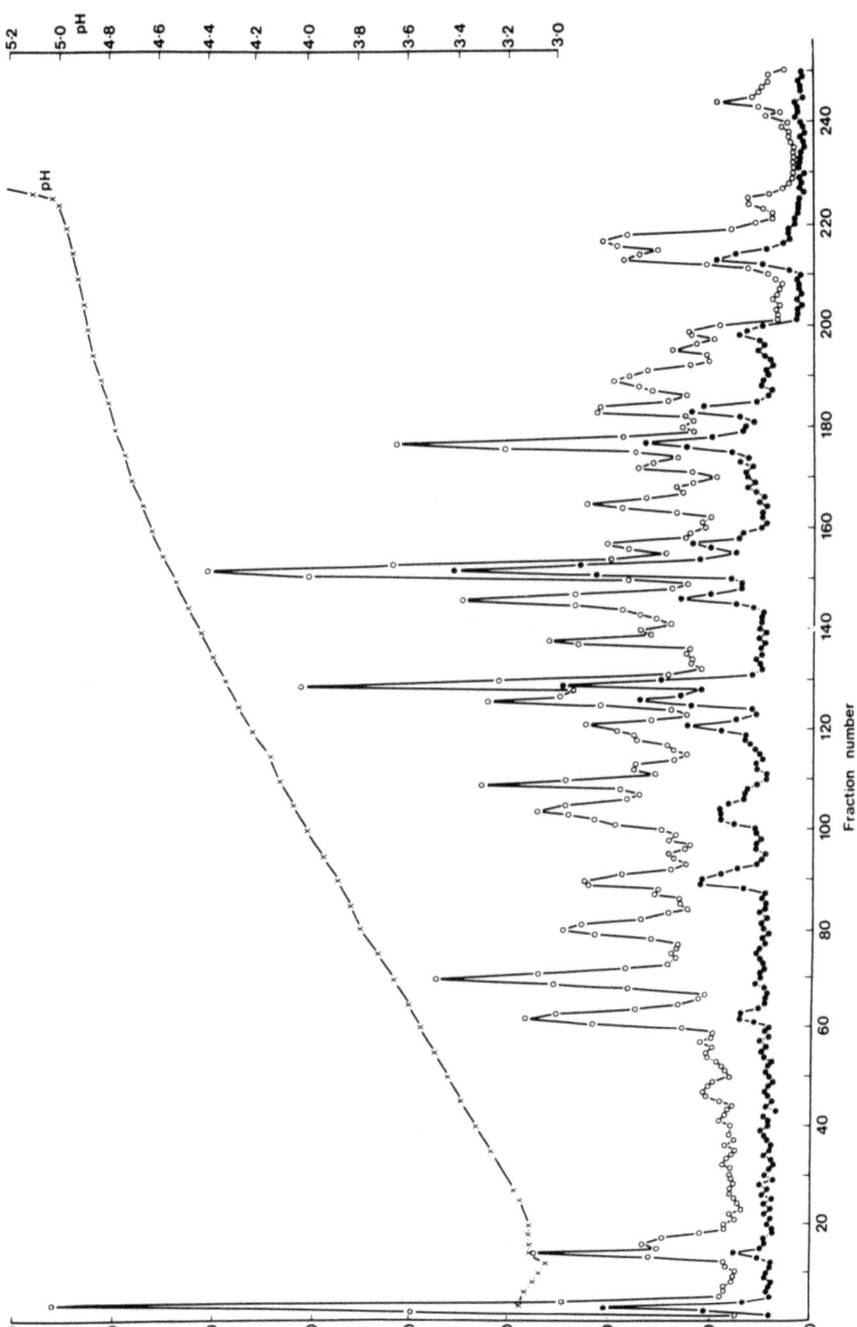

Figure 5. Comparison of tryptic peptide maps from [^{3}H]arginine-labeled K36.16 (*H-2*^{k}) precipitated by anti-H-2.4 (○) and [^{14}C]arginine-labeled H-2.4 from RAD.A-1 (*H-2*^{a}) (●). From Schmidt and Festenstein (1980).

sulfate gels were done using [^{3}H]arginine-labeled K36 glycoprotein, and three peaks were found with the anti-H-2.4 sera—one 70,000-, one 45,000-, and one 12,000-dalton. Absorption with BALB/c (*H-2*^{d}) as well as E♂G2 (*H-2*^{b}) substantially reduced the size of the 45,000-dalton peaks to about the same extent, while the 70,000-dalton peak was reduced only by the E♂G2 cells. These results indicate that the anti-H-2.4 sera probably contain, in addition to the expected anti-D^d activity, anti-viral antibody [E♂G2 carries the Gross cell-surface antigen (GCSA)]; BALB/c lymphoid cells removed the anti-H-2.4 activity, while E♂G2 removed not only gp70 but also viral gp45. The 12,000-dalton component is presumed to be β_2-microglobulin.

Further analysis of the 45,000-dalton product precipitated by anti-H-2.4 sera was made by tryptic digestion and peptide mapping (Fig. 5). A complicated map was obtained. All the peaks corresponding to a normal H-2.4 product were present both qualitatively and quantitatively. However, additional peaks, probably due to viral protein, were also present, and further experiments are in progress to find out whether they are derived from residues on the same or different molecules of the extra "H-2.4" product. Experiments are also being done to establish whether the H-2.4-like specificity on the K36 tumor has chemical properties similar to those of the H-2.4 products of normal cells (Schmidt and Festenstein, 1980).

3. Conclusions and Discussion

Several explanations for these results have already been discussed. In addition, Finberg *et al.* (1978) and other workers have suggested that viral products associate with syngeneic MHS determinants to provide "new" antigens and that these stimulate alloreactive effectors capable of cross-reacting with syngeneic cells. However, it is not clear from this proposal how autoreactivity could result from allostimulation, especially since Simpson *et al.* (1978) and others have shown that the H-2 restricted responses are highly specific and do not normally cross-react. Of all these possibilities, we favor the hypothesis that the reactivity against the K36 syngeneic tumor is directed against an H-2-like product and is the result of derepression of a silent H-2 gene. Such a hypothesis, which implies the presence and activation of silent H-2 genes of foreign haplotypes, can also explain the extremely high level of alloreactivity known to be present toward MHS antigens as compared with conventional antigens like bovine gamma globulin. This striking difference has intrigued immunobiologists for many years (see, for example, Simonsen, 1970; Jerne, 1971). If the derepression hypothesis is correct, it could be that genetically hyperreactive embryonic and tumor cells may be prone to express such histocompatibility determinants intermittently, so that primary sensitization against them has already been effected by birth (Festenstein, 1978). In this way, the individual could already have been primed against allodeterminants so that any H-2-like-carrying tumor will be readily eliminated. One consequence would be that only those tumors that do not express these determinants would escape from surveillance. In contrast, H-2 restricted responses against, say, TAA-controlled tumor growth could fail when there is loss of an important MHS K/D antigen.

Several criticisms have been leveled at the concept of derepressed H-2 antigens. It has been stated that:

1. TSTA are weak with respect to their ability to induce either cellular or humoral immunity and therefore these "TSTA" cannot be H-2 (Klein, 1978). While this may be true for some tumors, it is certainly not true for all systems, particularly for the murine sarcoma virus system (Levy, 1974), in which syngeneic histogenetic effects are clearly demonstrable.
2. H-2 congeneic strains were not used in several experimental systems. While this may be true for other experimental systems, in the K36 system reported here, congeneic strains were used, and non-H-2 antigens could be ruled out for both the histogenetic and the serological experiments, by the use of F_1 responders made with one partner of the strain of origin of the tumor.

Doubt has also been cast on the validity of the serological observations. In this context, Klein (1978), for example, emphasizes the need to avoid overinterpretation and to use antisera that have been carefully analyzed by extensive panel test and then rendered monospecific by carefully planned absorptions.

In our experiments on normal and neoplastic tissues with clearly defined antisera, we performed careful comparative tests using sera from several reputable different sources (Dr. Snell, Dr. Démant, Dr. Nathenson), including our own laboratory. The sera were extremely strong; were extensively panel-tested, absorbed, and diluted for specificity; and were used in a variety of serological tests including ^{51}Cr release—the standard test for normal lymphocytes. In this way and also by immunochemistry, great care was taken to ensure that the effects of contaminating antibodies did not obscure the results either directly or through modification of self by associative interactions. In addition, peptide mapping was used to obtain direct evidence for the molecular structures of the various precipitated gene products. This method, which has very high powers of resolution (Nathenson *et al.*, 1977), allows us to discriminate clearly between the likely patterns to be derived from products of (point) mutations and viral and other products and those of true H-2 alloantigens; evidence for the latter has already been obtained from our own experiments and presented above. In these experiments, we used different sublines as well as clones derived from the original tumor, which grows only in its strain of origin and in F_1 mice made with this strain. This speaks strongly against contamination with other laboratory cell lines.

H-2.4 ($H\text{-}2^d$) specificity is known to differ from H-2.23 ($H\text{-}2^k$) by at least 30–40% (Nathenson *et al.*, 1977). If the extra "H-2.4" were a point mutation at the K end, one would expect not more than 10% discordance between the mutant and the original strain, which is clearly not supported by the experimental data. The H-2 mutation data therefore support the gene cluster hypothesis for the extra specificities.

We have not yet found any convincing alternative explanation of the experimental data other than the repression–derepression hypothesis.

ACKNOWLEDGMENTS. We gratefully acknowledge the financial support of the Cancer Research Campaign of Great Britain, the German Research Council, D.G.F. (W.S.), and E.M.B.O. (C.T.).

References

Abstracts, Workshop on H-2 Antigens, London, England, April 29–May 3, 1979, *Immunogenetics* **9**:305–326, 1979.

Amos, D.B., 1971, Genetic control of the human HL-A histocompatibility system: Alternatives to the two sublocus hypothesis, *Transplant. Proc.* **3**:71.

Cikes, M., and Friberg, S., Jr., 1971, Expression of H-2 and Moloney leukaemia virus-determined cell-surface antigens in synchronized cultures of a mouse cell line, *Proc. Natl. Acad. Sci. U.S.A.* **6**:566.

Festenstein, H., 1978, *Natural Resistance Systems against Foreign Cells, Tumors and Microbes* (G. Cudkowicz, M. Landy, and G.M. Shearer, eds.), pp. 223–232. Academic Press, New York.

Festenstein, H., Schmidt, W., Testorelli, C., DeGiorgi, L., Marelli, O., Matossian-Rogers, A., and Atfield, G., 1979a, Immunogenetic and immunochemical studies of H-2 antigens of foreign haplotypes on tumor cells, *J. Immunogenet.* **6**:263.

Festenstein, H., Schmidt, W., Matossian-Rogers, A., deGiorgi, L., and Testovelli, C., 1979b, Nature of extra H-2 like antigenic specificities on tumor cells, in: *Current Trends in Tumour Immunology* (S. Ferrone, S. Govini, R. B. Herberman and R.A. Reisfeld, eds.), pp. 299-307, Garland STPM Press, New York.

Finberg, R., Burakoff, S.J. Cantor, H., and Benaceraff, B, 1978, Biological significance of alloreactivity: T cells stimulated by Sendai virus-coated syngeneic cells specifically lyse allogeneic target cells, *Proc. Natl. Acad. Sci. U.S.A.* **75**:5145.

Garrido, F., Schirrmacher, V., and Festenstein, H., 1976a, H-2-like specificities of foreign haplotypes appearing on a mouse sarcoma after vaccinia virus infection, *Nature (London)* **259**:228.

Garrido, F., Festenstein, H., and Schirrmacher, V., 1976, Further evidence for derepression of H-2 and Ia-like specificities of foreign haplotypes in mouse tumor cell lines, *Nature (London)* **261**:705.

Garrido, F., Schirrmacher, V., and Festenstein, H., 1977a, Studies on H-2 specificities on mouse tumor cells by a new microradioassay, *J. Immunogenet.* **4**:15.

Garrido, F., Schmidt, W., and Festenstein, H., 1977b, Immunogenetic studies on Meth.A-vaccinia tumor cells *in vivo* and *in vitro*, *J. Immunogenet.* **4**:115.

Hämmerling, G.J., Lemke, H., Hämmerling, U., Hohmann, C., Wallich, R., and Rajewsky, K., 1978, Monoclonal antibodies against murine cell surface antigens: Anti-H-2, anti-Ia and anti-T cells antibodies, in: *Current Topics in Microbiology and Immunology*, Vol. 81 (F. Melchers, M. Potter, and N. Werner, eds.), pp. 100–106, Springer-Verlag, Berlin, Heidelberg, New York.

Jerne, N.K., 1971, The somatic generation of immune recognition, *Eur. J. Immunol.* **1**:1.

Klein, J., 1973, H-2 mutations, *Adv. Immunol.* **26**:55.

Levy, J.P., 1974, Antigens associated with C type RNA virus induced tumors, in: *Progress in Immunology*, Vol. 3 (L. Brent and J. Holborow eds.), pp. 299–303, American Elsevier, New York.

Nathenson, S.G., Brown, J.L., Ewenstein, B.M., Nisizawa, T., Sears, D.W., and Freed, J.H., 1977, Structural differences between parent and variant H-2K glycoproteins from mouse strains carrying H-2 gene mutations, *Cold Spring Harbor Symp. Quant. Biol.* **41**:343.

Old, E.J., and Stockert, E., 1977, Immunogenetics of cell surface antigens of mouse leukaemia, *Annu. Rev. Genet* **17**:127.

Old, E.J., Boyse, E.A., and Stockert, E., 1965, The G (Gross) leukaemia antigen, *Cancer Res.* **25**:813–819.

Schmidt, W., and Festenstein, H., 1980, Serological and immunochemical studies of H-2 allospecificities on K36, a syngeneic tumour of AKR, *J. Immunogenetics* **7**:7.

Schmidt, W., Atfield, G., and Festenstein, H., 1979, Loss of H-2K^k gene product(s) from an AKR spontaneous leukaemia, *Immunogenetics* **8**:311.

Simonsen, M., 1970, On the nature and measurement of antigenic strength, *Transplant. Rev.* **3**:22.

Simpson, E., Mobraaten, L., Chandler, P., 1978, Cross-reactive cytotoxic responses. H-2 restricted are more specific than anti-H-2 responses, *J. Exp. Med.* **148**:1478.

Snell, G.D., 1979, The major histocompatibility complex: Its evolution and involvement in cellular immunity, *Harvey Lect.*

Testorelli, C., Marelli, O., Schmidt, W., and Festenstein, H., 1980, Changes in H-2 antigen expression on a murine spontaneous leukaemia (K36) detected by cell-mediated cytotoxicity assay, *J. Immunogenet.* **7**:19.

Workshop Issue, 1980, H-2 Antigens: Genetic Control and Expression on Normal, Tumour and Virally Infected Cells, London, England, April 29–May, 3, 1979, *J. Immunogenet.* **7**.

6

Hybrid Sterility Gene Located in the *T/t–H-2* Supergene on Chromosome 17

Jiří Forejt

1. Introduction

Recent advances in genetic analysis of the major histocompatibility systems of various species and the first successful attempts at molecular dissection of their products contrast with the limited knowledge concerning the biological function of this particular part of the eukaryotic genome. The major histocompatibility system of the mouse, the *H-2* system, adjoins closely the *T/t* genetic complex in chromosome 17. The *T/t* complex occupies a region of the chromosome 20 times longer than that pertaining to the *H-2* system, and controls a variety of vital functions necessary for the development of the organism and survival of the species.

In this chapter, the current ideas and available experimental evidence on the organization and function of the proximal part of chromosome 17, of which the *T/t–H-2* region is the main component, are brought together. Special attention is paid to *Hybrid-sterility-1* gene located inside this chromosome region. If the histocompatibility genes can be considered as safeguarding the uniqueness of unrelated individuals *within a species* by creating a histocompatibility barrier between them, then hybrid sterility genes can be described as serving a parallel function *between species in statu*

Jiří Forejt • Institute of Molecular Genetics, Czechoslovak Academy of Sciences, 142 20 Prague 4, Czechoslovakia.

nascendi. They create a fertility barrier between remote populations, thus safeguarding their uniqueness at the first stage of species diversification.

The presence of two most complex and polymorphic genetic systems of the murine genome in close proximity in chromosome 17 provokes some speculations about the possible nonrandomness of such association. The already-known building stones for a prospective hypothesis of this kind are being reexamined, and some new ones are introduced in this contribution.

2. Genetic Structure of Chromosome 17

2.1. Genetic Map of Chromosome 17

The best analyzed genome in mammals is that of the laboratory mouse (*Mus musculus* L.). The total length of the haploid genome can be estimated as 1300–1600 centimorgans (cM) from chiasma frequencies of meiotic chromosomes (Polani, 1972; Kyslíkovă and Forejt, 1972). This estimate is very close to 1290 cM (Roderick and Davisson, 1978), the sum of genetic distances between the 340 known gene loci.

Chromosome 17, the third smallest autosome of the murine haploid set, carries two complex and polymorphic genetic systems, the *T/t* complex and the *H-2* system. The latter represents a 0.5 to 1-cM-long part of the chromosome, while most of the *t* haplotypes of the *T/t* complex control by suppression of recombination a region of 15–20 cM in length, including the adjoining *H-2* system. Thus, all animals in natural populations with the recessive lethal *t* haplotype transmit the whole *t–H-2* region as a genetic unit undisturbed by recombination. At the population level, this particular organization of chromosome 17 is reflected in an extremely high linkage disequilibrium between the specific *H-2* and *t* haplotypes (Hammerberg and Klein, 1975a). Linkage relationships between gene loci of chromosome 17, with a recessive lethal *t* haplotype being either present or absent, are summarized in Fig. 1. The distance between centromere and *T/t* complex differs with the method used for its estimation. Forejt (1973) and Hammerberg and Klein (1975b) used a Robertsonian translocation (i.e., two telocentric chromosomes fused by their centromeres to give a single has been calculated from chiasma frequencies of chromosome 17 (see Section 2.4). Besides the *T* mutation, which causes a markedly shortened tail in *T*/+ heterozygotes, three other mutations, *Fused, Kinky,* and *Knobbly (Fu, Ki, Kb)* cause tail deformities and map near gene *tf* within the *T–H-2* region. The occurrence of four genes with a very similar type of mutant forms in a short chromosome segment could un-

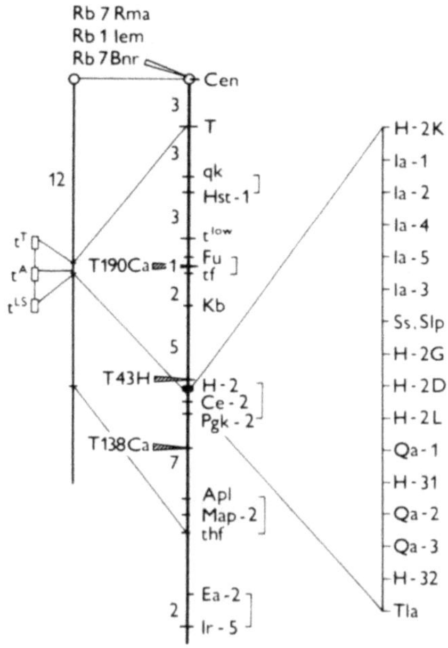

Figure 1. Genetic map of chromosome 17 of the mouse. The figures between gene symbols give the genetic distance in centimorgans (cM) in the presence (*left*) or absence (*right*) of *t* haplotypes. (*Cen*) Centromere; (*T*) *Brachyury* (short tail); *(qk) quaking; (Hst-1) Hybrid sterility-1; (t^{low}) low transmission ratio; (Fu) fused; (tf) tufted; (Kb) Knobbly; (H-2) histocompatibility-2; (H-2K, ^{-2}G, ^{-2}D, ^{-2}L, H-31, -32)* histocompatibility loci; (*Ia*) *I*-associated antigen loci; (*Ss, Slp*) *serum serological* and *sex-limited protein*; (*Qa*) *Q*-region antigen; *(Tla) thymus leukemia antigen; (Apl) acid phosphatase-liver; (Ce-2) liver catalase; (Pgk-2) phosphoglycerate kinase-2; (Map-2) mannosidase processing-2; (thf) thin fur; (Ea-2) erythrocyte antigen-2; (Ir-5) Immune response-5;* (Rb 7 Rma, Rb 1 Iem, Rb 7 Bnr) breakpoints of some Robertsonian translocations; (T190Ca, T43H, T138Ca) breakpoints of reciprocal translocations. *t* haplotype: (T) *T*-interaction factor; (A) Abnormal segregation factor; (LS) Lethality–sterility factor. The mutual order of gene loci in brackets is unknown. Based on data of Roderick and Davisson (1978), Beechey and Searle (1978), Klein, (1978), Lyon and Mason (1977), Hammerberg and Klein (1975a,b), Forejt (1972), Forejt and Gregorová (1977), and Forejt *et al.* (1978).

doubtedly have a bearing on the idea of nonrandom gene arrangement. However, since the test for allelism of the latter three mutations has not been done *(Kb* vs. *Fu, Ki)* or has given ambiguous results *(Fu* vs. *Ki),* any conclusion would still be premature.

The recessive mutation *tufted (tf)* affects the growth of hair in a characteristic wavy manner (Lyon, 1956). This mutation proved to be an invaluable tool in the genetic analysis of *t* haplotypes: the sterility and the lethality factors of the t^6 haplotype have been mapped in close proximity to this gene (see Section 2.3). The most proximal gene marker of chromosome 17 is *thin fur, thf,* another mutation that affects hair growth (Key and Hollander, 1972). The fine-genetic structure of the *H-2* system is presented in Fig. 1 in the arrangement suggested by Klein (1978).

Genes *Hst-1, qk,* and *Pgk-2* affect, and/or are expressed in, various stages of spermatogenic differentiation. They are discussed in greater detail in the following sections of this chapter. Two minor histocompatibility loci, *H-33* and *H-39,* have been described by Flaherty (1975) and Artzt *et al.* (1977). Their exact position on the chromosome is not known, but they map within the *T–H-2* chromosome region.

2.2. Are Genes of the *T–H-2* Region of Chromosome 17 Functionally Related?

The term "genetic system" refers to a set of closely linked and functionally related genes [for a discussion of histocompatibility genetic systems, cf. Bodmer (1977)]. The definition thus tacitly assumes a nonrandom arrangement of genes with respect to their function, a phenomenon not yet well documented in eukaryotic genomes. A piece of evidence has been gathered on the relatedness of gene products of the *H-2* system and of the major histocompatibility systems in general (Bodmer, 1977). One might wonder whether even the *T/t* complex codes for molecules engaged in functionally related processes and, moreover, whether both systems, the *T/t* and *H-2,* are related in a similar way or even form a functional unit, a "*T/t–H-2* supergene." The first step along this line of thinking was made by Snell (1968), who considered the close linkage of the *T/t* and *H-2* systems as a genetic device for maintaining heterozygosity of the *H-2* chromosome region. The forced heterozygosity at this chromosomal area was thought to act possibly through enhancing the chance of survival, particularly by providing resistance to the attacks of viral infections.

A much closer relationship between gene products of the *T/t* and *H-2* systems has been proposed by Gluecksohn-Waelsch and Erickson (1970) and Artzt and Bennett (1975). These authors suggested that the products of both systems, *T/t* and *H-2,* operate through the cell membrane, and furthermore that developmental abnormalities, resulting from homozygosity for certain *t* haplotypes, might be due to the failure of proper cell–cell interaction. If essentially correct, such hypotheses would impose far-reaching consequences on such diverse topics as embryonic and spermatogenic development, haploid gene expression, and organization of the eukaryotic genome. The concept of a *T/t–H-2* supergene, if confirmed in whatever form, would represent an unprecendented case in eukaryotes of nonrandom organization of genes with related functions, since it involves almost half of chromosome 17.

A strong mutual influence between the *T/t* and *H-2* systems can be envisaged without considering functional relatedness of the genes involved in both systems. Interlocking of presumably hundreds of genes, including *H-2* in a *t* haplotype by crossing-over suppression, should control spreading or elimination of a particular *H-2* haplotype according to the selectively advantageous or deleterious effect of the interlocked genes influencing such vital functions as embryonic development, fertility, and immune mechanisms (Forejt, 1976a).

2.3. *T/t* Complex

The *T/t* complex has been the subject of several recent reviews (Gluecksohn-Waelsch and Erickson, 1970; Braden, 1972; D. Bennett, 1975; Klein and Hammerberg, 1977); hence, only a short survey of properties of the *T/t* complex is presented here. However, three topics are discussed in greater detail for the sake of argument in the following discussion about the structure and function of the *T–H-2* chromosome region, namely, the effect of the *T/t* complex on male fertility, the attempts at immunogenetic ascertainment of the *T/t* gene products, and the genetic structure of *t* haplotypes.

The *T/t* complex occupies a relatively long region of the proximal part of chromosome 17 with loosely defined margins, especially at the centromeric side. The *T/t* complex comprises dominate *T* mutations (alleles), recessive *t* haplotypes (formerly *t* allelles), and the + allele. Animals with the *T/+ genotype* at the *T/t* complex are short-tailed, while with few exceptions, all *T/t* combinations cause taillessness. The *T/T* homozygotes die *in utero* between the 10th and 11th days of prenatal development. Mice +/+, *t/+*, and *t/t* (if viable) are normal-tailed; the only exception is the t^{AE5} allele, the homozygotes $t^{AE5/AE5}$ being short-tailed (Gluecksohn-Waelsch and Erickson, 1970).

Almost all *t* haplotypes extracted from natural populations of *Mus musculus* are recessive lethal (Dunn, 1964; Petras, 1967; Lewontin, 1962, 1968). The recessive lethal *t* haplotypes were assorted to six complementation groups (D. Bennett, 1975). Within a group, the *t* haplotypes do not complement each other; hence, they are assumed to be operationally identical. Among the groups, the t^1 haplotypes do complement; the $t^{1\text{-}1}/t^{1\text{-}2}$ compounds are viable. However, the complementation is in most instances imperfect, since in some combinations (e.g., t^{12}/t^0) as few as 18% of *t/t* animals survive. The degree of complementation depends on the particular combination of *t* haplotypes and on the influence of the genetic background (D. Bennett *et al.*, 1976; Klyde, 1970). The nature of incompleteness in complementation of the *t* haplotypes is still unclear.

Several semilethal *t* haplotypes (t^{sl}) have been extracted from wild mice. Only a certain part of t^{sl}/t^{sl} homozygotes survive, and no explanation for different action of the same t^{sl}/t^{sl} genotypes on embryonic development in individual animals is available (Johnston, 1968; D. Bennett *et al.*, 1969).

Viable *t* haplotypes arise as the result of exceptional recombination within a lethal *t* haplotype. Unlike t^1 or t^{sl} haplotypes with high transmission ratios (see below), the viable *t* haplotypes are transmitted from *t*/+ male heterozygotes in normal (= 0.5) or low (<0.5) ratios. They usually do not suppress recombination in the *T-tf* region, and *t/t* homozygotes are fertile in both sexes. Some confusion between properties of semilethal and viable *t* haplotypes has arisen due to the fact that before the semilethal *t* haplotypes were established as a separate group, some of them had been classified as viable [cf. t^{w2} in Dunn and Morgan (1953) and in D. Bennett *et al.* (1969)].

Recessive lethal *t* haplotypes have been found in natural populations of mice all over the world with gene frequencies between 0.20 and 0.50. They display a series of unique properties, the mechanism of none being clear so far, including *embryonic lethality* (mostly due to specific effects on the ectoderm and its derivatives), *distortion of segregation ratio* in heterozygous males, (so that 80–90% of progeny of *t*/+ males possess the *t*-bearing chromosome), and *suppression of recombination* between *T* and *H-2* loci (with the exception of the t^9 complementation group).

2.3.1. Effect of t Haplotypes on Male Fertility

Five different types of impairment of male fertility are under control by the *T/t* complex. In all cases, females of the same genotype display normal fertility.

1. Combination of two complementing recessive lethal *t* haplotypes, $t^{1\text{-}1}/t^{1\text{-}2}$, results in complete male sterility. Spermatogenesis is slightly disturbed (Bryson, 1944; Rajasekarasetty, 1954) or normal. The number of spermatozoa is not reduced, but their motility and morphology are abnormal (D. Bennett and Dunn, 1967). Electron microscopy revealed abnormalities in organization of spermatid microtubuli and irregularities of sperm heads in a fraction of spermatozoa (Olds, 1971a; Dooher and Bennett, 1977). The spermatozoa are unable to penetrate ova (Olds, 1971b).

2. Males homozygous for semilethal *t* haplotypes, t^{sl}/t^{sl}, are also completely sterile, with small testes and no spermatozoa in epididymides (Johnston, 1968; D. Bennett *et al.*, 1969). Abnormal spermatids showing irregularities in organization of microtubules are phagocytosed by Sertoli cells (Dooher and Bennett, 1974).

3. Reduced male fertility is characteristic for surviving T^{AE5}/t^{AE5} homozygotes. Part of the spermatids display a bizarre shape and undergo

necrosis. The motility of sperm is reduced. This exceptional *t* haplotype could resemble a semilethal *t* haplotype (only part of homozygotes survive) with incomplete spermatogenic arrest. If differs, however, in the phenotype, the $t^{AE\ 5}/t^{AE\ 5}$ homozygotes being short-tailed, and in the severe abnormalities of their lymphoid system (Vojtíšková *et al.*, 1976).

4. Partial failure of male fertility also results from combining a lethal or semilethal *t* haplotype with the viable one. Spermatogenesis has not yet been studied in these double heterozygotes (Dunn and Gluecksohn-Schoenheimer, 1950; Braden and Gluecksohn-Waelsch, 1958).

5. A new type of male quasi-sterility has recently been disclosed by Erickson *et al.* (1978). The authors studied interaction between T^{Orl} mutation presumably associated with interstitial deletion and t^0 and t^{12} haplotypes. The fertility of $T^{Orl}/+$ short-tailed males was unimpaired, in contrast to quasi-sterility of T^{Orl}/t^0 and T^{Orl}/t^{12} tailless males. The finding is interesting in that the genetic factor that in a hemizygous state causes quasi-sterility is apparently different from the LS factors (Lyon and Mason, 1977) responsible for sterility of t^0/t^{12} compounds.

2.3.2. *Attempts at Immunogenetic Ascertainment of T/t Gene Products*

There is no doubt that cell differentiation can be accompanied by differentiation of the cell membrane. The so-called differentiation antigens are by definition membrane antigens confined to one or a few types of cells or tissues (Boyse and Old, 1969). What is not *a priori* clear is whether the differentiation of cell surface is the cause or consequence of functional differentiation (Lengerová, 1977; Forejt and Lengerova, 1980). If the differentiation of a cell were connected with a change of a single gene activity, then it would be easy to postulate the causal relationship, but the problem is that cellular differentiation is obviously associated with the occurrence of a number of new gene products, part of which, at least, are the consequence of cell differentiation.

The first experimental evidence suggesting that the *T/t* complex codes for differentiation antigens was reported by D. Bennett and her coworkers (D. Bennett *et al.*, 1972; Yanagisawa *et al.*, 1974; Artzt and Bennett, 1977). Since the *T/t* complex also affects sperm, the authors began a search for possible cell-surface antigenic differences of sperm from males differing at the *T/t* complex. In analyses of the antisera, a number of technical pitfalls had to be circumvented, including the presence of natural autoantibodies in normal mouse serum reacting with sperm (Koo *et al.*, 1977), or low titer of specific antibodies; nevertheless, a series of antigenic specificities controlled by lethal *t* haplotypes has been reported (Artzt and Bennett, 1977).

Besides its phenotypic expression in male germ cells, the *T/t* complex governs various stages of embryonal development. The fetal cells might thus represent an alternative site of the possible *T/t* differentiation antigens. The employment of embryonal carcinoma—teratocarcinoma—cells instead of normal fetal cells enables one to produce an unlimited quantity of cells in the *in vitro* system (for reviews of the teratocarcinoma system, see Jacob, 1977; Gachelin, 1978). Hitherto, no observation has been published on teratocarcinoma derived from a mouse heterozygous for *t* haplotype, but some stimulating findings have been made with the F9 line of nullipotent primitive teratocarcinoma cells derived from the 129/Sv inbred male mouse (+/+ at *T/t* complex). Antisera of high titer and specificity were obtained by immunization of syngeneic 129/Sv recipients with irradiated F9 cells. The distribution of the antigen, which was designated "F9" in preimplantation embryos, and male germ cells was found to parallel the expression of the *t* haplotypes. However, the conclusion that the F9 antigen is coded for by a gene allelic to $t^{w\,32}$ (or t^{12}) (Artzt *et al.*, 1974) has not yet been confirmed; the original evidence was based on quantitative variation in the absorbing capacity of sperm from animals $t^{w\,32}/+$ and +/+ on a different genetic background.

Provided that the methodological difficulties are solved, e.g., by creating a series of teratocarcinoma lines carrying different *t* haplotypes or by preparing specific monoclonal antibodies against *T/t* determinants, then it might become feasible to investigate the presumed relationship between the observed cell-surface determinants and the function of the *T/t* complex in embryonic development and germ-cell differentiation.

Recent results of transplantations of t^1/t^1 embryos in an ectopic site and *in vitro* cultures of t^1/t^1 embryos indicate that at least some t^1 haplotypes are simply generalized cell lethals (Wudl and Sherman, 1976; Wudl *et al.*, 1977). If this mechanism of t^1/t^1 lethality turned out to hold generally, the assumption that the *T/t* complex governs cell organization in embryogenesis would require revision.

2.3.3. Genetic Structure of t Haplotypes

Our knowledge of the genetic organization of *t* haplotypes comes mainly from the analysis of the t^6 recessive lethal haplotype performed by Lyon and her co-workers (Lyon and Phillips, 1959; Lyon and Meredith, 1964a–c; Lyon and Mason, 1977; Lyon and Bechtol, 1977). The authors dissected the t^6 haplotype into individual factors by isolating the products of exceptional recombination in the *T-tf* region covered by cross-over suppression: $t^{h\,18}$ as the separated lethality–sterility factor (LS), t^{1ow} as the segregation distortion factor (A), and part of the viable haplotypes as the separated *T*-interaction factors (T). Thus, overwhelming evidence has been provided for the segmental nature of *t* haplotypes, the individual *t*-

factors being scattered over a chromosomal area of considerable length, extending from the *T* mutation to gene *tf*. Admittedly, however, the fine-genetic structure is still poorly understood. Lyon and Bechtol (1977) elaborated a model of the *t* haplotype structure postulating the presence in abnormal *t*-chromatin of at least three main regions carrying the aforementioned factors. According to this model, the *T* region is allelic with *T* mutation and the LS is closely linked to the *tf* gene (Fig. 1). The *A* region represents the most complicated part of the model, since in order to accommodate the experimental evidence, a complex pattern of interactions with the other two factors is to be postulated. The data of D. Bennett *et al.* (1976) are illuminating in this respect. A survey of the properties of 70 viable recombinant *t* haplotypes revealed that at least 50 of them lost a high segregation ratio. With 30 *t* haplotypes, the high transmission ratio returned to the normal 1:1, with 20 others it became low, and the remaining 20 were not sufficiently tested. Thus, all studies of viable *t* haplotypes revealed a rule that a single recombination event changes simultaneously all properties except for *T*-interaction of the parental t^1 haplotype.

Undoubtedly, the Lyon model provides a most valuable contribution to unraveling the genetic structure of t^1 haplotypes, since it permits one to formulate new questions that are amenable to experimental testing. A search could be directed particularly to the *tf-H-2* region covered by crossover suppression (Hammerberg and Klein, 1975b) to see which properties, if any, of t^1 haplotypes are affected by recombination within this region. Further useful information can be gained by deletion mapping (Erickson *et al.*, 1978) or by genetic analysis of the effect of partial trisomy of this chromosome region (Forejt *et al.*, 1978) (see Section 2.4.2).

2.4. Cytogenetics of Chromosome 17

For a long time, the cytogenetics of murine chromosomes had been neglected because of the uniform morphology of mitotic chromosomes and the absence of reliable cytological markers. After the discovery of new techniques of differential chromosome staining, each chromosome pair of the mouse was characterized by a unique pattern of transverse bands (Q or G banding) (Schnedl, 1971; Nesbitt and Francke, 1973). A chromosomal rearrangement can serve as a cytological marker of the particular chromosome site and simultaneously as a marker in the genetic map of the chromosome (Miller and Miller, 1975; Eicher and Washburn, 1978).

After G-band staining, chromosome 17 of the mouse displays 11 bands, 6 dark and 5 light ones (for nomenclature, see Nesbitt and Francke, 1973), and this "physical" map can be related, more or less exactly, to the genetic map of the chromosome (Fig. 2). Six reciprocal and

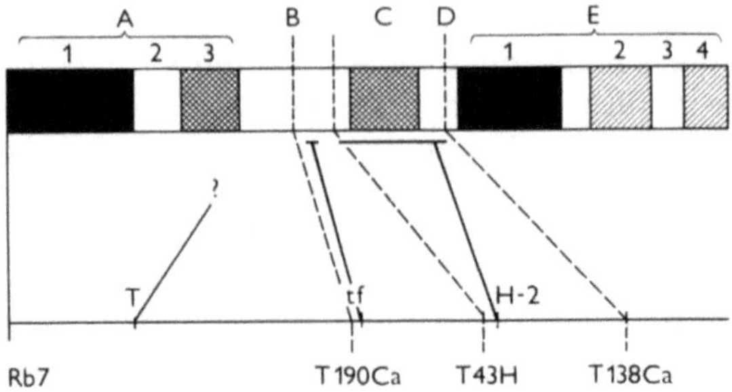

Figure 2. Relationship between cytological and genetic map of chromosome 17. G-band nomenclature according to Nesbitt and Francke (1973). The centromere occurs within the 17A1 band.

Robertsonian translocations involving chromosome 17, for which cytological and genetic data are available (Table 1), serve as markers cross-linking both maps. Thus, mapping of the *tf* gene on the cytological map of chromosome 17 is made possible by two translocations, T190Ca and T43H. The translocation break of the T190Ca translocation was situated proximally from *tf* (i.e., between *tf* and centromere) (Lyon, 1979). The breakpoint of the T43H translocation was placed distally from *tf* (Beechey and Searle, 1978; Forejt *et al.*, 1978), and both breakpoints were put into the 17B band on the cytological map. The gene locus for *tf* must therefore be located between both translocation breaks within the 17B band. Mapping of the *H-2* region on chromosome 17 is more complicated. Apparently, it could also be assigned to 17B, since no recombination between the T43H break and *H-2* takes place (Forejt *et al.*, 1978). On the other hand, the breakpoint of the T138Ca translocation has been found two bands distally, in 17D, yet the T138Ca break displays only 3% of

TABLE 1. Reciprocal and Robertsonian Translocations Involving Chromosome 17

Translocation	Chromosome breakpoints	Gene tag[a]	Comment	Reference
T(9;17)138Ca	9B 17D	*H-2* (3 cM)	—	Carter *et al.* (1955)
T(1;17)190Ca	1H5 17B	*tf* (0 cM)	Homozygotes lethal	Carter *et al.* (1955)
T(16;17)43H	16A 17B	*H-2* (0 cM)	Males sterile	Searle *et al.* (1978)
Rb(8.17)1Iem	8A 17A	*T*	—	Baranov and Dyban (1972)
Rb(16;17)7Bnr	16A 17A	*T* (4 cM)	—	Klein (1971)
Rb(2.17)11Rma	2A 17A	*T*		

[a]The gene tag is a gene marker nearest to the translocation breakpoint. The figure in parentheses is the distance in centimorgans between the two chromosome points.

recombination with *H-2* (Klein and Klein, 1972). The latter estimate seems to be more realistic for two reasons. First, suppression of recombination is likely to occur between the T43H break and *H-2* as a result of the centromeric interference phenomenon in translocated chromosome 16^{17}, where the *H-2* is brought to the close vicinity of centromere 16. Second, all translocations of chromosome 17 studied hitherto enhance the frequency of recombination in the interstitial segment by an unknown mechanism. Thus, recombination between *H-2* and the T138Ca breakpoint is most probably not reduced. The most likely location of the *H-2* system, then, could be in the 17D band (Fig. 2).

2.4.1. Recessive Lethal t Haplotypes Suppress Chiasma Formation in a Part of Chromosome 17 in Meiosis

Most t^1 haplotypes suppress recombination between *T* and *H-2* loci (D. Bennett, 1975; Klein and Hammerberg, 1977). The absence of crossovers can be due to true absence of crossing over, but recombination can also be envisaged to take place without crossovers being recovered (Forejt, 1972; Klein and Hammerberg, 1977). Experimental evidence of the effect of t^{12} and t^6 haplotypes on chiasma frequency of chromosome 17 supports the former alternative. Both *t* haplotypes suppress chiasma frequency in chromosome 17, and this suppression corresponds well to that of recombination frequency (Forejt, 1972; Forejt and Gregorová, 1977; Lyon and Glenister, 1977). The priniciple of the experiments is shown in Fig. 3, and the findings are summarized in Table 2. The results obtained by means of translocation T43H are particularly illuminating. The translocation break was situated in close proximity to the *H-2K* region of the *H-2* system (Forejt *et al.*, 1978), still under the recombination-suppression effect of the t^{12} haplotype. If the crossover-suppression effect extended proximally to the centromere of chromosome 17 in $+T43H/t^{12}+$ males, then no chiasma in the centromere 17–T43H region could be formed, and consequently no ChIV configurations could be found in spermatocytes of such mice (Fig. 3). We have, however, found 22% of spermatocytes with ChIV configuration indicating 11% of recombination between centromere 17 and the t^{12} haplotype. The data in Table 2 show that with a further two translocations, the results are essentially similar as far as the centromere–*t* haplotype distance is concerned.

The estimated recombination frequency between the centromere and the *t* haplotype has an important bearing on the predictable restrictions concerning the possible haploid *t* and *H-2* gene product expression on the sperm membrane. Figure 4 shows the scheme of differentiation of primary spermatocyte into mature sperm cells and the possible consequence of recombination between the centromere and a *t* haplotype. Obviously,

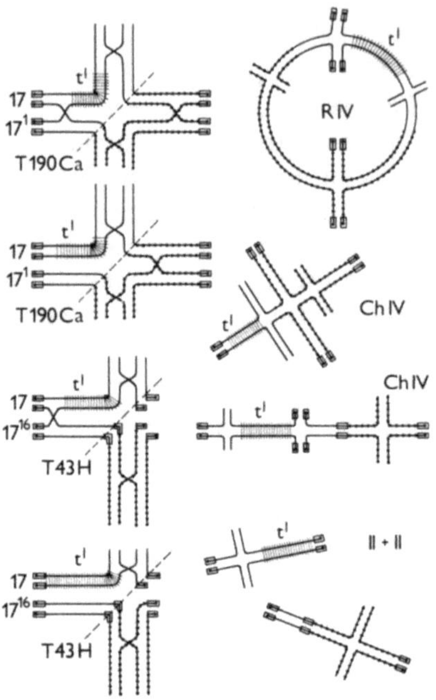

Figure 3. Principle of cytological estimation of crossing-over suppression by a *t* haplotype in chromosome 17. (Drawings are not to scale.) *Left:* Scheme of presumed homologous chromosome pairing—translocation cross—at pachytene of translocation heterozygotes is shown at the left. *Right:* Schemes of diakinesis–metaphase I translocation configurations, the frequency of which can be scored under the microscope (cf. Table 2). The occurrence of a translocation configuration—RIV, ChIV, II+II—depends on the formation of chiasmata in the relevant arm of the translocation cross. The bottom part of the figure illustrates the consequence of a hypothetical complete recombination suppression between centromere and T43H translocation break. The ChIV configurations cannot be expected to occur.

TABLE 2. Effect of *t* Haplotype on Chiasma Frequencies on Chromosome 17 of Male Translocation Heterozygotes

		Translocation configurations[b]						Recombination (%) from centromere to translocation break[c]
Expt.[a]	Genotype	RIV	ChIV	II+II[d]	Total	RIV %	ChIV %	
1	*T T190Ca/+ +*	212	144	23	379	56	—	28
	T T190Ca/t^{12}+	127	247	21	395	32	—	16
2	*T T138Ca/+ +*	263	149	37	449	59	—	29
	T T138Ca/t^{12}+	203	152	115	470	43	—	22
3	*+ T138Ca/+ +*	284	69	47	400	71	—	35
	t^6T138Ca/T+	162	55	181	398	41	—	20
4	*+T43H/T+*							
	+T43H/t^{121}+		276	124	400	—	69	34
	+ T43/x^{12}+		77	274	351	—	22	11

[a]Recalculated from: Forejt (1972), Expts. 1 and 2; Lyon and Glenister (1977), Expt. 3; and Forejt and Gregorová (1977), Expt. 4.

[b]In Expts. 1–3, spermatocytes at early and late diakinesis (not metaphase I) are included. Diakineses and metaphases I are included in Expt. 3.

[c]In expts. 1 and 4, the values of 16% and 11% reflect the recombination frequencies between centromere and the t^{12} haplotype. The values in Expts. 2 and 3 represent the minimum estimates of recombination between centromere and translocation break (see the text).

the haploid expression of the *t* haplotype can be expected if the relevant gene is transcribed in the course of spermatogenetic differentiation no earlier than at the spermatid stage. An earlier transcription in secondary spermatocytes would result in an expression of both allelic forms on sperm cells derived from primary spermatocytes where recombination took place between the centromere and the appropriate gene locus. The same idea can be applied to the occurrence of *H-2* gene products on the sperm. When considering 30% recombination between centromere and *H-2* (in the absence of t^1), 60% of spermatozoa would carry *H-2* products of both haplotypes present in the diploid precursor. However, a strong indication of *H-2* expression as early as in primary spermatocytes has been reported by several authors (Vojtíšková and Pokorná, 1972; Vojtíšková *et al.*, 1974; Fellous *et al.*, 1976; Erickson, 1977), and the presence of the F9 antigen—supposedly a product of the $+^{t^{12}}$ allele of the *T/t* complex—has been demonstrated in all forms of male germ cells starting from gonocytes (Gachelin *et al.*, 1976). All these observations make the haploid expression of *H-2* and *t* genes rather unlikely, even though not impossible. Provided that the cell-surface determinants display a fast turnover on the membrane of differentiating cells, and with the premise of gene transcription at the spermatid stage [which cannot be excluded (see, for example, Monesi, 1965; Moore, 1971; Kierszenbaum and Tres, 1975; Vandeberg *et al.*, 1976)], the haploid genes could be expressed, irrespective of the position of their loci on the chromosome, on the surface of sperm cells.

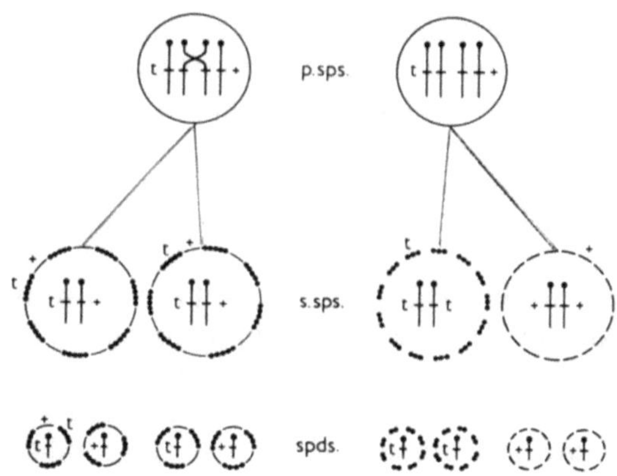

Figure 4. Expected consequence of crossing over between the centromere of chromosome 17 and one or more *t* genes controlling the presumed cell-surface antigen(s) on detection of haploid expression of this gene in secondary spermatocytes (s.sps.), spermatids (spds.), or sperm. For the sake of argument, the gene is considered to be expressed only in secondary spermatocytes. Further alternatives are discussed in the text. (p.sps.) Primary spermatocytes.

2.4.2. Phenotypic Expression of Abnormal Gene Dosage at the T/t–H-2 Supergene

The ultimate goal of the meiotic process is to precisely segregate the genetic material so that only one copy of each chromosome is present in the gamete. The mechanism is characterized by a remarkable frequency of errors, mainly chromosome nondisjunctions, of which trisomies alone are responsible for severe congenital defects in 0.3% of live births in man (Jacobs, 1972).

In the mouse, trisomy for the whole chromosome 17 invariably causes the death of embryos between the 8th and 10th days of embryonic development (Baranov and Dyban, 1972; Gropp, 1975); thus, of the known autosomal trisomies in the mouse, it is the earliest-acting one (Dyban and Baranov, 1978). Viable partial trisomy for the proximal part of chromosome 17 [viz., centromere 17–T190Ca breakpoint near gene *tf* (cf. Fig. 1)] and the small distal part of chromosome 1 (viz., T190Ca breakpoint–telomere of chromosome 1) has been observed by Lyon and Sayers, (1977). The partially trisomic animals arose through nondisjunction in a parent heterozygous for the T190Ca translocation. One of the tertiary trisomics died soon after birth; the other was a small and sterile male.

Recently, more than 40 viable and in most cases fertile animals with three doses of a part of chromosome 17 starting from the centromere up to the *H-2K* region have been prepared in our laboratory (Forejt, Gregorová, and Čapková, unpublished). All the animals carrying three doses of *T/t* complex genes arose from the product of adjacent-2 disjunction at meiosis of females heterozygous for the T43H translocation (Fig. 5), (cf. also Fig. 3). At birth and during the first 2 weeks of postnatal life, most of these trisomics were smaller than their normal sibs, and an undetermined number of them died before weaning. Later, however, the difference disappeared and the trisomics were phenotypically indistinguishable from their normal sibs.

Partial trisomy for chromosome 17 might prove useful as a tool in the genetic analysis of the *T/t* complex and in mapping the lethality effect of trisomy for the whole chromosome 17. The first observations seem promising; nevertheless, the entire project has been complicated by an unexpected finding of low transmission of the trisomic condition from parents to progeny. In all trisomics sufficiently tested so far (7 males and 7 females), the segregation ratio was significantly below 50%, ranging from 0 to 24%. The nature of the segregation distortion has not yet been studied. Hypothetically, it could operate through the embryonic or early postnatal losses, but the selection could take place already at the gametic level. The limited data available so far indicate that unlike the case with the t^1

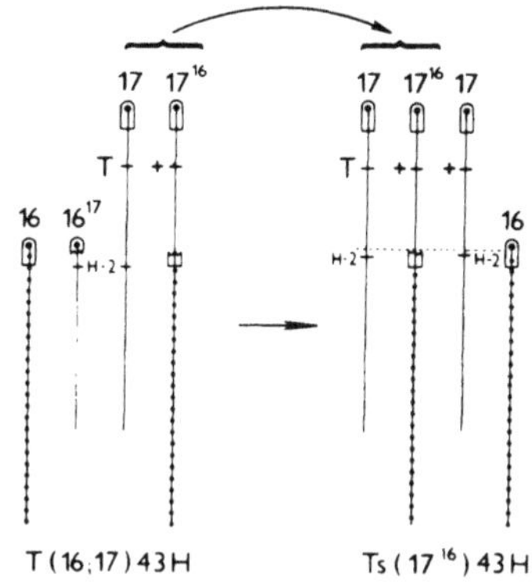

Figure 5. Scheme of chromosomes involved in balanced T(16;17)43H translocation and in the partial trisomy of chromosome 17. (Drawing is not to scale.) The translocation breaks are situated in centromeric heterochromatin (C-band) of chromosome 16 and near the *H-2* complex in chromosome 17. The trisomy for the proximal part of chromosome 17 is accompanied by monosomy for the proximal part of centromeric heterochromatin of chromosome 16, the site of nontranscribed, highly repetitive DNA.

haplotype, this segregation distortion operates in both sexes. There is little doubt at present that the *T/t* complex participates in the genetic control of a series of steps in embryonic and spermatogenic development (D. Bennett, 1964, 1975; Klein and Hammerberg, 1977; Gluecksohn-Waelsch and Erickson, 1970). Therefore, it was rather unexpected to find such a small phenotypic effect of trisomy for the *T/t*-bearing part of chromosome 17 on embryogenesis and male fertility, especially in light of the known fatal effect on embryonic development of trisomy for the whole chromosome 17.

Another puzzling observation of this type has been made by Lyon *et al.* (1972). The authors were able to distinguish, by appropriately chosen gene markers, the balanced combination of two complementary unbalanced gametes (i.e., with complementary duplications and deletions) that arose from the adjacent-2 disjunction in the T138Ca heterozygous parents. Animals that clearly arose from the egg with duplication of the *T-H-2* chromosome region, fertilized by sperm with deficiency (nullisomy) of the same part of chromosome 17, were recovered. From this observation, the conclusion can be drawn that starting from secondary spermatocytes, the genes belonging to the proximal part of chromosome 17 (centromere–*H-2*), including those of the *T/t* and *H-2* systems, are either silent or their activity is not essential for spermatogenic differentiation and sperm function in fertilization. Admittedly, the genetic defect of *T-H-2* nullisomic sperm could be compensated for by a transfer of the cell-membrane determinants or the information for their production through the intercellular bridges between spermatocytes and/or spermatids (Burgos and Fawcett, 1955; Fawcett, 1972). If this turns out to be the case and the phenomenon of interspermatocyte (spermatid) cooperation does exist, it would hardly be compatible with the haploid expression of the *t* haplotype on sperm (D. Bennett, 1975; Yanagisawa *et al.*, 1974).

3. *Hybrid Sterility-1* Gene in Chromosome 17

3.1. Sterility of Male Hybrids from Crosses between Laboratory and Wild Mice

The first stage in the creation of a new species begins, according to the allopatric hypothesis (Dobzhansky, 1951; Mayr, 1963), with spatial (geographic) isolation of a minor part of a species. The resulting breakdown of gene flow enables subsequent fixation of random genetic changes, some of which can eventually act as a genetic barrier between the main body of the species and the isolate, if the two come into contact again. Lewontin (1974) surveyed the available experimental evidence pertaining to various stages of species divergence and found it particularly scanty for the first stage. At present, obviously only two models are available. One example can be found in the paper of Prakash (1972), who observed complete male sterility of hybrids between females of Bogota populations of *Drosophila pseudoobscura* and males of the same species but from other localities. The second example of the initial phase of speciation has been described in our laboratory and concerns a partial reproductive isolation between certain laboratory and wild types of *Mus musculus* (Iványi *et al.*, 1969; Iványi and Micková, 1971; Forejt and Iványi, 1975; Pavljuková and Forejt, 1979, unpublished.

Hitherto, 66 males and 7 females of *Mus musculus* captured in 14 different localities have been sufficiently examined for their ability to produce sterile male hybrids in crosses with C57BL/10 inbred strain mice (abbreviated B10). The examined wild mice could be divided into three sets on the basis of whether their litters consist of (1) only sterile (set I), (2) only fertile (set II), or (3) both fertile and sterile male offspring (set III). Figure 6 shows a typical distribution of testes weights of hybrids from crosses between a wild male of set I and females of the B10 and C3H inbred strains. Variations in testes weight in such a type of hybrid fit well with the variation in fertility of the males (Forejt and Iványi, 1975). Thus, all (B10 × wild male) male hybrids are completely sterile with small testes and no sperms in epididymides, while fertile or quasi-fertile progeny are obtained from crosses of the same wild male with females of the C3H/Di inbred strain.

The sterility of male progeny of crosses between laboratory and wild mice corresponds to the definition of hybrid sterility formulated by Dobzhansky (1951), which states that two parental forms (symbolized as AA and BB) that are fertile *inter se* produce hybrids that are sterile (symbol AB). As shown in the following pages, the described hybrid sterility of (B10 × wild mice) males meets some additional criteria for being considered as a model of the incipient reproductive isolation mechanism of Lewontin's stage I of speciation (Lewontin, 1974).

With such a unique tool available, some old questions on the nature of the very beginning of species divergence could be reconsidered. For example, an estimate could be made of the degree of total genetic divergence between two partially isolated forms by means of electrophoretically distinguishable protein polymorphism. The idea of Mayr (1963) explaining reproductive isolation as an incidental byproduct of genetic "revolution" inside a small community of the isolate could be tested. Furthermore, the question could be asked about the number of genes engaged in the control of the reproductive isolation, and about the site and mechanisms of their action. All these problems represent *terra incognita* of speciation for which even such a favorite model of population genetics as the *Drosophila* species provided only incomplete answers or no information at all.

Another kind of question concerns the significance of the *Hybrid sterility-1* gene *(Hst-1)* in the genetic control of male sterility, its polymorphism, and its relationship to some other known genes of the *T/t-H-2* supergene.

Experimental analysis of some of the aforestated problems could be facilitated if a genetically defined stock of wild mice were available in the laboratory. For this purpose, production of seven inbred strains has been started. Each strain was founded from a single pair of wild mice of the same locality. The prospective male founders were first subjected to preliminary crosses with B10 inbred strain females, and only those producing sterile male progeny (set I; see above) were selected. The wild female mice were selected according to their ability to breed in captivity. Their classification to set I, II, or III was done afterward. Four strains failed to reproduce at some stage of inbreeding and were therefore eliminated. At present, three strains, PWB, PWD, and PWK, are being propagated, each in two separated sublines. All strains were tested in the course of inbreeding for their ability to produce sterile hybrid males when crossed with B10 inbred strain mice. All mice of the PWB, PWD, and PWK strains retained the genetic information for this type of hybrid sterility (Pavljuková and Forejt, 1978, unpublished).

3.2. Location of *Hybrid Sterility-1* Gene in the *T–H-2* Region of Chromosome 17

The hybrid sterility phenomenon is controlled by epistatic interaction of three or more genes, only one of which, the *Hst-1* gene, shows polymorphism in the tested inbred strains (Forejt and Iványi, 1975). Figure 6 shows that the same wild male produced sterile male progeny with B10 inbred strain females but fertile male progeny in crosses with C3H strain females. The *Hybrid sterility-1* gene has been defined as a gene the two allelic forms of which are responsible for the difference between the two

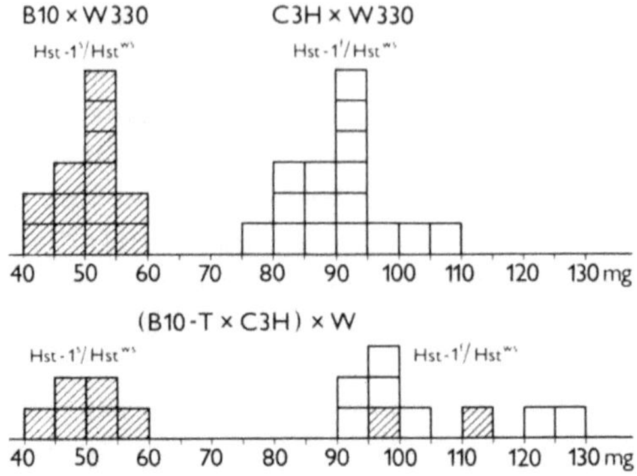

Figure 6. Example of distibutions of testes weights in (B10×W), (C3H×W), and [B10-*T*×C3H)*T*/+ × W] hybrids. Each square represents the wet weight of paired testes of a single male. The lower histogram shows a nonrandom distribution of testes weights of short-tailed males (*T*/+, hatched squares) that received the chromosome 17 of B10-*T* origin and normal-tailed males (+/+, open squares) with chromosome 17 of C3H origin. The wild male coded W330 and female W333, both captured in the Prague Zoo on March 29, 1974, were the founders of the PWB strain (see the text for details).

types of hybrids. In crosses of wild mice (set I) with (B10-*T*×C3H)F_1 animals, the male offspring that received chromosome 17 marked by *T* mutation of B10 origin were sterile, while animals with chromosome 17 of C3H origin were fertile. The three-point test cross showed that *Hst-1* was located between *T* and *H-2,* the distances being *T*—4.5 cM—*Hst-1*—13.5 cM—*H-2.* Results of this test cross and other different types of crosses (Forejt and Iványi, 1975; Pavljuková and Forejt, unpublished) have so far been compatible with the conclusion that the hybrid sterility phenomenon behaves as a single gene trait in all crosses where the "laboratory" and "wild" mice were crossed only once and the resulting hybrid progeny were examined. Three illustrative examples can be mentioned: (1) The animals of [(B10-*T*×C3H)*T*/+ × B10] BC_1 and BC_2 population were crossed with PWD, PWK, or original wild mice. Examination of the hybrid male progeny confirmed the single-gene assumption. (2) The wild-derived strains PWD and PWK were established from unrelated wild mice captured in two localities separated by 30 km ("Prague Zoo" and "Lhotka," respectively. When the (PWD×PWK) hybrids were crossed with B10 inbred mice or (B10-*T*×C3H) hybrids, the single-gene pattern of inheritance of the phenomenon was observed again. (3) Wild mice belonging to set III produced fertile and sterile male progeny in crosses with mice of the B10 inbred strain. Here again, the 1:1 ratio of both phenotypes was compatible with a single-gene hypothesis. The postulated Hst^w gene locus showed close linkage with *H-2* (recombination frequency of 8–

14%), and it has been tentatively concluded (hence the preliminary symbol Hst^{w}) that it could be identical with the *Hst-1* gene locus. Table 3 shows the allelic distribution at the *Hst-1* (Hst^{w}) gene in the examined inbred strains and wild mice.

The multigenic nature of hybrid sterility appeared immediately when the fertile hybrid females of laboratory and wild-derived parents [e.g., (B10 × PWD)] were crossed either to laboratory or to the wild-derived mice. Here, only a certain part of males that obtained a "sterile" combination of alleles at the *Hst-1* ($Hst\text{-}1^{s}/Hst^{ws}$) were actually sterile. The results are compatible with the assumption of at least two other independently segregating genes engaged in some kind of epistatic interaction with *Hst-1*. Unlike the *Hst-1*, which is polymorphic in both inbred strains and wild mice, the other two hybrid sterility genes are apparently monomorphic in both wild-derived and laboratory mice with different allelic forms fixed in homozygous state.

Polymorphism of the *Hst-1* (Hst^{w}) gene might be related to the forced heterozygosity of the proximal part of chromosome 17 maintained by t^{1} haplotypes. Admittedly, wild mice homozygous for Hst^{ws} and heterozygous for a t^{1} haplotype, $t^{1}Hst^{ws}/{+}Hst^{ws}$, as well as doubly heterozygous animals, $+Hst^{ws}/t^{1}\,Hst^{wf}$, have already been observed (Forejt and Iványi, 1975; Forejt and Pavljuková, unpublished). The observation raised two questions concerning the relationship between *t* haplotypes and the $Hst\text{-}1/Hst^{w}$ gene. First, the possibility may be considered that the *Hst-1* (Hst^{w}) gene is the separated sterility factor of *t* haplotypes. Both the *Hst-1* and the *t*-sterility factor have been mapped near the *tf* gene in the *T* -*H-2* chromosome region. Moreover, they are the only two known genes of the mouse genome that selectively affect male fertility and show polymorphism in wild populations. On the other hand, if the *Hst-1* or Hst^{w}

TABLE 3. Allelic Distribution at the *Hst-1* (Hst^{w}) Gene in Inbred Strains and Wild Mice

Allele symbol[a]	Mice of inbred strains or natural populations[b]
$Hst\text{-}1^{s}$	C57BL/10ScSnPh, B10.BR, B10.D2, BALB/c, DBA/1, AKR/J, A/Ph
$Hst\text{-}1^{f}$	C3H/Di, CBA/J P/J, I/St, F/St
Hst^{ws}	6 localities of Central Bohemia (39 mice); 1 locality of Jutland, Denmark (1 mouse); wild-mice-derived strains PWB, PWD, and PWK
Hst^{wf}	8 localities of Central Bohemia (35 mice); 1 locality of Jutland, Denmark (1 mouse); 1 locality of Great Gull Island, U.S.A. (3 mice)

[a]Only interaction of $Hst\text{-}1^{s}$ and Hst^{ws} causes sterility in $Hst\text{-}1^{s}/Hst^{ws}$ male hybrids. All other combinations result in fertile animals.
[b]In 6 localities, both types of Hst^{w} alleles were recovered. Thirteen wild mice were Hst^{ws}/Hst^{wf} heterozygotes.

were the *t*-sterility factors, then they would be expected to interact with the t^1 haplotype in $t^1/Hst\text{-}1^s$ or t^1/Hst^{ws} compounds and to induce male sterility. None of the six combinations tested affected male sterility (Forejt and Iványi, 1975). Another argument against identity of *Hst-1* and *t* sterility factors stems from the fact that $t^{1\text{-}1}/t^{1\text{-}2}$ sterility is clearly controlled by a single-gene interallelic interaction (or interaction of closely linked, pseudoallelic genes), whereas hybrid sterility is controlled by epistatic interaction of at least three independently segregating genes. The second question concerns the expected linkage disequilibrium between a particular allele of the Hst^w (*Hst-1*) gene and *t* haplotypes belonging to a single complementation group. This type of study could throw some light on the occurrence of *t* haplotypes and Hst^w alleles in mouse populations.

An attempt has been made to define the time and site of action of the *Hst-1* gene (Pavljuková, Vojtíšková, and Forejt, unpublished). Two "fertile" and two "sterile" genotypes were compared in four types of crosses (Table 4). The second and the third cross are particularly revealing, since the variation in fertility can be ascribed entirely to the effect of the *Hst-1* gene in this combination. The significant difference in testes weight between the two types of genotypes can be first observed at day 20 of postnatal development (Fig. 7). Cytological examination of preparations of testicular-cell suspensions disclosed the cause of reduced testis size of sterile hybrids; starting from day 13 of postnatal development, both types of fertile hybrids showed increasing numbers of primary spermatocytes at the pachytene stage, while this cell type was almost absent in prospectively fertile hybrids (Fig. 8). Thus, in this experiment, the interaction of $Hst\text{-}1^s$ and Hst^{ws} alleles resulted in blockage of transition of mitotically dividing spermatogonia into meiotically dividing primary spermatocytes at day 10 of postnatal development. The conclusion holds true for hybrids between the relevant inbred strain and the PWD or PWK wild-derived strain. When individual wild mice were tested, however, the arrest of spermatogenesis occurred in certain combinations clearly intrameiotically (Forejt and Ivanyi, 1975). Thus, for the time being, it would

TABLE 4. Preparation of Male Hybrids Differing in the $Hst\text{-}1/Hst^w$ Gene or in Genetic Background or in Both

Expt.	Genotype at the $Hst\text{-}1/Hst^w$ locus	Fertility of adult males
1 B10×PWK	$Hst\text{-}1^s/Hst^{ws}$	Sterile
2 [(B10-*T*×C3H)*T*/+ ×PWK] *T*/+	$Hst\text{-}1^s/Hst^{ws}$	Sterile
3 [(B10-*T*×C3H)*T*/+ ×PWK] +/+	$Hst\text{-}1^f/Hst^{ws}$	Fertile
4 [(B10-*T*×C3H)*T*/+ ×B10] *T*/+ and +/+	$Hst\text{-}1^s/Hst\text{-}1^{s(f)}$	Fertile

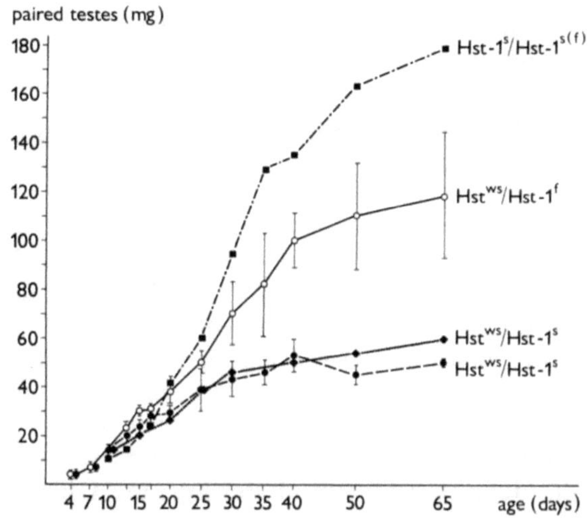

Figure 7. Mean testes weights of prospectively fertile and sterile hybrids between the 4th and 65th days of postnatal development. The means + 1 standard deviation are given for *T*/+ (●) and ++ (○) progeny of the [(B10-*T*×C3H)*T*/+ × PWK] cross (cf. Table 4).

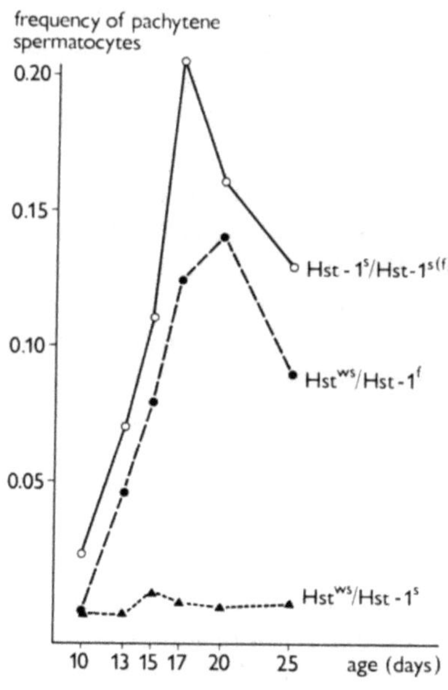

Figure 8. Frequency of pachytene spermatocytes in cytological preparations from testes of prospectively fertile (○,●) and sterile (▲) hybrids. See Table 4 for the origin of the hybrids examined.

be premature to speculate about the specific effect of the *Hst-1* gene on a particular differentiation step in spermatogenesis.

3.3. Is the *Hst-1* Gene Responsible for Variation in Spermatogenic Failure of Translocation Heterozygotes?

Certain chromosomal translocations in the heterozygous state cause arrest of spermatogenesis in the mouse and several other mammalian species studied (for reviews, see Searle, 1974; Searle *et al.*, 1978). Reciprocal translocation between murine chromosomes 14 15, T(14;15)6Ca (abbreviated T6), causes partial spermatogenic breakdown in the heterozygotes. The T6/T6 homozygotes of both sexes are, however, normally fertile. This translocation is amenable to genetic study, since it is available on the genetic background of the CBA inbred strain, CBA-T6/T6. In accord with the definition of hybrid sterility, the CBA and CBA-T6/T6 strains are fertile, while their hybrids display partial spermatogenic arrest. Thus, the (CBA×CBA-T6/T6)F_1 hybrids represent the most curious form of hybrid sterility attributable to a simple reciprocal chromosomal rearrangement. Cytogenetic analysis aimed at unraveling the chromosomal mechanism of this model of hybrid sterility (Forejt, 1974, 1979; Forejt and Gregorová, 1977) has indicated that the X chromosome inactivation during spermatogenic differentiation might represent the control mechanism that blocks spermatogenesis if certain chromosomal rearrangements are present.

A successful attempt to modify the extent of spermatogenic failure of T6 translocation heterozygotes by a genic factor has been made in a cross similar to that which disclosed the *Hst-1* gene, viz. CBA-T6/T6 × (B10-*T*×C3H)*T*/+. The male offspring that received $H\text{-}2^k$ and $+^T$ from the C3H parent were less severely affected than their brothers with $H\text{-}2^b$ and *T* of B10 origin, which had smaller testes and lower counts of spermatozoa in epididymides (Forejt, 1976b). The obvious question stimulated by this observation concerns a possible relationship between the *Hst-1* gene and the genetic factor [preliminary symbol: *Male sterility-1* (*Mst-1*)] responsible for variation in spermatogenic breakdown in T6 heterozygotes. In the chapter dealing with "strong" and "weak" races of *Drosophila pseudoobscura* and *D. persimilis*, Dobzhansky (1951) concluded that the building stones, the genetic elements from which the mechanism causing hybrid sterility could be built, are present already within a species. Thus, it would not be without precedent to find an isolating gene engaged in hybrid sterility that would operate within the species in modifying chromosomally determined spermatogenic failure. The first results of an experiment aimed at the elucidation of the question, however, indicate that the *Hst-1* and *Mst-1* genes affecting T6-determined partial male sterility can be separated by recombination within the *T-H-2* chromosome region (Forejt, Gregorová, and Čapková, 1979, unpublished).

3.4. Spermatogenic-Differentiation-Controlling Genes in Chromosome 17

Hst-1 and *Mst-1* genes and *t* haplotype sterility factors are obviously not the only genes of chromosome 17 that control spermatogenic differentiation (Fig. 9 and Table 5). The recessive gene *quaking,* closely linked to the *Hst-1* gene, causes, simultaneously, arrest of spermatogenesis in *qk/qk* homozygous males and deficient myelination in the central nervous system in animals of both sexes (W.I. Bennett *et al.*, 1971). Provided that *qk* is a point mutation, then its pleiotropy might indicate that the same gene product is engaged in differentiation of spermatogenic as well as neuroectodermic cells. This assumption might receive some indirect support from the available genetic and immunological evidence. From the genetic point of view, such a type of pleiotropic gene action is not unique, since the *t* haplotypes belonging to the t^{w1} complementation group and semilethal *t* haplotypes also affect both spermatogenesis and the normal development of the neural tube and brain (Klein and Hammerberg, 1977; D. Bennett, 1975). Another link, at the phenotypic level, between testicular and brain cells and preimplantation embryos can be seen in recently described differentiation antigens common to cell surfaces of all three origins (Goridis *et al.*, 1978). Location of genes coding these structures has not yet been reported.

It remains to be ascertained to what degree the arguments gathered here represent only artificially connected pieces of the incomplete mosaic of our knowledge of cellular differentiation and its genetic regulation. Investigation of the genetic structure of the *T/t-H-2* supergene and its effect on embryonic development and spermatogenic differentiation will certainly provide a new insight into these old questions.

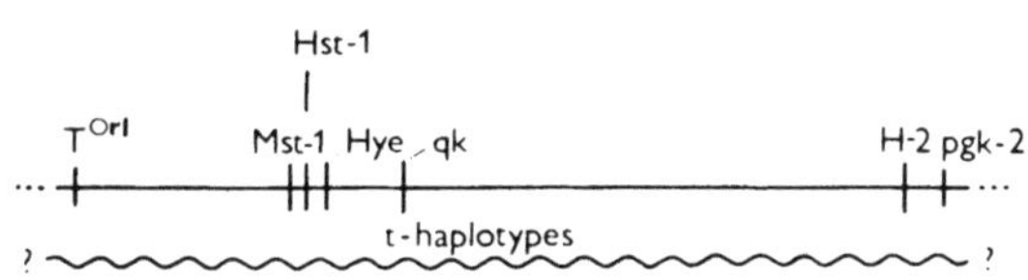

Figure 9. Genes of chromosome 17 known to be engaged in spermatogenic differentiation. The relative positions of the *Mst-1*, *Hst-1*, and *Hye* loci in respect to the centromere are based on preliminary results of recombination analysis.

TABLE 5. Inventory of *T/t—H-2*-Linked Genetic Factors Related to Spermatogenic Differentiation

Gene (genotype)	Phenotype expression	Reference
1. T^{Orl}/t^{12}, T^{Orl}/t^{6}	Male quasi-sterility.	Erickson *et al.* (1978)
2. *Mst-1*	Variable fertility. Modification of partial spermatogenic arrest of T6Ca translocation heterozygotes.	Forejt (1976a,b), Forejt *et al.* (1979, unpublished)
3. *Hst-1*	Male hybrid sterility. Premeiotic arrest.	Iványi *et al.* (1969), Forejt and Iványi (1975), Pavljukova *et al.* (1979, unpublished)
4. *qk*	Male sterility, recessive. Defect in spermatid differentiation.	W.I. Bennett *et al.* (1971)
5. *Hye*	Control of expressivity of H-Y differentiation antigen (testes-determining differentiation antigen).	Králová and Demant (1976), Králová and Lengerová (1979)
6. $t^{1\text{-}1}/t^{1\text{-}2}$	Male sterility. Defect in late spermatids and spermatozoa. Abnormal microtubuli, sperm head shape, and sperm motility.	Bryson (1944), Olds (1970), Dooher and Bennett, (1977)
7. t^{sl}/t^{sl}	Male sterility. No sperm. Abnormal microtubuli in spermatids.	Johnston (1968), Dooher and Bennett (1974)
8. t^{EA5}/t^{EA5}	Male quasi-sterility. Partial arrest at spermatid stage.	Vojtíšková *et al.* (1976)
9. t^{l}/t^{v}	Variable male fertility.	D. Bennett (1975)
10. $t^{12}/+$	t^{12}-controlled abnormal shape of sperm heads (15%; control, 1–3%).	Dooher and Bennett (1977)
11. *T/t*	Sperm- and embryonic-cell-specific differentiation antigens. Haploid expression (?).	Bennett *et al.* (1972), Yanagisawa *et al.* (1974), Artzt and Bennett (1977)
12. *T/t*	Structural or regulatory gene for Teratocarcinoma F9 antigen (?).	Artzt *et al.* (1974)

TABLE 5 *(continued)*

Gene (genotype)	Phenotype expression	Reference
13. *H-2*	Differential expression of H-2K, Ia, and H-2D antigens in germ-line cells: present on spermatocytes, spermatids, and spermatozoa; absent on spermatogonia.	Vojtíšková and Pokorná (1972), Erickson *et al.* (1977)
14. *pgk-2*	*Phosphoglycerate kinase-2* expression specific for spermatids and sperm.	Vandeberg *et al.* (1973), Vandeberg and Klein (1978), Erickson (1977)

References

Artzt, K., and Bennett, D., 1975, Analogies between embryonic (T/t) antigens and adult major histocompatibility (H-2) antigens, *Nature (London)* **256:**545.

Artzt, K., and Bennett, D., 1977, Serological analysis of sperm of antigenically cross-reacting T/t haplotypes and their recombinants, *Immunogenetics* **5:**97.

Artzt, K., Bennett, D., and Jacob, F., 1974, Primitive teratocarcinoma cells express a differentiation antigen specified by a gene at the T-locus in the mouse, *Proc. Natl. Acad. Sci. U.S.A.* **71:**811.

Artzt, K., Hamburger, L., and Flaherty, L., 1977, H-39, a histocompatibility locus closely linked to the T/t complex, *Immunogenetics* **5:**477.

Baranov, V.S., and Dyban, A.P., 1972, Embryonic damage of trisomic offsprings of mice with Robertsonian translocation (centric fusion) T1 Iem, *Arch. Anat. Histol. Embryol.* **63:**67 (in Russian).

Beechey, C.V., and Searle, A.G., 1978, Private communication, *Mouse News Lett.* **59:**20.

Bennett, D., 1964, Embryological effects of lethal alleles in the t-region, *Science* **144:**263.

Bennett, D., 1975, The *T*-locus of the mouse: A review, *Cell* **6:**441.

Bennett, D., and Dunn, L.C., 1967, Studies of effects of t-alleles in the house mouse on spermatozoa. I. Male sterility effect, *J. Reprod. Fertil.* **13:**421.

Bennett, D., Dunn, L.C., and Rynerson, D., 1969, Genetical and embryological comparisons of semilethal t-alleles from wild mouse populations, *Genetics* **61:**411.

Bennett, D., Goldberg, E., Dunn, L.C., and Boyse, E.A., 1972, Serological detection of a cell surface antigen specified by the T (Brachyury) mutant gene in the house mouse, *Proc. Natl. Acad. Sci. U.S.A.* **69:**2076.

Bennett, D., Dunn, L.C., and Artzt, K., 1976, Genetic change in mutations at the *T/t*-locus, *Genetics* **83:**361.

Bennett, W.I., Gall, A.M., Southward, J.L., and Sidman, R.L., 1971, Abnormal spermiogenesis in Quaking, a myelin-deficient mutant mouse, *Biol. Reprod.* **5:**30.

Bodmer, W.F., 1978, HLA: A super supergene, in: *Harvey Lectures 1976-1977*, pp. 91–138, Academic Press, New York.

Boyse, E.A., and Old, L.J., 1969, Some aspects of normal and abnormal cell surface genetics, *Annu. Rev. Genet.* **3**:269.

Braden, A.W.H., 1972, *T*-locus in mice: Segregation distortion and sterility in the male, in: *Proceedings of the International Symposium on the Genetics of the Spermatozoon* (R.A. Beatty and S. Gluecksohn-Waelsch, eds.), p. 289, Bogtrykkeriet Forum, Copenhagen.

Braden, A.W.H., and Gluecksohn-Waelsch, S., 1958, Further studies of the effect of the *T*-locus in the house mouse on male fertility, *J. Exp. Zool.* **138**:431.

Bryson, V., 1944, Spermatogenesis and fertility in *Mus musculus* as affected by factors at the T locus, *J. Morphol.* **74**:131.

Burgos, M.H., and Fawcett, D.W., 1955, Studies on the fine structure of the mammalian testis. I. Differentiation of the spermatids in the cat, *J. Biophys. Biochem. Cytol.* **1**:287.

Carter, T.C., Lyon, M.F., and Phillips, R.J.S., 1955, Gene tagged chromosome translocations in eleven stocks of mice, *J. Genet.* **53**:21.

Cattanach, B.M., 1978, Crossover suppression in mice heterozygous for tobacco mouse metacentrics, *Cytogenet. Cell Genet.* **20**:264.

Dobzhansky, T., 1951, *Genetics and the Origin of Species,* 3rd ed, Columbia University Press, New York.

Dooher, G.B., and Bennett, D., 1974, Abnormal microtubular systems in mouse spermatids associated with a mutant gene at the T-locus, *J. Embryol. Exp. Morphol.* **32**:749.

Dooher, G.B., and Bennett, D., 1977, Spermatogenesis and spermatozoa in sterile mice carrying different lethal T/t locus haplotypes: A transmission and scanning electron microscopic study, *Biol. Reprod.* **17**:269.

Dunn, L.C., 1964, Abnormalities associated with a chromosome region in the mouse, *Science* **144**:260.

Dunn, L.C., and Gluecksohn-Schoenheimer, S., 1950, Repeated mutations in one area of a mouse chromosome, *Proc. Natl. Acad. Sci. U.S.A.* **36**:233.

Dunn, L.C., and Morgan, W.C., 1953, Segregation ratios of mutant alleles from wild populations of *Mus musculus, Am. Nat.* **87**:327.

Dyban, A.P., and Baranov, V.S., 1978, *Cytogenetics of Development in Mammals,* Nauka, Moscow (in Russian).

Eicher, E.M., and Washburn, L.L., 1978, Assignment of genes to regions of mouse chromosome, *Proc. Natl. Acad. Sci. U.S.A.* **75**:946.

Erickson, R.P., 1977, Gene expression of a region of chromosome 17 during murine spermatogenesis, *J. Immunogenet.* **4**:353.

Erickson, R.P., Gachelin, G., Fellous, M., and Jacob, F., 1977, Absorption analysis of H-2D and K antigens on spermatozoa, *J. Immunogenet.* **4**:47.

Erickson, R.P., Lewis, S.E., and Slusser, K.S., 1978, Deletion mapping of the T-complex of chromosome 17 of the mouse, *Nature (London)* **274**:163.

Fawcett, D.W., 1972, Observations on cell differentiation and organelle continuity in spermatogenesis, in: *Proceedings of the International Symposium on the Genetics of the Spermatozoon* (R.A. Beatty and S. Gluecksohn-Waelsch, eds.), p. 37, Bogtrykkeriet Forum, Copenhagen.

Fellous, M., Ericksohn, R.P., Gachelin, G., Dubois, P., and Jacob, F., 1976, The time of appearance of Ia antigens during spermatogenesis in the mouse: Relationship between Ia antigens and H-2, beta-2 microglobulin and F9 antigen, *Folia Biol. (Prague)* **22**:381.

Flaherty, L., 1975, H-33—a histocompatibility locus to the left of the H-2 complex, *Immunogenetics* **2**:325.

Forejt, J., 1972, Chiasmata and crossing-over in the male mouse *(Mus musculus)*: Suppression of recombination and chiasma frequencies in the ninth linkage group, *Folia Biol. (Prague)* **18**:161.

Forejt, J., 1973, Centromere–T locus distance in the chromosome 17, *Mouse News Lett.* **49**:45.

Forejt, J., 1974, Nonrandom association between a specific autosome and the X chromosome in meiosis of the male mouse: Possible consequence of the homologous centromeres separation, *Cytogenet. Cell Genet.* **13**:369.

Forejt, J., 1976a, H-2-linked gene involved in modification of fertility of translocation carriers, *Folia. Biol. (Prague)* **22**:53.

Forejt, J., 1976b, Spermatogenic failure of translocation heterozygotes affected by H-2-linked gene in mouse, *Nature (London)* **260**:143.

Forejt, J., 1979, Meiotic studies of translocations causing male sterility in the mouse. II. Double heterozygotes for Robertsonian translocations, *Cytogenet. Cell Genet.* **23**:163.

Forejt, J., and Gregorová, S., 1977, Meiotic studies of translocations causing male sterility in the mouse. I. Autosomal reciprocal translocations, *Cytogenet. Cell Genet.* **19**:159.

Forejt, J., and Iványi, P., 1975, Genetic studies of male sterility of hybrids between laboratory and wild mice *(Mus musculus* L.). *Genet. Res.* **24**:189.

Forejt, J., and Lengerová, A., 1981, Membrane antigens as markers of cell differentiation and transformation, in: *Proc. XIV Int. Congress of Genetics* (in press).

Forejt, J., Gregorová, S., and Čapková, J., 1978, Private communication. Construction of a stock trisomic for T-t complex, *Mouse News Lett.* **59**:55.

Gachelin, G., 1978, The cell surface antigens of mouse embryonal carcinoma cells, *Biochim. Biophys. Acta* **516**:27.

Gachelin, G., Fellous, M., Guénet, J.L., and Jacob, F., 1976, Developmental expression of an early embryonic antigen common to mouse spermatozoa and cleavage embryos, and to human spermatozoa: Its expression during spermatogenesis, *Dev. Biol.* **50**:310.

Gluecksohn-Waelsch, S., and Erickson, R.P., 1970, The T-locus of the mouse: Implications for mechanisms of development, *Curr. Top. Dev. Biol.* **5**:281.

Goridis, C., Artzt, K., Wortham, K.A., and Schachner, M., 1978, Brain cell surface antigens on embryonal carocinoma cells, *Dev. Biol.* **65**:238.

Gropp, A., 1975, Chromosomal animal model of human disease: Fetal trisomy and developmental failure, in: *Teratology (C. Berry and D.E. Posville, eds.)*, pp. 17–31, Springer-Verlag, Berlin, Heidelberg, New York.

Gropp, A., Tettenborn, U., and Leonard, A., 1970, Identification of acrocentric chromosomes involved in the formation of "fusion" metacentrics in mice: Proposal for nomenclature of *M. poschiavinus* metacentrics, *Experientia* **26**:1018.

Hammerberg, C., and Klein, J., 1975a, Linkage disequilibrium between H-2 and t complexes in chromosome 17 of the mouse, *Nature (London)* **258**:296.

Hammerberg, C., and Klein, J., 1975b, Linkage relationships of markers on chromosome 17 of the mouse, *Genet. Res.* **26**:203.

Iványi, P., and Micková, M., 1971, Further studies on genetic factors in the ninth linkage group influencing reproductive performance in male mice in: *Proceedings of the Symposium on Immunogenetics of the H-2 System* (A. Lengerová and M. Vojtíšková eds.), pp. 104–119, S. Karger, Basel.

Iványi, P., Vojtíšková, M., Démant, P., and Micková, M., 1969, Genetic factors in the ninth linkage group influencing reproductive performance in male mice, *Folia Biol. (Prague)* **15**:401.

Jacob, F., 1977, Mouse teratocarcinoma and embryonic antigens, *Immunol. Rev.* **33**:3.

Jacobs, P.A., 1972, Human population cytogenetics, in: *Proceedings of the IVth International Congress on Human Genetics,* p. 232, Excerpta Medica, Amsterdam.

Johnston, P.G., 1968, Male sterility in mice homozygous for the T^{w2} allele, *Aust. J. Biol. Sci.* **21**:947.

Key, M., and Hollander, W.F., 1972, Thin fur, a recessive mutant of chromosome 17 of the mouse, *J. Hered.* **63**:97.

Kierszenbaum, A.L., and Tres, L.L., 1975, Structural and transcriptional features of the mouse spermatid genome, *J. Cell. Biol.* **65**:258.

Klein, J., 1971, Cytological identification of the chromosome carrying the IXth linkage group (including H-2) in the house mouse, *Proc. Natl. Acad. Sci. U.S.A.* **68:**1594.

Klein, J., 1978, H-2 mutations: Their genetics and effect on immune reactions, *Adv. Immunol.* **26:**55.

Klein, J., and Hammerberg, C., 1977, The control of differentiation by the T complex, *Immunol. Rev.* **33:**70.

Klein, J., and Klein, D., 1972, Position of the translocation break T/2:9/138Ca in linkage group IX of the mouse, *Genet. Res.* **19:**177.

Klyde, B.J., 1970, Selection in mice for change in viability of a semilethal genotype at the T locus, *J. Hered.* **61:**39.

Koo, G.C., Mittl, L.R., and Boyse, E.A., 1977, Antibody to testicular cells in the serum of normal mice, *Immunogenetics* **4:**213.

Králová, J., and Démant, P., 1976, Expression of the H-Y antigen on thymus cells and skin: Differential genetic control linked to K end of H-2, *Immunogenetics* **3:**583.

Králová, J., and Lengerová, A., 1979, H-Y antigen: Genetic control of the expression as detected by host-versus-graft popliteal lymph node enlargement assay maps between the T and H-2 complexes, *J. Immunogenet.* **6:**429.

Kyslíková, L., and Forejt, J., 1972, Chiasma frequencies in three inbred strains of mice, *Folia Biol. (Prague)* **18:**216.

Lengerová, A., 1977, *Membrane Antigens,* Gustav Fisher Verlag, Jena.

Lewontin, R.C., 1962, Interdeme selection controlling a polymorphism in the house mouse, *Am. Nat.* **96:**65.

Lewontin, R.C., 1968, The effect of differential viability on the population dynamics of t alleles ins the house mouse, *Evolution* **22:**262.

Lewontin, R.C., 1974, *The Genetic Basis of Evolutionary Change,* Columbia University Press, New York.

Lyon, M.F., 1956, Hereditary hair loss in the tufted mutant of the house mouse, *J. Hered.* **47:**101.

Lyon, M.F., and Bechtol, K.B., 1977, Derivation of mutant t-haplotypes of the mouse by presumed duplication or deletion, *Genet. Res.* **30:**63.

Lyon, M.F., and Glenister, P.H., 1977, Factors affecting the observed number of young resulting from adjacent-2 disjunction in mice carrying a translocation, *Genet. Res.* **29:**83.

Lyon, M.F., and Mason, I., 1977, Information on the nature of t-haplotypes from the interaction of mutant haplotypes in male fertility and segregation ratio, *Genet. Res.* **29:**255.

Lyon, M.F., and Meredith, R., 1964a, Investigations of the nature of t-alleles in the mouse. I. Genetic analysis of a series of mutants derived from a lethal allele, *Heredity* **19:**301.

Lyon, M.F., and Meredith, R., 1964b, Investigations of the nature of t-alleles in the mouse. II. Genetic analysis of an unusual mutant allele and its derivatives, *Heredity* **19:**313.

Lyon, M.F., and Meredith, R., 1964c, Investigations of the nature of t-alleles in the mouse. III. Short tests of some further mutant alleles, *Heredity* **19:**327.

Lyon, M.F., and Phillips, R.J.S., 1959, Crossing-over in mice heterozygous for t-alleles, *Heredity* **13:**23.

Lyon, M.F., and Sayers, I.M., 1977, Private communication, *Mouse News Lett.* **57:**17.

Lyon, M.F., Glenister, P.H., and Hawker, S.G., 1972, Do the H-2 and T loci of the mouse have a function in the haploid phase of sperm?, *Nature (London)* **240:**152.

Lyon, M.F., Evans, E.P., Jarvis, S.E., and Sayers, I., 1979, t-Haplotypes of the mouse may involve a change in intercalary DNA, *Nature (London)* **279:**38.

Mayr, E., 1963, *Animal Species and Evolution,* Harvard University Press, Cambridge, Massachusetts.

Miller, O.J., and Miller, D.A., 1975, Cytogenetics of the mouse, *Annu. Rev. Genet.* **9:**285.

Monesi, V., 1965, Synthetic activities during spermatogenesis in the mouse: RNA and protein, *Exp. Cell Res.* **39:**197.

Moore, G.P.M., 1971, DNA-dependent RNA synthesis in fixed cells during spermatogenesis in mouse, *Exp. Cell Res.* **68:**462.

Nesbitt, M.N., and Francke, U., 1973, A system of nomenclature for band patterns of mouse chromosome, *Chromosoma* **41:**145.

Olds, P.J., 1970, Effect of the T locus on sperm distribution in the house mouse, *Biol. Reprod.* **2:**91.

Olds, P.J., 1971a, Effect of the T locus on sperm ultrastructure in the house mouse, *J. Anat.* **109:**31.

Olds, P.J., 1971b, Effect of the T locus on fertilization in the house mouse, *J. Exp. Zool.* **177:**417.

Petras, M.L., 1967, Studies of natural populations of *Mus.* II. Polymorphism at the T locus, *Evolution* **21:**446.

Polani, P.E., 1972, Centromere localization at meiosis and the position of chiasmata in the male and female mouse, *Chromosoma* **36:**342.

Prakash, S., 1972, Origin of reproductive isolation in the absence of apparent genic differentiation in a geographic isolate of *Drosophila pseudoobscura, Genetics* **72:**143.

Rajasekarasetty, M.R., 1954, Studies on a new type of genetically determined quasi-sterility in the house mouse, *Fertil. Steril.* **5:68.**

Roderick, T.H., and Davisson, M.T., 1978, Private communication: Linkage map of the mouse, *Mouse News Lett.* **59:**5.

Schnedl, W., 1971, The karyotype of the mouse, *Chromosoma* **35:**111.

Searle, A.G., 1974, Nature and consequences of induced chromosome damage in mammals, *Genetics* **78:**173.

Searle, A.G., Beechey, C.V., and Evans, E.P., 1978, Meiotic effects in chromosomally derived male sterility of mice, *Ann. Biol. Anim. Biochem. Biophys.* **18**(2B):391.

Snell, G.D., 1968, The H-2 locus of the mouse: Observations and speculations concerning its comparative genetics and its polymorphism, *Fol. Biol. (Prague)* **14:**335.

Vandeberg, J.L., and Klein, J., 1978, Localization of mouse Pgk-2 gene at the D end of the H-2 complex, *J. Exp. Zool.* **203:**319.

Vandeberg, J.L., Cooper, D.W., and Close, P.J., 1973, Mammalian testis phosphoglycerate kinase, *Nature (London) New Biol.* **243:**48.

Vandeberg, J.L., Cooper, D.W., and Close P.J., 1976, Testis specific phosphoglycerate kinase B in mouse, *J. Exp. Zool.* **198:**231.

Vojtíšková, M., and Pokorna, Z., 1972. Developmental expression of H-2 antigens in the spermatogenic cell series: Possible bearing on haploid gene action, *Folia Biol. (Prague)* **18**:1

Vojtíšková, M., Pokorná, Z., Viklicky, V., Boubelík, M., and Hattikudur, N.S., 1974, The expression of H-2 and differentiation antigens on mouse spermatozoa, *Folia Biol. (Prague)* **20:**321.

Vojtišková, M., Viklický, V., Voráčová, B., Lewis, S.E., and Glueksohn-Waelsch, S., 1976, The effects of a t-allele (t^{AE5}) in the mouse on the lymphoid system and reproduction, *J. Embryol. Exp. Morphol.* **36:**443.

Wudl, L.R., and Sherman, M.I., 1976, *In vitro* studies of mouse embryos bearing mutations at the T locus: t^{w5} and t^{12}, *Cell* **9:**523.

Wudl, L.R., Sherman, M.I., and Hilmann, N., 1977, Nature of lethality of t mutations in embryos, *Nature (London)* **270:**137.

Yanagisawa, K., Bennett, D., Boyse, E.A., Dunn, L.C., and Dimeo, A., 1974, Serological identification of sperm antigens specified by lethal t-alleles in the mouse, *Immunogenetics* **1:**57.

7

Interspecies MHS Relationships Studied by Serological and Cellular Cross-Reactions

P. Ivânyi

1. Introduction

The major histocompatibility system (MHS) is an interrelated complex of genes located on a phylogenetically conserved chromosomal region involved in immunological processes. The gene products are transplantation antigens, Ia antigens, and complement factors. The precise relationship of these molecules to the multiple functions associated (in physiology and pathology) with the MHS is still unclear. It is characteristic of the MHS that an extensive series of alleles (a high degree of polymorphism) occurs at the individual gene loci.

This review will concentrate on the phylogenetic relationships among the MHS gene products mostly on the basis of serological studies. A high degree of structural homology emerges from amino acid sequence comparisons of human, mice, guinea pig, rat, and chicken MHS transplantation antigens. Therefore, xenoimmune anti-MHS sera cross-react widely with MHS structures of different species. This is not surprising, because interspecies homology has been found in different systems (e.g., immunoglobulins) with analogous consequences. The unique features of the MHS to which I shall refer are interspecies MHS serological cross-reactions defined by alloimmune sera. No other antigenic system has been

P. Ivânyi • Central Laboratory, Netherlands Red Cross Blood Transfusion Service; Laboratory of Experimental and Clinical Immunology, University of Amsterdam, Amsterdam, The Netherlands.

TABLE 1. Amino Acid Sequence of the NH_2 Terminal of Human, Murine, Rat,

Species	MHS Region	MHS Allele	Position 1	2	3	4	5	6	7	8	9	10	11	12
Human	*HLA-A*	*A2*	GLY	SER	HIS[b]	SER	MET	ARG	TYR	PHE	PHE	TYR	SER	VAL
		A9			HIS		MET		TYR	PHE	TYR			VAL
	HLA-B	*B7*	GLY	SER	HIS	SER	MET	ERG	TYR	PHE	TYR	THR	SER	VAL
	HLA	*B7+B12*	GLY	SER	HIS	SER	MET	ERG	TYR	PHE	PHE	THR	ALA	VAL
											ASP			MET
		A1+A2+		SER		SER	MET	ARG	TYR	PHE	PHE	THR	SER	VAL
		B8+B13								TYRTCTHR			SER	ALA
Mouse	*H-2K*	K^b		PRO	HIS	SER	LEU	ARG	TYR	PHE	VAL	THR	ALA	VAL
		K^d	MET		HIS		LEU	ARG	TYR	PHE		THR		
		K^k	GLY	PRO[c]	HIS	SER	LEU	ARG	TYR	PHE	HIS	THR	ALA	VAL
		K^q	GLY	PRO	HIS	SER	LEU	ARG	TYR	PHE	HIS	THR	ALA	VAL
		K^s					LEU	ARG	TYR	PHE	VAL		ALA	VAL
	H-2D	D^b		PRO				ARG	TYR				ALA	VAL
		D^d	MET		HIS		LEU	ARG	TYR	PHE	VAL	THR	ALA	VAL
		D^q		PRO				ARG	TYR	PHE			ALA	VAL
		D^s		ARG			LEU	ARG	TYR	PHE	VAL		ALA	VAL
Rat	*H-1*						LEU	ARG	TYR	PHE	TYR		ALA	VAL
							ILE							
Guinea pig	*GPLA*				HIS		LEU	ARG	TYR	PHE	TYR		PHE	VAL
							ILE						ALA	
Chicken	*B*	*WA*		LEU	HIS		LEU	ARG	TYR	ILE	PHE		ALA	
		WB		LEU	HIS		LEU	ARG	TYR	ILE			ALA	
		SC			HIS			ARG	TYR	PHE	ARG			MET

[a]For references, see Vitetta and Capra (1978), Coligan *et al.* (1978), and Maizels *et al.* (1979).
[b]Position 3 for A2 might be SER (cf. Allison *et al.*, 1978a).
[c]Position 2 for K^k might be SER (cf. Henriksen *et al.*, 1978).

described in which alloantibodies frequently detect polymorphism in phylogenetically widely different species. If we presume that the allotypic variants in each species are *generated by mutational events after speciation,* it is not easy to interpret the finding that alloimmune sera detect some kind of polymorphism across species barrier(s). A similarly puzzling phenomenon emerges from recently accumulated data that xenoimmune sera or cells detect alloantigenic differences in the immunized species.

Much of this review will be devoted to serological cross-reactions between the two best-defined MHSs, the *H-2* system in mice and the *HLA* system in humans. These cross-reactions have been studied mostly by the cytotoxic action of anti-H-2 sera on human cells.

Although the precise nature of the cytotoxic action of alloimmune sera on lymphoid cells of other species is not well understood, I shall uinea Pig, and Chicken Heavy-Chain MHS Antigens[a]

Position																		
13	14	15	16	17	18	19	20	21	22	23	24	25	26	27	28	29	30	31
SER	ARG	PRO	GLY	ARG	GLY	GLU	SER	ASX	PHE	ILE	ALA	VAL		TYR				
		PRO					PRO	PRO										
SER	ARG	PRO	GYL	ARG	GLY	GLU	PRO	PRO	PHE	ILE	ALA	VAL	GLY	TYR	VAL	ASP	GLN	THR
SER	ARG	PRO	GLY	ARG	GLY	GLU	PRO											
	ARG	PRO	GYL															
SER	ARG	PRO	GLY	LEU	GLY	GLU	PRO	ARG	TYR	MET	GLU	VAL	GLY	TYR	VAL			THR
	ARG	PRO		LEU			PRO	ARG	PHE					TYR				
SER	ARG	PRO		LEU		LYS	PRO	ARG	PHE					TYR				
SER	ARG	PRO		LEU		LYS	PRO	ARG	PHE	ILE		VAL		TYR	VAL			
	ARG			PHE				ARG	TYR					TYR	VAL			
	ARG	PRO		LEU			PRO	ARG	TYR					TYR				
THR	ARG	PRO		PHE			PRO	ARG	TYR					TYR				
	ARG	PRO		LEU				ARG	TYR	ILE		VAL		TYR	VAL			
	ARG			LEU				ARG	TYR			VAL		TYR	VAL			
									PHE	ILE	ALA	VAL		TYR	VAL			
		PRO							PHE			VAL		TYR				
		PRO		PRO		LEU			PHE					TYR				
		PRO																
									TYR									

refer to the phenomenon as interspecies MHS cross-reactions. I shall attempt to discuss the phenomenon in relation to other aspects of interspecies MHS relationships.

2. Comparative Gene Maps and Gene Orders of the MHS

The constituents of the MHS in several species seem to be firmly established: (1) two or more loci for Class I antigens (classic transplantation antigens); (2) two or more loci for Class II antigens (Ia or B-cell antigens); and (3) two or more loci for C′ factors and receptors.

The genetic length of the MHS chromosomal region is about 1 centimorgan. Consequently, the number of genes in this system is probably greater than is presumed at present. Genes located in the MHS chromosomal region represent a "system," because gene orders do not appear at random and because analogous linkage groups have been found in several species.

The two systems most studied are those of the *H-2* and *HLA*. The biochemical nature of H-2K and -D and HLA-A,B,C antigens is homologous. A 45,000-molecular-weight glycoprotein (the heavy chain) is noncovalently bound with the nonpolymorphic 12,000-molecular-weight β_2-microglobulin molecule (the light chain). The polymorphism is due to difference in amino acid sequences of the heavy chain (Table 1). Similar comparative data emerge for Ia antigens, although they have been less extensively studied hitherto.

In a number of species, an analogous MHS was found. The analogy concerns (1) the general organization of the chromosomal region and (2) the overall biochemical structure of the gene products, including (3) a striking homology in amino acid sequences of the major transplantation antigens.

Thus, the MHS represents an extensive chromosomal region unexpectedly well conserved during phylogenesis. I propose that the "boundaries" of the MHS could be defined by the interspecies comparative aspects: *genes (and functions) found to be closely linked with major transplantation antigens in more than one species belong to the MHS.*

The gene order follows the simplified "human *HLA* model" in several species:

cntr . . . . D . . . . B . . . . A . . .

C′-factors

In the mouse *H-2* system, the *I* region (analogous to *HLA-D*) and the *S*(*C′*) region occur between the two serologically defined loci *K* and *D*:

cntr . . . . K . . . . I . . . . S(C′) . . . . . . .D

It is presumed that an unknown accidental event at the chromosomal level translocated the *I* and *S* regions to the "wrong" place, i.e., between *K* and *D* (Fig. 1, alternative A). If the original gene order had been *I-S-K-D*, then *H-2K* becomes the analogue of *HLA-B* and *H-2D* becomes the analogue of *HLA-A*.

We propose an alternative possibility (Fig. 1, alternative B). Possibly, it is not the *I-S* segment that was placed unusually, but the *K* region that appeared on the "wrong" place. This hypothesis allows one to presume the original gene order as *I-S-D-K*. Now, *H-2D* is analogous to *HLA-B* and *H-2K* to *HLA-A* according to their positions on the gene maps.

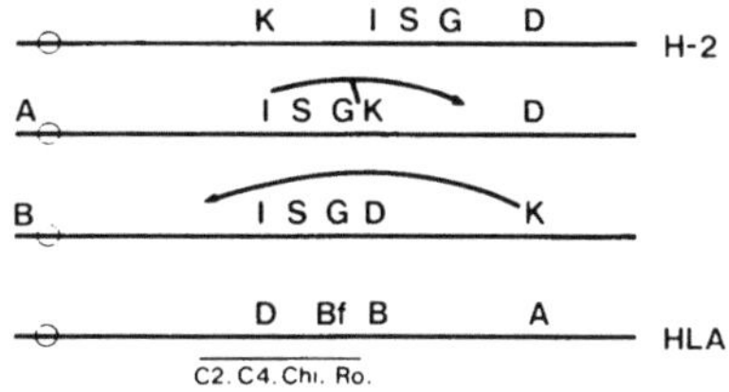

Figure 1. Two alternative *H-2*-region gene orders that occurred before a translocational event produced the *Mus musculus* exception for the MHS.

The following arguments favor the second possibility: (1) anti-H-2D^{d} antibodies cross-react with human cells having *HLA-B* locus antigens; (2) anti-H-2K^{f} antibodies cross-react with HLA-A2 antigen; and (3) anti-HLA-A2 antibodies cross-react with H-2K-end antigens (Sections 7.2–7.5).

Two major genes in the MHS of several species represent the backbone of MHS serology and formal genetics. However, neither *K*-ness and *D*-ness nor *HLA-A*-ness and -*B*-ness was found by amino acid sequence analysis of a series of *H-2* and *HLA* alleles (Maizels *et al.*, 1978). Nevertheless, it might be interesting if some kind of homology between the individual major loci among different species were confirmed.

3. Biochemical Evidence of Interspecies MHS Homology

The overall biochemical characterization (molecular weight, participation of sugars, conditions for solubilization) and the amino acid sequence analysis show that MHS antigens are homologous structures that developed from common precursor(s) (for references, see Table 1). Several amino acid positions in the first 20–30 thoroughly studied NH_2-terminal sequences are constant and identical in widely different species (human, rodent, chicken). This is an unprecedented degree of homology for a series of structures that exhibit that kind of extensive polymorphism. Although it is still in its preliminary stage (20–30 positions of about 300), this analysis allows the following conclusions: (1) there is a striking interspecies homology (common ancestry over more than 300 million years); (2) throughout different species, the same position might be found to exert marked conservation and variations; (3) the allelic products differ at multiple amino acid residues (complex allotypes) by about 10–20% of positions; (d) there is neither *K*-ness and *D*-ness nor *A*-ness and *B*-ness. Some *K* alleles differ more among each other than they differ from *D* alleles.

For the serological data, these findings can explain the interspecies serological cross-reactivity of xenoimmune sera as being due to antibodies directed against "common parts" of several alleles in different species. These common parts seem to be sufficiently frequent to ensure that most xenoimmune anti-MHS sera will react with all individuals of the immunizing species and those of different species. The biochemical data hitherto obtained do not explain how xenoimmune sera, produced in certain donor–recipient combinations, can detect polymorphism in other species or in the immunized species itself; neither do they explain how alloimmune sera might detect polymorphism across species barriers.

However, the biochemical data also do not explain the reaction pattern of alloimmune sera (in the immunized species) or the distinction between *H-2* private and *H-2* public specificities. K^k and K^q products do not differ in amino acid sequences hitherto analyzed, although they are clearly different serologically (Cook *et al.*, 1978). *H-2* mutants that cannot be distinguished serologically differ as to biochemical characterization (Brown and Nathenson, 1977). Possibly, further biochemical analysis will provide a final understanding of the serological data. However, as will be shown in later discussion, this might turn out not to be so, because the cross-reactivity pattern of alloimmune sera might be influenced by factors more complex than amino acid sequences. The protein structure might represent the backbone on which alterations occur that actually represent the complex target for alloimmune antibodies and cytotoxic T lymphocytes (CTL).

Owing to the physiological function of the MHS molecules, two kinds of MHS-region product might serve as target structures for antibodies or CTL: (1) the genetically coded and (2) the epigenetically (in physiology or pathology) altered, uncovered, exposed structure. Interspecies serological and cellular cross-reactions might reflect the existence of the latter.

The precise nature of alterations that might occur, owing to the function of the MHS antigens, is unknown. However, the conditions and end point(s) of an MHS antigen–antibody reaction, dependent on the ability of the former to cross-react with the latter, are multiple and complex. They might depend on the genetically coded structure itself or on processes that the antigen must undergo during its physiological (or pathological) ontogenetic development. Some of the potential variables will be mentioned: more or less exposure of the antigen at the cell membrane, masking of some parts by other membrane constituents or other type of dependence on different membrane structures (steric hindrance), direct molecular alterations, and production of new (hybrid) structures due to interaction with other molecules such as virus particles. Mutations have been described that are serologically not detectable by anti-mutant specific antibodies but only with alloimmune antibodies generated in third-party combinations against common parts of the antigen (J. Klein, 1978).

The activity of such antibodies with individual mutant strains might be dependent on regulatory changes influencing, for example, the exposure of the antigen at the cell membrane and its accessibility to some viral particles. The interpretation of the reaction becomes complex, because the component that decides the outcome of the serological reaction is not the major allele-specific epitope.

4. Structures that Cross-React with Transplantation Antigens Are Distributed Widely throughout Nature

Several observations suggest that structures cross-reacting with transplantation antigens are distributed widely throughout nature. Rodents immunized with *bacterial antigens* (e.g., streptococci of group A type) rejected allografts in an accelerated or white-graft manner (for a review, see Rapaport, 1972). *In vitro*, the cytotoxic action of anti-HLA sera was selectively blocked with a wide variety of bacterial products (Hirata and Terasaki, 1970; Mittal *et al.*, 1973c) or animal tissue extracts (Ratschko *et al.*, 1975), and some rabbit anti-*Klebsiella* sera reacted positively with HLA-B27 ankylosing spondylitis patients (Seager *et al.*, 1979). Artificial membrane vesicles (liposomes) containing HLA antigens have been shown binding to some strains of bacteria (Klareskog *et al.*, 1978a). Streptococcal infection was suggested as a cause of hyperacute renal allograft rejection (Dossetor *et al.*, 1978; Byrd *et al.*, 1978). The precise nature of these observations remains unclear.

A special relationship between a *parasite* and MHS antigens has been found for *Schistosoma mansoni*. The schistosomula, by the time they reach the lung stage, acquire on their tegumental surface specifically products of the *H-2K* and *I* regions. The same phenomenon occurs after cocultivation of parasite with mice lymphocytes *in vitro*. This situation seems to be a passive acquisition of MHS products by a parasite (Sher *et al.*, 1978). *Mycoplasma hyorhinis* isolated from a persistently infected murine lymphoblastoid cell line contained H-2K^{k} antigens possibly due to selective acquisitions of host-cell-membrane antigens (Wise *et al.*, 1978).

MHS–virus complexes (hybrid structures) have been described, and MHS antigens serve as virus receptors. These events are selective for individual viruses to different MHS antigens (see Section 7.9).

Heterophile antibodies are characterized by antigens shared in a rather unpredictable fashion by humans, animals, plants, and bacteria. Heterophile antibodies occur after allotransplantation or alloimmunization, and a possible role for them in alloimmune reactions has been suggested (Rapaport *et al.*, 1968; Kano *et al.*, 1975; Milgrom *et al.*, 1975; McDonald *et al.*, 1977; Milgrom and Zabriskie, 1977). The heterophile antibodies most frequently found in alloimmune sera reacted with extracts of bovine, sheep, and rat erythrocytes; Forssman, Paul–Bunnell, and blood-group-type antibodies seemed not to be involved in these reactions. Some anti-HLA sera from various sources also contain heterophile antibodies (Kano *et al.*, 1975). Rabbit heterophile antibodies (produced in the course of anti-IgD and A immunization) appeared to act on an *HLA-A2*-associated or -influenced antigen material (Smith *et al.*, 1974). Greatly different views have been expressed about the possible relationship of heterophile antibodies to histocompatibility antigens and their occurrence in alloimmune sera (Milgrom and Zabriskie, 1977).

Natural anti-human lymphocytotoxic antibodies are present in the sera of several species, mostly rodents. Some have been characterized as heat-labile autoantibodies (Herberman, 1969), some as directed against carbohydrate determinants (Kenneth *et al.*, 1976), and some as directed against a subpopulation of lymphoid cells (Budzko *et al.*, 1977). Species, as well as individual animals, varied in an unpredictable manner in the serum content of natural anti-human lymphocytotoxins. The titer of these antibodies was usually not higher than 1:4. The formation and specificity of these naturally occurring lymphocytotoxic antibodies are unclear. Sera from germ-free mice also contain natural anti-human lymphocytotoxins (Ferrone *et al.*, 1976).

From the many natural mice sera (NMS) studied on a panel of human cells, none had HLA specificity, although they detected some kind of differences on human lymphocytes. For example, many murine sera reacted with a frequency of about 20–30% with killing of 100% human blood lymphocytes at a serum dilution of 1:2–1:4 (Ferrone *et al.*, 1976). Mittal *et al.* (1973a,b) found anti-human natural lymphocytotoxins in a number of mammalian and avian species, some with high titers. However, none correlated with any HLA antigen. Nevertheless, the reaction patterns of 98 sera could be classified into five distinct lymphocyte groups. Some of the sera exerted a markedly high correlation coefficient (0.78–0.87) with the individual lymphocyte groups.

We examined a great number of NMS for cytotoxic action on human lymphocytes with the same results as those of the authors mentioned above. Anti-human lymphocytotoxins were mostly not detectable at a dilution of 1:2, although some had a somewhat elevated titer of 1:4–1:8 without apparent anti-HLA specificity. However, NMS of the BALB/c-H-2^{dm2} mutant strain were found to contain, about 25%, cytotoxic antibodies against human peripheral lymphocytes reacting to a titer of 1:100 with a 100% kill of human cells. The activity of these sera did not correlate with HLA antigens, although they detected some kind of polymorphism on human lymphocytes (Fig. 2). The nature of this "naturally" occurring antibody in murine sera with strong lymphocytotoxic reactions against human cells is under further investigation.

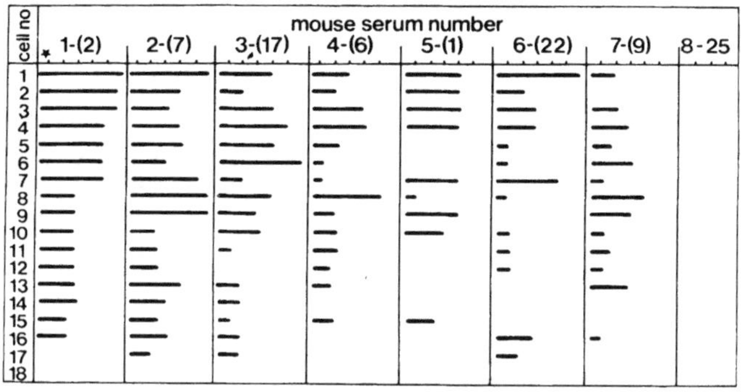

Figure 2. Natural anti-human lymphocytotoxic antibodies in the serum of 25 BALB/c-H-2^{dm2} mutant mice. Seven sera reacted positively. *Serial geometric serum dilutions (1 : 2–1 : 64). The end point is the last serum dilution with more than 50% cell kill.

Natural cytotoxic anti-HLA antibodies have been reported occasionally against HLA-A2 and B8 antigens in sera of human patients with multiple myeloma or gammopathy in the absence of known histoincompatible stimulation (Smith *et al.*, 1974). Natural anti-HLA-A2 antibodies characterized as cold IgM reacted only with A2 homozygous cells (Lepage *et al.*, 1976).

5. Interspecies MHS Relationships Detected by Xenoimmune Sera and Cells

Although MHS structures in different species are highly homologous, the complex molecule exerts sufficient interspecies differences to become a strong immunogen. Therefore, xenoimmune sera are expected to react either (1) with all or almost all MHS (Class I) products of the species from which the antigen was used for immunization, and with homologous products in different third-party species (xenoimmune sera against MHS common parts); or (2) with the allele-specific epitope used for immunization (allospecificity in xenoimmune sera). Obviously, most sera might be mixtures of both kinds of antibodies, although in some situations one of the two possibilities might be predominant.

The diverse data presented in the literature are exactly of the kind to be expected in view of the large diversity of strains and species used as responders and the differences in donor antigen sources, form of antigen presentation (whole cells, isolated cell membranes, or soluble preparations in various degrees of purity including highly purified heavy-chain material), mode of injection, immunization time schedules, and assays used for detection. However, still surprising is the sharp difference in conclusions claimed by several authors under analogous protocols. Whereas some sera are reported to represent a mixture of different kinds of antibodies (i.e., anti-common parts and anti-allele-specific epitopes), other sera contained no allospecificity, and yet others easily detected the allele-specific epitope of the immunogen. Probably more work will be needed before we can understand the role of the different variables involved in xenoimmunization experiments.

One of the variables noted only marginally in some works was the possible role of individual differences of animals within one species or even of individuals of one inbred strain. Specific anti-HLA-A9 antibodies can be obtained in rabbits by immunization with purified A9 substances from human serum. Individual rabbits differed greatly in their capacity to produce a specific anti-A9 antibody. This indicates that polymorphism at their own MHS structures might influence the outcome of immunization. However, breeding of selected good responders did not result in a progeny population of uniformly good responders (Ferrone *et al.*, 1977). This indicates that neither the immune response genes nor the antigen makeup of the recipients that might be decisive for the outcome of the immunization experiments reveals simple inheritance. Parham and Bodmer (1978) immunized a group of inbred BALB/c mice with purified HLA-A2 substance. Neither the individual clones examined from one mouse (see later) nor the individual BALB/c mice reacted identically to the injected material. These results are similar to our finding that an individual animal of one highly inbred strain produces anti-H-2 and anti-HLA antibodies of different specificities in the course of one immunization procedure (Ivânyi *et al.*, 1978a).

5.1. Xenoimmune Sera against MHS Common Parts

Common structures between H-2 and HLA antigens were detected by antisera produced in chicken against soluble H-2 and HLA substances (David *et al.*,1973). Rabbit sera against HLA common parts are reported by Batchelor (1969), Bachvaroff and Rapaport (1973), Cresswell and Ayres (1976), Sanderson (1977), and Wilson *et al.* (1978). These sera neither recognized allele-specific epitopes of the immunogen nor reacted specifically with HLA-A or -B series of antigens; hence no *A*-ness or *B*-ness could be demonstrated with xenoimmune sera, although in some experiments rabbits were immunized with highly purified A2 substance. Papain-solubilized HLA antigen preparations induced in rabbits antibodies against several distinct HLA common parts (Katagiri *et al.*, 1974; Nakamuro *et al.*, 1975). One of these was characterized as a "cryptic" HLA common antigenic determinant not present on intact HLA molecules and exposed or formed as a result of conformational changes resulting from the dissociation of a 33,000-dalton fragment from the rest of the original 48,000-dalton structure (Tanigaki *et al.*, 1974).

Similar studies have been performed with rabbit anti-mouse sera. Kvist *et al.* (1978a,b) extensively studied rabbit sera against highly purified papain-solubilized H-2^{d} antigens. The rabbit anti-H-2 antibodies reacted only with H-2-like material. Anti-β_2-microglobulin and anti-H-2 antibodies appeared as two distinct sets of non-cross-reacting antibodies. Anti-H-2^{d} sera were cytotoxic equally well for lymphoid cells of different H-2 types. However, only D^{d} cells (H-$2^{d,a,t2}$) were able to absorb all activity, whereas after absorption even with high doses of cells with *r,q,k,f,s* haplotypes, some anti-d activity remained. The rabbit anti-H-2 serum precipitated all H-2 material detectable by alloimmune sera. However, the alloimmune sera were not able to eliminate all molecules reactive with xenoimmune serum. Hence, lymphoid cells express additional H-2-like molecules not recognized by alloimmune sera. These might be (1) slightly deranged H-2 antigens or (2) similar but distinctly different molecules. This H-2-like material was present more on T than on B cells and displayed isoelectric focusing patterns similar to, if not identical with, H-2K and D antigens. The xenoimmune anti-H-2 serum cross-reacted with TL antigens and also detected similar yet distinct structures on F9 cells. The same serum precipitated membrane glycoproteins of 45,000 molecular weight, with electrophoretically identical mobility, from monkey, human, rat, guinea pig, pig, and cow (but not chicken) cells.

Morello *et al.* (1978) worked with analogous rabbit sera prepared against purified papain-solubilized H-2 antigens. The rabbit anti-H-2^{a} serum was equally cytotoxic against lymphocytes of various *H-2* haplotypes, but a light absorption (5×10^{6}) with cells belonging to any haplotype resulted in complete loss of the activity. No reaction was observed with F9 antigens by the immunofluorescent technique, and the slight cytotoxic action toward F9 cells seemed attributable to naturally occurring antibodies. The serum was absorbed completely by rat and partially by hamster, guinea pig, marmoset, kangaroo, and human cells. Interestingly, human cells revealed partial absorption against certain (but not all) *HLA* haplotypes. Consequently, this serum is unable to detect polymorphism in the antigen-donor species, although it will detect some polymorphism in a third-party (human) species.

Xenoimmune anti-HLA mouse sera were produced by immunization with syngeneic mouse–human hybrid cells containing human chromosome 6. These sera reacted only with mouse–human hybrid cells containing chromosome 6; lyso-strip experiments have shown that a common determinant of HLA-A and -B series antigens was the possible target. The serum, when tested by immuno-precipitation, reacted with antigens of 45,000 and 12,000 molecular weight and with several other proteins (Aden *et al.*, 1978).

5.2. Can Xenoimmune Sera Detect Allospecificity in the Antigen-Donor Species?

Interestingly, the murine *H-2* system, the first MHS to be discovered, was originally defined by a xenoimmune rabbit anti-mouse serum (Gorer, 1936) (for details, see Klein, 1975).

Several authors have demonstrated allospecificity in xenoimmune sera after quantitative absorptions or by simple serum-dilution tactics [rat anti-H-2 by D. H. Sachs *et al.* (1971, 1973); rabbit anti-H-2 by Staines *et al.* (1973); rabbit anti-Ag-B by Edwards *et al.* (1977) and Poloskey *et al.* (1975); rabbit anti-human by Einstein *et al.* (1971); Ferrone *et al.* (1972, 1975, 1977), Robb *et al.* (1975) Billing and Terasaki (1974), Reisfield *et al.* (1977), and Ferrone, (1978); monkey anti-human by Sanderson and Welsh (1973a,b, 1974)]. However, it is difficult to judge whether these sera contained distinct antibodies against one allele-specific major epitope or became only relatively (operationally) specific for the donor-specific immunogen (Staines *et al.*, 1973). The xeno-immune anti-mouse sera, which revealed specificity for the donor strain, were not tested extensively on a panel of other H-2 antigens. Thus, although after absorption the sera gained the ability to detect polymorphism among murine *H-2* haplotypes, it was not clear whether they became specific for one *H-2* gene product. Robb *et al.* (1975) refer to anti-HLA-A2 allospecificity in rabbit xenoimmune sera, although the sera also reacted with the cross-reacting A28 antigen and hence presumably with the common determinant of the two molecules. The most specific seems to be the rabbit anti-A9 serum prepared by immunization with A9 antigen purified from human serum or urine (see Ferrone *et al.*, 1975). However, A9 is actually a common determinant of A23 and A24, and thus possibly again the allele-specific major epitope is not the only target with which this serum reacts.

If the most restricted and monospecific anti-HLA antibodies and the ideally absorbed anti-H-2 sera represent the model of sera reacting with one allele-specific major epitope of the complex MHS molecule, I should be inclined to propose that none of the xenoimmune sera prepared by immunization with albeit highly purified MHS substances *in vivo* achieved a comparable level of specificity. Doubtless, some xenoimmune sera exert operational ability to recognize more specifically the donor immunogen than other allelic products (Sanderson and Thorsby 1977; Ferrone, 1978), but whether the nature of this specificity can be compared with that of the alloimmune sera remains an open question. Possibly, all xenoimmune sera react with common parts but some react with those that are more common than the others.

Hitherto, it seemed impossible to suggest some kind of generalization about the rules that regulate the outcome of MHS xenoimmunizations. It also remains unclear whether and to what extent the diversity of the published data reflects the variable influence of the MHS genotype of the immunized animals itself, due to (1) partial sharing of structures with the immunogen and (2) influences of immune-response genes, or whether the diversity of data is rather due to the multiple factors involved in the immunization procedure itself and the serological testing systems used.

Nevertheless, a number of xenoimmune sera have been used as immune reagents of great value for the isolation of MHS structures, and they will certainly be helpful for uncovering further unknown components of the MHS.

5.3. Can Xenoimmune Sera Detect MHS Polymorphism in Third-Party Species?

Xenoimmune sera against MHS structures are easily obtained; they (1) detect polymorphism or common parts in the antigen-donor species and (2) cross-react with third-party species. Because the MHS structures are highly polymorphic for every species, it becomes interesting to ask whether antibodies in Xenoimmune anti-MHS sera are able to detect some kind of polymorphism on targets of third-party species. Only very limited information of this kind is available.

Götze *et al.* (1972) have shown that some degree of specificity is involved in third-party interspecies cross-reactions. Rabbit sera against partially purified soluble HLA antigen reacted after selective absorptions with mouse cells bearing the products of D^d and K^b alleles. Furthermore, $H\text{-}2^a$ and $H\text{-}2^b$ cells selectively removed antibodies against *HLA-A* locus determinants. Indications were obtained for cross-reactivity between H-2^b and H-2^d vs. A2 and A10 antigens. However, the distinctions reported were made on a quantitative basis and mice with the same *H-2* haplotype did not give concordant results.

5.4. Can Xenoimmune Sera Detect MHS Polymorphism in the Immunized Species Itself?

If it is true not only that different species share the general homology of MHS structures but also that the intraspecies polymorphism is reflected by analogous determinants, then xenoimmune sera might detect some kind of MHS polymorphism when tested on a panel of targets of the immunized species itself. Preliminary data indicate that this is really so.

Götze *et al.* (1973) reported that mice sensitized against solubilized HLA antigens rejected allogeneic skin with significant acceleration and produced cytotoxic alloreactive antibodies. B10.BR ($H\text{-}2^k$) mice became allosensitized against B10.D2 ($H\text{-}2^d$) and B10 ($H\text{-}2^b$) antigens, whereas neither B10.D2 nor B10 mice became allosensitized under the same immunization conditions. Kren *et al.* (1976) reported on alloreactive antibodies in sera of Lewis rats sensitized with four different human cells. All recipients except one produced alloreactive hemagglutinating and cytotoxic antibodies, the latter being detectable less frequently and in lower titers. Lewis congenic strains with haplotype $H\text{-}1^{a,b,d,f,n,}$ reacted positively, $H\text{-}1^{c,h,w,}$ negatively. The strongest reactions were with $H\text{-}1^{d}$ erythrocytes (1:5000) and lymphocytes (1:16). The alloreactivity was absorbed completely with the human donor cells and only partially with third-party human cells.

Alloimmunity (mice) after xenosensitization (rat) was detected by CTL (Burakoff *et al.*, 1977b) (see Section 5.4).

We immunized two groups of 25 B10 mice with seven weekly intraperitoneal injections (1×10^6 cells per injection) of human lymphocytes and examined the individual sera for alloreactivity by the cytotoxicity test on a panel of murine lymph node cells. The sera of all individual mice were examined separately. Two different cell donors were used for the two recipient groups (*HLA-A28, A33, B21, B22, Cw3, DRw2, DRw5* and *HLA-A2, A3, B7, B18, DRw2, DRw4*) (Ivânyi and Boot, unpublished data).

Of the sera, 40% were negative, and 17% weakly positive, but 43% of the sera exhibited surprisingly strong alloimmune cytotoxic antibodies. Anti-Ia activity seemed not to be involved, because in high serum dilutions, 100% of mouse lymph node cells were killed. The different reaction patterns of the individual sera could not be related to the two human lymphocytes used for the two groups of recipient mice. All positive sera exhibited polymorphism on the panel of mice. In almost all positive sera, the specificity of the antibodies could be deduced from the reaction pattern on the panel of *H-2* haplotypes (Table 2). Anti-H-2^{r}, H-2^{k}, and H-2^{p} antibodies occurred most frequently, with 13, 12, and 5 positive sera, respectively; $H\text{-}2^{f}$, $H\text{-}2^{d}$, $H\text{-}2^{q}$, and $H\text{-}2^{s}$ haplotypes reacted with 4, 4, 3, and 1 sera, respectively. The positive reactions occurred mostly in different combinations, although some sera were positive only with $H\text{-}2^{k}$ (K^{k}, one serum) and $H\text{-}2^{r}$ (two sera). $H\text{-}2^{b}$ cells (on four different backgrounds) were always negative. Four representative examples are shown in Table 2. Evidently, a serum pool of all immunized mice would have resulted in a "low-titer/highly polyvalent" complex serum with very limited possibilities for further analysis.

The high degree of specificity against allogeneic targets in xenoimmune sera was a somewhat unexpected observation. Possibly we are facing the serological analogue of Burakoff's data on CTL specific for H-2 antigens after stimulation with rat cells.

It is difficult to speculate about the possible relationships of distinct

TABLE 2. Alloreactivity in Xenoimmune Sera[a]

Mouse strain	*H-2* haplotype	*K* and *D* allele		Serum number[b]			
				54-G-16	54-G-10	52-G-21	52-G-22
C57Bl/10	*b*	*b*	*b*	0	0	0	0
C57Bl/6	*b*	*b*	*b*	0	0	0	0
A.BY	*b*	*b*	*b*	0	0	0	0
C3H.B10	*b*	*b*	*b*	0	0	0	0
B10.D2	*d*	*d*	*d*	256	0	0	32
B10.D2(504)	*dml*	*d*	*d*	512	0	0	32
BALB/c	*d*	*d*	*d*	256	0	0	64
BALB/c-db	*dm2*	*d*	*d*	512	0	0	64
B10.A(5R)	*i5*	*b*	*d*	0	0	0	64
B10.AQR	*yl*	*q*	*d*	0	512	0	32
A.TFR2	*ap2*	*f*	*d*	0	0	1024	64
D2.GD	*g2*	*d*	*b*	256	0	0	0
C3H.OH	*o2*	*d*	*k*	128	0	0	0
B10.A(2R)	*h2*	*k*	*b*	0	1024	16	32
B10.AKM	*m*	*k*	*q*	0	256	16	64
B10.A	*a*	*k*	*d*	0	1024	64	256
C3H/J	*k*	*k*	*k*	0	128	4	64
AKR/J	*k*	*k*	*k*	0	512	64	64
B10.BR	*k*	*k*	*k*	0	256	32	128
B10.RIII	*r*	*r*	*r*	1024	1024	32	256
C3H.NB	*p*	*p*	*p*	256	0	32	64
DBA/1	*q*	*q*	*q*	0	256	0	32
B10.S	*s*	*s*	*s*	0	0	0	64
A.SW	*s*	*s*	*s*	0	0	0	32
B10.M	*f*	*f*	*f*	0	0	1024	0
H-2 specificities present:				K^d,r,p,	K^k,K^q,r,	K^k,K^f,p,r,	D^d,K^k,q, p,s,r,

[a]Cytotoxic antibodies were raised in the sera of 4 individual B10 mice immunized with human cells. All serum samples were examined after seven weekly intraperitoneal injections of 1×10^6 human cells.
[b]The results are the last dilutions at which the microcytotoxicity test with mice lymphnode cells was positive with more than 80% cell kill.

HLA antigens (on donor cells) to the H-2 specificities produced by the individual mice. In a parallel immunization experiment, as described above, B10.A (*H-2*[a]) mice did not produce alloimmune cytotoxic antibodies. This indicates the involvement of the *H-2* region for the immune response—due either to its antigen makeup or to immune-response regulation. More extensive immunization experiments, including purified antigens and several recipient strains, might provide a solution to this problem. Two alternative possibilities occur at this preliminary stage of our work: (1) human cells, by their cell-membrane product(s) from the *HLA* region, provide some kind of ***specific stimulation*** that is realized differently, although within the limits of a certain regulated variation, by individual mice of one inbred strain; or (2) human cells, not dependent specifically on their *HLA*-region products, provide some kind of ***nonspecific activation*** of the silent potential of individual mice, based on a predetermined clonal preference for the production of certain types of alloreactive antibodies. Better knowledge of the mechanism of induction and fine specificity involved in the alloreactivity of xenoimmune sera and cells might become a powerful instrument for an understanding of the biological role of the MHS.

5.5. Interspecies Relationships for B-Cell Antigens

Biochemical evidence also shows homology between Class II MHS antigens in different species (*HLA-DR* or *H-2I* region Ia or B-cell antigens). Of the four loci coding for Ia antigens in mice, the *I-A* region seems analogous to *HLA-DR* because of its major role in both B-cell serology and mixed-lymphocyte culture (MLC) genetics. However, preliminary amino acid residue comparisons show that *H-2I-E/C* (and not *I-A*) subregion products are homologous to *HLA-DR* (Cook *et al.*, 1977; Silver *et al.*, 1977; McMillan *et al.*, 1977, 1978; Allison *et al.*, 1978b).

Initial steps were performed with interspecies serological work analogous to that for MHS Class I antigens. Several authors have shown that rabbits immunized with either H-2I or HLA-DR purified antigens are able to produce ***xenoimmune*** anti-B cell antibodies. Such sera were helpful for the study of new subloci of the human *HLA-D* region (Tosi *et al.*, 1978) and identification of Ia antigens on a small population of human T lymphocytes (Fu *et al.*, 1978). The specificity of xenoimmune rabbit anti-Ia^k antibodies was evidently directed against distinct ***common parts*** of mouse Ia antigens because some third-party strains absorbed all activity; donor-halotype-specific (anti-Ia.2) antibodies could not be detected (Parish and McKenzie, 1978). Similar results were obtained with rabbit anti-HLA-DR sera (Klareskog *et al.*, 1978b; Solheim *et al.*, 1978), although 6 of 31 rabbit sera showed preferential reactivity with cells bearing the donor-specific DR antigen (Solheim *et al.*, 1978).

Alloimmune mouse anti-Ia sera reacted with rat Ia antigens, although no polymorphism for rat Ia antigens was detected when mouse sera were tested on three rat strains. Interestingly, the rat Ia antigens detected by the mouse alloimmune anti-Ia sera were on molecules separable from the rat Ia antigens detected by rat alloimmune antibodies. Thus, the presence of at least two *Ia* subloci in rats was suggested: (1) one for the shared structure involved in the reaction with both mouse and rat alloimmune anti-Ia sera and (2) one for the structure that reacted only with rat alloimmune anti-Ia sera (D.H. Sachs *et al.*, 1977; Shinohara *et al.*, 1978).

Alloimmune mouse anti-Ia sera reacted only weakly or negatively with human T cells, although they reacted positively with human peripheral-blood B cells (Ivânyi *et al.*, 1977). These preliminary results were recently confirmed by testing of A.TH anti-A.TL (I^s anti-I^k) sera from individual immunized mice on human B and T cells (table 3). Sera from some alloimmunized individual mice exerted a surprisingly high cytotoxic titer on human B cells and revealed polymorphism. Sera with the highest anti-B cell titers also reacted with T cells, although in a very low titer. The specificity of these reactions is now under study. Sera produced in the opposite direction (A.TL anti-A.TH) were practically negative although produced in a parallel experiment under the same immunization conditions.

5.6. Interspecies Cross-Reactivity of Serum Serological Protein

Borovska *et al.* (1971) tested rabbit antisera against the mouse serological (Ss) serum protein for cross-reactivity with the sera of seven different species (human, cattle, horse, pig, guinea pig, rabbit, and rat);

TABLE 3. Cytotoxic Effect of Alloimmune Murine Anti-Ia Antibodies on Human B Cells[b]

Human cell number and DRw type	Anti-Ia (anti-I^k) mouse serum number[b]					
	1-5-9	2-5-8	3-5-36	4-4-12	5-5-12	6-5-15
1. 6/7	1024	64	16	4	0	0
2. 1/4	256	32	32	0	8	4
3. 2/7	128	32	2	0	0	0
4. 1/2	128	32	4	0	0	0
5. 2/5	64	16	16	0	0	0
6. 5/7	128	32	8	2	16	0
7. 5/7	32	128	4	0	0	0

[a]Donor: A.TL (I^k); recipients: A.TH (I^s).
[b]Serum numbers 1–6 represent samples of serum from individual recipient mice after 18 weeks of immunization. The results are the highest serum dilutions with more than 80% cell kill.

positive reactions were found only with the sera of rats. Ss protein cross-reactions now need reconsideration because the Ss protein was found to be a part of the complement system (Demant *et al.*, 1973).

5.7. Hybridoma Products from Xenoimmune Cells

The fusion of murine myeloma cells with spleen cells from immunized mice resulted in the possibility of deriving continuous hybrid cell lines, hybridomas. The spleen cells for such lines can be selected so that the multispecific response to a complex immunogen becomes resolved into a set of monospecific responses due to the preparation of a number of clones that each secrete one monoclonal antibody.

Parham and Bodmer (1978) immunized BALB/c mice with purified papainsolubilized HLA-A2 antigen. The serum antibodies reacted without apparent anti-A2 specificity. From a number of hybridomas on continued growth, obtained from three immunized BALB/c mice with the highest antibody titer, 14 cultures retained strong activity and were selected for further study. All were inhibited by A2 antigen but not by β_2-microglobulin. However, 10 of the 14 clones reacted equally well to all human cells; hence, they probably recognize antigenic determinants common to all HLA-A,B,C antigens. Four reagents revealed a polymorphic reaction pattern, but only one was specific for A2. The anti-H-2 specificity reported was excellent, and also negative with the strongly cross-reacting A28 antigen. A2 homozygous and heterozygous individuals were distinguishable. Three hybridoma products probably recognize cross-reacting antigenic determinants that A2 antigens share with other HLA-A,B,C antigens. Interestingly, one seemed to react with most *A*-locus antigens; if confirmed, this would indicate serologically defined HLA-A series common determinants. Such a bipartite feature was not noted for H-2K and -D or HLA-A and -B series antigens by biochemical studies. It seems interesting that individual cell clones obtained from spleen cells of genetically identical individuals reveal all the features of xenoimmune anti-MHS sera discussed in the previous sections: (1) anti-HLA activity without any specificity, (2) anti-HLA activity to common parts that exert some polymorphism, and (3) anti-HLA activity that corresponds exactly to one of the allele-specific epitopes (A2).

Lampson *et al.* (1978) followed the xenoimmune response of spleen cells by cultures *in vitro* (not hybridomas) of mice immunized with whole human cells. Of 167 culture fluids, 141 contained antibodies to human cells, but only 3 showed specificity for HLA antigens. All three were able to discriminate between A2+ and A2− cells. However, these antibodies also recognized the strongly cross-reacting HLA-A28 antigen, and it was not possible to prepare a monospecific serum to either of the two antigens. Hence, the antibodies were directed against the cross-reactive common part of A2 and A28 antigens and not to the allele-specific epitope.

When spleen cells from rat immunized with mouse spleen cells were fused and cloned, from a number of hybrid clones monoclonal antibodies were obtained that recognized four types of antigens: (1) a heterophilic, Forssman-like antigen, (2) a 210,000-molecular-weight cell-surface protein, (3) a minor component of two polypeptides of 190,000 and 105,000 molecular weight, and (4) a glycolipid component present on red cells and thymocytes. However, non detected polymorphic murine antigens (Springer *et al.*, 1978). Similarly, hybridomas of mouse spleen cells immunized with human cells produced clones that made anti-β_2-microglobulin and other antibodies to human lymphocyte antigens suspected to react with lymphocyte surface Ig or Epstein–Barr-virus-dependent antigens (Trucco *et al.*, 1978). Thus, after immunization with whole xenogeneic cells, antibodies to non-MHS structures seem to dominate the immune response. This is in contrast with reports that in cellular tests [MLC and cell-mediated lympholysis (CML)], MHS structures dominate the xenoimmune response (see the next section).

5.8. Xenogeneic Cellular Responses (Primed-Lymphocyte Test and Cell-Mediated Lympholysis)

Lindahl and Bach (1976) studied the response of human lymphocytes to mouse cells in the primed-lymphocyte test (PLT). Human lymphocytes recognized, by a strong secondary response, only those murine lymphocytes that had the *I-A* region structure of the original stimulator cell. Thus, the same order of relative importance and specificity was found in xenogeneic and allogeneic PLTs. Analogous results were obtained by Boylston and Anderson (1978) and Carnaud *et al.* (1977), including those from the human anti-mouse graft-vs.-host assay.

Lindahl and Bach (1975), Carnaud *et al.* (1977), and Klajman *et al.* (1978) studied the CML of human cells sensitized with mouse cells. Human effector cells recognized primarily products of the *H-2K* and *D* regions; only target-cell *K* or *D* alleles identical with that of the sensitizing mouse strain were killed by the human xenosensitized lymphocytes. An identical situation was found in the rat-vs.-mouse combination (Ginsburg, 1968; Burakoff *et al.*, 1977a). Mice cytotoxic T cells were also induced by purified HLA antigens; the xenogeneic cytotoxic cells demonstrated specificity, although a low level of cross-reactive lysis occurred (Engelhard *et al.*, 1978).

The same repertoire of T cells was involved in allogeneic and xenogeneic cellular responses (Burakoff *et al.*, 1978). Probably the common denominator of the aforementioned findings is the high frequency of immunocompetent cells (1–3%) potentially reactive to alloantigens. This high level of preferential readiness to react specifically against alloantigens seems also to be reflected in the xenogeneic cellular responses. Indeed, the cross-reactive structure in different species was also found with cellular techniques. Martinis and Bach (1977a,b) sensitized human lymphocytes with a pool of 20 allogeneic stimulator cells: monkey, dog, and cattle (but, surprisingly, not mouse) cells induced significant restimulation. Lymphocytes from some rhesus monkeys restimulated human cells specifically for LK1 (Dw3). Alloimmune anti-H-2 mouse sera were found to strongly inhibit human MLC reactions (Sula et al., 1977).

Extremely puzzling results on the specificities involved were obtained by Burakoff *et al.* (1977b). When mice were sensitized with rat cells, CTL were generated that reacted specifically with the immunizing strain. However, these xenogeneically sensitized mice CTL also exerted allogeneic CML activity by killing of mouse cells with $H\text{-}2^{k}$ or $H\text{-}2^{r}$ targets, whereas $H\text{-}2^{s}$ and $H\text{-}2^{q}$ targets remained negative. Cold-target-inhibition studies showed that distinct clones were present for each allogeneic target in the xenogeneically stimulated mouse. A simple explanation of the *specificity* of the allogeneic kill after xenogeneic sensitization would be that the sensitizing cells shared MHS antigenic components with $H\text{-}2^{k,r,}$ but not (or less) with $H\text{-}2^{s,q,}$. However, this explanation seems unlikely because the same pattern of allogeneic CML was observed after stimulation of one mouse-strain with three different rat-strain cells.

For the specificity pattern of MHS cross-reactions in the model presented by Burakoff *et al.* (1977b), there emerges the crucial question: what kind of structure, common to three different xenogeneic rat MHS haplotypes selected by chance, was responsible for an identical alloreactive reaction pattern in the responder mouse strain? This might be a biologically important structure, whatever its nature. If we have not to presume that only an MHS-coded common structure, conserved or developed by chance, can explain the specificity of alloimmunity after xenogeneic stimulation, some other *raison d'être* must be involved in the regulation of the specific relationship observed. Because a specific relationship among MHS and virus structures has been documented (see later), we propose that a virus structure associated with several rat MHS haplotypes is responsible for the occurrence of an identical reaction pattern in the xenoimmunized mouse cells. Consequently, cross-reacting virus particles were associated with the positive mouse *H-2* haplotypes ($H\text{-}2^{k,r,}$ and partially $H\text{-}2^{d}$) and absent from the responder $H\text{-}2^{b}$ and the negative strains ($H\text{-}2^{s,q,}$).

6. Primate–Human Relationships

From man's closest living relatives, the great apes, the chimpanzees, MHS was elaborated in most detail (Balner *et al.*, 1970, 1978; Balner, 1977; van Rood *et al.*, 1972; Schreuder *et al.*, 1975; Metzgar and Seigler, 1970, 1972). A system homologous to that of the *HLA* system was found with two loci for Class I antigens. The two loci are designated *ChLA-A* and -B, and six to seven alleles were described for each of the two loci. Serologically, the *ChLA-A* locus antigens cross-react with *HLA-A* and CHLA-B with *HLA-B*. Probably the separation of the *A* and *B* loci occurred before man and chimp diverged.

Alloimmune human sera detect polymorphism on chimp cells and chimp alloimmune sera detect polymorphism on human cells. Some sera were absorbed completely with positively reacting cells of the other species and revealed typing results practically identical with those from alloimmune sera in panel studies. The best examples of possible identity are *HLA-A11/ChLA-A108* and *HLA-B17/ChLA-B125*. The same holds for Bw4 and Bw6 (4a, 4b) in both species. Other cross-reactions are less perfect in absorption and panel studies. It is not clear whether this selection has biological implications or is due to chance, owing to the somewhat limited number of individuals available for testing from the *Pan troglodytes* species. Interestingly, of the seven HLA antigens most cross-reactive with ChLA antigens, four were found to cross-react also with H-2 sera, namely, A11, Aw31, B17, and B37 (see Section 7.5).

The *HLA/ChLA* relationship enables one to test the crucial question of whether the respective gene products are identical in both species or whether the similarity is so close that the biochemical differences cannot be ascertained serologically. This latter possibility has to be tested by comparison of amino acid sequences and tryptic peptide profile characteristics. It would be useless to raise possible speculations about the consequences of either possibility until such work is accomplished. However, the elucidation of this situation must have important consequences for our understanding of MHS interspecies relationships. Bruce and Ayala (1978) commented on the high level of similarity in protein chemistry among man and primates (the difference being not greater than that between morphologically indistinguishable sibling species of *Drosophila* flies) as an argument in favor of the view that the considerable differences in morphology and behavior are due primarily to changes in gene regulation rather than to changes in structural gene loci.

A different situation occurs among other primate and monkey species. Neither chimp nor human alloimmune sera exhibited reaction patterns on gorilla or orangutan cells that would allow us to presume identical structures, although significant correlations were found (Bw4, Bw6, B12, B7). The same holds for reactions with several monkey species, including rhesus monkeys. However, in practically all interspecies relationships (some more and some less phylogenetically distant), alloimmune sera detected polymorphism in other species. A comparable degree of similarity to that between chimp and human, indicative of identity, was found between rhesus monkeys and stumptail macaques, two species with origins in adjacent geographical areas and apparent morphological similarity (Balner, 1977).

In this complex situation, where close phylogenetic relationship appears in parallel with either close similarity or real structural identity in products of polymorphic gene loci, only biochemical analysis can provide further contributions to the final evaluation of the biological meaning of the serological observations. We are facing the possibility that some gene products of gene loci that exert a high level of polymorphism will be found identical in closely related species. Moreover, whenever the phylogenetic relationship becomes more distant, the gene products are evidently *not identical*, although alloimmune antibodies produced in one species detect polymorphism in another species, albeit among much more distant species, say, mouse, cattle, and man. If the positively reacting cells are not able to absorb all antibodies, the cross-reactivity is not due to sharing of major allele-specific epitopes but to common structures that appear to spread across species barriers. This situation will be discussed on the model of MHS cross-reactions among widely distant species. However, the serological data elaborated on the model of interspecies relationships among outbred individuals contain numerous problems that make final conclusions difficult. The alloimmune sera raised between outbred individuals might contain antibodies directed against more than one MHS gene product. However, some well-controlled monospecific sera seem to contain antibodies against only one *HLA* gene product.

The MHS antigens most cross-reactive among the different primate and monkey species and man were Bw4 and Bw6 (4a4b) (Balner, 1977; Bright and Balner, 1976). This phenomenon revealed several pecularities: (1) chimp anti-4a4b sera reacted on monkeys more broadly than did human anti-4a4b; (2) individual human or chimp anti-4a4b sera did not react identically; (3) in monkeys, there was a lack of *4a4b* heterozygotes, in contrast to the excess of 4a4b heterozygotes in humans. All these findings led to the conclusion that the determinants (4a4b) detected in monkeys by human and chimp sera represent common determinants of a nature similar, but not identical, to that of their human and chimp counterparts. I propose the view that these cross-reactions observed were due rather to "remnants" of original structures (phylogenetically conservative common parts) than to new structures that developed after speciation.

Indications were found for associations of certain rhesus *RhLA-B* locus antigens (RhLA-B9, B3, B22 and B6, B19, B27) with human (and chimp) anti-4a and anti-4b sera, respectively. In other terms, the anti-4a4b sera reacted preferentially with rhesus cells bearing certain antigens of the *RhLA-B* locus series antigens. However, the panel of target cells was too limited for the evaluation of the real significance of these findings (Bright and Balner, 1976). If confirmed, this finding would be analogous to the reaction pattern of anti-H-$2D^d$ sera that correlate with a number of *HLA-B* locus antigens included in the Bw4 (4a) supertypic specificity (see Section 7.8 and Fig. 5.)

In conclusion, the human–primate cross-reactions represent the most challenging possibility for testing whether individuals of different species contain structurally identical antigens coded by highly polymorphic series of allelic genes. However, this conclusion must await detailed biochemical analysis of the two structures to be compared.

7. Alloimmune Sera Detect MHS Polymorphism across Species Barriers

7.1. Introduction

The unique feature of the interspecies MHS relationship is that alloimmune antibodies against polymorphic differences in one species are able to detect polymorphism in another, distant species. No other antigenic system is known in which alloimmune antibodies frequently detect polymorphism across species barriers. Blood groups or Ig allotypes cannot be detected in one species by alloimmune sera produced in another species; in contrast, the polymorphism of the *HLA* system could have been discovered by murine alloimmune H-2 sera if tested on human cells after Gorer and O'Gorman (1956) introduced the cytotoxic test for *H-2* serology (see Figs. 3–5).

Biochemical evidence shows a high degree of evolutionary conservation in the structure of MHS antigens of distant species separated by millions of generations (see Table 1). This explains why xenoimmune sera react with MHS structures of different species. However, there is still no biochemical explanation for specific relationships between individual allelic products of different species. If it could be shown that, for example, the *H-2*K^f gene product is very much more closely similar to the *HLA-A2* gene product, or if any other biochemical finding were to explain the specificity of the hitherto observed interspecies cross-reactions, this would promote the explanation for the phenomenon of "xenoreactivity in alloimmune" sera.

Only a few proposals have been offered as explanations for the specific activity of alloimmune sera across species barriers. Bodmer (1973) found the surprising phenomenon of interspecies serological cross-reactions by alloimmune sera to imply that the polymorphic differences now found predate the evolutionary separation of distant species. Because this cannot be easily accommodated by present genetic concepts, he proposed a new genetic model for MHS, presuming that "perhaps the serologically detected allelic differences are actually the products of different, closely linked genes, and the genetic polymorphism is for the control of whichever of the genes is expressed." If this be so, identical or closely similar gene products might be preserved and expressed in any species.

The following possibilities were listed by Ivaskova *et al.* (1975) and Ivanyi (1978a) for H-2/HLA cross-reactions: (1) There is a biochemical similarity due to common origin or to accidental events. (2) Anti-H-2 sera contain an antibody against an unknown component of the H-2 system that cross-reacts with homologous structures of the HLA system. (3) Because some H-2 sera react with all human cells, species-specific determinants, strongly influenced in expression by *HLA* haplotypes, might be the target structure. It remains unclear why such antibodies would be generated during H-2 alloimmunization. (4) Anti-common-part H-2 antibodies react with analogous human structures that occur in linkage disequilibrium and/or under quantitative regulation of HLA antigens. (5) Analogous virus particles, incorporated in the genome or otherwise associated with the expression of MHS antigens, might be the ultimate reason for the observed cross-reactions.

For the xenoreactivity (anti-rat) of alloimmune murine anti-Ia antibodies, D.H. Sachs *et al.* (1977) proposed two alternatives: (1) convergent evolution with random appearance of structurally similar alloantigens in different species or (2) divergent evolution with incomplete conservation of shared antigenic determinants that reflect common primordial sequences.

Suffice it to say that no conclusive explanation has hitherto been found for the serological MHS cross-reactions detected by alloimmune sera. Before I describe the phenomenon in more detail, let me introduce a view on the possible origin of allele-specific (anti-private) and anti-common-part (anti-public) antibodies in H-2 sera. It might be important to know which of the two is involved in interspecies serological cross-reactions.

It is presumed that MHS polymorphism developed from precursor substances by mutational events. *H-2* mutations are the model of such diversification. The average *H-2* mutation rate has been estimated as 4 ×

10^{-5} per locus per gamete. This is 1–3 levels higher than for other murine genes (J. Klein, 1978). The *H-2K*^{b} gene seems to be the most mutable mammalian gene (2.2×10^{-4}).

H-2 mutations generate diversification. If we imagine the schematic model of the originally limited mouse population to be homogeneous for its MHS, (1) the "first" gain mutation produced the first detectable allele-specific (private) antigen, whereas (2) the "first" loss mutation made possible the detection of the respective common part—the first public antigen.

Biochemical evidence shows that some parts of the MHS proteins are highly conservative. Possibly there are some highly variable positions or regions in the frame of the 300-amino-acid-chain molecule, while other parts might be almost or completely invariable. This distinction might parallel the existence of (1) the anti-H-2 antibodies directed against the allele-specific determinants and (2) the antibodies directed against determinants common to several allelic products. If so, which of the two kinds of antibodies is responsible for the interspecies cross-reactions detected with allo-immune sera? I propose the view that (1) if the allele-specific antibodies are responsible for the cross-reactions, then these detect identical or analogous mutational events, whereas (2) if the anti-common-part antibodies are responsible for the cross-reactions, than we detect rather "remnants" of the original common-core substance. This classification is somewhat schematic, because the common parts (public antigens) detected by cross-reactions of alloimmune sera within one species are partially different in different alleles. However, the possible existence of two kinds of target structures with *different evolutionary histories* and probably also *different functional roles* must be stressed.

7.2. Xenoactivity in Alloimmune Rabbit, Rat, Cattle, Murine, and Human Sera

Abeyounis and Milgrom (1969) and Albert *et al.* (1969) were the first to show that alloimmune post posttransplantation rabbit sera detect *H-2*-associated and *HLA*-associated polymorphism in mice and humans. Anti-mouse activity could be absorbed with *H-2*^{k} cells of three different genetic backgrounds, whereas two strains with *H-2*^{b} haplotypes failed to absorb. In humans, the rabbit sera followed the segregation of *HLA* haplotypes in family studies without correlation with any particular HLA antigen. Important details were reported in these initial studies: (1) The donor rabbit always absorbed all activity, whereas some (but not all) unrelated rabbits absorbed as well. We can presume that unrelated rabbits did not share the MHS haplotype. Thus, although the anti-donor specific antibodies remained in the serum, anti-human activity was absorbed. (2)

In some paired experiments, both partners produced anti-H-2^{k} antibodies. Hence, the rabbit has some, but not all, H-2^{k} antigens. Apparently the rabbits had neither the whole "*H-2*^{k} haplotype" nor the allele-specific major epitope.

Anti-human cytotoxins have been found in alloimmune cattle (Iha *et al.*, 1973), rat H-1 (J.A. Sachs and Kren, 1976), and murine H-2 sera (Ivaskova *et al.*, 1972; Pellegrino *et al.*, 1974); in the latter report, the MHS of both species was well defined for the first time. The reaction pattern of cattle and murine sera was indicative of correlations with HLA antigens or haplotypes or both. Third-party rat cells completely absorbed anti-human activity; third-part cow cells could not absorb all the anti-human activity. Pellegrino *et al.* (1974) and Colombani *et al.* (1977) detected polymorphism on murine cells with HLA sera; this approach is much more difficult because of the high titer of natural anti-mouse antibodies in normal human sera (1:10–20). Pellegrino and co-workers showed that anti-HLA sera detect polymorphism on mouse cells with the help of absorptions. Using hyperimmune sera from multitransfused patients, Colombani and co-workers obtained cytotoxicity on mouse cells safely above the level of natural antibodies (<1:1000). The 11 strong sera all revealed polymorphism due to *H-2* differences. However, none exerted clear-cut correlations of anti-HLA antibodies to certain H-2 antigens. Eluates obtained from murine lymphocytes revealed anti-HLA-A2 specificity, identical with the specificity originally defined in the antiserum. One serum, studied on recombinant strains, reacted with *H-2K* locus product(s). Thus, an anti-*HLA-A* locus antibody revealed H-2K specificity. However, murine cells negative in cytotoxicity absorbed and eluted antibodies of the same specificity.

7.3. Cytotoxic Activity of Anti-H-2 Sera on Human Lymphocytes: H-2/HLA Cross-Reactions

We shall summarize here data from a long-term study in which the basic approach was the analysis of specificities involved in the cytotoxic action of congenic anti-H-2 sera on human peripheral-blood lymphocytes.

Because the murine strains differed only in the *H-2* region, and the reaction pattern of the anti-H-2 sera correlated with the presence of certain HLA antigens (dependent on the mouse donor–recipient combination), the designation H-2/HLA cross-reactions (H-2/HLA CR) will be used, although the precise nature of the phenomenon is not fully understood.

Studies on H-2/HLA CR were initiated in 1968 owing to the belief in the existence of one evolutionary homologous MHS in every species (Ivânyi, 1970; Ivaskova *et al.*, 1972). Because of the availability of an extensive series of anti-H-2 sera and a large panel of *HLA*-typed individuals, a great number of congenic anti-H-2 sera were tested by the routine *HLA* microcytotoxicity test on human lymphocytes. The technique, as used in numerous *HLA* laboratories, was applied without modification. All sera were tested in 6–10 serial geometric dilutions. Most sera analyzed had a titer 1:16++++ on human lymphocytes. However, many of the H-2 sera had a titer of greater than 1:100 and still produced 100% cell kill. Exceptional sera had a titer of about 1 : 1000. The H-2 immunizations were performed by weekly intraperitoneal injections of lymphoid cells in the dose 1 donor/10 recipients (spleen+lymph node+thymus cells) (Ivaskova *et al.*, 1975). In all work until 1977, we examined anti-H-2 sera, which always represented a pool obtained from several individual mice from one inbred strain. In recent work, we used only sera obtained from individual mice (Ivânyi *et al.*, 1978a).

7.4. Screening for Anti-H-2 Sera with Cytotoxic Activity against Human Cells

Which anti-H-2 sera exert cytotoxic effects on human cells? The question is crucial because if only certain H-2 alloimmunizations result in the production of anti-human cytotoxic activity, this would be the clue for an understanding of the mutual relationship between certain H-2 and HLA antigens. However, there is no clear answer to this question, although a great number of combinations has been tested. In general, we found that anti-H-$2^{f,p,s,d,}$ sera became more easily cytotoxic for human cells than anti-H-$2^{b,k,}$ sera. Lists of H-2 sera with anti-human cytotoxic activity have been published (Ivoskova *et al.*, 1972, 1974, 1975, 1976; Ivaskova and Ivânyi, 1974; Ivânyi *et al.*, 1978a; Pellegrino *et al.*, 1974) (see also Tables 4 and 5). However, other reports, as well as ours, about the presence or absence of anti-human activity in different H-2 sera cannot be taken as conclusive, because of the particular dynamics of the occurrence of anti-human activity in H-2 sera. Figure 3 shows that anti-human activity occurs much later than do anti-H-2 antibodies. Many laboratories would stop with the preparation of the H-2 serum at immunization week J (see Fig. 3) with a very high alloimmune titer (after 10 weekly injections) and collect a large serum pool that might be found negative for human cells. However, after 2 further weeks of immunization, strong anti-human activity was found in these sera.

The second point to which we turned our attention only recently was the great variation among individual mice of one inbred strain in their ability to produce anti-human activity in the course of H-2 immunization. After 19 weeks of immunization ($D^d \rightarrow D^b$) about 1/4 of the individual mice sera was completely negative, 2/4 were weak or medium strong, and

1/4 was strongly positive (i.e., high titers and high reaction frequencies). This is in sharp contrast with the observation that almost all individual mice sera become strongly positive against the donor strain after a few weeks of immunization with a difference in *K*- or *D*-locus alleles (Ivânyi *et al.*, 1978a; Ivânyi and de Greeve, 1978).

In general, analogous problems do not occur in the preparation of H-2 sera with anti-donor activity. However, difficulties of similar nature

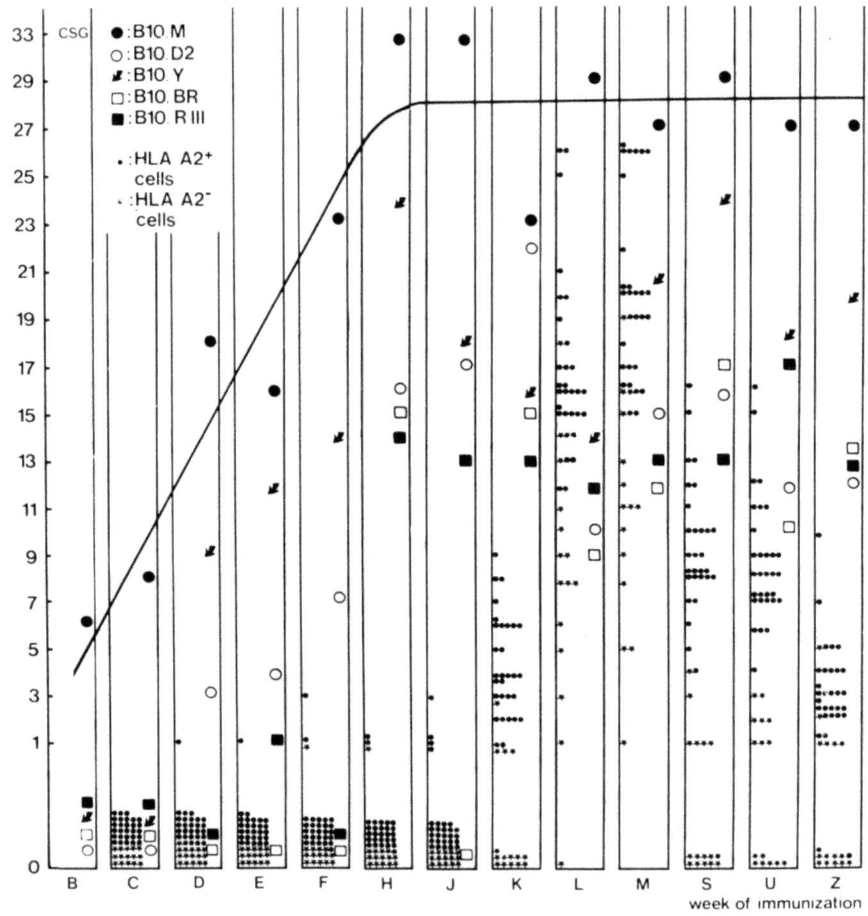

Figure 3. Specificity of anti-H-2 and anti-human cytotoxic antibodies during long-term allo-immunization. Recipients: (B10×A.SW)F_1 (*H-2*^{b}/*H-2*^{s}); donors: B10.M (*H-2*^{f}). (CSG) Cytotoxicity scoring grade; (B-Z) weeks of immunization; last week when recipients were injected was week N. Every week, a serum pool obtained from the bleeding of 5–15 mice was tested. (——) CSG for the donor B10.M strain.

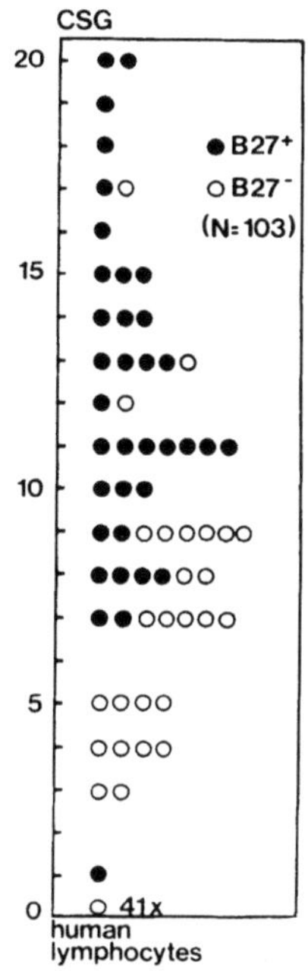

Figure 4. H-2/HLA cross-reactions. Cytotoxic effect of anti-H-2p serum on human lymphocytes. Of the 103 cells tested, 24 were from patients with ankylosing spondylitis, 18 from patients with juvenile rheumatoid arthritis, and 61 from normal patients. (CSG) Cytotoxicity scoring grade.

do occur with the production of anti-H-2 antibodies against determinants common to several H-2 alleles.

7.5. The Reaction Patterns of Anti-H-2 Sera Correlate Strongly with the Presence of Certain HLA Antigens

H-2 sera can be subdivided into two categories: (1) sera strongly positive with some cells and less positive or negative with other cells, but without correlation to any HLA antigen; and (2) sera with low or high correlations to certain HLA antigens.

The variables are (1) the donor–recipient combination and (2) the time in the course of immunization at which the serum is examined. The example in Fig. 3 shows that all samples significantly correlated with the presence of HLA-A2. However, (1) samples J and K were weak and reacted at dilutions of 1:4–1:8 only with some few A2 cells; (2) samples L and K were very strong and reacted positively with almost all human cells, but significantly more strongly with A2 cells; and (3) samples S, U, V, and Z were weaker, but reacted positively almost exclusively with A2 cells. Sample U separated, without exception, A2+ from A2− cells, although we do not expect the small difference in the cytotoxicity scoring grades (CSG 3 and CSG 5) to be reliably reproducible. Similar degrees of correlation were found for other HLA antigens (Fig. 3–5). Absorptions

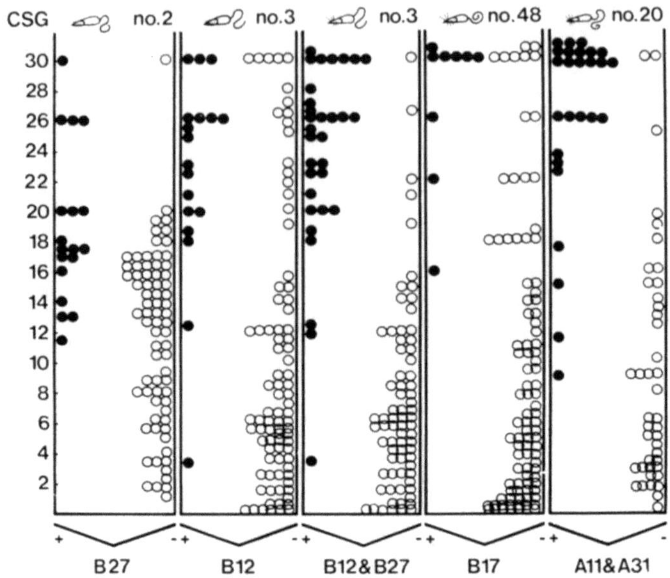

Figure 5. H-2/HLA cross-reactions. Cytotoxic effect of four individual mice sera on a panel of human lymphocytes. Donor: B10.A; recipient B10.A(4R); ($D^b \rightarrow D^d$). All samples of serum were from one bleeding after 19 weeks of immunization. (CSG) Cytotoxicity scoring grade.

cannot basically change this situation, i.e., the number of exceptions. However, by the appropriately selected borderlines (high and low CSG), significant correlation coefficients as high as 0.80–0.90 were obtained. Table 4 gives a list of the best associations found, and examples are shown in Figs. 3–5.

The overall results obtained from the works on serologically defined H-2/HLA CR are summarized in Table 5, in the form of the H-2/HLA chart. The chart was compiled on the basis of (1) data about *H-2* haplotypes of the mouse strains used for the production of the anti-H-2 sera that showed significant associations with HLA antigens; (2) absorption experiments of H-2 sera with mouse cells and subsequent retesting on human cells; and (3) the significant associations of the H-2 sera with HLA antigens. The chart can be read as follows (e.g., rows 2 and 1): the $H\text{-}2^d$ haplotype (row 2) contains, at its K end, structures that cross-react (weakly) with HLA-A2, and at its D end, structures that cross-react (strongly) with B27, B12, B37, and A11 and/or Aw31; the $H\text{-}2^b$ haplotype (row 1) does not contain these structures. This chart attempts to summarize serological data and does not imply structural relationships.

The $H\text{-}2^f$ serum, which correlated with HLA-A2 (see Fig. 3), was

TABLE 4. List of Anti-H-2 Sera That Showed the Highest Correlations with Certain HLA Antigens[a]

Donor strain and *H-2* haplotype	Recipient strain and *H-2* haplotype	Highest correlation with HLA antigen
C3H.NB $H\text{-}2^{p}$	(C3H – A.CA)F_1 ($H\text{-}2^{k}$ – $H\text{-}2^{f}$)	B27
A.CA $H\text{-}2^{f}$	(C3H – A.SW)F_1 ($H\text{-}2^{k}$ – $H\text{-}2^{s}$)	B7
B10.M $H\text{-}2^{f}$	(B10 – A.SW)F_1 ($H\text{-}2^{b}$ – $H\text{-}2^{s}$)	A2
B10.Y $H\text{-}2^{p}$	(B10.M – A)F_1 ($H\text{-}2^{f}$ – $H\text{-}2^{a}$)	A9
B10.A $H\text{-}2^{a}$ (D^{d})	B10.A(4R)[b] $H\text{-}2^{h4}$(D^{b})	B27, B12, B17, B37, (Bw4?), A11, Aw31

[a]From Ivaskova and Ivânyi (1974), Ivaskova *et al.* (1974, 1975, 1976), and Ivânyi *et al.* (1978a,b).
[b]Highest correlations observed with sera from individually tested recipient mice.

TABLE 5. H-2/HLA Chart[a]

	H-2 specificity							
	K-end		Not mapped			D-end		
	37	8	f	p	p	D^{d}		
	HLA antigens							
H-2 haplotype	A2	A2	B7	B27	A9	Bw4[b]	A11	Aw31
b	–	–				–	–	–
d	–	±				+	+	+
f	+	+	+	–	–			
k	–	±	–	–				
p	+	+		+	+			
q	–	–						
s	–	–	–					
a (k/d)	–	±			–	+	+	+
h4 (k/b)	–	+				–	–	–

[a]Cross-reactivity present (+), weak (±), or absent (–).
[b]The assignment of Bw4 interprets the finding that individual (D^{b} anti-D^{d}) sera correlated with B27, B12, B17, B37; these antigens are all included in Bw4.

tested extensively on individuals of four populations (Czech, French, Siberian Mongoloid, and Cuban) and on several groups of diseased individuals with the same result in all groups ($N = 1063$, $r = 0.73$). Family studies have shown that the high CSG segregates with A2 (Ivaskova *et al.*, 1975). The correlations observed revealed higher values in children then in adults, mainly because of more "false" positives in the latter. Among juvenile rheumatoid arthritic patients, boys reacted more frequently by a higher CSG than girls; in accord with this possibility, an increasing tendency of CSG with male puberty was found (Macurova *et al.*, 1976). These preliminary results support the idea that *HLA*-associated membrane structures responsible for the reaction with anti-H-2 sera differ in their expressivity, dependent on sex and age. MHS relationships to hormone metabolism have been reviewed by Ivânyi (1978a).

7.6. Absorption and Lyso-Strip Experiments

Absorption and lyso-strip experiments indicate that mice antibodies are not directed against the allele-specific major epitope of the HLA antigen.

Absorptions with low doses of A2 cells ($5–10 \times 10^6$) eliminated from the anti-H-2^f serum first the activity against A2 negative cells; with higher doses ($80–100 \times 10^6$), the CSG rapidly declined against A2 cells. With increasing doses of A2-negative cells, first the "false-positive" reactions (i.e., high CSG with A2-negative cells) gradually disappeared, but there was also a gradual decrease of CSG for A2 cells (thus, the number of "false-negative" reactions gradually increased); however, even 500×10^6 A2-negative cells could not absorb all activity against the most strongly reacting A2 human cells. Hence, the specificity for A2 is involved on a somewhat quantitative basis (Ivaskova *et al.*, 1975; Ivânyi *et al.*, 1976). It seems that a substance present on all human cells is responsible for the cytotoxic action of the H-2 serum, and its quantity is regulated by certain HLA antigens. This structure can be a part of the normal or altered HLA molecule itself, an HLA-associated virus particle, or a structure coded by another gene. However, it cannot be the allele-specific major epitope of an HLA antigen. Nevertheless, it is noteworthy that (dependent on the mouse donor–recipient combination in the H-2 congenic alloimmunization) different anti-H-2 sera are in that way correlated with several different HLA antigens.

Lyso-strip experiments. Human cells *HLA-B17* were rendered resistant to lysis with human anti-B17 serum. Such cells became completely or partially resistant to the cytotoxic action of those individual H-2 sera that correlated with B17. This shows that the target for human and murine sera was present on the same molecule. Converse tests (redistribution with anti-H-2 and testing for lysis with anti-HLA) could not yet be accomplished because we could not elaborate conditions for complete resistance to lysis with H-2 sera although 90% of lymphocytes showed cap formation after redistribution with H-2 sera. However, partial resistance to lysis produced by H-2 sera reduced the sensitivity to HLA antibodies (Ivânyi and van Mourik, unpublished results).

7.7. Are Antibodies against the Allele-Specific Epitope (Anti-Private) or against Common Parts (Anti-Public) Responsible for the Cytotoxic Action on Human Cells?

There are three sources of evidence that anti-H-2 common-part antibodies are responsible for the cytotoxic action of the H-2 sera on human cells:

1. In the course of alloimmunization, the anti-donor mouse activity (anti-private) appears much earlier than the anti-human activity. Figure 3 shows that samples with the highest anti-donor titers are still negative with human cells. The anti-human activity develops last, at the time when the serum reveals the broadest cross-reactivity pattern.

2. Certain third-party mouse-strain cells are equally able to absorb all anti-human activity from the H-2 serum as donor-strain cells. Thus, from the anti-H-2^{f} serum, mouse cells with *H-2*^{f}, *H-2*^{p}, and *H-2*^{w7p} haplotypes were able, with the same doses (10–15 $\times$ 10^{6}), to absorb all anti-human activity. The absorption capacity of the mouse cells mapped the anti-HLA-A2-correlated activity in the K-end (Ivânyi *et al.*, 1976).

3. When the cytotoxic activity of H-2 serum against human cells was eliminated by absorption with strongly reacting human cells, the mouse serum still retained its ability to react strongly with the donor strain cells.

These findings strongly support the view that anti-H-2 private (i.e., donor-specific) antibodies are not responsible for the cytotoxic action of the H-2 sera on human cells. This means that mouse and man do not share homologous allele-specific major epitopes of the respective classic transplantation antigens. This finding must strongly influence further speculation about the structural basis and biological role of the H-2/HLA CR.

7.8. Individual Mice of One Inbred Strain Produce Anti-H-2 and Anti-HLA Antibodies of Different Specificites

All serological *H-2* work (see J. Klein, 1975; Ivânyi and Egorov, 1975; Snell *et al.*, 1976; Festenstein and Dêmant, 1978), including our previously described work, was performed with anti-H-2 sera that represented serum pools constituted from several immunized recipient mice. When we changed this approach and began to work with sera from individual immunized mice, we found ourselves in a rather changed situation (Ivânyi *et al.*, 1978a, 1979; Ivânyi and de Greeve 1978). In the course of H-2 immunization, although directed only against differences coded by one *H-2 region* ($D^d \rightarrow D^b$), individual mice produced anti-H-2 and anti-HLA antibodies of different specificities. Of 50 individual sera tested, almost all were strongly positive with the donor strain. However, the individual sera differed greatly in the degree and specificity of the cross-reactivity pattern on a series of allogeneic targets. Some reacted only with the donor strain (operationally monospecific sera), others with 1–3 other haplotypes (oligospecific sera), and some were highly cross-reactive with a great number of third-party cells (the test panel was extended by wild mice). Some serum patterns (types of cross-reactivity) were much more frequent than others. The specificity of the cross-reactivity pattern of the individual sera was remarkably constant during a long alloimmunization

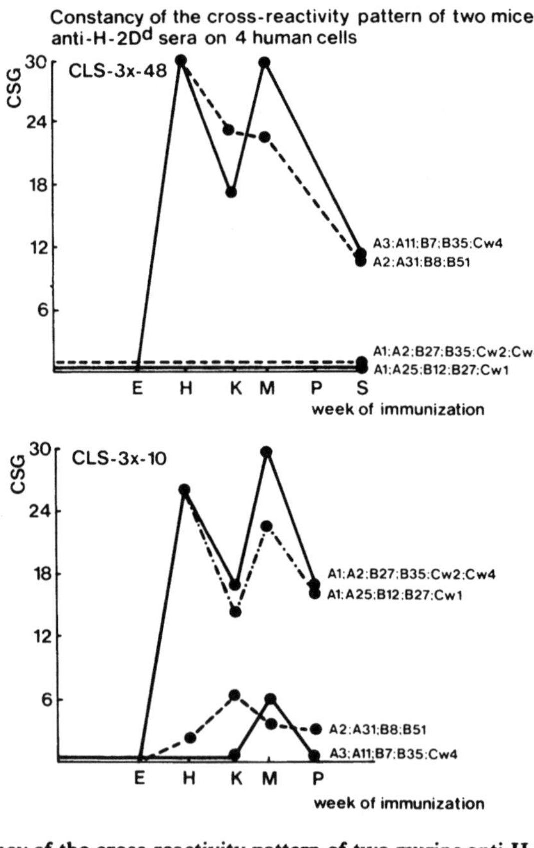

Figure 6. Constancy of the cross-reactivity pattern of two murine anti-H-2D^d sera on four human cells.

period (Fig. 6) (Breuning and Ivânyi, unpublished results). Although the mechanism responsible for the generation of this kind of diversity in antibody production is unknown, we presume that on the basis of clonal preference (or dominance), individual mice differ in their ability to produce cross-reacting anti-H-2 antibodies.

When the same set of alloimmune sera was tested for H-2/HLA CR on human lymphocytes, the same phenomenon was found in an even extended form. The individual sera differed greatly in their cross-reactivity on human cells. Some were completely negative, some strongly positive and reactive with a high (70–90%) proportion of human individuals. Some revealed HLA correlations of magnitude similar to that of other previously tested serum pools. In the combination B10.A donor, B10.A(4R) recipient ($D^d \rightarrow D^b$), the individual sera correlated with the presence of B27, B17, B12, B37, A11, and Aw31. None of the sera still behaved as a monospecific typing reagent (see Fig. 5). Because all *HLA-B*-locus antigens that correlated with the cytotoxic action of the anti-D^d sera are included in the supertypic specificity Bw4 (4a), we presume that the individual mice dissect the complex nature of this antigen. Because, in the same donor–recipient combination, sera also occurred that correlated with A11 and Aw31, we presume that these two antigens share some structural components with Bw4. Alternatively, another product of the *H-2D* end might be responsible for the occurrence of anti-HLA-A-locus antibodies.

We have seen the same phenomenon in a further three combinations (Ivânyi *et al.*, 1979, and unpublished data). In the combination BALB/c donor vs. BALB/c-H-2^{dm2} (loss mutant) recipient, several individual sera contained an unexpected specificity reacting with K^k antigens. Some of these sera were also positive with human cells, although the specificity did not correlate with any HLA antigen. Although the effect was not sufficiently understood, we demonstrated that H-2 sera produced in recipients with a loss mutation exerted a cytotoxic effect on human cells.

After preliminary work with individual mouse anti-H-2 sera, in contrast to H-2 serum pools, we believe that this approach might be interesting both for the analysis of MHS targets and for immunological problems of anti-H-2 antibody formation. First, the individual sera are helpful in dissecting the complex nature of MHS antigens. Second, this approach might extend understanding in the general field of generation of diversity in antibody production (Jerne, 1971). The extensive polymorphism of MHS alleles at several loci provides a unique series of more or less cross-reactive structures that might serve for studies on the extent of diversity in antibody specificity that occurs among genetically identical individuals of one highly inbred strain. For the study of generation of diversity in antibody production, the existence of H-2/HLA CR helps us to extend the series of cross-reacting targets to a very high number. There is no other source for such an extensive series of naturally ocurring cross-reactive antigens.

7.9. Hypothesis for the Explanation of H-2/HLA Cross-Reactions

During alloimmunization, antibodies are produced first against *H-2* structures that developed, probably by mutation(s), after speciation. These allele-specific *H-2* epitopes have a very low frequency in the wild-mouse population (Ivânyi, 1978b; J. Klein *et al.*, 1978). The new structures are not present in the recipient, and recognition results in strong and quick antibody production. Only donor-strain *H-2*-identical cells are able to absorb these antibodies. These (anti-private) antibodies do not cross-react across species barriers.

However, there is also a second type of MHS difference between the donor and recipient. This possibly concerns the more conservative common part(s) of the roughly 300-amino-acid residues of the MHS polypeptide. The recipient might have lost some structural information for, and/or contain partially changed or altered common parts of, the MHS antigen. The reasons for variation in common structures might be different: loss mutations, deletions, or regulatory changes of expressivity or alterations due to incorporation or complexing with virus particles. Some common structures might become exposed only on altered molecules. Similar or identical common parts can occur in 20–60% of wild mice (Mickova and Ivânyi, 1976; Ivânyi, 1978b). Sera raised against the wild-type parental strain in the $H\text{-}2^{dm2}$ ($H\text{-}2^{db}$) loss mutant recognize common structures in a very high percentage of other inbred and wild mice. Some common structures, because of their masked or hidden nature, are recognized only after prolonged alloimmunization. Antibodies against them can be absorbed as well, or sometimes even better, by cells of third-party strains (Ivânyi *et al.*, 1979). These might be antibodies against the evolutionarily most conservative part(s) of the H-2 molecule. Comon structures might be shared, with only minor alterations among a high number of different individuals of the species.

I hypothesize that H-2 antibodies, which occur at the later stages of hyperimmunization among H-2 congenic strains, and which are directed against the evolutionarily most conservative part of the H-2 molecule, are responsible for the cytotoxic action of H-2 sera on human cells. These antibodies are believed to react with structurally and functionally analogous common structures of HLA antigens on human lymphocytes. The crucial problem here is: why do they, at least in some cases, correlate so clearly with some HLA antigens? I presume that by an unknown mechanism, HLA common structures are qualitatively and/or quantitatively influenced by the *HLA-A-* and *B*-locus allele-specific major epitope, to become specifically more or less exposed or sensitive to the action of the murine antibody. This relationship, whether structural or regulatory, is of major interest for further research.

What kind of HLA common structure, specifically regulated by the major epitope, might be the target of the cytotoxic action of the H-2 sera (i.e., anti-public H-2 antibodies)? And why do different, albeit "non-cross-reacting," major epitopes of H-2 and HLA molecules (e.g., K^f and A2) contain, express, or regulate for expression certain cross-reactive structures?

1. The cross-reactions might be due to remnants of some most conservative MHS common structures that are present by chance. The allele-specific major epitope of the HLA antigen, by its regulatory influence, exposes to the cell surface certain HLA common structures or certain parts of one common structure.

2. The cross-reactions might be due to analogous virus particles specifically complexed with certain HLA antigens; similarly, virus-complexed H-2 common-part structures are involved in the generation of the respective antibodies. MHS antigens serve as specific virus receptors, and/or virus particles might occur specifically complexed with, or incorporated into, H-2 structures (for details, see later). The unanswered question remains: do virus structures serve as targets for cytotoxic action of H-2 sera on human peripheral-blood lymphocytes?

3. The cross-reaction might be due to analogously altered MHS structures. Several results support the notion that the functional role of the MHS antigens is to interact with foreign antigens, under natural conditions mostly with viruses. This might be regulated by the allele-specific epitope, but carried out by the conservative common part.

Presumably, analogous cross-reacting virus particles produce identical or analogous changes or alterations in H-2 and HLA common structures. The specificity of this MHS–virus relationship is regulated by the allele-specific H-2- and HLA-antigen major epitope. Thus, some H-2 and HLA antigens will be preferentially related to certain virus structures. This specific antigen–virus relationship is the explanation of the significant correlation of certain H-2 sera with individual HLA antigens, and the target for the antibody (in both mice and humans) is conservative common parts, altered by the complexed virus structure.

The nature of the interaction between virus and MHS antigens, although under intensive study, is still unclear. We list here, in brief, data on widely different models and techniques that might provide some understanding for MHS cross-reactions.

T cells, which have become specific (anti-virus) CTL, recognize the virus in relation to MHS antigens (for a review, see Doherty *et al.,* 1976) either by dual recognition of virus and MHS molecules or by recognition of hybrid structure(s) between the virus and MHS product (altered self). Bubbers *et al.* (1978) offered the notion that "such H-2/virus molecular complex may serve not only as a target antigen for H-2 restricted T lymphocytes but also as a stimulating antigen in the generation of these cells." I hypothesize that in the course of prolonged immunization, antibodies can be generated that recognize the existence of such virus-altered MHS structures. Anti-H-2L^d sera were found that were able to distinguish lymph-node cells between murine leukemia virus (MuLV)-positive and -negative C57B1/10 mice (Ivânyi *et al.*, 1979).

MHS structures can serve as virus receptors (Helenius *et al.*, 1978). Complexes between viral proteins and human, mice, or rat MHS antigens were isolated by affinity chromatography or immunoprecipitation (Gooding and Edidin, 1974; Callahan and Allison, 1978; Helenius *et al.*, 1978; Kvist *et al.*, 1978c) or visualized by cocapping experiments (Schrader *et al.*, 1975; Bourguignon *et al.*, 1978). The virus–MHS interaction, at least in some examples, is specifically selective, because selective cocapping (Bubbers and Lilly, 1978; Zarling *et al.*, 1978) as well as nonrandom inclusion of K and D antigens in virus particles was found (Bubbers and Lilly, 1977; Blank and Lilly, 1977; Bubbers *et al.*, 1977, 1978; Gomard *et al.*, 1977a,b). Some viruses seem to recognize determinants that are common to different histocompatibility antigens in different species (Helenius *et al.*, 1978).

Virus or virus-like particles have been observed on lymphoid or other normal cells (Milner *et al.*, 1976; Collins *et al.*, 1977; McClintock *et al.*, 1977; Takemoto *et al.*, 1978). Viral proteins (Helenius *et al.*, 1978) or viral antibodies inhibit the action of anti-H-2 antibodies (Henning *et al.*, 1976). Mutual influences on their expressivity indicate a close relationship between virus and MHS antigens (see Ehrnst and Sundqvist, 1976, Haspel *et al.*, 1977). *H-2* haplotypes influence the mottled expression of ecotropic MuLV (Tucker *et al.*, 1977; Melief *et al.*, 1978). Interestingly Datta *et al.* (1978) found genetic differences unrelated to *H-2* among *H-2*-congenic mice due to virus integration into germ-line genes during early stages of the development of the congenic strain. The role of *H-2* in allowing this situation to occur remains uncertain.

H-2 sera contain anti-virus antibodies that produce anomalous reactions on tumor and lymphoid cells (Nowinski and Kachler, 1974; Ihle *et al.*, 1974; P.A. Klein, 1975; Nowinski and Klein, 1975; Milner *et al.*, 1976). Some of these reactions might be directed against virus-altered and/or virus-complexed MHS products. As an alternative to the theory of derepression of silent genes, such antibodies have been proposed to be responsible for unexpected reactions of H-2 sera on virus-infected or tumor cells (Garrido *et al.*, 1976; Meschini and Parmiani, 1978; Flaherty and Rinchik, 1978; Ivânyi *et al.*, 1979; Schirmacher *et al.*, 1978). Syngeneic rat sera against adenovirus-transformed cells precipitate MHS antigens in a ternary complex with a 19,000-dalton virus-coded cell-surface antigen (Kvist *et al.*, 1978c).

The type of hormone dependence for expressivity of some virus proteins (Obata *et al.*, 1978) might be analogous to similar indications for the human cell target of H-2 antibodies (Macurova *et al.*, 1976).

T cells stimulated by syngeneic cells coated with Sendai virus specifically lyse allogeneic cells (Finberg *et al.*, 1978; Burakoff *et al.*, 1978). These were initial studies, and the specificity of the allogeneic cross-kill was tested on a limited number of targets. Possibly, different viruses will produce different specificity patterns of cross-kill. If so, this might serve as the cellular analogy of the hypothesis about the role of MHS–virus complexes in the generation of the serological cross-reactivity that extends across species barriers. It was noticed by Finberg *et al.* (1978) that very high levels of cytolytic activity must be attained for the observation of cross-reactivity; this is in line with our results that strong and long-term hyperimmunization is required for alloimmune sera to become xenoreactive.

HLA restriction of human anti-viral cytotoxic T lymphocytes has been reported (McMichael, 1978). Efficient lysis of target cells occurred when HLA-A1, A3, B.7, B8, B27, and B21 were shared with the CTL, but when HLA-A2 was the only shared antigen, lysis was minimal, although this deficiency associated with A2 was not absolute. If a virus-complexed or -altered HLA structure is needed as a target for the killer CTL, individual HLA antigens might be found differentially accessible for this sort of alteration dependent on the specificity of the virus.

The hypothesis that virus-altered or -complexed, evolutionarily conservative structures are the targets in interspecies MHS cross-reactions detected by alloimmune sera has been presented here only in preliminary form, owing to the absence of a number of direct proofs. However, it remains clear that there is no certain explanation for the observation of xenoreactivity in alloimmune sera and for alloreactivity in xenoimmune sera. The hypothesis that H-2 antibodies react with evolutionarily conservative MHS (HLA) common structures, altered or otherwise selectively associated with virus particles under the regulatory influence of the allele-specific major epitope, might be neglected were another more reasonable hypothesis presented. The only published hypothesis for the unexpected serological MHS cross-reactions is that of Bodmer (1973) on series of closely linked silent genes that predate evolutionary separation and the derepression of which is under the control of regulatory genes. This possibility remains an alternative. However, we have not found that identical or cross-reactive "private" antigens are involved in the H-2/

HLA CR. I also feel unable to accommodate our serological findings with present data about the primary structure of the MHS proteins (for a review, see Vitetta and Capra, 1978). These data show remarkable evolutionary conservation in the structure of the MHS proteins; however, interspecies MHS cross-reactions, which we are trying to understand, detect polymorphism across species barriers with the help of alloimmune sera directed against minor allotypic differences. Possibly some more complete analysis of several alleles in different species will finally indicate a kind of fine-structural relationship among the products of different alleles in different species that will specifically correlate with the serological cross-reactions. Thus, we hope that the hypothesis presented herein may at least initiate a search for more direct evidence that would elucidate the remarkable phenomenon of serological MHS cross-reaction.

MHS proteins are complex antigens with mutual differences in a number of amino acid substitutions (complex allotypes). The allele-specific major epitopes behave as simple Mendelian traits and can be used as extremely useful markers in population genetics and for identification of individuals. Intraspecies and interspecies MHS cross-reactions represent lasting obstacles for operational "typing" but nevertheless attract continuous interest as a phenomenon inherent to the system. Recent data have accumulated in favor of the view that the functional role of the MHS antigens is to serve as cross-reactive targets.

8. Summary

The MHS is an interrelated complex of genes located on a phylogenetically conserved chromosomal region. At the chromosomal level, with some exceptions, the individual genes occur in the same order in different species. Comparative biochemical analysis shows a great degree of evolutionary conservatism. These data still do not provide the bases for a reasonable explanation of the experimental findings about cross-reactions across species barriers. The crucial puzzling points of MHS cross-reactions are the *specificities* involved in xenoreactivity of alloimmune sera or cells and alloreactivity of xenoimmune sera or cells. (In the mouse–human model, H-2 sera detect HLA polymorphism on human cells, and human cells evoke H-2 antibodies in murine sera.)

It is presumed that the function of MHS antigens is to become altered and/or complexed by virus particles and other foreign antigenic material. The hypothesis is offered that the alterations or complexes might occur on evolutionarily conservative parts of the protein molecule under the selectively regulatory role of the allele-specific major epitope. Antibodies (as well as CTL) produced against virus-altered or -complexed MHS structures are able to cross-react with analogous structures presented by a series of allelic products of the species itself or by MHS structures across species barriers. Therefore, xenoreactivity occurs in alloimmune sera and alloreactivity in xenoimmune sera.

ACKNOWLEDGMENT. This research was supported by the Foundation for Medical Research (FUNGO).

References

Abeyounis, C.J., and Milgrom, F., 1969, Tissue isoantigens shared by rabbits and mice, *Transplant. Proc.* **1:** 556–559.

Aden, D.P., Mausner, R., and Knowles, B.B., 1978, Production of HLA antibody in mice immunised with syngeneic mouse-human hybrid cells containing human chromosome 6, *Nature (London)* **271:** 375–377.

Albert, E., Kano, K., Abeyounis, C.J., and Milgrom, F., 1969, Detection of human lymphocyte isoantigens by rabbit homotransplantation sera, *Transplantation* **8:** 446–471.

Allison, J.P., Ferrone, S., Walker, L.E., Pellegrino, M.A., Silver, J., and Reisfeld, R.A., 1978a, Partial amino acid sequence of HLA-A9 antigen purified with a specific xenoantiserum, *Transplantation* **26:**451–454.

Allison, J.P., Walker, L.E., Russell, W.A., Pellegrino, M.A., Ferrone, S., Reisfeld, R.A., Frelinger, J.A., and Silver, J., 1978b, Murine Ia and human DR antigens: Homology of amino-terminal sequences, *Proc. Natl. Acad. Sci. U.S.A.* **75:** 3953–3956.

Bachvaroff, R., and Rapaport, F.T., 1973, Immunological studies of the relationship between HL-A and species-specific antigenic sites on the human lymphocyte surface, *Transplantation* **15:**586–593.

Balner, H., 1977, The major histocompatibility system of subhuman primate species, in: *The Major Histocompatibility System in Man and Animals* (D. Götze, ed.), pp. 79–127, Springer-Verlag, Berlin.

Balner, H., van Leeuwen, A., van Vreeswijk, W., Dersjant, H., and van Rood, J.J., 1970, Leukocyte antigens of chimpanzees and their relation to human HL-A antigens, *Transplant. Proc.* **4:** 454–462.

Balner, H., van Vreeswijk, W., Roger, J.H., and D'Amaro, J., 1978, The major histocompatibility complex of chimpanzees: Identification of several new antigens controlled by the A and B loci of ChLA, *Tissue Antigens* **12:** 1–18.

Batchelor, J.R., 1969, The relationship between HL-A specificity and a human species antigen, *Transplantation* **7:**554–561.

Billing, R.J., and Terasaki, P.I., 1974, Rabbit antisera to HL-A9 isolated from normal serum, *Transplantation* **17:**231–234.

Blank, K.J., and Lilly, F., 1977, Evidence for an H-2/viral protein complex on the cell surface as the basis for the H-2 restriction of cytotoxicity, *Nature (London)* **269:**808–809.

Bodmer, W.F., 1973, A new genetic model for allelism at histocompatibility and other complex loci: Polymorphism for control of gene expression, *Transplant. Proc.* **4:**1471–1475.

Borovska, M., Korinek, J., Vaclavikova, I., and Démant, P., 1971, Ss protein: Search for cross-reacting substances in different species, *Folia Biol. (Prague)* **17:**283–285.

Bourguignon, L.Y.W., Hyman, R., Trowbridge, I., and Singer, S.J., 1978, Participation of histocompatibility antigens in capping of molecularly independent cell surface components by their specific antibodies, *Proc. Natl. Acad. Sci. U.S.A.* **75**:2406–2410.

Boylston, A.W., and Anderson, R.L., 1978, Human–mouse mixed lymphocyte cultures, *Immunology* **35**:455–461.

Bright, S., and Balner, H., 1976, The antigens 4a and 4b in rhesus monkeys and stumptailed macaques, *Tissue Antigens* **8**:261–271.

Brown, J.L., and Nathenson, S.G., 1977, Structural differences between parent and mutant H-2K glycoproteins from two H-2K gene mutants: B6.C-H-2^{ba} (HzI) and B6-H-2^{bd} (M505), *J. Immunol.* **118**:93–102.

Bruce, E.J., and Ayala, F.J., 1978, Humans and apes are genetically very similar, *Nature (London)* **276**:264–265.

Bubbers, J.E., and Lilly, F., 1977, Selective incorporation of H-2 antigenic determinants into friend virus particles, *Nature (London)* **226**:458–459.

Bubbers, J.E., and Lilly, F., 1978, Anti-Friend virus antibody-induced resistance of friend virus-infected spleen cells to lysis mediated by anti-H-2 antisera, *Cancer Res.* **38**:2722–2728.

Bubbers, J.E., Blank, K.J., Freedman, H.A., and Lilly, F., 1977, Mechanisms of the H-2 effect on viral leukemogenesis, *Scand. J. Immunol.* **6**:535–539.

Bubbers, J.E., Chen, S., and Lilly, F., 1978, Nonrandom inclusion of H-2K and H.2D antigens in Friend virus particles from mice of various strains, *J. Exp. Med.* **147**:340–351.

Budzko, D.B., Kierszenbaum, F., and Waksman, B.H., 1977, Cytotoxic effects of normal sera on lymphoid cells. III. Selective killing of mouse T cells by normal guinea pig serum, *J. Immunol.* **119**:381–386.

Burakoff, S.J., Dorf, M.E., and Benacerraf, B., 1977a, Specificity of rat xenogeneic cell-mediated cytolysis for the products of the K and D loci of the mouse H-2 complex, *J. Immunol.* **118**:1795–1798.

Burakoff, S.J., Ratnofsky, S.E., and Benacerraf, B., 1977b, Mouse cytolytic T lymphocytes induced by xenogeneic rat stimulator cells exhibit specificity for H-2 complex alloantigens, *Proc. Natl. Acad. Sci. U.S.A.* **74**:4572–4576.

Burakoff, S.J., Finberg, R., Glimcher, L., Lemonnier, F., Benacerraf, B., and Cantor, H., 1978, The biologic significance of alloreactivity: The ontogeny of T-cell sets specific for alloantigens or modified self antigens, *J. Exp. Med.* **148**:1414–1422.

Byrd, L.H., Cheigh, J.S., Stenzel, K.H., Tapia, L., Aronian, J., and Rubin, A.L., 1978, Association between *Streptococcus faecalis* urinary infections and graft rejection in kidney transplantation, *Lancet* **2**:1167–1169.

Callahan, G.N., and Allison, J.P., 1978, H-2 antigens on a murine lymphoma are associated with additional proteins, *Nature (London)* **271**:165–167.

Carnaud, C., Fadaï-Ghotbi, M., Lesavre, P., and Bach, J.F., 1977, Education of human lymphocytes against mouse cells: Specific recognition of H-2 antigens, *Eur. J. Immunol.* **7**:81–85.

Coligan, J.E., Kindt, T.J., Ewenstein, B.M., Uehara, H., Nisizawa, T., and Nathenson, S.G., 1978, Primary structure of murine major histocompatibility complex alloantigens: Amino acid sequence studies of cyanogen bromide fragments of the H-$2K^{b}$ glycoprotein, *Proc. Natl. Acad. Sci. U.S.A.* **75**:3390–3394.

Collins, G.J., Bolio, L.D., Denny, T.P., and Bolognesi, D.P., 1977, Specificity and distribution of the determinants of the major glycoprotein (gp71) of murine oncornaviruses as detected by an *in vitro* cytotoxicity assay, *J. Natl. Cancer Inst.* **59**:99–106.

Colombani, J., Colombani, M., Degos, L., David, C.S., and Shreffler, D.C., 1977, Reactivity of anti-HLA sera against mouse lymphocytes, *Tissue Antigens* **9**:111–120.

Cook, R., Vitetta, E.S., Capra, J.D., and Uhr, J.W., 1977, The partial amino acid sequence of a murine Ia molecule: Lack of homology between murine I-C^d and human P29, *Immunogenetics* **5**:437–443.

Cook, R.G., Vitetta, E.S., Uhr, J.W., Klein, J., Wilde, C.E., and Capra, J.D., 1978, Structural studies on protein products of murine chromosome 17, *J. Immunol.* **121**: 1015–1019.

Cresswell, P., and Ayres, J.L., 1976, HLA antigens: Rabbit antisera reacting with all A series or all B series specificities, *Eur. J. Immunol.* **6**:82–88.

Datta, S.K., Tischlis, P., Schwartz, R.S., Chattopadhyay, S.K., and Melief, C.J.M., 1978, Genetic differences unrelated to H-2 in H-2 congenic mice, *Immunogenetics* **7**:351–365.

David, C.S., Klein, J., and Schreffler, D.C., 1973, Serologic homology between H-2 and HL-A system, *Transplant. Proc.* **5**:461–466.

Doherty, P.C., Blanden, R.V., and Zinkernagel, R.M., 1976, Specificity of virus-immune effector T cells for H-2K or H-2D compatible interactions: Implications for H-antigen diversity, *Transplant. Rev.* **29**:89–124.

Dossetor, J.B., Schlaut, J., Olson, L.A., and Zabriskie, J.B., 1978, Streptococcal infection as a cause of hyperacute renal allograft rejection, *Transplant. Proc.* **10**:483–487.

Démant, P., Capkova, J., Hinzova, E., and Voracova, B., 1973, The role of the H-2 linked Ss-Slp region in the control of mouse complement, *Proc. Natl. Acad. Sci. U.S.A.* **70**:863–864.

Edwards, P.A., Kunz, H.W., and Gill, T.J., 1977, Genetic studies in inbred rats. VIII. The production of xenoantisera against Ag-B histocompatibility antigens, *J. Immunogenet.* **4**:53–60.

Ehrnst, A., and Sundqvist, K.G., 1976, The mechanisms of appearance of viral glycoproteins at the cell surface membrane, *Exp. Cell Biol. 44*:198–225.

Einstein, A.B., Mann, D.L., Gordon, H.G., Trapani, R.J., and Fahey, J.L., 1971, Heterologous antisera against specific HLA antigens, *Transplantation* **12**:299–304.

Engelhard, V.H., Strominger, J.L., Mescher, M., and Burakoff, S., 1978, Induction of secondary cytotoxic T lymphocytes by purified HLA-A and HLA-B antigens reconstituted into phospholipid vesicles, *Proc. Natl. Acad. Sci. U.S.A.* **75**:5688–5691.

Ferrone, S., 1978, The major portion of rabbit antibody of serum HLA-A9 antigens is directed to allospecificity, *Tissue Antigens* **12**:153–155.

Ferrone, S., Natali, P.G., Hunter, A., Terasaki, P.I., and Reisfeld, R.A., 1972, Immunogenicity of soluble HLA alloantigens, *J. Immunol.* **108**:1718–1722.

Ferrone, S., Pellegrino, M.A., Billing, R., Terasaki, P.I., and Reisfeld, R.A., 1975, Production of anti-W24 xenoantisera in rabbits, *Tissue Antigens* **5**:41–47.

Ferrone, S., Pellegrino, M.A., and Mittal, K.K., 1976, Natural antibodies to human lymphocytes in murine strains, *J. Natl. Cancer Inst.* **56**:75–78.

Ferrone, S., Mittal, K.K., Pellegrino, M.A., Allison, J.P., and Reisfeld, R.A., 1977, Immunogenicity of HLA antigens purified from serum, *Transplantation* **23**:7–15.

Festenstein, H., and Démant, P., 1978, *HLA and H-2 Basic Immunogenetics, Biology and Clinical Relevance,* Edward Arnold, London.

Finberg, R., Burakoff, S.J., Cantor, H., and Benacerraf, B., 1978, Biological significance of alloreactivity: T cells stimulated by Sendai virus-coated syngeneic cells specifically lyse allogeneic target cells, *Proc. Natl. Acad. Sci. U.S.A.* **75**:5145–5149.

Flaherty, L. and Rinchik, E. 1978, No evidence for foreign H-2 specificities on the EL4 mouse lymphoma, *Nature (London)* **273**:52–53.

Fu, S.M., Chiorazzi, N., Wang, C.Y., Montazeri, G., Kunkel, H.G., Ko, H.S., and Gottlieb, A.B., 1978, Ia-bearing T lymphocytes in man, *J. Exp. Med.* **148**:1423–1428.

Garrido, F., Schirrmacher, V., and Festenstein, H., 1976, H-2 like specificities of foreign haplotypes appearing on a mouse sarcoma after vaccinia virus infection, *Nature (London)* **259:**228–229.

Ginsburg, H., 1968, Graft vs. host reaction in tissue culture. I. Lysis of monolayers of embryo mouse cells from strains differing in the H-2 histocompatibility locus by rat lymphocytes sensitized *in vitro*, *Immunology* **14:**621–630.

Gomard, E., Duprez, V., Henin, Y., and Levy, J.P., 1977a, Relationships between H-2 and viral antigens in murine oncornavirus-induced tumors, *J. Immunogenet.* **4:**35–45.

Gomard, E., Duprez, V., Reme, T., Colombani, M.J., and Levy, J.P., 1977b, Exclusive involvement of H-2D^b or H-2K^d product in the interaction between T-killer lymphocytes and syngeneic H-2^b or H-2^d viral lymphomas, *J. Exp. Med.* **146:**909–922.

Gooding, L.R., and Edidin, M., 1974, Cell surface antigens of a mouse testicular teratoma, identification of an antigen physically associated with H-2 antigens on tumor cells, *J. Exp. Med.* **140:**61–78.

Gorer, P.A., 1936, The detection of antigenic difference in mouse erythrocytes by the employment of immune sera, *Br. J. Exp. Pathol.* **17:**42–50.

Gorer, P.A., and O'Gorman, 1956, The cytotoxic activity of isoantibodies in mice, *Transplant. Bull.* **3:**142–143.

Götze, D., Ferrone, S., and Reisfeld, R.A., 1972, Serologic cross-reactivity between H-2 and HL-A antigens. I. Specific reactivity of rabbit anti-HL-A sera against murine cells, *J. Immunol.* **109:**439–450.

Götze, D.B., Lee, S., Ferrone, S., Pellegrino, M.A., and Reisfeld, R.A., 1973, Cross-reactivity between HL-A and H-2 antigens. II. Allogeneic sensitization by xenogeneic soluble lymphocyte antigens (HL-A), *Transplant. Proc.* **1:**467–470.

Haspel, M., Pellegrino, M.A., Lampert, P.W., and Oldstone, M.B.A., 1977, Human histocompatibility determinants and virus antigens: Effect of measles virus infection on HLA expression, *J. Exp. Med.* **146:**146–156.

Helenius, A., Morein, B., Fries, E., Simons, K., Robinson, P., Schirrmacher, V., Terhorst, C., and Strominger, J.L., 1978, Human (HLA-A and HLA-B) and murine (H-2K and H-2D) histocompatibility antigens are cell surface receptors for Semliki Forest virus, *Proc. Natl. Acad. Sci. U.S.A.* **75:**3846–3850.

Henning, R., Schrader, J.W., and Edelman, G.M., 1976, Antiviral antibodies inhibit the lysis of tumour cells by anti-H-2 sera, *Nature (London)* **263:**689–691.

Henriksen, O., Robinson, E.A., and Appella, E., 1978, Structural characterization of H-2 antigens purified from mouse liver, *Proc. Natl. Acad. Sci. U.S.A.* **75:**3322–3326.

Herberman, R.B., 1969, Cytolysis of human cells by antibodies in normal rabbit serum, *Transplantation* **8:**813–820.

Hirata, A.A., and Terasaki, P.I., 1970, Cross-reactions between streptococcal M proteins and human transplantation antigens, *Science* **168:**1095–1096.

Iha, T.H., Gerbrandt, G., Bodmer, W.F., McGary, D., and Stone, W.H., 1973, Cross-reactions of cattle lymphocytotoxic sera with HL-A and other human antigens, *Tissue Antigens* **3:**291–302.

Ihle, J.N., Hanna, M.G., Roberson, J.E., and Kenney, F.T., 1974, Autogenous immunity to endogenous RNA tumor virus, identification of antibody reactivity to select viral antigens, *J. Exp. Med.* **139:**1568–1581.

Ivanyi, P., 1970, The major histocompatibility antigens in various species, *Curr. Top. Microbiol. Immunol.* **53:**1–90.

Ivânyi, P., 1978a, Some aspects of the H-2 system, the major histocompatibility system in the mouse, *Proc. R. Soc. Lond. Ser. B* **202:**117–158.

Ivânyi, P., 1978b, Studies on histocompatibility antigens and hybrid sterility gene in wild mice: A short survey, in: *Origins of Inbred Mice* (H.C. Morse, ed.), pp. 657–665. Academic Press, New York.

Ivânyi, P., and de Greeve, P., 1978, Individual mice of one inbred strain produce anti-H-2 antibodies of different specificities, in: *Origins of Inbred Mice* (H.C. Morse, ed.), pp. 633–655, Academic Press, New York.

Ivànyi, P., and Egorov, I.K., 1975, *Immunogenetics of Histocompatibility; HLA and H-2*, Nauka, Moscow (in Russian).

Ivânyi, P., Pavljukova, H., and Ivaskova, E., 1976, H-2/HLA cross-reactions, absorption analysis of cytotoxic antihuman activity in anti-H–2 mouse sera, *Transplantation* **6:**612–618.

Ivânyi, P., Gyodi, E., Gyorffy, Gy., Pavljukova, H., Ivaskova, E., and Petranyi, Gy., 1977, Cytotoxic effect of anti-H-2 and anti-Ia anti-sera on human B and T cells, *Scand. J. Immunol.* **6:**431–437.

Ivânyi, P., van den Berg-Loonen, E.M., and de Greeve, P., 1978a, Individual mice of one inbred strain produce anti-H-2 and anti-HLA antibodies of different specificities, *Tissue Antigens* **12:**32–38.

Ivânyi, P., van den Berg-Loonen, E., and de Greeve, P., 1978b, Anti-H-2D^d antibodies cross-react with HLA-A11 and Aw31, *Tissue Antigens* **11:**439–442.

Ivânyi, P., Melief, C.J.M., de Greeve, P., and van Mourik, P., 1979, Individual mice recognize the complex nature of H-2 antigens; unexpected reactions (anti-K^k) in anti-BALB/c-H-2^d sera produced in the BALB/c-H-2^{db} mutant, *Transplant. Proc.* **9:** 642–646.

Ivaskova, E., and Ivânyi, P., 1974, Cytotoxic effect of anti-H-2 sera on human lymphocytes: Association with HL-A7 and W27, *Folia Biol. (Prague)* **20:**283–285.

Ivaskova, E., Dausset, J., and Ivânyi, P., 1972, Cytotoxic reactions of anti-H-2 sera with human lymphocytes, *Folia Biol. (Prague)* **18:**194–197.

Ivaskova, E., Macurova, H., Bavorova, H., Mickova, M., and Ivânyi, P., 1974, Cross-reactions of mouse anti-H-2 sera with human HL-A antigens, *Haematologia* **8:**273–279.

Ivaskova, E., Ivanyi, P., Mickova, M., and Démant, P., 1975, Cross-reactions between the major histocompatibility system of man and mice (HL-A and H-2): Cytotoxic action of anti-H-2 sera on lymphocytes, *Tissue Antigens* **6:**286–311.

Ivaskova, E., Ivânyi, P., Bavorova, H., and Egorov, I.K., 1976,Cross-reactions of some anti-H-2^p sera with HL-A9, *Folia Biol. (Prague)* **22:**58–59.

Jerne, N.K., 1971, The somatic generation of immune recognition, *Eur. J. Immunol.* **1:**1–19.

Kano, K., Loza, U., Gerbasi, J.R., and Milgrom, F., 1975, Studies on heterophile antibodies in transplantation sera, *Transplantation* **19:**20–26.

Katagiri, M., Tanigaki, N., Kreiter, V.P., and Pressman, D., 1974, Common antigenic structures of HLA antigens. III. An HL-A common antigenic marker closely associated with HL-A alloantigenic activity and detected by use of rabbit anti-rhesus monkey cell membrane antibodies, *Immunology* **27:**487–500.

Kenneth, T.H., Fairbrother, T., Hampshire, B., and Bodmer, W.F., 1976, The specificity of naturally occurring heterophile antibodies in normal rabbit serum, *Tissue Antigens* **8:** 21–28.

Klajman, A., Becker, M., Farkash, R., and Steiner, Z., 1978, Xenogenic response of human peripheral blood lymphocytes against murine cells *in vitro*, *J. Immunol. Methods* **24:**9–18.

Klareskog, L., Banck, G., Forsgren, A., and Peterson, P.A., 1978a, Binding of HLA antigen-containing liposomes to bacteria, *Proc. Natl. Acad. Sci. U.S.A.* **75:**6197–6201.

Klareskog, L., Trägardh, L., Lindblom, J.B., and Peterson, P.A., 1978b, Reactivity of a rabbit antiserum against highly purified HLA-DR antigens, *Scand. J. Immunol.* **7:**199–208.

Klein, J., 1975, *Biology of the Mouse Histocompatibility-2 Complex*, Springer-Verlag, New York.

Klein, J., 1978, H-2 mutations: Their genetics and effect on immune functions, *Adv. Immunol.* **26**:55–146.

Klein, J., Duncan, W.R., Wakeland, E.K., Zaleska-Rutczynska, Z., Huang, H.J.S., and Hsu, E., 1978, Characterization of H-2 haplotypes in wild mice, in: *Origins of Inbred Mice* (H.C. Morse, ed.), pp. 667–687, Academic Press, New York.

Klein, P.A., 1975, Anomalous reactions of mouse alloantisera with cultured tumor cells, *Immunol.* **115**:1254–1260.

Kren, V., Sachs, J.A., and Bishop, C.E., 1976, Studies on the homology between human and rat MHS. 1. Allogeneic affect of xenogeneic rat anti-human immunization, *Folia Biol. (Prague)* **22**:60–62.

Kvist, S., Klareskog, L., and Peterson, P.A. 1978a, Identification of H-2 and Ia-antigen analogues in several species by immunological cross-reactions of xenoantisera, *Scand. J. Immunol.* **7**:447–452.

Kvist, S., Östberg, L., and Peterson, P.A., 1978b, Reactions and cross-reactions of a rabbit anti-H2 antigen serum, *Scand. J. Immunol.* **7**:265–276.

Kvist, S., Östberg, L., Persson, H., Philipson, L., and Peterson, P.A., 1978c, Molecular association between transplantation antigens and cell surface antigen in adenovirus-transformed cell line, *Proc. Natl. Acad. Sci. U.S.A.* **75**:5674–5678.

Lampson, LA., Levy, R., Grumet, F.C., Ness, D., and Pious, D., 1978, Production *in vitro* of murine antibody to a human histocompatibility alloantigen, *Nature (London)* **271**: 461–462.

Lepage, V., Degos, L., Dausset, J., and Dehay, C., 1976, A "natural" anti-HLA-A2 antibody reacting with homozygous cells, *Tissue Antigens* **6**:139–142.

Lindahl, K.F., and Bach, F.H., 1975, Human lymphocytes recognise mouse alloantigens, *Nature (London)* **254**:607–609.

Lindahl, K.F., and Bach, F.H., 1976, Genetic and cellular aspects of xenogeneic mixed leukocyte culture reaction, *J. Exp. Med.* **144**:305–318.

Macurova, H., Ivaskova, E., Havelka, S., and Ivânyi, P., 1976, HL-A antigens in juvenile rheumatoid arthritis, *J. Immunogenet. 3*:229–236.

Maizels, R.M., Frelinger, J.A., and Hood, L., 1978, Partial amino acid sequences of mouse transplantation antigens, *Immunogentics* **7**:425–444.

Martinis, J., and Bach, F.H., 1977a, Human LD antigens are present on xenogeneic cells, *Nature (London)* **266**:540–542.

Martinis, J., and Bach, F.H., 1977b, LD sharing between species. *Transpl. Proc.* **9**:1235–1237.

McClintock, P.R., Ihle, J.N., and Joseph, D.R., 1977, Expression of AKR murine leukemia virus gp71-like and Balb(x) gp71-like antigens in normal mouse tissues in the absence of overt virus expression, *J. Exp. Med.* **146**:422–434.

McDonald, B.L., Hawkins, B.R., Dawkins, R.L., and Davey, M.G., 1977, Characterization of human heterophile antibodies apparently induced by allo-immunization, *Vox Sang.* **33**:143–149.

McMichael, A., 1978, HLA restriction of human cytotoxic T lymphocytes specific for influenza virus, *J. Exp. Med.* **148**:1458–1467.

McMillan, M., Cecka, J.M., Murphy, D.B., McDevitt, H.O., and Hood, L., 1977, Structure of murine la antigens: Partial NH_2-terminal amino acid sequences of products of the I-E or I-C subregion, *Proc. Natl. Acad. Sci. U.S.A.* **74**:5135–5139.

McMillan, M., Cecka, J.M., Murphy, D.B., McDevitt, H.O., and Hood, L., 1978, Partial amino acid sequences of murine Ia antigens of the I-EC^{d} subregion, *Immunogenetics* **6**:137–147.

Melief, C.J.M., Vlug, A., Barendsen, W., De Bruyne, C., and Molenaar, J.L., 1978, Ecotropic type C RNA virus expression and its consequences in congenic resistant C57BL

mice, in: *Advances in Comparative Leukemia Research 1977* (Bentvelzen A., ed.), pp. 78–83, Elsevier/North-Holland, Amsterdam.
Meschini, A., and Parmiani, G., 1978, Anti-H-2 alloantibodies elicited by syngeneic immunizations with a chemically induced fibrosarcoma, *Immunogenetics* **6:**117–123.
Metzgar, R.S., and Seigler, H.F., 1970, Tissue antigens of man and chimpanzees: Their role in xenografting, *Transplant. Proc.* **2:**463–467.
Metzgar, R.S., and Seigler, H.F., 1972, Species-distribution and evolutionary development of HLA antigens, in: *Transplantation Antigens* (B.D. Kahan and R.A. Reisfeld, eds.), pp. 209–224, Academic Press, New York.
Mickova, M., and Ivânyi, P., 1976, Study of H-2 antigens of wild mice (*Mus musculus* L.), *Folia Biol. Prague* **22:**169–189.
Milgrom, F., and Zabriskie, J.B., 1977, Workshop on cross-reacting antigens, *Transplant. Proc.* **9:**1281–1285.
Milgrom, F., Kano, K., Fjelde, A., and Bloom, M.L., 1975, Heterophile antigen and antibodies in transplantation and tumors, *Transplant. Proc.* **7:**201–207.
Milner, R.J., Henning, R., and Edelman, G.M., 1976, Identification of the murine leukemia viral antigens detected on mouse cells by H-2 alloantisera, *Eur. J. Immunol.* **6:**603–607.
Mittal, K.K., Ferrone, S., Mickey, M.R., Pellegrino, M.A., Reisfeld, R.A., and Terasaki, P.I., 1973a, Serological characterization of natural antihuman lymphocytotoxic antibodies in mammalian sera, *Transplantation* **16:**287–294.
Mittal, K.K., Ferrone, S., Mickey, M.R., Pellegrino, M.A., Reisfeld, R.A., and Terasaki, P.I., 1973b, Specificity of lymphocytotoxic anti-human antibodies in normal rabbit sera, *Tissue Antigens* **3:**88–94.
Mittal, K.K., Terasaki, P.I., Springer, G.F., Desai, P.R., McIntire, F.C., and Hirata, A.A., 1973c Inhibition of anti-HL-A alloantisera by glycoproteins, polysaccharides, and lipopolysaccharides from diverse sources, *Transplant. Proc.* **5:**499–506.
Morello, D., Gachelin, G., Dubois, P., Tanigaki, N., Pressman, D., and Jacob, F., 1978, Absence of reaction of xenogenic anti-H-2 serum with mouse embryonal carcinoma cells, *Transplantation* **26:**119–125.
Nakamuro, K., Tanigaki, N., and Pressman, D., 1975, Common antigenic structures of HLA antigens. VI. Common antigenic determinants located on the 33,000 dalton alloantigenic fragment portion of papain-solubilized HL-A molecules, *Immunology* **29:**1119–1132.
Nowinski, R.C., and Kachler, S.L., 1974, Antibody to leukemia virus: Widespread occurrence in inbred mice, *Science* **185:**869–871.
Nowinski, R.C., and Klein, P.A., 1975, Anomalous reactions of mouse alloantisera with cultured tumor cells. II. Cytotoxicity is caused by antibodies to leukemia viruses, *J. Immunol.* **115:**1261–1268.
Obata, Y., Stockert, E., Yamaguchi, M., and Boyse, E.A., 1978, Source and hormone-dependence of GIX-gp70 in mouse serum, *J. Exp. Med.* **147:**793–798.
Parham, P., and Bodmer, W.F., 1978, Monoclonal antibody to a human histocompatibility alloantigen, HLA-A2, *Nature (London)* **276:**397–399.
Parish, C.R., and McKenzie, I.F.C., 1978, A detailed serological analysis of a xenogeneic anti-Ia serum, *Immunogenetics* **6:**183–196.
Pellegrino, M.A., Ferrone, S., Mittal, K.K., Götze, D., Terasaki, P.I., and Reisfeld, R.A., 1974, Cross-reactivity between human and murine lymphocyte antigens. III. Reactivity of H-2 allo- and xenoantisera with human lymphoid cells, *Immunogenetics* **1:**158–173.
Poloskey, P.E., Kunz, H.W., and Gill, T.J., 1975, Genetic studies in inbred rats. V. Xenoantisera against two major histocompatibility antigens raised by immunization with red cells, *J. Immunogenet.* **2:**189–197.
Rapaport, F.T., 1972, The biological significance of cross-reactions between histocompati-

bility antigens and antigens of bacterial and/or heterologous mammalian origin, in: *Transplantation Antigens* (B.D. Kahan and R.A. Reisfeld, eds.), pp. 182–208, Academic Press, New York.

Rapaport, F.T., Kano, K., and Milgrom, F., 1968, Heterophile antibodies in human transplantation, *J. Clin. Invest.* **47**:633–642.

Ratschko, K.W., Stamm, H., Westphal, E., and Muller-Ruchholtz, W., 1975, Search for HLA antigenic determinants in bacteria and rodents, *Z. Immunitaetsforsch.* **148**:407–410.

Reisfeld, R.A., Pellegrino, M.A., and Ferrone, S., 1977, The immunologic and molecular profiles of HLA antigens isolated from urine, *J. Immunol.* **118**:264–269.

Robb. R.J., Humphreys, R.E., Strominger, J.L., Fuller, T.C., and Mann, D.L., 1975, Rabbit anti-HL-A2 sera, *Transplantation* **19**:445–447.

Sachs, D.H., Winn, H.J., and Russell, P.S., 1971, The immunologic response to xenografts, *J. Immunol.* **107**:481–492.

Sachs, D.H., McKenzie, I.F.C., Winn, H.J., and Russell, P.S., 1973, Serologic distinction between soluble species-specific and strain-specific transplantation antigens, *Transplant. Proc.* **5**:477–480.

Sachs, D.H., Humphrey, G.W., and Lunney, J.K., 1977, Sharing of Ia antigens between species. I. Detection of Ia specificities shared by rats and mice, *J. Exp. Med.* **146**:381–393.

Sachs, J.A., and Kren, V., 1976, Studies on the homology between human and rat MHS. 2. Cytotoxic action of congenic rat alloimmune H-1 sera with human lymphocytes, *Folia Biol. (Prague)* **22**:62–64.

Sanderson, A.R., 1977, HLA "help" for human B2-microglobulin across species barriers, *Nature (London)* **269**:414–417.

Sanderson, A.R., and Thorsby, E., 1977, Anti-MHC xenoantisera and alloterminology, *Transplantation* **23**:525–526.

Sanderson, A.R., and Welsh, K.I., 1973a, HL-A specific antibodies by immunization of *Macaca irus* (Cynomologous) monkeys with purified HL-A substances, *Transplant. Proc.* **5**:471–475.

Sanderson, A.R., and Welsh, K.I., 1973b, HL-A reagents from primates. I. Antigen preparation, immunization, and preliminary analysis of sera, *Transplantation* **16**:304–312.

Sanderson, A.R., and Welsh, K.I., 1974, Further studies with HL-A reagents raised in primates: Analysis of the human HL-A2/HL-A28 cross-reaction, *Transplant. Proc.* **2**:163–167.

Schirmacher, V., Marxen, I., and Robinson, P., 1978, Characterization of antigens on murine tumor cells reacting with alloantisera against foreign H-2 specificities: Analysis by absorption with purified murine leukemia virus and normal lymphoid cells of different H-2 haplotypes, *Z. Immunitaetsforsch.* **155**:155–168.

Schrader, J.W., Cunningham, B.A., and Edelman, G.M., 1975, Functional interactions of viral and histocompatibility antigens at tumor cell surfaces, *Proc. Natl. Acad. Sci. U.S.A.* **72**:5066–5070.

Schreuder, I., van Leeuwen, A., and Balner, H., 1975, A further study on the detection of HLA-like antigens in a colony of chimpanzees, in: *Histocompatibility Testing 1975*, pp. 130–135, Munksgaard, Copenhagen.

Seager, K., Bashir, H.V., Geczy, A.F., Edmonds, J., and Vere-Tyndall, A., 1979, Evidence for a specific B27-associated cell surface marker on lymphocytes of patients with ankylosing spondylitis, *Nature (London)* **277**:68–70.

Sher, A., Hall, B.F., and Vadas, M.A., 1978, Acquisition of murine major histocompatibility complex gene products by schistosomula of *Schistosoma mansoni*, *J. Exp. Med.* **147**:46–57.

Shinohara, N., Lunney, J.K., and Sachs, D.H., 1978, Sharing of Ia antigens between species. II. Molecular localization of shared ia determinants implies the existence of more than one *I* sublocus of the rat MHC, *J. Immunol.* **121**:637–640.

Silver, J., Russell, W.A., Reis, B.L., and Frelinger, J.A., 1977, Chemical characterization of murine Ia alloantigens determined by the I-E/I-C subregions of the H-2 complex, *Proc. Natl. Acad. Sci. U.S.A.* **74**:5131–5134.

Smith, G., Walford, R.L., and Fishkin, B., 1974, Antibody specificity for HL-A in human myeloma sera and immune rabbit sera, *Tissue Antigens* **4**:595–600.

Snell, G.D., Dausset, J., and Nathenson, S., 1976, *Histocompatibility*, Academic Press New York.

Solheim, B.G., Fuks, A., Smith, L., Strominger, J.L., and Thorsby, E., 1978, Possible detection of HLA-DR alloantigenic specificities in man with unabsorbed rabbit antisera, *Scand. J. Immunol.* **8**:15–20.

Springer, T. Galfrê, G., Secher, D.S., and Milstein, C., 1978, Monoclonal xenogenic antibodies to murine cell surface antigens: Identification of novel leukocyte differentiation antigens, *Eur. J. Immunol.* **8**:539–551.

Staines, N.A., O'Neill, G.J., and Davies, D.A.L., 1973, Xenoantisera against lymphoid cells: Specificity and use in monitoring purification of mouse and human histocompatibility antigens, *Tissue Antigens* **3**:1–21.

Sula, K., Rychlikova, M., and Ivânyi, P., 1977, Alloimmune anti-H-2 mouse sera inhibit human mixed lymphocyte reactions, *Folia Biol. (Prague)* **23**:263–272.

Takemoto, L.J., Fox, C.F., Jensen, F.C., Elder, J.H., and Lerner, R.A., 1978, Nearest-neighbor interactions of the major RNA tumor virus glycoprotein on murine cell surfaces, *Proc. Natl. Acad. Sci. U.S.A.* **75**:3644–3648.

Tanigaki, N., Katagiri, M., Nakamuro, K., Kreiter, V.P., and Pressman, D., 1974, Common antigenic structures of HLA antigens. II. Small fragments derived from papain-solubilized HL-A antigen molecules, *Immunology* **26**:155–168.

Tosi, R., Tanigaki, N., Centis, D., Ferrara, G.B., and Pressman, D., 1978, Immunological dissection of human Ia molecules, *J. Exp. Med.* **148**:1592–1611.

Trucco, M.M., Stocker, J.W., and Ceppellini, R., 1978, Monoclonal antibodies against human lymphocyte antigens, *Nature (London)* **273**:666–668.

Tucker, H.G., Weens, J., Tsichlis, P., Schwartz, R.S., Khiroya, R., and Donnelly, J., 1977, Influence of H-2 complex on susceptibility to infection by murine leukemia virus, *J. Immunol.* **118**:1239–1243.

van Rood, J.J., van Leeuwen, A., and Balner, H., 1972, HL-A and ChL-A: Similarities and differences, *Transplant. Proc.* **4**:55–62.

Vitetta, E.S., and Capra, J.D., 1978, The protein products of the murine 17th chromosome: Genetics and structure, *Adv. Immunol.* **26**:147–193.

Wilson, L.A., Cowdery, J.S., and Gallaspy, G.T., 1978, Xenoantibody directed against molecular components of the HLA system, *Transplantation* **25**:73–79.

Wise, K.S., Cassell, G.H., and Acton, R.T., 1978, Selective association of murine T lymphoblastoid cell surface alloantigens with *Mycoplasma hyorhinis*, *Proc. Natl. Acad. Sci. U.S.A.* **75**:4479–4483.

Zarling, D.A., Keshet, I., Watson, A., and Bach, F.H., 1978, Association of mouse major histocompatibility and Rauscher murine leukaemia virus envelope glycoprotein antigens on leukaemia cells and their recognition by syngeneic virus-immune-cytotoxic T-lymphocytes, *Scand. J. Immunol.* **8**:497–508.

8

The *DR* Region of *HLA*

Serological Analysis

A.H. Johnson, R. Hartzman, and D.B. Amos

1. Introduction

Following the finding by van Leeuwen *et al.* (1973) that antisera that blocked mixed-lymphocyte reactivity (MLR) were reactive with only a small proportion of blood lymphocytes, many other investigators have developed methods for examining and categorizing the antigen(s) involved. These antigens are present on B lymphocytes and have been designated HLA-DR for HLA-D related. Technical developments include the removal of antibodies to *HLA-A, -B* and *-C* allelic products by absorption with platelets that do not have DR (B-cell) antigens (van Rood *et al.*, 1975a) and enrichment of the lymphocyte population for "B" lymphocytes by adsorption onto anti-F(ab')$_2$-coated surfaces (Mage *et al.*, 1977; Grier *et al.*, 1977), differential sedimentation after rosetting T lymphocytes with sheep red cells (van Rood *et al.*, 1975a; Terasaki *et al.*, 1978), or differential adherence to nylon wool (Danilovs *et al.*, 1979; Lowry *et al.*, 1978).

In 1977, an international exchange of antisera allowed a comparison of reactivities of many random panel donors and of a limited number of members of families. The data were analyzed by the World Health Organization HLA Nomenclature Committee, and the main conclusions drawn

A.H. Johnson • Department of Pediatrics, Division of Immunologic Oncology, Georgetown University School of Medicine, Washington, D.C. 20007. R. Hartzman • Department of Pediatrics, Division of Immunologic Oncology, Georgetown University School of Medicine, Washington, D.C. 20007; and the Naval Medical Research Institute, Bethesda, Maryland 20014. D.B. Amos • Division of Immunology, Department of Microbiology, Duke University Medical Center, Durham, North Carolina 27710.

were that seven specificities were well enough defined to be allocated a provisional (workshop or "w") designation and that these could be allelic products of a single locus, *HLA-DR,* for *HLA-D*-related. The specificities were designated DRw1–7 and the assignments were made so that there was a correspondence, in Caucasians, between *DR* and *D* alleles on the *HLA* haplotype. Three additional specificities designated during the 1977 workshop as wIa8, wIa4 × 7, and WIAA were also examined, but the data were considered inadequate for even a provisional designation to be given.

The Oxford analysis made a number of assumptions in assigning specificities. In particular, it was assumed that similarities among certain groups of sera were due to cross-reactivity. While we agree that cross-reactivity is an important problem, data from our laboratory and from others suggest that there are three additional sources of difficulty in assigning specificities: (1) Some of the antisera contain more than one antibody. These antibodies are not necessarily cross-reactive. (2) There is more than one determinant on each DR (or DR-like) molecule. Some antibodies may identify determinants common to two or more alleles. An analogous situation has been shown for the HLA-B product, where Bw4/6 and LHe sites coexist with the subtypic specificities (Cresswell and Ayres, 1976; Kostyu *et al.,* 1980). (3) Some antisera define unique antigens that were not identified by Oxford and do not define, necessarily, alleles at one locus.

From the onset, there were three main sources of difficulty with the assignment of DR specificities. First, reproducibility was not entirely satisfactory even in the laboratories selected as giving the best correlation in blind duplicates. Second, there was both a lack of good fit for a single locus based on Hardy–Weinberg analysis and also a high frequency (21%) of haplotypes with more than one DR specificity. Third, the Japanese data showed absence of some DR specificities and the existence of apparent new alleles in Japanese (Sasazuki *et al.,* 1978). The significant ($p < 1\%$) departure from Hardy–Weinberg equilibruim and the coexistence of more than one apparent specificity on a haplotype was dismissed in the joint report as being caused by "technical reasons" and by extensive cross-reactivity between some specificities (mainly DRw4, 5, and 6) (Pickbourne *et al.,* 1978).

We believe that there is now overwhelming evidence that the original interpretation (i.e., all DR specificities are allelic products of a single locus) was wrong, and that there is evidence for at least two *DR*-like loci in the *HLA-D/DR* region of the haplotype. Evidence comes from four main lines of investigation: indirect immunoprecipitation (Mann *et al.,* 1979), immunochemical findings of molecular heterogeneity (Tosi *et al.,* 1978), serological data from random panels (Tosi *et al.,* 1978; Ward *et al.,*

1978), and the reactions of clones of hybridomas (Levy *et al.*, 1979). We wish to add further serological evidence and to discuss the probability of two or more *DR* loci.*

While there are many advantages to the massive generation of data that occurs during an international workshop, there are disadvantages, primarily from having to pool data because the mass of information is too great to be analyzed in detail; consequently, fine points are obscured or overlooked in the analysis. Thus, we have analyzed our own data collected during and after the 1977 workshop. We believe our data are informative in a way the pooled workshop data cannot be, for several reasons.

1. Our method of B-cell enrichment, adapted by Mann from procedures developed for the mouse by Mage *et al.* (1977) and further refined in our laboratory (Grier *et al.*, 1977), is based on positive selection of Ig+ lymphocytes. This is more efficient than elimination of T-cell rosettes and gives a more consistent cell population. Only data from individual preparations with more than 85% B lymphocytes (as judged by reactivity with a heterologous anti-DR standard serum) were included in the analyses. This restriction avoided problems caused by contaminating T cells, which appear to have a low density of DR antigens on their surface (Mann and Sharrow, 1980) and can cause false-negative reactions (Zmijewski *et al.*, 1977), or of theophylline-sensitive Ia-positive T cells, which although infrequent have a high antigen content (Shuurman *et al.*, 1979).

2. The use of a shorter complement-incubation time (60 min vs. 120 min) than that of the standard procedure of the 7th International Workshop eliminated many cross-reactivities that complicated the analysis of data from other participating laboratories. For example, B cells from 20 individuals were tested by our shorter complement incubation and by the longer workshop time. Analysis of this data sample reveals that the longer incubation time develops additional reactions not seen with the shorter time (unpublished observations).

3. Approximately 85% of our tests were performed in duplicate. Whenever significant discrepancies were noted, the typing was repeated a third time.

4. Approximately 50% of all typings were read independently by two individuals. Additional wells were spot-checked, especially where duplicate tests showed differences.

5. Comparisons between the assignment of DR specificities given by the Oxford computer and our local B-cell specificity (DuB) assignments

*Findings from our laboratories (Market and Cresswell, *Proc. Natl. Acad. Sci.* **10:**6101, 1980) have now provided chemical evidence for the existence of at least three separate DR-like products coded for on a single haplotype.

(Ward *et al.*, 1978) showed excellent agreement ($r > 0.8$) except for DRw4 ($r = 0.77$), DRw6 ($r = 0.64$), and wIa8 ($r = 0.66$). In addition, in seven of eight instances, the correlations (*r* values) between the two most highly correlated antisera on our local cell panel were higher than the *r* values between the two most highly correlated antisera reported by the workshop analysis on data from selected laboratories.

2. Serological Complexity of DRw4, DRw5, and DRw6

In the past year, we have undertaken an intensive examination of the less well defined specificities: DRw4, DRw5, and DRw6. These DR specificities are serologically complex, and at least six unique serological reaction patterns can be identified (Table 1). Each of these patterns has been observed to segregate with a single *HLA* haplotype in at least one family. The patterns are reproducible on different days and are found in panel donors as well as in families. Reference cells defining each of these "specificities" were included in the lymphocyte panel used to test American Workshop (Phase II) antisera. Each specificity was also recognized with Phase II antisera, thus confirming the discrete differences with additional sera not selected by us (Johnson and Ward, 1979; Grier *et al.*, 1979).

2.1. DuB15 (wIa4×7)

One of the six specificities is DuB15 (now officially designated DRw9, following the 8th Workshop). This pattern of reactivity was recognized by the Oxford analysis but was regarded as cross-reactivity and designated wIa4×7. DuB15 has been extensively analyzed both by serology and by the primed-lymphocyte test (PLT) (Johnson *et al.*, 1978). All individuals available to us and typing as DRw4 were positive with 7th Workshop antisera reacting with DuB15 (Table 1). However, individuals we have classified as DuB15 do not react with DRw7 antisera and show only weak, occasional reactions with two of the DRw4 antisera (7w059 and 7w037). Lymphocytes from DRw7-positive individuals reacted to recognizing DuB15, while 7w057 failed to react with DRw7-positive individuals. The phenotype frequency of DuB15 in our panel is low ($f = 0.15$).

A family with an HLA-B/D recombinant was informative for the segregation of DuB15 (Table 2). DuB15 segregates with the maternal *d* haplotype and independently from DRw7. Specific primed cells could be generated against the *DwX, DuB15* haplotype using appropriate family members as stimulating cells and homozygous typing cells (HTC) as responders in the primary phase. All family members positive for DuB15,

TABLE 1. Serological Complexity of DRw4, 5, and 6: Reactivity of 7th Workshop Sera

DuB specificity	Workshop specificity	DuB15 wIa4×7				DRw4				DRw5				DRw6						DuB31						HLA-D type
		056[a]	057	038	115	059	129	106	037	074	155	126	094	075	111	157	046	179	144	045	099	104	039	102	097	
DuB15	wIa4×7	+	+	+	+	−	−	±	−	−	−	−	±	−	−	−	−	−	−	±	−	±	−	±	−	−
	DRw4	+	+	+	+	+	+	+	+	−	−	−	+	−	−	−	−	−	−	−	+	+	+	+	−	4
DuB47	DRw(4,5)	−	−	−	−	+	+	+	±	+	+	+	+	+	+	+	+	+	+	+	+	+	+	+	+	5
	DRw5	−	−	−	−	±	−	−	−	+	+	+	+	+	±	±	−	−	−	+	+	+	±	+	+	5
DuB31		−	−	−	−	−	±	+	−	−	−	−	+	+	±	+	−	−	−	+	+	+	±	+	+	−
	DRw6	−	−	−	−	−	−	−	−	−	−	−	±	+	+	+	+	+	+	−	−	−	−	−	+	6

[a]Serum number as designated by the 7th International Workshop.

Table 2. Segregation of DuB15

		HLA-A	HLA-C	HLA-B	HLA-DR	HLA-D	DuB15-PLT[a]	DRw4 059[b]	DRw4 129	DRw4 106	DRw4 037	DuB15 056	DuB15 057	DuB15 038	DuB15 115	DRw7 051	DRw7 077	DRw7 069	DRw7 054	DRw7 052
Father	*a*	1	−	7	w2	w2	−	−	−	−	−	−	−	−	−	−	−	−	−	−
	b	2	−	51	w2	−		−	−	−	−	−	−	−	−	−	−	−	−	−
Mother	*c*	w30	−	w44	w7	w7	++	−	−	−	−	±	−	±	±[c]	+	+	+	+	+
	d	26	−	w38	DuB15	−		−	−	±	−	+	+	+	+	−	−	−	−	−
Ch 1	*b*	2	−	51	w2	−	−	−	−	−	−	−	−	−	−	−	−	−	−	−
	c	w30	−	w44	w7	w7		−	−	−	−	±	−	±	±	+	+	+	+	+
Ch 2[d]	*b*	2	−	51	w2	−	++	−	−	−	−	−	−	−	−	−	−	−	−	−
	c/d	w30	−	w44	DuB15	−		−	−	±	−	+	+	+	+	−	−	−	−	−
Ch 3	*b*	2	−	51	w2	−	++	−	−	−	−	−	−	−	−	−	−	−	−	−
	d	26	−	w38	DuB15	−		−	−	±	−	+	+	+	+	−	−	−	−	−
Ch 4	*a*	1	−	7	w2	w2	++	−	−	−	−	−	−	−	−	−	−	−	−	−
	d	26	−	w38	DuB15	−		−	−	±	−	+	+	+	+	−	−	−	−	−
Ch 5	*b*	2	−	51	w2	−	++	−	−	−	−	−	−	−	−	−	−	−	−	−
	d	26	−	w38	DuB15	−		−	−	±	−	+	+	+	+	−	−	−	−	−

[a](+ +) Restimulation in secondary phase (> 70% of positive control) of a cell primed against the *Dw* − , *DuB15* haplotype; (−) no restimulation. Combinations used in the primary phase: (1) responder, Dw7 HTC; stimulator, mother; and (2) responder, Dw2 HTC; stimulator, Ch 4.
[b]Serum number as assigned by the 7th International Workshop.
[c]Deduced from segregation patterns.
[d]HLA-B/D recombinant.

including the HLA-B/D recombinant, restimulated PLT cells made against the *DwX-DuB15* haplotype (Table 2). Two unrelated individuals positive for DuB15 (*Dw3, DRw3, DuB15* and *Dw2, DRw2, DuB15*) restimulated these PLT cells to a level equal to restimulation by family members; other unrelated individuals lacking DuB15 failed to do so.*

2.2. DRw4

DRw4-positive individuals, even cells homozygous for DRw4, do not react with antisera used to define DRw5 or DRw6, but do react with 7th Workshop sera used to define DuB15. The frequency of DRw4 was 3% in our reference panel: DRw4 segregated independently in two reference families. Segregation of DRw4 in one family is shown in Table 3. (Recently available DuB15 antisera do not react with DRw4-positive cells.)

2.3. DuB47 (DRw4, 5)

In one of our HLA recombinant reference families, DRw4 and DRw5 segregate together on a single *HLA* haplotype. We identify this specificity as DuB47. DuB47-positive individuals HLA-D type as a probable Dw5 with HTC. DuB47-positive cells are characteristically positive with DRw4 antisera, but not with DuB15 (wIa4 × 7) antisera. The segregation patterns in the family are given in Table 4. DuB47 segregated with the *HLA-B* end of the *HLA* complex. The frequency of DuB47 in our mainly Caucasian reference panel is 0.9%.

2.4. DRw5

DRw5 is defined here by the antisera used during the Oxford workshop. We agree that this specificity is unique. DRw5 has been seen to segregate as a single specificity in two of our reference families. One, shown in Table 3, had DRw4 and DRw5 segregating independently and with no apparent cross-reactivity. In this family, Ch3 is a paternal HLA-A/B recombinant. A second family with DRw5 is shown in Table 4.

2.5. DuB31

DuB31 (Ward *et al.*, 1978; Johnson and Ward, 1979) was originally defined by a cluster of antisera not recognized in the Oxford analysis.

*Subsequently, during the 8th International Workshop, the DuB15 specificity was well defined by several antisera and was officially designated DRw9. In addition, at least one homozygous typing cell (8w316) gives typing responses with DRw9-positive individuals and serologically similar B-cell types.

TABLE 3. Segregation of DRw4 and DRw5

							DuB15				DRw4				DRw5				DRw6					
		HLA-A	HLA-C	HLA-B	HLA-DR	HLA-D	056[a]	057	038	115	059	129	106	037	074	155	126	094	075	111	157	046	144	179
Father	*a*	w24	w2	27	w4	w4	+	+	+	+	+	+	+	+	−	−	−	+	−	−	−	−	−	−
	b	2	w5	w44	w5	w5	−	−	−	−	±	−	−	−	+	+	+	+	+	+	+	−	−	−
Mother	*c*	1	−	8	w7	w7	−	−	−	−	−	−	−	−	−	−	−	−	−	−	−	−	−	−
	d	3	−	7	w2	w2	−	−	−	−	−	−	−	−	−	−	−	−	−	−	−	+	+	+
Ch 1,2	*a*	w24	w2	27	w4	w4	+	+	+	+	+	+	+	+	−	−	−	+	−	−	−	−	−	−
	d	3	−	7	w2	w2	−	−	−	−	−	−	−	−	−	−	−	−	−	−	−	+	+	+
Ch 3[b]	*a/b*	2	w2	27	w4	w4	+	+	+	+	+	+	+	+	−	−	−	+	−	−	−	−	−	−
	d	3	−	7	w2	w2	−	−	−	−	−	−	−	−	−	−	−	−	−	−	−	+	+	+
Ch 4,5	*b*	2	w5	w44	w5	w5	−	−	−	−	±	−	−	−	+	+	+	+	±	±	+	−	−	−
6,7	*d*	3	−	7	w2	w2	−	−	−	−	−	−	−	−	−	−	−	−	−	−	−	+	+	+
Ch 8,9	*a*	w24	w2	27	w4	w4	+	+	+	+	+	+	+	+	−	−	−	+	−	−	−	−	−	−
	c	1	−	8	w7	w7	−	−	−	−	−	−	−	−	−	−	−	−	+	+	+	−	−	−

[a]Serum number as assigned by the 7th International Workshop.
[b]HLA-A/B recombinant.

TABLE 4. Segregation of DuB47 (DRw4,5)

		HLA-A	HLA-C	HLA-B	HLA-DR	HLA-D	DuB15				DRw4				DRw5				DRw6					
							056[a]	057	038	115	059	129	106	037	074	155	126	094	075	111	157	046	144	179
Father	*a*	28	–	w44	DuB47	(w5)[c]	–	–	–	–	+	+	+	±	+	+	+	+	+	+	+	?	?	?
	b	2	w4	w35	w2	(w2)[c]	–	–	–	–	–	–	–	–	–	–	–	–	–	–	–	+	+	+
Mother	*c*	3	–	7	w2	w2	–	–	–	–	–	–	–	–	–	–	–	–	–	–	–	+	+	+
	d	(3)	w4	w35	w1	w1	–	–	–	–	–	–	–	–	–	–	–	–	–	–	–	–	–	–
Ch 1	*a*	28	–	w44	DuB47	w5	–	–	–	–	+	+	+	±	+	+	+	+	+	+	+	?	?	?
	c	3	–	7	w2	w2	–	–	–	–	–	–	–	–	–	–	–	–	–	–	–	+	+	+
Ch 2	*b*	2	w4	w35	w2	(w2)	–	–	–	–	–	–	–	–	–	–	–	–	–	–	–	+	+	+
	c	3	–	7	w2	w2	–	–	–	–	–	–	–	–	–	–	–	–	–	–	–	+	+	+
Ch 3[b]	*a/b*	28	w4	w35	w2	(w2)	–	–	–	–	–	–	–	–	–	–	–	–	–	–	–	+	+	+
	c	3	–	7	w2	w2	–	–	–	–	–	–	–	–	–	–	–	–	–	–	–	+	+	+

[a]Serum number as assigned by the 7th International Workshop.
[b]HLA-A/B recombinant.
[c]Gives equivocal double normalized values (DNV).

Antisera in this cluster were apparently multispecific and reacted with either DRw4 or DRw5 or with DRw3, DRw5, DRw6, and DRw8. This specificity has been determined to be strongly represented in other populations (Grier *et al.*, 1979). Independent segregation of DuB31 is shown in Table 5. The paternal *a* haplotype types serologically as DRw5, while the maternal *d* haplotype types serologically as DuB31. Three children in this family received the *a* and *d* haplotypes *(Dw-, DRw5/Dw-, DuB31)*.*

DRw serology of 7th Workshop HTC shows patterns similar to those in Table 1 [for comparison, see Table 3.26 of the joint report on cellular typing (Festenstein and Oliver, 1978)]. HTC for Dw1, 2, 3, 4, and 7 gave internally consistent reactions with the antisera best defining the corresponding DRw specificity. The HTC available to the 7th International Workshop for Dw5 gave poor internal correlation of HTC and complex serological patterns. B-cell typing data with workshop antisera are given in the joint report for five cells that were submitted to the workshop as Dw5 HTC (7w522, 7w554, 7w555, 7w523, 7w553). None of these five cells gave the same B-cell serological pattern. HTC 7w523 and 7w553 were two of the three HTCs that gave the "best" definition of Dw5. HTC 7w523 lacked the corresponding DRw5 antigen. It reacted weakly with one DRw4 antiserum (7w106), two DRw5 antisera (7w074, 7w094), and two DRw2+6 antisera (7w075, 7w111). DuB31-positive cells also give positive reactions with all but one, 7w074, of the antisera that react with HTC 7w523 (see Table 1). HTC 7w553 typed serologically identical to the DRw5 pattern shown in Table 1. HTC 7w554 most closely fits the DuB47 (DRw4, 5, 6) pattern. One HTC, 7w522, typed serologically as DRw4. HTC 7w555 was positive for two DR specificities. These serological differences among Dw5 HTC emphasize the complexity of the D/DR region.

3. Serological Evidence for a Second Allelic Series

A local antiserum, MAX, has been particularly informative in identification of a second B-cell allelic series. Antiserum MAX was produced by immunizing a father (*A2, B8, CwX, DRw6, Dw6/A3, B7, CwX, DRw2, Dw2*) against lymphocytes from his son having the same *A2, B8* haplotype and a maternal *Aw31, B14, Cw8, DRw7, Dw7* haplotype. Initially, we

*All DuB31-positive cells reacted with one possibly operationally monospecific antiserum (8w719) in the 8th International Workshop. Several DRw7 antisera also reacted with DuB31-positive cells. This specificity was designated 8w13 in the pre-workshop analysis but not considered well enough defined to be given an official DR designation. One HTC (8w319) gave typing responses with most individuals typing as DuB31.

TABLE 5. Segregation of DRw5 and DuB31

		HLA-A	HLA-C	HLA-B	HLA-DR	HLA-D	DRw4 059[a]	DRw4 129	DRw4 106	DRw4 037	DRw5 074	DRw5 155	DRw5 126	DRw5 094	DRw6 075	DRw6 111	DRw6 157	DRw6 046	DRw6 144	DRw6 179	DuB31 045	DuB31 099	DuB31 104	DuB31 106	DuB31 039	DuB31 091	DuB31 097
Father																											
	a	w30	w4	w53	w5	–	±	–	–	–	+	+	+	+	+	+	+	–	–	–	+	+	+	+	+	+	+
	b	–	–	7	w2	w2	–	–	–	–	–	–	–	–	–	–	–	+	+	+	–	–	–	–	–	–	–
Mother																											
	c	3	–	7	w2	w2	–	–	–	–	–	–	–	–	–	–	–	+	+	+	–	–	–	–	–	–	–
	d	1	w4	w35	DuB31	–	–	–	±	–	–	–	–	+	+	±	+	–	–	–	+	+	+	+	+	+	+
Ch 1	b	–	–	7	w2	w2	–	–	–	–	–	–	–	–	–	–	–	+	+	+	–	–	–	–	–	–	–
	d	1	w4	w35	DuB31	–	–	–	+	–	–	–	–	+	+	±	+	–	–	–	+	+	+	+	+	+	+
Ch 2	b	–	–	7	w2	w2	–	–	–	–	–	–	–	–	–	–	–	+	+	+	–	–	–	–	–	–	–
	d	1	w4	w35	DuB31	–	–	–	+	–	–	–	–	+	+	±	+	–	–	–	+	+	+	+	+	+	+
Ch 3	b	–	–	7	w2	w2	–	–	–	–	–	–	–	–	–	–	–	+	+	+	–	–	–	–	–	–	–
	d	1	w4	w35	DuB31	–	–	–	+	–	–	–	–	+	+	±	+	–	–	–	+	+	+	+	+	+	+
Ch 4	a	w30	w4	w53	w5	–	±	–	+	–	+	+	+	+	+	±	+	–	–	–	+	+	+	+	+	+	+
	d	1	w4	w35	DuB31	–	–	–	–	–	–	–	–	+	+	±	+	–	–	–	+	+	+	+	+	+	+

[a] Serum number as assigned by the 7th International Workshop.

observed that lymphocytes from one of our reference panel donors, Daw *(DRw6, DRw7)*, would remove activity only for himself and his mother, but for no other DRw7 panel member tested. Other DRw7 cells remove activity for Daw as well as for all other DRw7 cells. In addition, the antiserum reacted with the majority (but not all) DRw3-positive cells. These data suggested to us the presence of two antibodies against two antigenic determinants, although cross-reactivity as the explanation could not be ruled out.

Quantitative absorption studies were performed (McKeown and Johnson, 1979). Absorption experiments were also performed using enriched B cells (>90% B cells as judged by an anti-DR heterologous control) from Daw- and several DRw7-positive individuals. As few as 1×10^7 B cells/100 μl from Daw or any "typical" DRw7-positive individual could remove activity for Daw. A quantity of 2×10^7 DRw7-positive B cells was required to remove all activity for DRw7-positive individuals other than Daw. Up to 3×10^7 B cells from Daw removed no activity for any typical DRw7- or DRw3-positive panel members. Lymphoblastoid cell lines (LCL) made from *Dw3/DRw3* (PALA-AMO) and from *Dw7/DRw7* (BURK-HSU) HTC were also used in quantitative absorption experiments. As few as 1×10^6/100 μl antiserum of the *Dw7/DRw7* LCL removes all activity for Dw7-, for Daw-, and for DRw3-positive individuals. Likewise, 1×10^6/100 μl antiserum of the *Dw3/DRw3* LCL removes all activity for DRw3-positive individuals. However, up to a total of $5 \times 10^6 \times$ *Dw3/DRw3* LCL/100 μl antiserum in five sequential absorptions failed to remove any activity for Daw or for any "typical" DRw7.

Such absorption results argue against cross-reactivity as the explanation but do not rule it out, since quantitatively more antigen is required to remove a cross-reactive antibody (Eguro *et al.*, 1973). However, five sequential absorptions should have produced a noticeable effect (Yunis *et al.*, 1972). We therefore concluded that cross-reactivity was an unlikely explanation for the results. We preferred to interpret the results as being due to the presence of two determinants on the DRw7 and DRw3 cells used for absorption. Thus cells would share one common determinant, and each would possess a unique determinant. Antiserum MAX would have at least two antibodies, one against the common determinant and one against the determinant unique to the DRw7 antigen.

The common determinant detected by antiserum MAX may be identical to MB2 in the allelic series proposed by Duquesnoy (Duquesnoy *et al.*, 1979), although our local definition of the MB2 antigen is more narrow. Antiserum MC-2 (7w127) from Dr. Fuller shows almost an identical reactivity pattern to MAX absorbed with Daw to remove the DRw7 and leave the antibody against the common determinant ($r = 0.99$; $N = 231$).

4. Discussion

While much remains to be done to resolve the complexity of B-cell antigens, the data suggest that the haplotype carries at least two *DR* loci. The same statement can be made for the Dw determinant loci, since frequent examples of stimulation of homozygous typing cells (HTC) of one D type with HTC of the same general D classification have been noted (van Rood *et al.*, 1976; DuPont *et al.*, 1976). Gene duplication has been cited as a cause for the genetic complexity of the major histocompatibility complex (MHC). Thus, duplication of *DR* and of *D* would not be surprising. In the mouse, genes coding for the serological polymorphism of Ia antigens are found in the *I-A* and in the *I-E/C* region of the MHC (Cook *et al.*, 1979). In his original publications, van Rood equated DR specificities with *D* alleles and believed that the sera were detecting the *D*-locus product (van Rood *et al.*, 1975b). We doubted this because we could easily identify individuals having one *D* allele but having a completely different DR specificity (Ward *et al.*, 1978). Lack of correspondence between *D* and *DR* types is also common in non-Caucasians (Saszuki *et al.*, 1978). However, we originally overlooked the possibility that there could be at least two loci, each with two domains, one recognized functionally as a *D* allele and one serologically as *DR*. If these represent two domains of the same molecule coded for by two adjacent genes, recombination between them would be rare.

If there are, as we believe, at least two DR antigens and two D specificities per haplotype, there must have been gene duplication, and there are three obvious ways in which the genetic information could be carried. (1) D and DR could be coded for by separate genes, each having been duplicated to give at least two *D* loci and two *DR* loci per haplotype. In this hypothesis, the *D*-locus product has not yet been isolated. (2) D and DR could be on different chains of what is now recognized as the DR molecule. This requires that a second signal be generated by the stimulating cell, since the isolated DR product is nonstimulatory. Two α chains and two β chains would be coded for. (3) D and DR could be attributes of different domains of one of the chains, presumably the α chain. This would require that two genes code for one protein molecule and that the gene doublet would be duplicated.

No single measure will resolve the identity of the D–DR determinants. Resolution of the DR specificities into two DR allelic series is the first essential, since recombinants between the two *DR* loci will be missed until this is done. Definition of the DR allelic series will then give better resolution of the role of D and DR in PLT priming and their role as targets for cytotoxic T lymphocytes (CTL). Identification of the second signal for

D-locus priming might enable us to isolate a biologically active *D*-locus product and thus allow us to determine whether D and DR are really products of one locus.

Thus, the simplest model we propose would have at least two D–DR doublets. One method for resolving this, namely, immunoprecipitation, has been successful in the hands of others, insofar as showing the existence of two DR-like molecules (Tosi *et al.*, 1978; Mann *et al.*, 1979). Blocking studies by van Leeuwen *et al.* (1973) suggest but do not prove the close association on the cell surface of D and DR because of the findings of Flaherty and Zimmerman (1979) that two or more discrete membrane molecules may migrate together on the cell surface in the presence of antibody directed against one of the molecules. Further studies of other cell types, e.g., macrophages, and of other ethnic groups might be informative.

We believe that DR typing will be resolved by the elimination of antisera containing more than one antibody, by selective absorption as we have performed with serum MAX, by the procurement of additional antisera, and by the introduction of monoclonal antibodies. The number of loci in the *D/DR* region and their interrelationships to each other, both structurally and functionally, must be resolved to give greater precision to disease-association studies and a better knowledge of functioning of this complex region.

ACKNOWLEDGMENTS. We are greatly indebted to Dr. Peter Cresswell for his helpful comments and to Ms. Janice Kerber for her patience in coping with numerous alterations to the text. This work was supported in part by U.S.P.H.S. Grant No. GM-10356 and by Naval Medical Research and Development Command Research Task Number ZF 58.524.013.1035. The opinions and assertions contained herein are the private ones of the writers and are not to be construed as official or reflective of the views of the Navy Department or the naval service at large.

References

Cook, R.G., Vitetta, E.S., Uhr, J.W., and Capra, J.D., 1979, Structural studies of the murine Ia alloantigens. V. Evidence that the structural gene for the I-E/C beta polypeptide is encoded within the I-A subregion, *J. Exp. Med.* **149:**981.

Cresswell, P., and Ayres, A., 1976, HLA antigens: Rabbit antisera reacting with all A series or all B series specificities, *Eur. J. Immunol.* **6:**82.

Danilovs, J., Terasaki, P.I., Park, M.S., and Ayoub, G., 1978, B lymphocyte isolation by thrombin-nylon wool, 8th International Histocompatability Workshop Newsletter No. 6.

Duquesnoy, R.J., Marrari, M., and Annen, K., 1979, Identification of an HLA-DR-associated system of B cell alloantigens, *Transplant. Proc.* **11:**1757.

Dupont, B., Yunis, E.J., Hansen, J.A., Reinsmoen, N., Succi-Foca, N., Mickelson, E., and Amos, D.B., 1975, Evidence for three genes involved in the expression of the mixed lymphocyte culture reaction, in: *Histocompatability Testing 1975* (F. Kissmeyer-Nielsen, ed.), p. 547, Munksgaard, Copenhagen.

Eguro, S.Y., Dorf, M.E., and Amos, D.B., 1973, Cross-reactions of HLA antibodies. VI. Dissection of a complex serum, *Tissue Antigens* **3:**195.

Festenstein, H., and Oliver, R.T.D., 1978, Cellular typing, in: *Histocompatibility Testing 1977* (W.F. Bodmer *et al.*, eds.), pp. 85–156, Munksgaard, Copenhagen.

Flaherty, L., and Zimmerman, D., 1979, Further study of the mapping of surface antigens of mouse thymocytes, *Proc. Natl. Acad. Sci. U.S.A.* **76:**1990.

Grier, J.O., Abelson, L.A., Mann, D.L., Amos, D.B., and Johnson, A.H., 1977, Enrichment of B lymphocytes using goat anti-human $F(ab')_2$, *Tissue Antigens* **10:**236.

Grier, J.O., Ruderman, R.J., and Johnson, A.H., 1979, HLA-DR profile in Lumbee Indians of North Carolina, *Transplant. Proc.* **11:**1767.

Johnson, A.H., and Ward, F.E., 1979, Serological complexity of B cell specificities associated with HLA-Dw5, *Transplant. Proc.* **11:**1761.

Johnson, A.H., Pappas, F., Ward, F.E., Amos, D.B., and Hartzman, R.J., 1978, DuB15: A B-cell specificity in the HLA-D, DR region, *Transplant, Proc.* **10:**805.

Kostyu, D.D., Cresswell, P., and Amos, D.B., 1980, A public HLA antigen associated with HLA-A9, Aw32 and Bw4, *Immunogenetics* **10:**433.

Levy, R., Lampson, L.A., Dilley, J., and Fox, R., 1979, Human lymphoid cell surface antigens as defined by monoclonal antibodies, *J. Supramol. Struct., Suppl.*, 3., p. 304 (Abstract No. 798).

Lowry, R.P., Person, A.E., Gaguen, J.E., Carpenter, C.B., and Garvoy, M.R., 1978, Technical modifications for antibody-dependent-cell-mediated cytotoxicity versus T and B lymphocytes: T- and B-cell separation by nylon wool columns, *Transplant. Proc.* **10:**833.

Mage, M.G., McHugh, L., and Rothstein, T.L., 1977, Mouse lymphocytes with and without surface immunoglobulin: Preparative scale separation in polystyrene tissue culture dishes coated with specifically purified anti-immunoglobulin, *J. Immunol. Methods* **15:**47.

Mann, D.L., and Sharrow, S., 1980, HLA-DRw alloantigens can be detected on peripheral blood T lymphocytes, *J. Immunol.* **125:**1889.

Mann, D.L., Kaufman, J., Orr, H., Robb, R., and Strominger, J., 1979, Serologic and structural studies of DR-related antigens, *Transplant. Proc.* **11:**668.

McKeown, P.T., and Johnson, A.H., 1979, Identification of a DRw7 variant, *Transplant. Proc.* **11:**1764.

Pickbourne, P., Piazza, A., and Bodmer, W.F., 1978, Population analysis, in: *Histocompatibility Testing 1977* (W.F. Bodmer *et al.*, eds.), pp. 259–278, Munksgaard, Copenhagen.

Sasazuki, T., Kohno, Y., Iwamoto, I., Tannimura, M., Naito, S., Kashiwagi, N., Itakura, K., Aizawa, M., Hasegawa, T., Miyajima, T., Akiyama, N., Juji, T., Tsuji, K., Sekiguchi, S., Yoshida, T.O., Akaza, T., Matsuyama, M., and Toyda, K., 1978, Japanese Regional Report: The relationship between HLA-D and WIA specificities in the Japanese population, in: *Histocompatibility Testing 1977* (W.F. Bodmer *et al.*, eds.), pp. 489–498, Munksgaard, Copenhagen.

Schuurman, R., Matheson, D., Gelfand, E.W., and Dosch, H., 1979, Identification of Ia determinants on a subpopulation of human peripheral blood T-lymphocytes, *Fed. Proc. Fed. Am. Soc. Exp. Biol.* **38:**1423 (abstract).

Terasaki, P.I., Bernoco, D., Park, M.S., Ozturk, G., and Yuichi, I., 1978, Microdroplet testing for HLA-A, -B, -C and -D antigens, *Am. J. Clin. Pathol.* **69:**103.

Tosi, R., Tanigaki, N., Centis, D., Ferrara, G.B., and Pressman, D., 1978, Immunological dissection of human Ia molecules, *J. Exp. Med.* **148:**1592.

van Leeuwen, A., Schuit, H.R.E., and van Rood, J.J., 1973, Typing for MLC (LD). I. The selection of non-stimulator cells (MISIS) and fluorescence antibody studies, *Transplant. Proc.* **5:**1539.

van Rood, J.J., van Leeuwen, A., Keuning, J.J., and Bluse van Oud Alblas, A., 1975a, The serological recognition of human MLC determinants using a modified cytotoxicity technique, *Tissue Antigens* **5:**73.

van Rood, J.J., van Leeuwen, A., Parlevliet, J., Termijtelen, A., and Keuning, J.J., 1975b, LD typing by serology. IV. Description of a new locus with three alleles, in: *Histocompatibility Testing 1975* (F. Kissmeyer-Nielsen, ed.), pp. 629–636, Munksgaard, Copenhagen.

van Rood, J.J., van Leeuwen, A., Termijtelen, A., and Keuning, J.J., 1976, B-cell antibodies, Ia-like determinants, and their relation to MLC determinants in man, *Transplant. Rev.* **30:**122.

Ward, F.E., Johnson, A.H., Amos, D.B., and Zmijewski, C.M., 1978, Human B cell antigens: A description of 34 specificities identified with 7w sera, in: *Histocompatibility Testing 1977* (W.F. Bodmer *et al.*, eds), pp. 529–542, Munksgaard, Copenhagen.

Yunis, E.J., Amos, D.B., Eguro, S.Y., and Dorf, M.E., 1972, Cross reactions of HLA antibodies, *Transplantation* **14:**474.

Zmijewski, C.M., Kelley, M.A., and Ozida, L., 1977, The effect of "T"-cells on the serologic detection of "B"-cell alloantigens, *Tissue Antigens* **10:**237.

9

The Genetics of B-Cell Alloantigens

Dean L. Mann

1. Introduction

Reagent development over the last several years has made possible the identification of a series of alloantigens expressed preferentially on B lymphocytes (Mann *et al.*, 1975a; Winchester *et al.*, 1975). These antigens may be considered differentiation antigens in that other subpopulations appear to express the antigens detected readily on B cells. These subpopulations are monocytes and, under the right circumstances, T cells (Mann and Sharrow, 1980). The role of the B-cell antigens in the immune response remains to be determined; however, if these antigens are similar to the Ia antigens of mice, they may be implicated in or identify immune response genes.

It has been well documented that these antigens are controlled by the major histocompatibility complex in man. Early studies from this laboratory (Mann *et al.*, 1975b) and elsewhere (Barnstable *et al.*, 1976) have demonstrated that these antigens are inherited and are under the genetic control of genes linked to the genes controlling the HLA-A, -B, -C antigens. There is in addition evidence to suggest that these antigens may play a role in the mixed-lymphocyte response. Prior to the serological description of these antigens, it was demonstrated (Amos and Bach, 1968) that a locus mapping separately from the *HLA-A*, *-B*, and *-C* genetic regions controlled the ability of lymphocytes to stimulate in mixed-lymphocyte reactions. These antigens have come to be known as the Dw antigens. Using lymphocytes well-defined for their capability to stimulate in mixed-

Dean L. Mann • Immunology Branch, National Cancer Institute, National Institutes of Health, Bethesda, Maryland 20205.

lymphocyte reactions, and thus having assigned Dw antigens specificities, it has been possible to identify serologically antigens that show a high degree of correlation with the ability to stimulate in mixed-lymphocyte reactions (van Rood *et al.*, 1975). These antisera thus detect antigens known as the DRw antigens.

There is inferential evidence that in addition to the loci controlling the expression of the B-cell alloantigens, there may be additional genes that control the expression of B-cell alloantigens. We have previously reported (Mann *et al.*, 1976) the observation that in HLA-AB recombinant families, certain antisera react in a pattern suggesting that there are genes controlling the expression of the B-cell alloantigens that are linked to the *HLA-A* locus. There is preliminary evidence from other laboratories suggesting that the Dw antigens and the DRw antigens are not identical due to the lack of concomitant serological reactions with known DRw antigens and the ability to stimulate in mixed-lymphocyte reactions.

We will present evidence in this chapter that strongly suggest that more than one locus controls the expression of the B-cell alloantigens. The implication from these studies is that there may be at least two loci with alleles at these loci that provide the genetic control of B-cell alloantigens. This evidence will be presented in two parts. In the first part, data are presented that demonstrated that at least three DRw antigens are inherited in families. Another family study is presented wherein it appears that there is a crossover in the genetic region relegated to the control of B-cell alloantigens. In addition to the aforementioned evidence, immunoprecipitation analysis of solubilized B-cell membranes demonstrated the presence of at least three gene products that have the molecular characteristics of the B-cell alloantigens.

2. Family Studies

B-cell typing was performed by methods previously described (Nelson *et al.*, 1977) and was done briefly as follows: Whole peripheral-blood lymphocytes were isolated by Ficoll–Hypaque sedimentation. After extensive washing with phosphate-buffered saline, pH 7.4, the monocytes were removed from the lymphocyte preparation with 1-hr. incubation with carbonyl iron. The lymphocyte population was again subjected to Ficoll–Hypaque sedimentation. The B cells were isolated using goat anti-human IgG (Fab_2) plastic-coated surfaces. The typing antisera used in these studies were kindly provided by a number of investigators. These antisera were known to detect the DRw antigens as assigned by the 7th International Workshop. In addition to these antisera, we have developed a panel of our own sera that in some instances correlate in their reactivity pattern with the antisera known to detect DRw antigens. However, in some instances, these antisera appear to react discordantly with the serological reactions that demonstrate the presence of DRw antigens, and thus appear to be detecting other B-cell alloantigens.

The observation that antisera may be detecting B-cell antigens that are products of more than one locus came in our studies with two disease populations, Sicca syndrome (Moutsopoulos *et al.*, 1978) and systemic lupus erythematosus (Reinertsen *et al.*, 1978). In these studies, it was clearly demonstrated that there occurred in the diseased population a consistent pattern of reactivity of antisera that was different from that of the DRw antigens. The best example of this was in our studies with the patient population having systemic lupus erythematosus. In these studies, it was observed that a majority of the patients had DRw2 or DRw3 antigens, or both. In addition, it was observed that several antisera reacted with a high degree of frequency in this patient population. These antisera showed no correlation of reaction with the DRw specificity detected in this patient population or in the normal population. The two antisera showing increased frequency of reactivity were Ia AGS and Ia 715. Antiserum Ia 715 showed a correlation with DRw6 in the normal population; however, it reacted with 75% of the disease population and only 14% of the normal population. These antisera were used in family studies. An example of one such family is illustrated in Table 1. This table shows the pattern of inheritance of the HLA-A, -B antigens as well as the DRw

TABLE 1. Family Study Demonstrating Inheritance of Three "DRw" Antigens

	HLA-A, -B	DRw	Reactive antisera having other DRw associations
Mother	A28, B51	7	
	A1, B8	3	Ia AGS, Ia 715
Father	A3, B35	6	
	A29, B12	4	
Offspring			
1 and 2	A29, B12	4	
	A1, B8	3	Ia AGS, Ia 715
3	A24, B12	4	
	A28, B51	7	
4	A3, B35	6	
	A1, B8	3	Ia AGS, Ia 715

Correlations between antisera Ia AGS and Ia 715 and DRw specificities in a nonrelated population:

	DRw1	DRw2	DRw3	DRw4	DRw5	DRw6	DRw7	DRw8
Ia AGS	—	0.48	—	—	—	0.32	—	—
Ia 715	0.31[a]	0.34	—	—	—	0.41	—	—

[a]Coefficient of contingency.

specificities as assigned by the reactivity patterns with the sera known to detect DRw specificities. The reactivity pattern of the antisera mentioned above, Ia AGS and Ia 715, is also shown in this table. These two antisera reacted with the mother and three of the four offspring and followed the inheritance of the haplotype *HLA-A1, B8, DRw3.* As is shown at the bottom of Table 1, these antisera showed no correlation with either the DRw3 or in fact in three instances the other DRw antigen inherited in the other haplotype in the offspring. These data strongly suggest that in addition to the DRw3 antigen, there was an additional antigen or antigens that could not be accounted for by the simple interpretation of two DRw specificities, and thus alleles at a single locus.

During the 7th International Workshop, antisera were distributed to a number of investigators for population and family studies. We utilized these antisera in the study of several families. An observation was made in one family suggesting a crossover or recombinant in the genetic region controlling the DRw specificities. These results are illustrated in Table 2. The father, mother, and offspring are listed across the top of the table. The HLA haplotype as assigned by the serological reactions to detecting HLA-A, -B is illustrated by assigning the four haplotypes in this family as haplotype *A* and *B* in the father and haplotype *C* and *D* in the mother. The pattern of inheritance of these haplotypes is illustrated for the five offspring. The specific HLA-A and -B antigens are noted in footnote *b*. The assignment of DRw specificity, based on the serological reactions of the B cells isolated from the members of this family, is illustrated together with the specific sera reacting with each member of the family. After obtaining

TABLE 2. Family Study Demonstrating Probable DRw Recombinant

	Father		Mother		Offspring									
					1		2		3		4		5[a]	
HLA haplotype[b]	*A*	*B*	*C*	*D*	*A*	*C*	*A*	*C*	*A*	*D*	*B*	*C*	*B*	*C*
DRw	3	4	5	2	3	5	3	5	3	2	4	5	4/3	5
Antisera reactions used to assign DRw specificities[c]	26	59	74	17	26	74	26	74	26	17	59	74	59	74
	24	37	126	16	24	126	24	126	24	16	37	126	37	126
	95	38	155	15	95	155	95	155	95	15	38	155		155
	32			21	32		35		32	21			95	
												32		

[a] Recombinant.
[b] *A*: AW32, B39; *B*: A2, B8; *C*: Aw25, B7; *D*: A1, Bw15.
[c] Numbers designate 7th International Workshop sera and DRw assignments based on workshop analysis.

the results of the workshop, we were able to assign the DRw specificities to each member of the family. The father's DRw type was 3 and 4; the mother's was 2 and 5. The serological reactions occurring with the B cells from offspring 5 did not fit with the paternal *B* haplotype as it was inherited in the other members of the family. The 7th International Workshop sera 59, 37, and 38 reacted with the cells from the father and also reacted with the cells obtained from Offspring 4. Only two of these sera reacted with Offspring 5, these being sera 59 and 37. In addition to the reactions of these two sera with Offspring 5, sera 95 and 32 reacted with this individual's B cells. In the analysis of the other members of the family, these antisera reacted in a pattern consistent with the inheritance of the paternal haplotype *A* in three members of the family and also in the father. The most logical interpretation of these results is that there was a crossover in the genetic region that controlled the expression of the DRw antigens. In our experience, antisera 95 and 32 react in a relatively broad fashion and appear to contain two antibodies or at least are cross-reactive with other specificities. Serum 95 has been studied in some depth and appears to have significant correlations with the presence of the DRw3, 5, and 6 antigens. If one argues for the presence of one locus with multiple alleles, it would be impossible for a serum to show positive correlations in reactivity patterns with three DRw specificities. It is our view that the most reasonable explanation for this reactivity pattern is that there are genes sometimes closely linked (linkage disequilibrium) to the DRW3, 5, and 6 antigens, and thus, the serum detects not the DRW3, 5, or 6 antigens, but an antigen controlled by another locus. While the foregoing argument is speculative, the rationale seems to fit and explain the observed reactivity patterns noted in this family study.

3. Immunoprecipitation Studies

Further evidence to substantiate the hypothesis that at least two loci control the expression of the DRw antigens was observed with immunoprecipitation of solubilized B-cell antigens from a long-term lymphoid-tissue-culture cell line, JY. This cell line is known to be homozygous *HLA-A2, B7,* and *DRw4, DRw6.* In brief, the technique used in this study is as follows: The lymphoid-tissue-culture cell line was grown in the presence of tritiated leucine, and the membrane components solubilized with NP-40. The solubilized material was then exposed to a concanavalin A/Sepharose 4B column and the adhered material eluted with α-methyl mannoside. A 100-μm aliquot of the eluted material was incubated with the appropriate anti-DRw antiserum or normal human serum and subjected to precipitation with the *Staphylococcus* A (Cowan strain) organism. The antigen–antibody complex adhering to the *staphylococcus* organism was then eluted by boiling in sodium dodecyl sulfate in the presence of mercaptoethanol. The eluted material was then electrophoresed on 10% polyacrylamide gels, and the gels were sectioned in 2-ml slices and counted in a beta counter. This technique is detailed elsewhere, as are the electrophoretic patterns of the precipitates (Nilsson *et al.*, 1977). When the antiserum was reactive with the components in the NP-40-solubilized material, materials electrophoresed as having molecular weight of 34,000 and 29,000 daltons. Table 3 illustrates the results of the immunoprecipitation data for single precipitates and sequential precipitation. All reactions were first cleared with normal human serum, and no radioactive peaks were seen in the polyacrylamide gel electrophoresis. This is designated in the table as a negative result. After first being cleared with a normal human serum, the DRw antisera, the DRw6 antiserum, and an antiserum showing positive correlations with DRw3,5,6, as well as a heterologous anti-B cell serum, all showed patterns consistent with the reactions of 34,000- and 29,000-dalton-molecular-weight components. When the solubilized material was reacted with the antiserum detecting DRw4, this antigen was completely cleared, and the remaining material reacted with either the DRw6 serum or the DRw3,5,6 antiserum and the hetero-anti-B cell serum. Anti-DRw6 serum removed activity for this specificity in reprecipitation attempts with anti-DRw6 serum, but did not remove the reactivity of the anti-DRw4 serum and the anti-DRw3,5,6 serum. When the DRw3,5,6 antiserum was used in the initial immunoprecipitation, the DRw4 antiserum precipitated antigenic material and no precipitates were seen with the initial antiserum or the antiserum detecting DRw6. The

TABLE 3. Two-Stage Immunoprecipitation of NP-40-Solubilized Antigens from Lymphoblastoid-Cell line JY (*DRw4, 6*) and Resulting Polyacrylamide Gel Electrophoresis Patterns

Antiserum used in first or clearing precipitate	Antiserum used in second precipitate[a]				
	NHS	DRw4	DRw6	DRw3,5,6	Hetero-anti B
NHS	−	+	+	+	+
DRw4	−	−	+	+	+
DRw6	−	+	−	+	+
DRw3,5,6	−	+	−	−	+
DRw4 + DRw6	−	−	−	+	+
DRw6 + DRw3,5,6	−	+	−	−	+
DRw4 + DRw3,5,6	−	−	−	−	+/−

[a]No radioactive peaks seen on 10% polyacrylamide gel electrophoresis; (+) radioactive peaks of approximately 34,000 and 28,000 daltons.

heteroantiserum in this instance also showed a pattern of positive reaction.

Combinations of antisera were then used in the first precipitation or clearing reaction, and subsequent precipitation was then performed with the individual antisera. When the antisera detecting DRw4 and DRw6 were used in combination in the initial precipitation reaction, the DRw3,5,6 antiserum showed a positive pattern, as did the heteroantiserum. The initial combination of DRw6 and DRw3,5,6 resulted in remaining activity that could be precipitated by antisera detecting DRw4 as well as the hetero-anti-B cell serum. When the DRw4, DRw3,5,6 antisera combination was used, subsequent reactions with the individual antisera showed no precitation pattern; however, the hetero-anti-B cell serum showed small radioactive peaks in the region of the 29,000- and 34,000-dalton molecular weights. Our interpretation of the results illustrated in Table 3 is as follows: Antiserum DRw3,5,6 shares an antibody with the more specific DRw6 antiserum. This antiserum cleared the solubilized material for the DRw6. However, the DRw6 antiserum did not clear for the DRw3,5,6 antiserum or the DRw4 antiserum. This could not be explained by cross-reactivity, since the antiserum with multiple specificities did not clear for the DRw4 specificity and the DRw4 antiserum did not clear for the antiserum detecting antigens DRw3,5,6. When combinations of sera were used in the clearing reactions and individual sera were used in the second precipitation, the results presented above were confirmed. We conclude from these studies that three molecular components represent at least two genetic loci.

4. Discussion

The serologically detectable DRw antigens were developed on the basis of B-lymphocyte typing of cells that have been characterized for the *D*-locus specificity. The D specificity is defined by mixed-lymphocyte reactions. Whether or not it is a molecular entity is an open question. Attempts to isolate the cell-membrane component that causes stimulation in mixed-lymphocyte reactions have not been successful. There appears to be only one major locus that affects stimulation in mixed-lymphocyte reactions, and therefore the serological correlate, DRw, has been assumed to be identical to the *D* locus. This assumption is based on the observation that a number of sera react in a manner such that a high degree of correlation of reactivity exists between the serologically detectable antigen and the ability to stimulate in mixed-lymphocyte reactions. This, of course, does not preclude the possibility that other loci may determine control of the expression of the B-lymphocyte antigens. If the major histocompatibility complex of man is similar to that in mice and one can draw an analogy, one would assume that there is more than one locus controlling the expression of B-cell antigens.

The observations cited in this paper strongly suggest that at least another locus in addition to DRw controls the expression of these antigens. The family studies that have been done and that are illustrated in this paper suggest this possibility in that three "DRw" antigens could be defined. Another observation that has been made is that when typing a homogeneous population of individuals, the Pima Indians, a majority of these patients typed for the three DRw specificities. That is to say, antisera detecting DRw specificities as defined in a Caucasian population (non-American Indian) show a specific pattern of reactivity that is different from the pattern in which the sera were originally defined. The most logical explanation for this is another locus. There is the possibility that these reactions could be ascribed to cross-reactivity.

The family studies wherein a crossover appears in the genetic region that controls the expression of the DRw specificities obviates in some sense the argument for cross-reaction. Such a family is illustrated in Table 2. Similar observations have been made in other laboratories, from which it has been reported that the D antigen does not segregate with the corresponding serological reaction. This implies a crossover between the *D* region and the *DRw* region. As more sera and specific serological reagents are developed, it is most probable that additional crossovers will be detected.

The immunoprecipitation data are probably the most convincing evidence that more than one locus controls the expression of the DRw or B-cell antigens. The ability to isolate three components having the same molecular weights from a single cell source strongly suggests the presence of an additional locus. Recently, Tosi *et al.* (1978) have made similar observations using sera in immunoprecipitation studies. These studies clearly demonstrate the presence of antigens in addition to DRw.

In summary, three lines of evidence strongly suggest that more than one locus controls the expression of the B-cell or human Ia-like antigens. This evidence is provided by family studies, family studies wherein an apparent crossover appears outside the *HLA* and *B* region, and biochemical studies using immunoprecipitation techniques.

References

Amos, D.B., and Bach, F.J., 1968 Phenotypic expression of the major histocompatibility locus in man (HL-A): Leukocyte antigens and mixed leukocyte culture reactivity, *J. Exp. Med.* **128**:623.

Barnstable, C.J., Jones, E.A., Bodmer, W.F., Bodmer, J.G., Arce-Gomez, B., Snary, D., and Crumpton, M.J., 1976, Genetics and serology of HLA linked Ia antigens, *Cold Spring Harbor Symp. Quant. Biol.* **41**:443.

Mann, D.L., and Sharrow, S.O., 1980, DRw antigens can be detected on human peripheral blood T lymphocytes, *J. Immunol.* **125**:1889.

Mann, D.L., Abelson, L., Harris, S., and Amos, D.B., 1975a, Detection of antigens specific for B-lymphoid cultured cell lines with human alloantisera, *J. Exp. Med.* **142**:84.

Mann, D.L., Abelson, L., Henkart, P., Harris, S., and Amos, D.B., 1975b, Specific human B lymphocyte alloantigens linked to HLA, *Proc. Natl. Acad. Sci. U.S.A.* **72**:5103.

Mann, D.L., Abelson, L., Harris, S., and Amos, D.B., 1976, Second genetic locus in the HLA region for human B cell alloantigens, *Nature (London)* **259**:143.

Moutsopoulos, A.M., Chused, T.M., Johnson, A.H., Knudsen, B., and Mann, D.L., 1978, B-lymphocyte alloantigens in sicca syndrome, *Science* **199**:1441.

Nelson, D.L., Strober, W., Abelson, L.D., Bundy, B.M., and Mann, D.L., 1977, Distribution of alloantigens on human Fc receptor bearing lymphocytes: The presence of B-cell alloantigens in sIg positive but not sIg negative lymphocytes, *J. Immunol.* **118**:943.

Nilsson, S., Schwartz, B.D., Wavdal, M., Green, I., Cullen, S., and Mann, D.L., 1977, Human alloantiserum precipitates Ia-like molecules from chronic lymphocytic leukemia cell, *J. Immunol.* **118**:1271.

Reinertsen, J., Klippel, J., Johnson, S.H., Steinberg, A., Decker, J., and Mann, D.L., 1978, B lymphocyte alloantigens associated with systemic lupus erythematosus, *N. Engl. J. Med.* **299**:515.

Tosi, R., Tanigaki, N., Centis, D., Farrara, G.B., and Pressman, D., 1978, Immunological dissection of human Ia molecules, *J. Exp. Med.* **148**:1592.

van Rood, J.J., van Leenwen, A., Kenning, J.J., and Blusse van Ond Alblus, A., 1975, The serologic recognition of the human MLC determinants using a modified cytotoxicity technique, *Tissue Antigens* **5**:73.

Winchester, R.J., Fu, M., and Wernet, P., 1975, Recognition by pregnancy serum of non-HLA alloantigens selectively expressed on B lymphocytes, *J. Exp. Med.* **141**:924.

10

Serological Testing of the HLA Antigens

Problems and Approaches to Standardization

Kamal K. Mittal and Daljit Kaur

1. Introduction

In recent years, the demand for HLA testing has increased greatly, to the extent that it has outpaced the capacity of HLA-typing laboratories to adequately fulfill this need. This is due, in part, to an increasing application of HLA typing not only to organ and tissue transplantation, but also to granulocyte and platelet transfusion (Mittal *et al.*, 1976). To provide optimally HLA-matched platelets to various thrombocytopenic patients, it is necessary that large numbers of potential donors be HLA-phenotyped prospectively.

The recently discovered associations of HLA antigens with certain diseases have introduced the application of HLA typing in the diagnosis and prognosis of these diseases and to related genetic counseling (Mittal, 1976, 1977). Among the major types of associations are the following: (1) B27 is strongly associated with spondylitic syndromes, and it is suspected that this antigen is fairly directly involved in the pathogenesis of these diseases; (2) Dw3 and B8 appear to be associated with certain autoimmune diseases, possibly through positive linkage disequilibrium with defective immune-response genes; and (3) genes controlling the elaboration of complement components, C2 and C4, are linked to those of the HLA system, and the genetically caused deficiencies of these complement components can be traced in families through HLA genotyping (Mittal, 1977).

Kamal K. Mittal and Daljit Kaur • Division of Blood and Blood Products, Bureau of Biologics, Food and Drug Administration, Bethesda, Maryland 20205.

Another rapidly increasing use of HLA genotyping is in paternity determination. Because of its profound polymorphism, the HLA system is uniquely powerful in resolving questions of paternity with a high degree of certainty (Terasaki, 1978).

The application of HLA testing in these various clinical and medicolegal situations makes it necessary that the interlaboratory variations in HLA testing be at least minimized if not altogether eliminated. Interlaboratory comparability in HLA phenotyping is essential if donors typed in one laboratory are to be made available to recipients typed in another laboratory through regional or national collaboration.

That HLA serology is extremely complex is well known. At present, the generally accepted criterion for determining the presence of an antigen in an individual is that the donor cells react with a majority of the available antisera of the corresponding specificity. Unfortunately, when tested with several antisera of a given specificity, cells from different unrelated individuals possessing the corresponding antigen often react similarly, but not identically. Since standard antisera do not exist for any of the HLA specificities, and the various laboratories do not use the same typing antisera, significant differences may be found among different laboratories in the phenotyping of a given individual. This difficult situation has developed because HLA antigens behave as molecules with multiple determinants, and each HLA antigen appears to consist of a family of numerous similar but nonidentical "variants." Such intraspecificity variation is not limited to any one ethnic group, and may be accentuated by ethnic differences. Further, sharing of determinants between allelic HLA antigens is thought to be the cause of the extensive serological cross-reactivity of the HLA system, a phenomenon that further complicates the serological patterns.

This intrinsic complexity of HLA serology, and its important applications to human welfare, necessitate that some national or international standards for HLA typing be developed. A number of modifications of the basic lymphocyte-typing technique are in wide use, and no well-defined standards exist for any of the reagents used in this test. The inherent characteristics of the HLA molecules have led to great difficulty in the production of monospecific HLA-typing antisera by deliberate immunization. The majority of antisera currently in use have low titers and are only operationally monospecific for their respective specificities. Some steps toward standardization of these reagents appear overdue (Mittal, 1978).

We discuss here in: (1) the unique serological and genetic characteristics of the HLA antigens; (2) the methods of procurement and characterization of HLA antisera; (3) the determination of HLA phenotypes; and (4) the approaches to standardization of HLA typing.

2. Serological and Genetic Complexities of the HLA Antigens

The HLA antigens are known to be serologically complex molecules (Legrand and Dausset, 1972, 1974; Mittal *et al.*, 1970, 1971; van Rood and Eernisse, 1968; Svejgaard and Kissmeyer-Nielsen, 1968; Amos and Yunis, 1968; Ceppellini *et al.*, 1967). This complexity is easily recognized through a wide variety of reaction patterns seen between antisera and cells of the same HLA specificity (Mittal *et al.*, 1970, 1971). It is widely known that different individuals, all possessing the same alloantigen, do not react uniformly with an antiserum of the corresponding specificity. Also, different antisera, operationally monospecific for an HLA antigen, do not react uniformly with the lymphocytes of an individual possessing the corresponding HLA alloantigen (Mittal *et al.*, 1968, 1970, 1971; van Rood and Eernisse, 1968; Amos and Yunis, 1968; Ceppellini *et al.*, 1967). These differences are due primarily to the multivalent or multideterminant nature of the HLA antigens.

2.1. Multivalence of HLA Antigens

Each HLA antigen, as currently defined, is a multivalent cluster of possibly several antigenic determinants (or haptens). Each of these clusters (called HLA antigens) differs from the others in the number and the type of determinants that it consists of. The immunogenicity of a cluster toward a host may vary depending on: (1) the size and the type of the antigenic cluster; (2) the degree of sharing of determinants between the immunogen and the host; and (3) the immune responsiveness of the immunized host, which is in turn controlled by several factors including immune-response genes.

For convenience, different-sized clusters of antigenic epitopes may be defined simply as follows: (1) *supertypic* or multigenic cluster—a broad cluster of determinants that is the product of two or more allelic *HLA* genes; (2) *typic* or single-genic cluster—a cluster of determinants that is the product of a single *HLA* gene; and (3) *subtypic* or subgenic cluster—a determinant or a small cluster of determinants that is the product of a nonallelic subdivision of a single *HLA* gene.

The great diversity in the specificity of antibodies produced against these multivalent structures may be examined as follows: First, each of the three major types of clusters—supertypic, typic, and subtypic—is capable of producing allogeneic antibodies that will react specifically with the given combination of determinants in the immunizing cluster. Second, an antiserum against a supertypic cluster may react with cells from all those persons possessing one or more of the typic or subtypic clusters included in the immunizing supertypic cluster. Similarly, antibodies against a typic cluster may react with cells from all those persons possessing one or more of the epitopes included in the immunizing typic cluster. Third, in certain circumstances, a single epitope or a small group of them may be immunogenic enough to induce a subtypic antibody. This antiserum may react with cells from all those individuals who possess the immunizing epitope(s) either as a part of the same HLA antigen presented by the immunizing donor or as a part of a different HLA antigen.

Antigens 4a (Bw4) and 4b (Bw6) are the original examples of two supertypic specificities (van Rood and Eernisse, 1968). Since then, several other antigens have been widely recognized as supertypic in nature, e.g., A9, A10, Aw19, B5, B12, Bw16, Bw21, Bw22, and others. It is important to recognize that several alleles together behave as a single allele in their genetic transmission at the population level. It is for this reason that the current definition of an HLA antigen as "typic" remains genetically valid even though antisera may be subsequently found that permit splitting of a previously recognized typic antigen into two new typic specificities. This consequently changes the status of the previous "parent" specificity from typic to supertypic.

2.2. Cross-Reactivity of Allelic HLA Antigens

It is widely known that certain allelic HLA antigens demonstrate serological cross-reactivity (Mittal, 1975; Legrand and Dausset, 1974; Mittal and Terasaki, 1974; Svejgaard and Kissmeyer-Nielsen, 1968). This cross-reactivity may be unidirectional or bidirectional (Mittal, 1975). Further, different antisera of an HLA specificity may cross-react with none, one, or several allelic antigens, and different donors carrying a cross-reactive antigen do not necessarily cross-react comparably with an antiserum having a cross-reactive specificity (Snell *et al.*, 1976; Mittal, 1975). Various combinations of cross-reactive antigens and antibodies of *HLA* loci *A* and *B* are summarized in Fig. 1.

The actual mechanism behind serological cross-reactivity of the *HLA* system is not known. It appears clear that any two cross-reactive antigens must share certain antigenic epitopes or determinants in order to cross-react with an antiserum of the alternate specificity (Reisner *et al.*, 1976). Further, this sharing may be either of two types: (1) it may permit sufficient binding between an antigen and the alternate antibody to cause cell death in the presence of complement or (2) it may produce a relatively weak binding, which permits only adsorption of the alternate antibody onto the cells carrying the antigen, and does not lead to cell death in the presence of complement [cytotoxicity-negative/adsorption-positive (CYNAP)]. The CYNAP may vary from total to partial (Ferrone *et al.*, 1967).

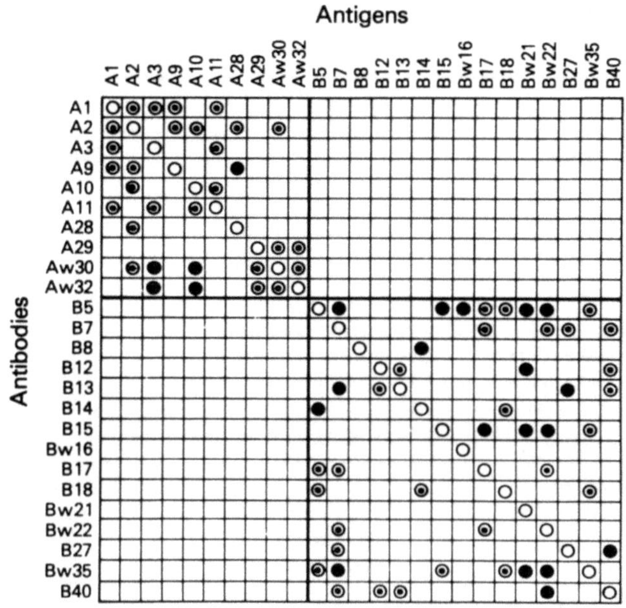

Figure 1. Cross-reactions between allelic antigens of *HLA* loci *A* and *B* as determined by inhibition of specific antisera by platelets of known HLA phenotype (Mittal, 1975). Two-way cross-inhibition of antisera of either specificity by platelets possessing antigen of the other specificity (symmetrical cross-reactivity); (●) one-way cross-inhibition (asymmetrical cross-reactivity); (○) specific inhibition of an antiserum by platelets possessing the corresponding antigen (control). No cross-reactivity was observed between antibodies specific for one locus and antigens of the other locus.

In addition, depending on the number and type of shared antigenic determinants, either immunization with a cross-reactive antigen may evoke no antibody response in a host or the antibody produced may be reactive only in a subtypic manner, i.e., it reacts only with those determinants that are not shared between the immunogen and the host. Since this sharing of determinants may vary in the number of shared determinants from one to several, and in the type of combination of determinants from one to another, the antibodies produced against the same alloantigen may differ from one immunized host to another. The phenomenon of cross-reactivity of the HLA antigens may thus be explained in two different ways (Table 1), as discussed below.

2.2.1. *Theory of Shared Supertypic Specificities*

This theory is based on the association of two or more typic antigens with a supertypic antigen. Thus, in the example in Table 1 (Theory 1), an

TABLE 1. An Example Illustrating Two Theories for the Phenomenon of Cross-Reactivity

Theory 1. Sharing of supertypic cluster

Typic antigen		*Supertypic clusters*
A1	may coexist with	a and b
A3	may coexist with	a and c
A11	may coexist with	b and c
A1, A3, and A11	may coexist with	d

1. Anti-a will make A1 and A3 appear cross-reactive.
2. Anti-b will make A1 and A11 appear cross-reactive.
3. Anti-c will make A3 and A11 appear cross-reactive.
4. Anti-d will make A1, A3, and A11 appear cross-reactive.

Theory 2. Sharing of subtypic determinants

Typic antigen		*Subtypic determinants*
A1	may consist of	a, b, c, and d
A3	may consist of	a, b, e, and f
A11	may consist of	c, d, e, and f

1. Anti-a, -b, -ab will make A1 and A3 appear cross-reactive.
2. Anti-c, -d, -cd will make A1 and A11 appear cross-reactive.
3. Anti-e, -f, -ef will make A3 and A11 appear cross-reactive.
4. Anti-ac, -ace, -abcdef, etc., will make A1, A3, A11 appear cross-reactive.
   (A host will not make antibodies against determinants he or she possesses.)

antibody against the supertypic cluster "a" will make antigens A1 and A3 appear cross-reactive because both A1 and A3 are included in the supertypic cluster "a."

2.2.1. Theory of Shared Subtypic Determinants

This theory is based on the sharing in common of one or more subtypic (subgenic) determinants between two or more typic antigens. Again, in the example of Table 1 (Theory 2), Anti-a will make A1 and A3 appear cross-reactive because the epitope "a" is shared in common by the two typic antigens A1 and A3.

2.3. Linkage Disequilibrium of Linked *HLA* Genes

If given genes of two different but linked loci occur together on the same chromosome as often as the product of their individual gene frequencies, they are considered to be in linkage equilibrium. However, if the two linked genes occur together either more or less frequently than the product of their gene frequencies, then they are considered to be in positive or negative linkage disequilibrium, respectively. The two types of disequilibria may be expressed as positive or negative deltas ($\tilde{\Delta}$), which reflect preferential gametic association or repulsion of the linked genes, respectively. Positive linkage disequilibria observed among genes of *HLA-A*, *-B*, and *-C* loci among 511 healthy, unrelated, North American Caucasoids of the Washington, D.C., metropolitan area are given in Table 2 and Fig. 2. Gametic associations between genes of the *B* and *DR* loci, based on preliminary data from 83 of these 511 individuals, are included in Fig. 2. These results appear to suggest that most of the positive linkage disequilibrium in the *HLA* region of white Americans is centered around the *B* locus (Fig. 2). Two significant gametic associations, between DRw1 and Bw35, and between DRw7 and B12, observed in the French popula-

TABLE 2. Positive Linkage Disequilibrium ($\tilde{\Delta}$) between HLA loci *A*, *B*, and *C* in 511 North American Caucasians (per Thousand)[a]

Gene combination	HF[b]	$\tilde{\Delta}$	t[c]	Gene combination	HF[b]	$\tilde{\Delta}$	t[c]
Loci *A* and B				Loci *A* and *C*			
A1-B8	68	55	8.5	A2-Cw3	63	21	2.7
A29-B12	22	17	4.2	A9-Cw4	26	14	2.7
A3-B7	31	20	3.9	A2-Cw1	18	9	2.4
A26-Bw16	13	11	3.2	A2-Cw5	11	6	2.3
A26-Bw38	11	10	3.2	Aw23-Cw4	6	5	2.3
A10-Bw38	12	10	3.0	Aw24-Cw4	18	10	2.2
A9-Bw49	9	8	2.9				
A25-Bw18	9	8	2.8	Loci *B* and *C*			
Aw30-B13	8	8	2.8				
A11-Bw35	18	11	2.7	Bw35-Cw4	88	75	10.5
A10-Bw16	14	10	2.7	B15-Cw3	63	52	8.3
A29-Bw44	11	9	2.7	B40-Cw3	42	33	6.2
A2-B15	37	15	2.5	B12-Cw5	13	10	3.5
A2-B27	19	10	2.5	B27-Cw1	13	12	3.5
A10-B18	12	9	2.5	Bw22-Cw3	16	12	3.4
A9-Bw21	12	8	2.3	B27-Cw2	11	10	3.2
Aw33-B14	6	5	2.3	Bw54-Cw3	9	8	3.0
A28-B15	11	8	2.2	Bw44-Cw5	6	5	2.2
Aw24-Bw16	11	7	2.0	B17-Cw5	7	6	2.1
A28-B14	8	6	2.0	B37-Cw6	5	4	2.1
A11-Bw22	7	5	2.0	Bw22-Cw1	5	5	2.0

[a]All calculations were made as described before (Mittal, 1976).
[b](HF) Per-thousand frequency of a haplotype.
[c]t = $\tilde{\Delta}$/standard error of $\tilde{\Delta}$. Values of 2 or greater than 2 indicate significant positive linkage disequilibrium.

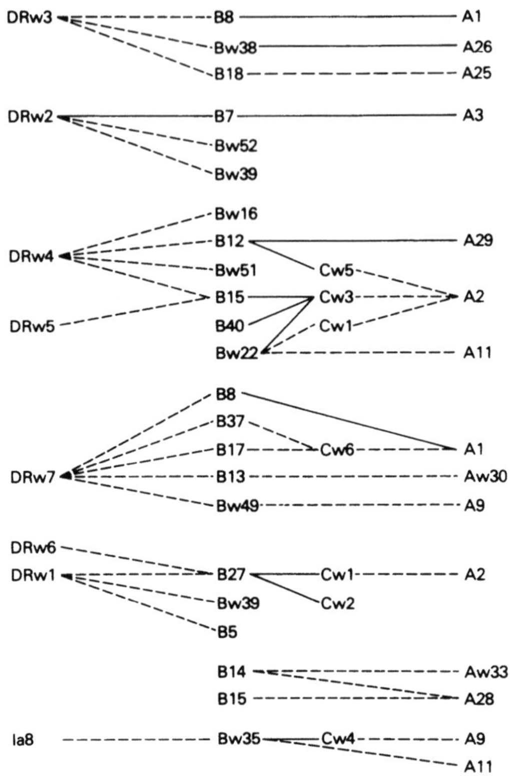

Figure 2. A model of positive linkage disequilibria (or gametic associations) between HLA genes of 511 healthy, unrelated, North American Caucasoids. (————) Strong positive linkage disequilibrium, (— — —) less significant gametic association. (Gametic associations between genes of the *DR* and *B* loci are based on preliminary data from 83 individuals.)

tion (Dausset *et al.*, 1978), were not detected in these 83 individuals. However, a positive gametic association between DRw7 and B12 has been observed in an international pool of 623 unrelated Caucasians (Thompson *et al.*, 1978).

Antiserum specific for one antigen (e.g., A1) of such a pair of antigens (e.g., A1 and B8) may appear specific for both specificities because most members of the cell panel may either possess or lack both antigens simultaneously due to their positive linkage disequilibrium. In such circumstances, it is very important to examine the reactivity of an antiserum against cell donors who possess one and not the other of the two antigens in question. Without such an evaluation, an antiserum may be erroneously identified as multispecific (Mittal *et al.*, 1970).

3. Procurement and Characterization of HLA Antisera

The multideterminant nature of the HLA molecules, and the sharing of determinants among different HLA antigens, are perhaps the two most basic reasons for a majority of the difficulties encountered in the production and characterization of HLA-typing antisera.

3.1. Procurement of Antisera

All the HLA-typing antisera currently in use around the world are essentially allogeneic. The HLA antibodies in these antisera are primarily immunoglobulins of the IgG class, although occasionally traces of IgM antibodies may also be present (Ahrons and Glavind-Kristensen, 1971). Most of these HLA antisera come from women who have had one or more pregnancies or from persons who have received allotransfusions or allotransplants. They are therefore available in limited quantities. So far, only a very small proportion of useful antisera have resulted from immunization of allogeneic (Ferrara *et al.*, 1978) or xenogeneic (Ferrone *et al.*, 1977; Einstein *et al.*, 1971) hosts.

In all the situations of alloimmunization described above, a certain proportion of hosts may never produce any detectable HLA antibody, while others may produce sequentially "broader" antisera such that the reactivity of the antibody that appeared early during immunization is always included in the "broad" reactivity of the antiserum that appears later. The antisera from such hosts may thus contain several different populations of progressively broader antibodies. Xenogeneic hosts respond primarily to species-specific antigens; however, progress is being made in the production of HLA antibodies in animals by the use of purified HLA antigens for immunization, followed by extensive absorption of the resulting antisera (Wilson *et al.*, this volume).

Development of cell-fusion techniques, to produce hybrid cell lines secreting monoclonal antibodies against histocompatibility antigens (Galfre *et al.*, 1977), holds great promise for the future development and refinement of HLA serology. This method could permit unlimited production of one type of antibody by a hybrid clone, originally elicited by a nonpurified mixture of histocompatibility antigens.

3.2. Characterization of HLA Specificity in an Antiserum

Thorough characterization of the HLA specificity in an antiserum requires determination of: (1) the presence of lymphocytotoxic antibodies in the antiserum; (2) the antiserum's titer and strength index (percentage of all antigen-positive donors whose cells demonstrated 80% or greater cell death over negative controls); (3) the association of the antiserum's reaction pattern with a common antigen among the positive donors; (4) the mutually exclusive (or allelic) behavior of the pattern as revealed by Mendelian segregation in family studies, and by the "triplet test" (a test in which an antiserum suspected to detect a new allotypic specificity does not result in production of three allelic antigens for an *HLA* locus in any of the panel members); and (5) cross-reactivity of the antiserum with allelic antigens, or reactivity with antigens that may be in linkage disequilibrium.

3.2.1. Lymphocytotoxicity and Titer

The first step in serological evaluation of an antiserum is the determination of whether it reacts adequately with cells from any person. Since several HLA antigens occur with extremely low frequencies, and are occasionally restricted to certain ethnic groups, it is essential that an antiserum of unknown specificity be examined (screened!) against a panel of cell donors adequately representative of all HLA specificities. Selwood (1972) has shown how variation of samples may affect the accuracy of determining the specificity of an antiserum. In a system as polymorphic as *HLA*, with diverse antigen frequencies within and among various ethnic groups, only a very large panel of random cell donors will be adequately representative of the general population for all the HLA specificities. However, for purposes of initial antiserum evaluation, a highly selected panel of as few as 40–100 donors may provide adequate representation of virtually all the HLA specificities.

The second step consists in titrating the antiserum against reactive donor cells. The importance of this step lies in the fact that it is frequently not possible to remove "extra" antibodies from an antiserum by adsorption without also losing or at least weakening the desired reactivity. It is often possible, however, to dilute out the "extra" reactivity without diminishing the desired specific reactivity (Mittal *et al.*, 1970).

3.2.2. Statistical Associations of Reactions

After an unknown antiserum has been tested with a panel of cells, its reaction pattern may be compared either with patterns simultaneously produced by antisera of known HLA specificities or with the HLA phenotypes of various panel members.

At present, no single antiserum is nationally or internationally considered a standard measure of any known HLA specificity. The main criteria for determination of an antigen on the cells of a donor are that the donor cells react with most of the best available antisera of that specificity and that the cells possess no more than two typic specificities of any given locus. Therefore, until standard HLA antisera are agreed on, it appears more appropriate to compare the reaction pattern of an antiserum with the phenotypes of the cell panel than to compare it with the pattern of any known antiserum. Further, it is obviously desirable to select only those antisera that are strongly reactive with a majority of the antigen-positive cell donors.

3.2.3. Determination of HLA Specificity

Once it is established that an antiserum reacts with cells of only some of the panel members, most of whom share a given HLA specificity, that specificity may be tentatively assigned to the antiserum. Further confirmation of the specificity is achieved by testing the antiserum with additional donors of known phenotypes. In the absence of standard typing antisera and donor cells, it is important to test such an antiserum with cell donors of diverse ethnic origins, so as to learn more about its stability and reaction characteristics.

If the antiserum appears to react with only a few of the donors possessing a typic HLA specificity, it becomes crucial to ascertain whether this potentially "short" split, included under a well-defined HLA specificity, is indeed a typic split or is merely a subtypic split. If it is a typic split, it will demonstrate Mendelian segregation in double-backcross families without suggesting three alleles for the same locus. However, this type of family testing may often be greatly hampered by lack of an adequate number of appropriate families. Although the absolute proof of discovering a new allelic or typic split must always come from studies of the new antisera with double-backcross families, additional antisera that define the same specificities may be discovered through the use of cell panels well characterized with the primary antisera. We have utilized this latter approach in characterizing specificities in 176 antisera of the 7th International Histocompatibility Workshop (Mittal *et al.*, 1977, 1978). Although all the 176 Workshop Antisera were examined by the standard lymphocyte-microcytotoxicity test (Mittal, 1978; Mittal *et al.*, 1968) against a panel of 177 unrelated normal donors, results of 42 selected antisera are given here to demonstrate the usefulness of this method of analysis. Reaction patterns for these 42 antisera are displayed as serographs in Fig. 3 and 4.

A serograph is a display of reactions for antisera of related specificities against lymphocytes from donors possessing the corresponding antigens. In such a display, it is possible to compare the reactions of many

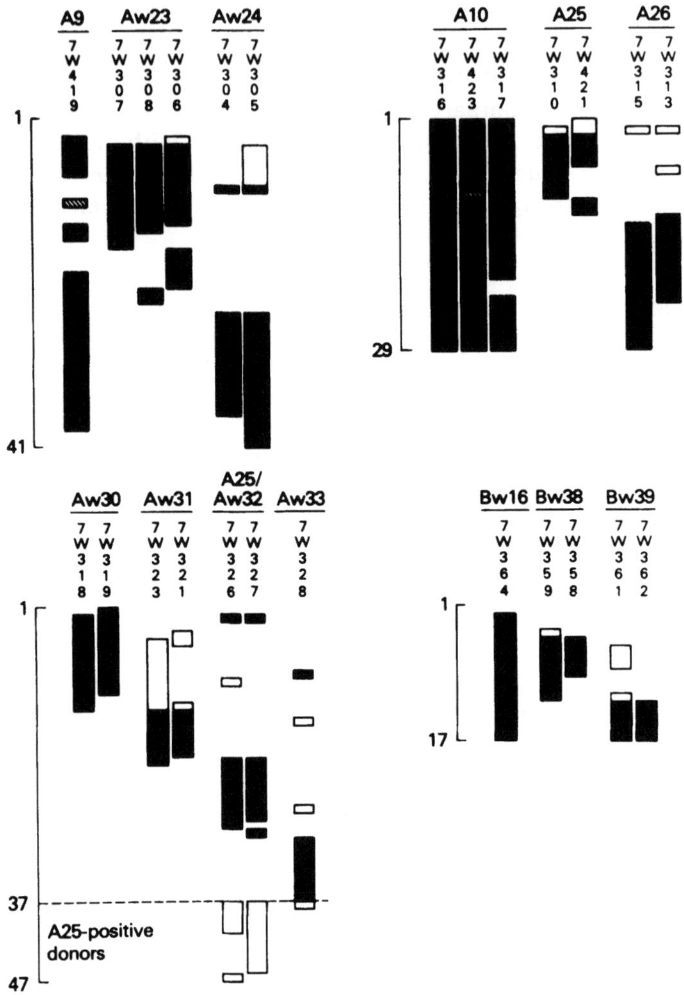

Figure 3. Splitting of four supertypic clusters (A9, A10, Aw19, and Bw16) by the 7th International Workshop Antisera. (■) Antiserum reactions with cell donors *possessing* the corresponding antigen; (□) reactions with donors *lacking* the corresponding antigen; (▨) the combination was "not tested." The scale at the side indicates the total number of cell donors included in the serograph.

antisera with each other and with the antigens in the cell panel. Thus, the degree of concordance between the reactions of an antiserum and the presence of corresponding and/or cross-reactive antigen(s) in the cell donors, or the presence of a unique pattern possibly detecting an undiscovered antigen, may be recognized. The serographs in Fig. 3 show examples of four supertypic clusters, A9, A10, Aw19, and Bw16:

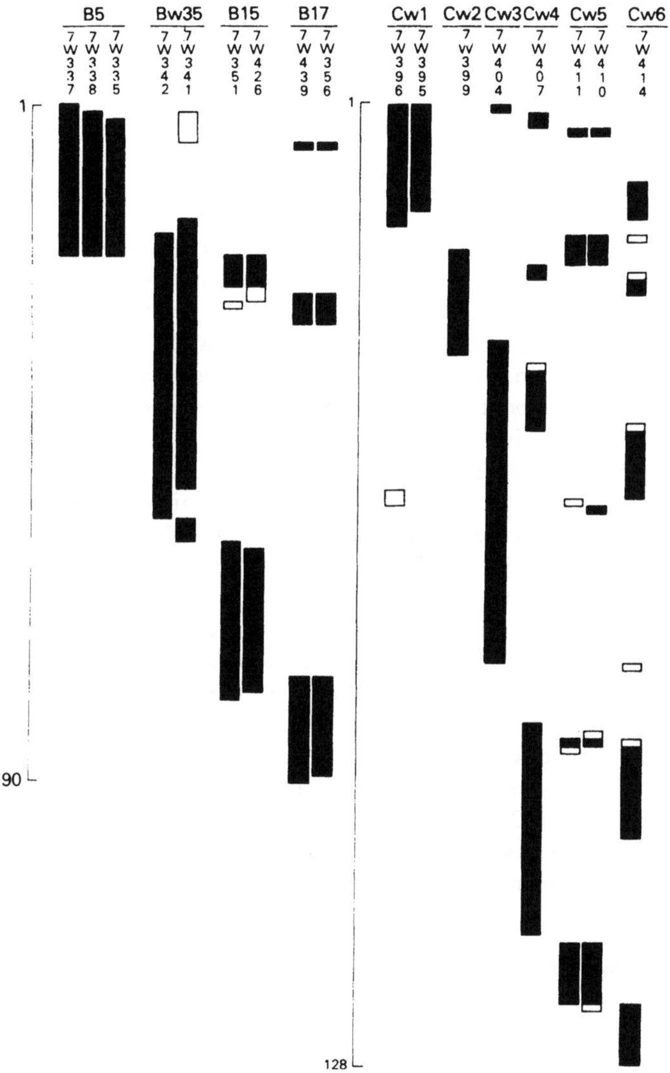

Figure 4. Definition of specificities in the *4C* complex and of the *C*-locus antigens by antisera of the 7th International Histocompatibility Workshop. (■) Reactions with donors *possessing* the corresponding antigen; (□) reactions with donors *lacking* the corresponding specificity (which may be a result of cross-reactivity or of a second specificity in the antiserum). The scale at the side indicates the number of cell donors included in the serograph.

A9 Cluster: Although this cluster appeared reasonably well split into Aw23 and Aw24, the A9 antiserum (7W419) did not react with all the A9-positive cells in the panel, and appeared to react preferentially with Aw24-positive donors. Although the three Aw23 antisera reacted identically with 10 of the 22 Aw23-positive cell donors, they reacted differently with the remaining 12 Aw23-positive donors.

A10 Cluster: Antigen A10 was well recognized by three antisera, which reacted identically with 26 of 29 A10-positive donors. This cluster was reasonably well split into A25 and A26. An A26 antiserum (7W315) cross-reacted with four of 12 A29-positive donors.

Aw19 Cluster: Typic subdivisions of Aw19 appeared to have a mutually exclusive relationship, although Aw30 and Aw31 were not adequately distinguished in a monospecific manner by the antisera of these specificities. Further, one Aw32 antiserum (7W326) appeared to cross-react (weaker reactions) with some of the A25-positive cell donors, while the other (7W327) appeared to be duospecific because it reacted strongly with 9 of 10 A25-positive donors.

Bw16 Cluster: The Bw16 antigen in the cell panel was fairly well recognized by antiserum 7W364, and this supertypic antigen was split into Bw38 and Bw39 by shorter antisera. Two donors whose cells reacted with the Bw16 antiserum, but not with either Bw38 or Bw39 antiserum, may possess a third split of Bw16.

With the use of a well-typed panel, antisera with overlapping specificities in the *4C* complex (Payne *et al.*, 1978) can be separated clearly into B5, B15, B17, and Bw35 (Fig. 4). Similarly, antisera containing specificities for the *C*-locus antigens can be separated from each other (Fig. 4). It is noteworthy, however, that of the 128 donors utilized in defining *C*-locus antigens, only 3 appeared to express "triplets," i.e., three antigens of this locus. Moreover, all 3 donors reacted with the same two Cw4 (7W407) and Cw6 (7W414) antisera, which may suggest a cross-reactivity in these antisera with the alternate antigen.

4. Determination of HLA Antigens on Lymphocytes

The HLA antigens of an individual are generally detected by a lymphocyte-microcytotoxicity test. Since each HLA antigen consists of a family of similarly reacting "variants," the assignment of an HLA antigen to an individual is based on the reactivity of donor lymphocytes with a majority of antisera of that specificity. Certain technical and clinical factors may also significantly influence the reaction patterns such that the cells from a donor appear to have gained or lost certain antigens.

4.1. Technical Variables

The determination of HLA antigens on lymphocytes can be influenced both by the use of lymphocytes from different tissues of a host and by variations in methodology.

4.1.1. Sources of Lymphocytes

The T cells usually comprise a majority (range 65–85%) of the lymphocytes circulating in the peripheral blood, the most common source of cells used for HLA testing. An increase in the proportion of B lymphocytes in the test-cell suspension could result in the detection of additional antigens due to contaminating anti-HLA-DR antibodies in the HLA-A, -B, and -C typing antisera. This increase in B lymphocytes might occur due to either inherent individual variation or the use of cells from lymphoid tissues such as lymph nodes, spleen, and bone marrow. Since the DR antigens, unlike the *A*, *B*-, and *C*-locus antigens, do not contain β_2-microglobulin, it is possible to differentiate between their reactions by demonstrating that avian anti-β_2-microglobulin blocks reactions of the *A*-, *B*-, and *C*-locus antigens, but does not block those of the DR antigens. It will be necessary to use an anti-β_2-microglobulin of avian origin because antibodies from avian species can fix only avian complement and will therefore not activate rabbit complement in the lymphocyte-microcytotoxicity test (Bernoco *et al.*, 1976; Poulik *et al.*, 1974; Rice, 1948).

4.1.2. Variations in Methodology

The endpoint of the most commonly used HLA-typing method is cell death. This makes the HLA-typing method greatly vulnerable to false reactions with even minor alterations in the methodology.

Differences in the methods of lymphocyte isolation or of storage, such as by freezing, may alter the ratio of B and T cells in the cell suspension. Variations in the sensitivity to complement-mediated cell death may be seen with cells originating from different tissue sources, and especially with cultured cells.

4.2. Clinical Variables

Difficulties in the determination of HLA antigens in clinical situations may arise from the pathological changes of the disease itself, or they may be iatrogenic.

4.2.1. *Influence of Disease*

An absolute or relative lymphopenia as may arise in various leukemias, or granulocytosis, may give rise to difficulties in isolation and testing of lymphocytes. The HLA testing may also be complicated by gross changes in lymphocyte subpopulations, such as the predominance of B-lymphocyte-derived cells in chronic lymphatic leukemia. It is possible that new antigens are acquired, or the existing ones are altered, as a result of neoplasia or changes mediated by infection. However, the extent to which HLA ("self") antigens may be altered by non-HLA ("non-self," e.g., microbial) antigens through somatic association or other mechanism is not known (Snell, 1978; Zinkernagel and Doherty, 1975; Jerne, 1971). Whether aging results in loss or gain of any antigens also remains to be established.

4.2.2. *Iatrogenic Effects*

Immunosuppressive therapy can result in profound lymphopenia, and cytotoxic drugs may enhance the susceptibility of lymphocytes to cytolysis (Bach, 1975). Both these changes may create problems during HLA testing. The presence of lymphocytes of different genetic constitutions in an individual may result in either the detection of additional antigens or the apparent loss of antigens. This situation may occur as a result of transfusions, bone marrow transplantation, or an intermingling of fetal circulations *in utero*. Unequal recombination may also result in gain or loss of antigens.

5. Approaches to Standardization of HLA Typing

Due to serological and genetic complexities, standardization of HLA typing will require attention to at least three different areas: (1) development of a single, simple HLA-typing procedure; (2) development of specificity and potency requirements for acceptable HLA-typing antisera; and (3) development of criteria for the assignment of HLA antigens, i.e., for HLA phenotyping.

5.1. Standardization of the HLA-Typing Procedure

The lymphocyte-microcytotoxicity test as used for HLA typing is vulnerable to a number of technical problems. A change in either incubation period or incubation temperature alone can significantly alter the reaction patterns. Perhaps the single most significant technical variable is the pooled rabbit serum utilized as a source of complement (Ferrone, 1977). Depending on a number of factors, such as the "natural" antibody content, a given pool of rabbit serum may vary in strength from very weak to very strong. Weak complement will lead to false-negative reactions and excessively strong complement may lead to false-positive reactions.

To develop some uniformity in HLA phenotyping by the various laboratories, it is essential that the HLA methodology be standardized. Some progress in this direction has already been made through the efforts of a large group of investigators (Mittal, 1978). So far, only the method of typing for antigens of *HLA* loci *A*, *B*, and *C* has been standardized, and even this only in broad terms. Much improvement remains to be made with regard to standardization of complement, an important component of this test. Efforts are underway to standardize the methodology of B-cell (DR) typing. Whether or not serologically detected DR antigens are the same as mixed leukocyte culture (MLC)-detected D antigens remains to be resolved. If not, then the D-typing technique will also require standardization.

5.2. Standardization of the HLA-Typing Antisera

One of the important problems of HLA serology is to identify standard HLA-typing antisera. The multivalent nature of typic HLA antigens has the effect of generating a wide array of antisera that, although "operationally" monospecific for the same specificity, do differ from one another in reaction patterns. Difference at a single epitope in the immunogens, or sharing of a different epitope of an immunogen with different immunized hosts, may be enough to make two antisera appear as though they are reacting with closely related "variants" of the same mosaic or typic HLA specificity. How then does one identify a standard HLA-typing reagent? In 1976, the Bureau of Biologics of the Food and Drug Administration held a workshop, which resulted in certain recommendations about the definition of good or acceptable HLA-typing antisera (Mittal, 1978). It was recommended that the cell panel used in the evaluation of an antiserum consist of nearly 150 cell donors selected in a manner such that it includes no fewer than 10% and no more than 60% of individuals who possess the antigen of the same specificity as the antiserum. The recommended requirement for potency was that an antiserum produce 80% or greater increase in cell death over baseline with at least 70% of the donors possessing the antigen of the corresponding specificity. The recommended requirement for specificity was that an antiserum produce no more than 3% discrepant positive reactions with antigen-negative donors and no more than 14% discrepant negative reactions with antigen-positive donors (Mittal, 1978). However, an ideal antiserum would be one that produces 100% strong reactions (80% or greater cell death over baseline) and does not produce any discrepant reactions. The possibility of minimal technical variation alone requires that the definition of a standard antiserum be sought somewhere between the ideal (or best) and the acceptable (or good). Further, this definition may vary from specificity to specificity, and may be upgraded frequently as more precise antisera for a given specificity become available.

Great progress has been made in identifying the most useful HLA antisera by extensive collaboration of the various investigators through frequent regional, national, and international HLA workshops, which permit exchange of typing antisera as well as cells. In addition, these workshops have allowed various HLA-typing laboratories to standardize the phenotypes of their local cell panels.

The difficult nature of this task may be appreciated through the data given in Table 3. Of the 176 antisera utilized in the 7th International Histocompatibility Workshop, only 26 (15%) of the antisera met both the potency and the specificity requirements. Only 10 of these 26 antisera produced a correlation coefficient of 0.95 or greater. The specificity and potency data of these 10 antisera are given in Table 3. Only one antiserum, 7W439, behaved as an ideal antiserum; i.e., it produced 100% strong reactions and did not produce a single discrepant reaction against a panel of 177 cell donors.

TABLE 3. Examples of Monospecific Antisera Utilized in the 7th International Histocompatibility Workshop[a]

Workshop antiserum no.	Antigen-positive donors[b]	Potency: Strength index[c]	Specificity: False reactions (%)		r value[f]	Assigned specificity
			F-neg[d]	F-pos[e]		
7W303	42	83	2	0	0.98	A1
7W316	29	97	0	1	0.98	A10
7W423	28	93	0	1	0.98	A10
7W317	29	93	7	0	0.96	A10
7W338	21	76	10	0	0.95	B5
7W379	28	75	4	0	0.98	B7
7W324	5	80	0	0	1.00	B13
7W393	15	93	7	0	0.96	B14
7W351	25	84	0	1	0.98	B15
7W439	20	100	0	0	1.00	B17

[a]All antisera were tested with a panel of 177 normal donors (143 Caucasian, 21 black, and 13 other).
[b]Number of donors possessing antigen corresponding to the specificity assigned to a given antiserum.
[c]Percentage of all antigen-positive donors who demonstrated 80% or greater cell death over negative controls.
[d]Percentage of false-negative reactions with "antigen-positive" donors.
[e]Percentage of false-positive reactions with "antigen-negative" donors.
[f]Coefficient of correlation between reactions of Workshop Antisera and antigens of cell donors.

5.3. Development of HLA-Phenotyping Criteria

It is obviously unrealistic to look for criteria for HLA phenotyping in the absence of any standard typing antisera or cells. It is pertinent, however, to consider what will be required to eventually standardize HLA phenotyping.

Criteria for assignment of HLA antigens to cell donors would require some indication of (1) the methodology used for typing; (2) the quality and minimum numbers of antisera utilized for each HLA specificity; and (3) the minimum strength of reactivity of at least a certain proportion of specific antisera of a specificity used in the test. Further, it would be important to deal with detection of more than two antigens at any given locus. Some consideration would have to be given to cross-reactivity of the allelic HLA antigens. These are obviously difficult problems, and standard criteria for HLA phenotyping will evolve only as our understanding of these problems improves. How soon monoclonal antibodies against these complex antigenic structures (Parham and Bodmer, 1978; Galfre *et al.*, 1977) will begin to play a role in the standardization of HLA serology remains to be seen.

References

Ahrons, S., and Glavind-Kristensen, 1971, Cytotoxic HLA antibodies: Immunoglobulin classification, *Tissue Antigens* **1:**129.

Amos, B., and Yunis, E., 1968, Human leukocyte antigenic specificity HL-A3: Frequency of occurrence, *Science* **165:**300.

Bach, J.F., 1975, *The Mode of Action of Immunosuppressive Agents* (A. Neuberger and E.L. Tatum, eds.), pp. 1–374, North-Holland, Amsterdam.

Bernoco, D., Bernoco, M., Ceppellini, R., Poulik, M.D., van Leeuwen, A., and van Rood, J.J., 1976, B cell antigens of the HLA system: A simple serotyping technique based on non-cytotoxic anti-β_2-microglobulin reagents, *Tissue Antigens* **8:**253.

Ceppellini, R., Curtoni, E.S., Mattiuz, P.L., Miggiano, V., Scudeller, G., and Serra, A., 1967, Genetics of leukocyte antigens: A family study of segregation and linkage, in: *Histocompatibility Testing 1967* (E.S. Curtoni, P.L. Mattiuz, and R.M. Tosi, eds.), pp. 149–187, Munksgaard, Copenhagen.

Dausset, J., Legrand, L., Lepage, V., Contu, L., Marcelli-Barge, A., Wildloecher, I., Benajam, A., Meo, T., and Degos, L., 1978, A haplotype study of HLA complex with special reference to the HLA-DR series and to Bf, C2 and Glyoxalase I polymorphisms, *Tissue Antigens* **12:**297.

Einstein, A.B., Mann, D.L., Gordon, H.G., Trapani, R., and Fahey, J.L., 1971, Heterologous antisera against specific HLA antigens, *Transplantation* **12:**299.

Ferrara, G.B., Tosi, R., Longo, A., Castellani, A., Viviani, C., and Carmainati, G., 1978, A safe blood transfusion procedure for immunization against major histocompatibility complex determinants in man, *Transplantation* **26:**150.

Ferrone, S., 1977, Rabbit complement in the lymphocytotoxicity test, *Tissue Antigens* **9:**223.

Ferrone, S., Tosi, R.M., and Centis, D., 1967, Anticomplementary factors affecting the lymphocytotoxicity test, in: *Histocompatibility Testing 1967* (E.S. Curtoni, P.L. Mattiuz, and R.M. Tosi, eds.), pp. 357–364, Munksgaard, Copenhagen.

Ferrone, S., Mittal, K.K., Pellegrino, M.A., Allison, J.P., and Reisfeld, R.A., 1977, Immunogenicity of HLA antigens purified from serum, *Transplantation* **23**:7.

Galfre, G., Howe, S.C., Milstein, C., Butcher, G.W., and Howard, J.C., 1977, Antibodies to major histocompatibility antigens produced by hybrid cell lines, *Nature (London)* **266**:550.

Jerne, N.K., 1971, The somatic generation of immune recognition, *Eur. J. Immunol.* **1**:1.

Legrand, L., and Dausset, J., 1972, Serological evidence of the existence of several antigenic determinants (or factors) on the HLA gene products, in: *Histocompatibility Testing 1972* (J. Dausset and J. Colombani, eds.), pp. 441–453, Munksgaard, Copenhagen.

Legrand, L., and Dausset, J., 1974, The complexity of the HLA gene product, *Tissue Antigens* **4**:329.

Mittal, K.K., 1975, Cross-reactivity of monospecific anti-HL-A antisera, *Vox Sang.* **29**:418.

Mittal, K.K., 1976, The HLA polymorphism and susceptibility to disease, *Vox Sang.* **31**:161.

Mittal, K.K., 1977, Possible mechanisms for association of HLA antigens and disease, in: *HLA and Malignancy*, (G.P. Murphy, E. Cohen, J.E. Fitzpatrick, and D. Pressman, eds.), pp. 39–51, Alan R. Liss, New York.

Mittal, K.K., 1978, Standardization of the HLA typing method and reagents, *Transplantation* **25**:275.

Mittal, K.K., and Terasaki, P.I., 1974, Serological cross-reactivity in the HLA system, *Tissue Antigens* **4**:146.

Mittal, K.K., Mickey, M.R., Singal, D.P., and Terasaki, P.I., 1968, Serotyping for homotransplantation. XVIII. Refinement of microdroplet lymphocyte cytotoxicity test, *Transplantation* **6**:913.

Mittal, K.K., Rossen, R.D., and Butler, W.T., 1970, Evaluation of HLA serum specificity and lymphocyte reactivity, in: *Histocompatibility Testing 1970* (P.I. Terasaki, ed.), pp. 343–349, Munksgaard, Copenhagen.

Mittal, K.K., Mickey, M.R., and Terasaki, P.I., 1971, Heterogeneity of HL-A specificities shown by platelet complement fixation, *Tissue Antigens* **1**:279.

Mittal, K.K., Ruder, A., and Green, D., 1976, Matching of histocompatibility (HL-A) antigens for platelet transfusion, *Blood* **47**:31.

Mittal, K.K., Fraize, L.E., and Kaur, D., 1977, Strength and specificity in the workshop HLA antisera, *Tissue Antigens* **10**:186.

Mittal, K.K., Fraize, L.E., and Kaur, D., 1978, Specificity and potency in the workshop HLA antisera, in: *Histocompatibility Testing 1977* (W.F. Bodmer, J.R. Batchelor, J.G. Bodmer, H. Festenstein, and P.J. Morris, eds.), pp. 578–580, Munksgaard, Copenhagen.

Parham, P., and Bodmer, W.F., 1978, Monoclonal antibody to a human histocompatibility alloantigen, HLA-A2, *Nature (London)* **276**:397.

Payne, R., Amos, B., Kostyu, D., Engelfriet, C.P., van den Berg-Loonen, P.M., Curtoni, E.S., and Richiardi, P., 1978, Subdivisions of the HLA-B5 and Bw35 complex, *Tissue Antigens* **11**:302.

Poulik, M.D., Ferrone, S., Pellegrino, M.A., Sevier, D.E., Oh, S.K., and Reisfeld, R.A., 1974, Association of HLA antigens and β_2-microglobulin: Concepts and questions, *Transplant. Rev.* **21**:106.

Reisner, E.G., Legrand, L., and Dausset, J., 1976, Specificities shared between HLA-A3 and HLA-A11 detected by Fab'$_2$ blocking, *Immunogenetics* **3**:233.

Rice, C.E., 1948, Inhibitory effects of certain avian and mammalian antisera in specific complement fixation systems, *J. Immunol.* **59**:365.

Selwood, N.H., 1972, Definition of specificity and the analysis of HL-A reagents by a computerised numerical method, *Tissue Antigens* **2:**147.

Snell, G.D., 1978, T cells, T cell recognition structures, and major histocompatibility complex, *Immunol. Rev.* **38:**3.

Snell, G.D., Dausset, J., and Nathenson, S., 1976, The HLA complex: Serology and genetics, in: *Histocompatibility*, pp. 181–247, Academic Press, New York.

Svejgaard, A., and Kissmeyer-Nielsen, F., 1968, Cross-reactive human HLA iso-antibodies, *Nature (London)* **219:**868.

Terasaki, P.I., 1978, Resolution by HLA testing of 1,000 paternity cases not excluded by ABO testing, *J. Family Law* **16:**543.

Thompson, J.S., Severson, C.D., Mickey, M.R., Braun, W.E., and Gatti, R.A., 1978, HLA-A, B, and D associations with B-cell antigen DRw7, *Tissue Antigens* **12:**350.

van Rood, J.J., and Eernisse, J.G., 1968, The detection of transplantation antigens in leukocytes, *Semin. Hematol.* **5:**187.

Zinkernagel, R.M., and Doherty, P.C., 1975, H-2 compatibility requirement for T-cell-mediated lysis of target cells infected with lymphocytic choriomeningitis virus, *J. Exp. Med.* **141:**1427.

11

Carbohydrate-Defined Antigens Controlled by the *I* Region

C.R. Parish and I.F.C. McKenzie

1. Introduction

The *I*-region-associated (Ia) antigens of the mouse represent a highly polymorphic system of antigens that are coded for by a cluster of genes located within the *H-2* complex (Shreffler and David, 1975; C.S. David, 1976). The possibility that these Ia antigens actually represent the product of immune-response *(Ir)* genes is still an unresolved issue. However, the Ia antigens undoubtedly play a role in mixed-lymphocyte reactions (MLRs) (R.H. Schwartz *et al.*, 1976a; Okuda *et al.*, 1977; Okuda and David, 1978) and T cell–macrophage interactions (R.H. Schwartz *et al.*, 1976b, 1978). They are also associated with several immunoregulatory molecules, such as helper factors (Armerding *et al.*, 1974; Munro and Taussig, 1975; Howie and Feldmann, 1977) and suppressor factors (Tada *et al.*, 1976; Thèze *et al.*, 1977) of antibody formation and suppressor factors of contact sensitivity (Greene *et al.*, 1977) and MLRs (Rich *et al.*, 1977).

It is generally accepted that the Ia antigens represent a family of glycoprotein molecules of molecular weight 58,000 daltons, which can be dissociated into two nonidentical polypeptide chains of molecular weight 33,000 and 25,000 daltons (Cullen *et al.*, 1976). The antigenic determinants of these molecules appear to reside in their protein portion. However, we have recently obtained evidence that suggests that the *I* region controls a

C.R. Parish • Department of Microbiology, John Curtin School of Medical Research, Australian National University, Canberra, A.C.T. 2601, Australia. I.F.C. McKenzie • Department of Medicine, Austin Hospital, Heidelberg, Victoria 3084, Australia.

second family of antigens that express carbohydrate-defined antigenic determinants. This chapter will summarize the evidence that suggests that this second family of Ia antigens exists in both mouse and man. The chemical and biological properties of these antigens will also be discussed and their possible biological relevance considered.

2. Evidence for Carbohydrate-Defined Ia Antigens in Mice

2.1. Serum Inhibition Studies

Initially, it was found that mouse serum could inhibit the binding of cytotoxic Ia antisera to mouse spleen cells (Parish *et al.*, 1976a; Callahan *et al.*, 1976). By testing of serum from a wide range of mouse strains, this inhibition was shown to be *I*-region-specific (Parish *et al.*, 1976a). It was originally thought that the inhibitory material in serum represented glycoprotein Ia antigen that had been shed by cells. However, the evidence now suggests that a new class of carbohydrate-defined Ia antigen is involved. First, the bulk of the Ia antigenic activity in serum was dialyzable (Parish *et al.*, 1976a) and fractionated with serum oligosaccharides and glycolipids (Parish *et al.*, 1976c). Second, Ia antigenicity was destroyed by neuraminidase digestion or periodate oxidation, but was resistant to pronase treatment (Parish *et al.*, 1976c). These results suggested that the Ia antigens in serum were carbohydrate, rather than protein, in nature. This conclusion was supported by recent experiments that suggest that the Ia antigenic activity is associated with certain serum gangliosides (Parish *et al.*, 1977; Higgins and Parish, 1980).

2.2. Xenogeneic Antiserum Studies

With the demonstration that normal mouse serum contained a dialyzable form of Ia antigen, attempts were made to produce xenogeneic antisera against these molecules. The immunization protocol used was to simply immunize rabbits with normal mouse serum and absorb the resultant antiserum with exhaustively dialyzed mouse serum (Parish *et al.*, 1976a). This protocol reproducibly resulted in antibodies directed against a family of low-molecular-weight antigens in serum. In contrast, several attempts at raising antibodies in rabbits against semipurified Ia antigens from serum (e.g., crude oligosaccharide fraction from serum) failed completely (Jackson *et al.*, 1977).

A xenogeneic antiserum was then rigorously tested to determine whether it did, indeed, recognize *I*-region-controlled antigens. A summary of the evidence in favor of this antiserum's reacting with Ia antigens is presented in Table 1. It can be seen that the cellular distribution of the antigens recognized by the rabbit antiserum resembles that of Ia antigens detected by alloantisera (Shreffler and David, 1975; Hämmerling, 1976; Cowing *et al.*, 1978). Cell absorption and strain distribution studies indicated that the rabbit antiserum recognized a polymorphic series of antigens (Table 1). Some of these antigens had a strain-distribution pattern similar to that of Ia antigens delineated by alloantisera (e.g., Ia specificities 1, 3, 7, 15, and 17) (Parish and McKenzie, 1978a). However, it has become increasingly apparent that additional antigens are recognized by the rabbit antisera that do not correlate with known Ia specificities, the implications of which will be discussed in more detail later in this chapter.

A backcross study formally demonstrated identity, or close linkage, of the genes coding for the antigens detected by the rabbit antiserum and the Ia antigens distinguished by alloantisera (Table 1). Blocking and cocapping studies at the cell surface also indicated identity, or close association, at the molecular level of conventional Ia antigens and the antigens recognized by the rabbit antiserum (Table 1).

TABLE 1. Summary of Evidence That Rabbit Antiserum Recognizes Murine *I*-Region-Controlled Antigens

Evidence	Reference
1. Cellular distribution of antigen:	
a. Carried by most B cells (90% in spleen).	Parish *et al.* (1976a)
b. Carried by a subpopulation of peripheral T cells (30–50% in spleen).	Parish *et al.* (1976a)
c. Carried by macrophages.	Unpublished
d. Absent from red blood cells, platelets, brain, liver (?), and kidney.	Parish and McKenzie (1978a)
2. Strain-distribution pattern of reactivity—antiserum recognizes a polymorphic system of antigens, some specificities correlating with known Ia antigens.	Parish and McKenzie (1978a)
3. In a backcross, antigens recognized by rabbit antiserum segregate with H-2 and Ia antigens.	Parish and McKenzie (1978a)
4. Reciprocal blocking between rabbit antiserum and mouse anti-Ia sera.	Parish *et al.* (1976a)
5. Cocapping of antigens recognized by rabbit antiserum and mouse anti-Ia sera.	Parish *et al.* (1978)
6. Rabbit antiserum gives same results as mouse anti-Ia sera in serum and sugar inhibition studies.	Parish *et al.* (1976a,b), McKenzie *et al.* (1977), Parish and McKenzie (1977a)

Finally, the rabbit antiserum gave results similar to those of mouse alloantisera in serum inhibition studies (Table 1). In particular, the antigens recognized by the rabbit antiserum appeared to be carbohydrate in nature and very similar to the serum-borne antigens detected by mouse anti-Ia sera. This conclusion was based on: (1) the cofractionation on paper and thin-layer chromatograms of the serum antigens detected by xenogeneic and allogeneic antisera (Parish *et al.*, 1976c, 1977); (2) the destruction of the antigens recognized by the rabbit antiserum by neuraminidase and periodate, but not by pronase (Parish *et al.*, 1976c); and (3) the ability of similar sugars to inhibit the binding of both rabbit antibodies and mouse anti-Ia antibodies to lymphocytes (McKenzie *et al.*, 1977) (see also below).

It should be emphasized at this point that the xenogeneic antisera discussed above are directed exclusively against a family of carbohydrate-defined Ia antigens. There is no evidence that these sera react with polypeptide antigens on the cell surface (e.g., C.S. David *et al.*, 1977; Parish *et al.*, 1978).

2.3. Sugar Inhibition Studies

If a family of carbohydrate-defined Ia antigens exists, then it would be predicted that monosaccharides and oligosaccharides should specifically inhibit the binding of anti-Ia antibodies to lymphocytes. Sugar inhibition studies revealed that this was indeed the case. In these inhibition experiments, allogenic and xenogeneic anti-Ia sera were absorbed and/or tested on target cells selected so that only a limited spectrum of Ia specificities would be observed, i.e., putative Ia specificities 1, 3, 7, and 15. It should be emphasized, however, that these specificity numbers may be misleading, since they are based predominantly on protein-defined Ia antigens; hence the "Ia-like" nomenclature in Table 2.

The sugar inhibition studies (McKenzie *et al*,, 1977) revealed that the immunodominant sugars in the following Ia specificities are (Table 2): (1) "Ia.1-like": *N*-acetyl-D-mannosamine; (2) "Ia. 3-like": α-D-galactose; (3) "Ia.7-like": L-fucose; and (4) "Ia.15-like": *N*-acetyl-D-glucosamine.

TABLE 2. Nature of Several Carbohydrate-Defined Ia Antigenic Specificities

Specificity	Immunodominant sugar
"Ia. 1-like"	*N*-Acetyl-D-mannosamine
"Ia. 3-like"	α-D-Galactose
"Ia.7-like"	α1–2 L-Fucose (probably linked to β1–4 galactose)
"Ia.15-like"	*N*-Acetyl-D-Glucosamine (probably β-linked and intrachain)

Comparable results were obtained whether xenogeneic or allogeneic anti-Ia sera were used (McKenzie *et al.*, 1977). A more detailed analysis of the structure of Ia specificities "7" and "15" was obtained by using a range of human milk oligosaccharides as inhibitors. It was found that Ia.7 probably represents α1–2 linked L-fucose and the *N*-acetyl-D-glucosamine of Ia.15 is most likely intrachain and β-linked to neighboring sugars (Parish *et al.*, 1977; Parish and McKenzie, 1977b).

It is noteworthy that the Ia specificities carried by one haplotype (namely, I^k) were examined in the sugar inhibition studies. This may explain the association of different immunodominant monosaccharides with each specificity examined. Consistent with this interpretation are preliminary studies that implicate D-galactose in determinants associated with "Ia.8" and "Ia.9."

2.4. Effect of Glycosidases on Ia Antigenicity

If allogeneic anti-Ia sera contain antibodies against carbohydrate-defined antigens, then one would expect to both destroy and reveal antigenic specificities by treating cells with glycosidases, analogous to the studies of ABO blood groups (Hakomori and Kobata, 1974). Recently, we have obtained evidence that suggests that neuraminidase (NA) treatment of murine spleen cells reveals Ia antigenic specificities that are not normally expressed by the cells (Parish *et al.*, 1980). Furthermore, NA treatment resulted in a partial loss of Ia antigens from spleen cells. A summary of the results of the NA study is presented below.

1. Following treatment with NA, spleen cells gained unexpected reactivities with anti-Ia sera. For example, NA-treated A.TH spleen cells reacted quite strongly with A.TH anti-A.TL (anti-I^k, S^k, G^k) sera (Fig. 1). In contrast, normal A.TH serum reacted only weakly with NA-treated A.TH cells (Fig. 1). This result indicated that the phenomenon was not simply due to natural antibodies present in all mouse sera against NA-exposed antigens, similar to the T-antigen system in man (Rogentine and Plocinik, 1974; Springer and Desai, 1977). When a range of alloantisera were tested on NA-treated splenocytes, only antisera against the *I* region, particularly the *I-A* subregion, exhibited strong reactivity. Thus, Fig. 1, anti-K^k, anti-I-J^k and anti-I-J^k, I-E/C^k sera did not bind to NA-treated A.TH spleen cells, whereas an anti-I-A^k, I-B^k, I-J^k serum reacted to a high titer.

2. The NA-exposed antigens exhibited a restricted cellular distribution, being expressed on more than 90% of splenic B cells and from 40 to 50% of splenic T cells. Few, if any, null cells in spleen display the antigen.

3. Cell absorption studies confirmed the direct testing experiments

described in (1). For example, absorption of an A.TH anti-A.TL serum with NA-treated A.TH spleen cells significantly reduced the reaction of this antiserum with certain target cells. In contrast, no detectable absorption of the antiserum was seen with untreated A.TH spleen cells.

4. A range of proteolytic enzymes (e.g., pronase, trypsin, elastase, bromelain), phospholipase-C treatment, and periodate oxidation did not expose "new" Ia antigens on spleen cells. Furthermore, the production of "new" Ia antigens by NA was blocked by free sialic acid, which suggested that contaminating enzymes in the NA preparation were not involved in new-antigen exposure.

5. Sugar inhibition studies revealed that the NA-exposed antigens were carbohydrate in nature, since D-galactose effectively inhibited the binding of antibodies to the new antigens (Table 3). However, the proportion of α- and β-linked D-galactose residues involved depended on the target cell used and the anti-Ia serum tested (Table 3).

6. Absorption of anti-Ia sera with normal spleen cells obtained from

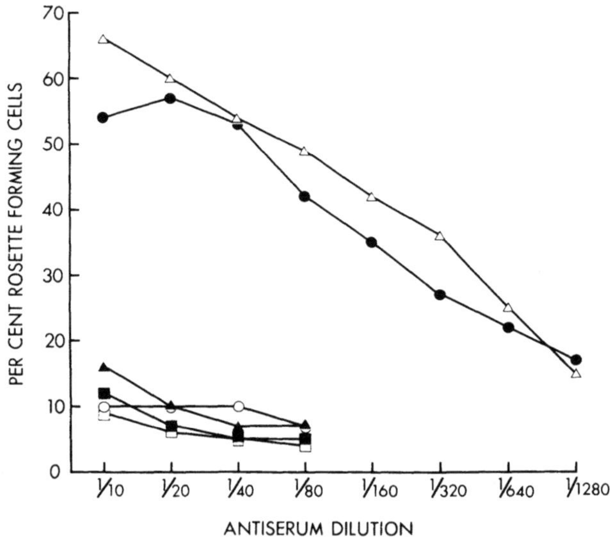

Figure 1. Ability of neuraminidase (NA) treatment to expose new antigens that can be detected by anti-Ia sera. Spleen cells from A.TH mice were incubated with NA (50 U/ml, 37°C, 30 min, pH 6.5) prior to reaction with serial dilutions of the different antisera. Binding of antibodies to the splenocytes was detected by a rosetting assay (Parish and McKenzie, 1978b). Sera used were normal A.TH (○), A.TH anti-A.TL (anti-I^k, S^k, G^k) (●), (B10.HTT × A.SW)F_1 anti-A.TL (anti-I-A^k, I-B^k, I-J^k) (Δ), B10.S (7R) anti-B10.S (9R) (anti-I-J^k, I-E/C^k) (▲), A.TL anti-A.AL (anti-K^k) (□), and (B10.HTT × BALB/c)F_1 anti-B10.S (9R) (anti-I-J^k) (■). The sera used did not react with untreated A.TH spleen cells (titers <1:10).

TABLE 3. Sugar Inhibition of Reaction of Anti-Ia Sera with Neuraminidase-Treated Spleen Cells

		Antibody titer[a]	
Sugar	Concn. (mg/ml)	A.TH anti-A.TL[b] on NA-treated A.TH	A.TL anti-A.TH[b] on NA-treated CBA/H
Nil	—	120	160
D-Glucose[c]	10	120	160
D-Galactose	10	20	40
Lactose (β-D-galactose)	10	10	60
Melibiose (α-D-galactose)	10	40	10
Lactose Melibiose	5	<5	5

[a] Antibody titers were measured by rosetting assay (Parish and McKenzie, 1978b) and represent dilution of antiserum at which 20% of spleen cells formed rosettes. Respective antisera had titers of less than 5 on untreated targets.
[b] Spleen cells treated with 50 U/ml NA at pH 6.5 for 30 min at 37°C.
[c] Also, no inhibition was observed with 10 mg/ml of L-fucose, *N*-acetyl-D-glucosamine, D-galactose, *N*-acetyl-D-galactosamine, D-mannose, or *N*-acetyl-D-mannosamine.

C57B1/10 congenic mice of different *H-2* haplotype in some cases resulted in removal of the antibodies that reacted with NA-treated spleen cells. Thus, antibodies in an A.TH anti-A.TL serum against NA-treated A.TH spleen were almost completely absorbed by *k* and *r* haplotypes, partially absorbed by *b, d,* and *q* haplotypes, and not absorbed by *f, p,* and *s* haplotypes. From an examination of the absorption results, sugar inhibition studies, and anti-Ia sera reactions, it seems likely that several antigenic specificities are being exposed by NA. Furthermore, although some of the NA-exposed antigens appear to be associated with the Ia.3 and 15 specificities, additional antigens are involved that do not correlate with any previously described Ia specificities.

7. Finally, as well as exposing new antigens, NA treatment did result in a partial loss of Ia antigens from spleen cells, which was detected by both direct testing and cell absorption analyses.

Collectively, the data presented in (1)–(7) are consistent with the notion that NA clips off terminal sialic acid residues from carbohydrate-defined Ia antigens on the cell surface and exposes subterminal sugars that resemble antigens expressed by strains bearing other *H-2* haplotypes.

2.5. Importance of Antisera and Assay Systems

At this point, it should be noted that some workers, using inhibition assays, have been unable to confirm that Ia antigens exist in appreciable amounts in normal mouse serum (C.S. David *et al.,* 1977). This discrepancy can probably be explained by the assay system used and the antisera examined. The following points can be made:

1. Alloantisera contain antibodies against *both* the carbohydrate-defined antigens discussed above *and* the glycoprotein Ia antigens described by others (Cullen *et al.*, 1976). Thus, unless antibodies against the carbohydrate antigens are predominant in alloantisera, inhibition assays would not detect this family of antigens in serum. In contrast, the xenogeneic antisera contain *only* antibodies against the carbohydrate series of Ia antigens; thus, clear-cut inhibition would be detected with these antisera.

2. Other laboratories have exclusively used complement-mediated lysis of lymphocytes by alloantisera to detect Ia antigens. This assay method has the disadvantage that non-complement-fixing antibodies would not be detected. The fact that cytotoxicity does not necessarily correlate with the activity (serological or other) of antisera is most clearly demonstrated by monoclonal alloantibodies, which frequently do not fix complement (McKenzie, unpublished), and by the rabbit antibodies against the carbohydrate-defined Ia antigens, which are poor complement fixers (McKenzie and Parish, unpublished). We now routinely use rosette-forming-cell assays to detect the binding of both xenogeneic (Parish *et al.*, 1976a) and allogeneic (Parish and McKenzie, 1978b; Sandrin *et al.*, 1978) anti-Ia antibodies to lymphoid cells. These binding assays detect all antibody categories and confirm, via inhibition studies, that Ia antigenic activity is present in mouse serum (Parish *et al.*, 1978).

3. Finally, it should be emphasized that in our hands, several assay systems in different laboratories have given comparable results and have supported our contention that carbohydrate-defined Ia antigens exist, e.g., xenogeneic vs. allogeneic anti-Ia sera, cytotoxic vs. rosette-forming-cell assays, and others. In addition, using inhibition assays, other workers have demonstrated that Ia antigens are in serum (Callahan *et al.*, 1976).

3. Isolation and Chemical Nature of Carbohydrate-Defined Ia Antigens

3.1. Low-Molecular-Weight Ia Antigens in Serum

A procedure has been devised for isolating the bulk of the low-molecular-weight Ia antigen in mouse serum (Parish *et al.*, 1976c). The method entails precipitation of serum proteins by $(NH_4)_2\ SO_4$, extraction of the antigenic activity from the supernatant with organic solvents, and further fractionation of the material on paper chromatograms. This procedure results in high yields of the antigen from serum as detected both by inhibition of xenogeneic and allogeneic antisera and using either cytotoxicity or rosetting assays.

Several lines of evidence, which are summarized below, now suggest that the low-molecular-weight Ia antigens in serum are gangliosides, i.e., water-soluble glycosphingolipids that contain sialic acid.

1. The Ia antigens contain a sugar moiety, since both concanavalin A (specific for glucose and sterically related sugars) and *Lotus tetragonolobus* (specific for L-fucose) lectins bound the antigen (Parish *et al.*, 1976c).

2. Similarly, the antigenic determinants of the serum Ia molecules appear to be carbohydrate in nature, since Ia antigenicity was destroyed by either periodate oxidation or neuraminidase treatment, but was untouched by pronase (Parish *et al.*, 1976c).

3. The mobility of the antigens on paper chromatograms developed with ethyl acetate (5)–glacial acetic acid (1)–pyridine (5)–water (3) was high (R glucose = 0.4), which suggested that glycolipids rather than free oligosaccharides were involved (Parish *et al.*, 1976c, 1977).

4. When the antigen preparation was subjected to thin-layer chromatography (TLC) in chloroform (60)–methanol (45)–water (10), antigenic activity was found to be associated with several spots that stained for both carbohydrate and lipid (Higgins and Parish, 1980). In fact, these TLC studies have begun to suggest that a number of different gangliosides, which carry separate antigenic specificities, are present in the antigen preparation.

5. When mouse serum was fractionated on a KBr density gradient, the bulk of the antigenic activity was recovered in the lipoprotein fraction (Parish *et al.*, 1977). This result is consistent with the Ia antigens in serum being glycolipids and suggests that the glycolipids either are forming micelles in serum or are weakly associating with serum lipoproteins, as has been observed for some blood-group glycolipids (Marcus and Cass, 1969). The demonstration by others that Ia antigen in mouse serum is associated with high-density lipoproteins (Callahan *et al.*, 1976) supports the latter suggestion.

3.2. High-Molecular-Weight Ia Antigens in Serum

At this point, it should be noted that more than 95% of the Ia antigenic activity in mouse serum appears to be present as the low-molecular-weight (ganglioside) form. However, a small proportion (<5%) of the Ia antigenic activity in serum, particularly from mitogen-injected mice, is nondialyzable and is actually associated with a 500,000-molecular-weight glycoprotein that has an α_2-macroglobulin-like electrophoretic mobility (Jackson *et al.*, 1977). Table 4 compares the properties of the low-molecular-weight and high-molecular-weight Ia antigens in serum.

Both forms of serum Ia appear to carry the same antigenic specificities, since they cross-inhibit anti-Ia antibodies. However, it is still uncertain whether the α_2-macroglobulin antigen has noncovalently bound gly-

TABLE 4. Comparison of Two Forms of Carbohydrate-Defined Ia Antigens Detected in Mouse Serum

Property	Low-mol.-wt. antigen	High-mol.-wt. antigen
Proportion of Ia antigenic activity in serum	90–99%	1–10%
Chemical nature	Glycosphingolipid (ganglioside)	Glycoprotein (α_2-macroglubulin)
Mol. wt.	2000–5000	500,000
Origin	T cell (Ly 1$^+$)	T cell (Ly?)
Secretion stimulated by mitogens	Yes	Yes
General	May associate with lipoproteins or form micelles in serum.	Non-Ig in nature

colipid Ia or has been directly glycosylated with carbohydrate-defined Ia antigens.

Which form of the carbohydrate-defined Ia antigens is present on the lymphocyte surface is still uncertain. However, the inability of rabbit antisera against the carbohydrate-defined Ia antigens to immune-precipitate any glycoproteins from lymphocyte cell membranes (C.S. David *et al.*, 1977; B.D. Schwartz and Cullen, 1978; Parish *et al.*, 1978) suggests that the ganglioside form of the antigen is expressed on lymphoid cells.

4. Comparison of Carbohydrate-Defined and Protein-Defined Ia Antigens

4.1. General Considerations

There is now ample evidence that murine anti-Ia sera react with a family of glycoprotein molecules on the lymphocyte surface, which have molecular weights of approximately 58,000 daltons and consist of two nonidentical polypeptide chains of 33,000 and 25,000 daltons molecular weight, respectively (Cullen *et al.*, 1976). When we initially observed that anti-Ia sera contained antibodies against a number of carbohydrate-defined antigens, we proposed that the antigenic determinants of the glycoprotein Ia antigens resided in their carbohydrate portion (McKenzie *et al.*, 1977). We also suggested that the oligosaccharide Ia antigens in serum may have arisen from proteolytic cleavage of the glycoprotein Ia antigens (Parish *et al.*, 1976c). However, this interpretation was made untenable by the following evidence that the polypeptide portion of the glycoprotein Ia antigens carries the antigenic activity:

1. The antigenicity of the glycoprotein Ia.7 specificity was destroyed by pronase treatment, but was resistant to neuraminidase digestion (Cullen *et al.*, 1975). Furthermore, glycopeptides isolated from pronase digests of the Ia.7 glycoprotein did not appear to bind to anti-Ia antibodies (Cullen *et al.*, 1975).

2. The carbohydrate portion of the Ia glycoprotein molecule closely resembles that of the H-2 antigens (Freed and Nathenson, 1977a,b). Also, although the glycoprotein Ia antigens carried variable amounts of sialic acid, antigenic specificity did not appear to correlate with sialic acid composition (Freed and Nathenson, 1977a,b). Monosaccharides were also unable to inhibit the precipitation of the glycoprotein Ia by alloantisera (Freed and Nathenson, 1977a).

3. The amino acid sequences of different Ia glycoproteins appear to correlate with antigenic specificity. For example, comparative ion-exchange chromatography of tryptic peptides of Ia glycoproteins suggested a correlation between sharing of tryptic peptides and sharing of serological specificities (Cullen *et al.*, 1976; Freed and Nathenson, 1977a; Freed *et al.*, 1978). Similarly, sequencing studies indicated both haplotype-associated and subregion-associated differences in the amino acid sequences of the 33,000-molecular-weight (α) and 25,000-molecular-weight (β) polypeptide chains of glycoprotein Ia (Cecka *et al.*, 1977; Silver, 1977; Silver *et al.*, 1977; McMillan *et al.*, 1977).

The simplest means of reconciling our results with data described above is that two distinct families of alloantigens are controlled by the murine *I* region—one family expresses protein-defined determinants and the other has carbohydrate-defined antigenic specificities (Parish *et al.*, 1978). Consistent with this interpretation is the inability of a rabbit antiserum, directed exclusively against the carbohydrate-defined antigens, to immune-precipitate glycoprotein Ia from lymphocyte cell membranes (C.S. David *et al.*, 1977; B.D. Schwartz and Cullen, 1978; Parish *et al.*, 1978). An important implication of this interpretation is that most, if not all, mouse anti-Ia sera probably contain antibodies against *both* families of antigens.

Table 5 compares the properties of the carbohydrate-defined and protein-defined Ia antigens. Although the table is self-explanatory, certain points warrant discussion. First, the carbohydrate-defined Ia antigens already appear to express a high polymorphism. On the basis of sugar inhibition studies (McKenzie *et al.*, 1977) and the analysis of a xenogeneic antiserum against these antigens (Parish and McKenzie, 1978a), at least six or seven different specificities are expressed by the $H\text{-}2^k$ haplotype alone. Some of these specificities exhibit a strain-distribution pattern similar to that of known glycoprotein Ia antigens (Parish and McKenzie, 1978a), whereas the neuraminidase studies described earlier in this chapter appear to reveal unique specificities. At this time, a nomenclature problem exists. The specificity designations of the carbohydrate-defined antigens obviously need to be separated from the Ia glycoprotein antigens. However, a reliable method of preparing alloantisera exclusively against the carbohydrate-defined antigens is essential before firm specificity numbers can be quoted. In addition, the location within the *I* region of the genes controlling the carbohydrate antigens is still unclear. It seems likely that the *I-A* subregion controls most of the antigens, with the possible involvement of the *I-E/I-C* subregion (Parish *et al.*, 1976a; McKenzie *et al.*, 1977; Parish and McKenzie, 1978a), but the evidence is incomplete. An interesting speculation at this point is that the *I-J* subregion may also control a family of carbohydrate-defined antigens, since attempts to isolate glycoprotein antigens from the cell surface with anti-I-J sera have been unsuccessful (J. Freed, personal communication).

Recent experiments suggest that in contrast to the protein-defined Ia

TABLE 5. Comparison of Properties of Carbohydrate-Defined and Protein-Defined Ia Antigens

Property	Carbohydrate-defined Ia antigens	Protein-defined Ia antigens
Chemical nature	Glycosphingolipid[a] (gangliosides)	Glycoprotein
Antigenic determinants	Defined by sugars.	Defined by protein.
Mol. wt.	2000–5000	58,000 (two chains: 33,000 and 25,000)
Polymorphism	High	High
Cellular distribution	90% of B cells, subpopulations of T cells and macrophages	90% of B cells, subpopulations of T cells and macrophages
Levels in serum	High (T-cell-derived)	Low
Strong MLR determinant?[b]	No (?)	Yes

[a] A small proportion (1–10%) of this antigen associates with α_2-macroglobulin in serum [Jackson *et al.* (1977) and Table 4].
[b] See the data in Table 6.

TABLE 6. Inhibition of Mixed-Lymphocyte Reactions by Different Anti-Ia Sera [a]

Stimulator spleen cells	Antiserum added	Antiserum during culture[b] cpm[d]	Antiserum during culture[b] Inhibition (%)	Cells preincubated with antiserum[c] cpm[d]	Cells preincubated with antiserum[c] Inhibition (%)
A.TH	—	7,461 ± 928	—	14,225 ± 1376	—
A.TL	—	55,650 ± 2265	—	45,825 ± 3068	—
A.TL	Normal A.TH	60,583 ± 2755	0	45,609 ± 2025	0.7
A.TL	Normal A.TL	57,920 ± 2757	0	43,761 ± 1652	6.5
A.TL	A.TH anti-A.TL	5,208 ± 312	104.7	7,973 ± 354	119.8
A.TL	A.TL anti-A.TH	48,287 ± 1171	15.3	41,552 ± 2062	13.5
A.TL	Control rabbit[e] anti-Ia^k	57,566 ± 1464	0	28,549 ± 1975	54.7
A.TL	Rabbit anti-Ia^k	54,313 ± 3452	2.8	32,748 ± 2853	41.4

[a]MLR between 5×10^6 Ig^-A.TH spleen cells and 5×10^6 2000-rad-irradiated stimulator spleen cells. After 4 days' culture, each treatment was pulsed for 18 hr with 0.5 μCi/well of [^{125}I]-UdRib.
[b]Ig fraction isolated from antisera and 1% serum concentration added to cultures.
[c]Stimulator cells preincubated with 2.5% concentrations of mouse sera and 25% concentrations of rabbit sera and washed prior to culturing.
[d]Means ± standard error of triplicate cultures.
[e]Rabbit anti-Ia^k from which all anti-Ia antibodies had been absorbed.

antigens, the carbohydrate-defined Ia antigens are not major lymphocyte-activating determinants (Table 5). The data in favor of this statement are presented in Table 6. The experimental protocol was to examine the ability of a rabbit antiserum directed against the carbohydrate-defined Ia antigens to block an *I*-region-induced MLR. It can be seen in Table 6 that the rabbit antiserum showed no specific blocking of the MLR (any inhibition observed was also obtained with control serum), whereas alloantisera completely inhibited the response in a specific manner. The mouse antisera had anti-Ia titers 10- to 20-fold higher than the rabbit antiserum. However, sufficient rabbit antiserum was used in the preincubation experiment to rule out the possibility of too low a concentration of blocking antibody.

4.2. Genetic Implications

The genetic implications of the claim that the *I* region controls families of protein-defined and carbohydrate-defined antigens should be considered. First, if carbohydrate-defined Ia antigens exist, then the *I*-region genes controlling these antigens probably code for glycosyltransferases.

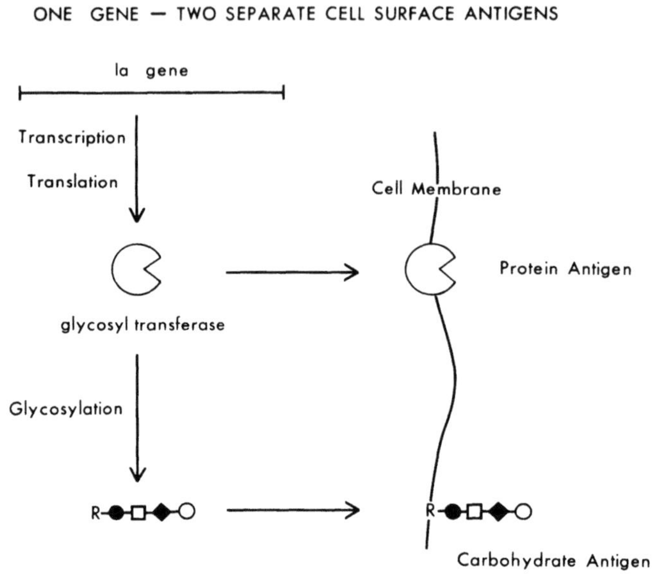

Figure 2. A possible mechanism whereby one *Ia* gene could produce both the protein-defined and the carbohydrate-defined Ia antigens.

It is possible, but less likely, that the *I* region codes for regulators of glycosylation rather than the glycosyltransferases themselves. Second, it is probable that the *I* region contains at least two families of genes, one coding for the protein-defined Ia antigens and the other coding for glycosyltransferases. If this is indeed the case, eventually recombinant mouse strains should be identified that separate these two gene families. Third, on a more speculative note, it is feasible that one family of genes could control both forms of Ia antigen. This hypothesis is depicted in Fig. 2 and suggests that the primary structural product of each *Ia* gene is a glycosyl transferase. Thus, two separate Ia antigens, which are expressed in the cell membrane, can be produced by each *Ia* gene—the glycosyltransferase itself (i.e., the protein Ia antigen) and the carbohydrate side chain that the transferase produces (i.e., the carbohydrate Ia antigen). Experiments are in progress to test this hypothesis.

5. Biological Properties of Carbohydrate-Defined Ia Antigens in Serum

5.1. Origin

Soon after the detection of Ia antigens in serum, it became apparent that their production was, in some way, T-cell-dependent (Parish *et al.*,

1976b). This conclusion was initially based on *in vivo* studies that revealed that T-cell-deprived mice lacked serum Ia antigens (Parish *et al.*, 1976b). Furthermore, the depression of serum Ia levels by anti-lymphocyte serum treatment, but not by adult thymectomy, implicated long-lived, recirculating T cells in secretion (Parish *et al.*, 1976b). Subsequent *in vitro* studies with fractionated spleen-cell populations demonstrated that Ia secretion was dependent on an Ig^-, Thy-1^+, nonadherent cell (i.e., T lymphocyte), which was Ly-1^+, Ly-2^- and Ia^- (Parish *et al.*, 1976b; McKenzie and Parish, 1976). The simplest interpretation of these results is that Ly-1^+, Ly-2^- and Ia^- T cells secrete the carbohydrate-defined Ia antigens. However, it is still possible that this T-cell subpopulation induces other cells to secrete the antigen, although if this were the case, the secreting cell would need to be a null cell (non-T or -B) that was nonadherent and lacked surface Ia antigens. In addition, *in vitro* secretion was measured over such a short time span (<6 hr) that cell collaboration seems to be most unlikely.

5.2. Influence of Mitogens and Antigens on Serum Levels

It was found that certain immunization procedures resulted in dramatic increases in serum Ia levels. In particular, every mitogen tested stimulated Ia secretion (up to 125-fold increase in serum levels), irrespec-

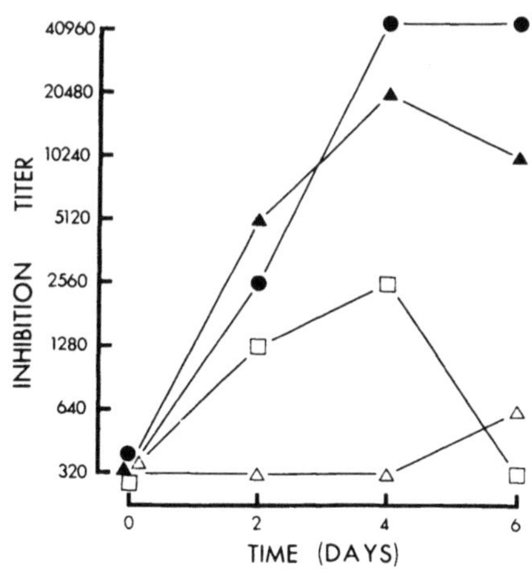

Figure 3. Content of Ia antigen in the sera of CBA/H mice at various times after intraperitoneal injection with saline (△), phytohemagglutinin (▲), *Escherichia coli* lipopolysaccharide (●), or concanavalin A (□). A 50-μg dose of mitogen was injected and serum Ia levels measured by an inhibition assay using an A.TH anti-A.TL (anti-Ia^k) serum (Parish *et al.*, 1976a). Data reproduced from Parish and McKenzie (1977a) with permission of the publishers.

tive of whether they are mitogenic for T or B cells (Parish and McKenzie, 1977a). The time course of appearance of Ia antigens in serum after mitogen injection is depicted in Fig. 3. In a similar manner, all T-independent antigens examined significantly augmented serum Ia concentrations, although they did vary substantially in their ability to activate secretion; e.g., polymerized flagellin induced a 100-fold increase, whereas polyvinyl pyrrolidone produced only a 3-fold augmentation (Parish and McKenzie, 1977a). Alloantigens presented in a graft-vs.-host reaction were also potent stimulators of Ia secretion (Parish *et al.*, 1976b). On the other hand, T-dependent antigens, unless injected in large amounts, produced no detectable changes in the serum levels of Ia antigens (Parish and McKenzie, 1977a). Thus, there seems to be an inverse relationship between the T dependence of an antigen (or mitogen) and its ability to stimulate release of Ia antigens, even though cell-separation studies indicated that mitogens and T-independent antigens triggered T lymphocytes to secrete the antigens (Parish and McKenzie, 1977a). This observation suggested that T cells (memory T cells?) require little or no cell division after antigen stimulation before they release Ia antigens. The findings also led us to propose that perhaps antibody responses to all antigens are T-dependent, but antigens simply vary in the efficiency with which they activate T cells to produce helper factors (Parish and McKenzie, 1977a).

5.3. Serum Levels during Different Disease States

Since mitogens and T-independent antigens substantially augment the concentrations of carbohydrate-defined Ia antigens in serum, it was of interest to assess the influence of different infectious agents on serum Ia levels. Table 7 summarizes the results we have obtained with viral, bacterial, and protozoal infections and also with tumors (Parish *et al.*, 1979). It is clearly apparent that different disease states resulted in substantial enhancement or suppression, or both, of serum Ia concentrations. At present, it is difficult to interpret these results in detail, since, although Ly-1$^+$, Ly-2$^-$, Ia$^-$ T cells are implicated in Ia secretion (McKenzie and Parish, 1976), this cell-surface phenotype does not discriminate between helper T cells and T cells that mediate delayed-type hypersensitivity (DTH) reactions (Cantor and Boyse, 1975; Vadas *et al.*, 1976). It seems reasonable, however, to interpret serum Ia levels as a measure of general T-cell activation. Consistent with this interpretation was the observation that *P. yoelii*, a malarial parasite that stimulates prolonged T-cell proliferation (Jayawardena *et al.*, 1975; Freeman and Parish, 1978), augmented serum Ia levels, whereas *P. berghei*, a form of the parasite that suppresses T-cell division (Jayawardena *et al.*, 1975; Freeman and Parish, 1978), suppressed Ia secretion (Table 7).

TABLE 7. Levels of Carbohydrate-Defined Ia Antigens in Mouse Serum during Different Infections

Pathogen	Dose	Serum Ia antigen levels[a]	
		Above normal	Below normal
Lymphocytic choriomeningitis virus	2000 LD_{50}, i.v.[b]	+++ (day 5)	++ (day 9)
Listeria monocytogenes	10^3 organisms, i.v.	No	+++ (day 6)
Brucella abortus	5 × 10^5 organisms, i.v.	++ (day 7)	No
Malaria			
P. berghei	10^4 parasitized red blood cells, i.v.	No	++ (day 15)
P. yoelii	Same	++ (day 6)	No
Syngeneic tumors	10^6 cells, subcutaneously	+ (day 2)	+++ (>day 7)

[a](+, ++, +++) Extent of elevation or depression of Ia levels; day in parentheses is the day after infection that maximum elevation or depression of serum Ia levels occurred.
[b]LD_{50} when injected intracerebrally into mice.

The ability of lymphocytic choriomeningitis virus to both augment and suppress serum Ia levels during the course of infection is intriguing (Table 7), augmentation corresponding with maximal viremia and suppression with the peak cytotoxic T-cell response (Dunlop and Blanden, 1977). Similarly, the rapid suppression of Ia production by tumors is striking, and may be related to the well-documented immunosuppression of T cells by tumors (Kilburn *et al.*, 1974).

The two bacterial infections examined, *Listeria* and *Brucella*, produced very different effects on serum Ia levels (Table 7), even though both bacteria preferentially grow inside macrophages. This difference may be a reflection of the relative persistence of the two infections—*Listeria* is an acute infection, whereas *Brucella* chronically infects macrophages (Cheers and Pagram, 1979).

5.4. Ontogeny

When the time of appearance of Ia antigens in serum was measured, it was found that fetal serum contained little or no Ia antigen, whereas 2 days after birth, newborn mice expressed adult levels of antigen in their serum (Fig. 4). The ontogeny experiment presented in Fig. 4 was designed in such a way that only paternally derived Ia antigens were detected in serum. Thus, the serum Ia antigens must be synthesized by the newborn

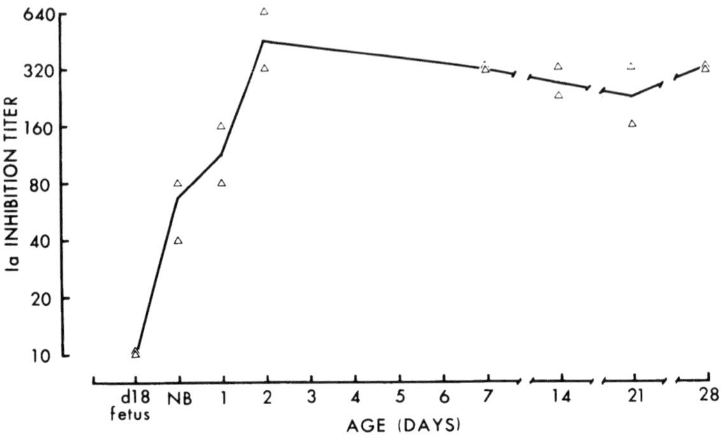

Figure 4. Appearance of Ia antigens in mouse serum with age. Concentrations of Ia antigen were measured by an inhibition assay using a xenogeneic anti-Ia serum (Parish *et al.*, 1976a). To ensure that only paternally derived Ia antigens were detected, BALB/c (Ia.3 −) females were mated with C57Bl/6 (Ia.3 +) males, and Ia antigen in the serum of the offspring was measured by performing the inhibition assay with DBA/1 (Ia.3 +) target cells. With this arrangement, only C57Bl/6-derived Ia antigens (an "Ia.3-like" specificity) were detected. Each point represents an inhibition titer for a single animal. (NB) Newborn.

mice rather than being transferred, via milk, from mother to offspring. It also appears, from analysis of maternally derived Ia antigens, that serum-borne Ia does not cross the placenta (Parish, unpublished).

Although Ia production is T-dependent (Parish *et al.*, 1976b; McKenzie and Parish, 1976), the onset of Ia secretion in newborn mice appears to precede the development of T-helper-cell function, since antibody responses to T-dependent antigens appear only after 3 days of age (Hardy *et al.*, 1976) and take several weeks to mature to adult levels (Spear and Edelman, 1974; Hardy *et al.*, 1976; Rabinowitz, 1976). However, this lack of T–B collaboration in neonates may be due to macrophage dysfunction resulting from immaturity (Hardy *et al.*, 1973), incorrect lymphoid-tissue architecture (Friedberg and Weissman, 1974), or the presence of nonspecific suppressor T cells (Mosier *et al.*, 1977), rather than to a deficiency of helper T cells. On the other hand, there is still no firm evidence that helper T cells secrete the carbohydrate-defined Ia antigens; another functional subpopulation of Ly-1^{+}, Ly-2^{-}, Ia^{-} T cells may be involved (McKenzie and Parish, 1976).

The levels of Ia antigen in mouse serum remain remarkably constant with age, no significant changes in inhibition titer being observed up to 2 years of age. However, there was some decline (from 2- to 8-fold) in serum levels after 2 years (Parish, unpublished). This constant background stimulation of T cells to secrete Ia antigens is surprising and may reflect a response against "self" rather than exogenous antigens, analogous to the situation with B cells (Dresser, 1978; Steele and Cunningham, 1978).

6. Detection of a Similar System of Antigens in Man

An advantage of raising xenogeneic anti-Ia sera is that antisera can be simply produced against Ia-like determinants in a wide range of different species. In fact, using immunization procedures virtually identical to those described for the mouse (Parish *et al.*, 1976a) (i.e., by immunizing rabbits with whole serum in adjuvant and absorbing the antiserum with dialyzed serum), we have produced antisera to a similar set of cell-surface and serum molecules in man, rats, guinea pigs, sheep, and cattle. The rabbit antisera made against the serum of each of these species share the following common properties: (1) reaction, by rosetting, with a proportion of peripheral-blood lymphocytes (PBL), analogous to the percentage of B cells present (that these are B cells has not been shown in all the species listed); (2) reaction with a low-molecular-weight molecule (dialyzable) in whole serum; and (3) present in a polymorphic form in that the antisera recognize multiple specificities that are carried by different individuals of the species. The approach should be of considerable value in producing anti-Ia sera in species where genetic analysis is difficult. In this review, we will concentrate on the data obtained from studies in man, which parallel to a great extent the studies described thus far in inbred mice.

6.1. Production and Testing of Antisera

Antisera have been produced by immunizing rabbits with whole human serum in Freund's complete adjuvant and then absorbing the antiserum with dialyzed human serum obtained from the same donor (Sandrin *et al.*, 1979a,b). Since rabbits vary in their antibody response to serum components, the volume of dialyzed serum used for absorption was calculated on the basis of the amount of nondialyzed serum required to totally absorb the serum. The absorbed antisera contain few, if any, cytotoxic antibodies for lymphocytes, and therefore binding of antibodies to lymphoid cells was assessed by a rosetting assay using sheep anti-rabbit-Ig-coupled erythrocytes (Parish *et al.*, 1976a; Sandrin *et al.*, 1979a,b). Assays using protein A–red cell complexes are not suitable for human studies, since human B cells bind protein A (Sandrin, unpublished). Different antisera have been produced against more than 20 individuals, and each yielded similar, but unique findings, to be detailed below.

6.2. Tissue Distribution

The antisera produced against an individual's serum reacted, after absorption, with that individual's PBL, but mostly with the B-cell fraction, although there was some T-cell reactivity. There was also reactivity with some null cells (E^-Ig^-), although most, but not all, of this reaction was removed by exposing these cells to carbonyl iron. The reaction of a typical antiserum against the serum donor's cells is shown in Table 8. Comparison of the tissue distribution of a xenogeneic anti-Ia serum is made with that of an anti-DRW serum, and it is clear that both sera have a similar cell distribution pattern (Table 9). This comparison extends to tests on platelets and red cells (Table 9), where both antisera are nonreactive. In addition, serum inhibition studies performed with both xenogeneic and allogeneic sera indicate that both sera detect antigenic specificities present in normal human serum (Table 9).

6.3. Evidence That Xenogeneic Antisera Recognize DRW (Ia) Specificities

The similarities between the findings obtained with several xenogenic antisera and DRW sera (the human equivalent of the mouse Ia system) are listed in Table 9. The almost identical tissue distribution has been de-

TABLE 8. Cellular Reactivity of Human Xenogeneic and Allogeneic Anti-Ia Sera

Target cell[a]	Xenogeneic antiserum (% RFC)[a,b]	DRW antiserum (% lysis)[b]
Peripheral blood lymphocytes (PBL)	13	20
T cells (E^+Ig^-)	7	<5
B cells (E^-Ig^+)	87	100
Null cells (E^-Ig^-)	21	30
Macrophage (carbonyl iron) depleted null cells	6	10

[a](RFC) Rosette-forming cells; (E^+) sheep-erythrocyte-rosetting PBL; (Ig^+) PBL that rosette for surface immunoglobulin. The PBL were prepared on Isopaque–Ficoll (IF) and E-RFC formed and also separated on IF into E^+ and E^-cells. The E^- cells were further fractionated by forming Ig^+ RFC and again separating into E^-Ig^+ and E^-Ig^- fractions on IF. These cells were then exposed to carbonyl iron to remove macrophages.

[b]Corrected for background levels: 0–2% for RFC, 0–10% for cytotoxicity.

TABLE 9. Comparison of the Reactivities of Xenogeneic Anti-Ia Sera and Allogeneic Anti-Ia (DRW) Sera in Man

Property	Anti-DRW	Xenogeneic anti-Ia
1. Cellular distribution		
B cells	+	+
Some T	+	+
Null	±	±
Platelets, red blood cells	−	−
Serum	+	+
2. Coded for by HLA-linked genes		
Family studies	+	+
Cocaps with β_2 microglobulin.	−	−
Cocaps with anti-DRW/ xenogeneic antisera.	Cocaps with xenogeneic antisera	Cocaps with anti-DRW antisera
3. Polymorphism	Present	Present
4. Blocking studies	DRw antisera and xenogeneic anti-Ia sera reciprocally block each other.	

scribed above. The further similarities are: (1) In family studies, xenogeneic anti-Ia sera have been shown to segregate with HLA-A and HLA-B specificities, and further mapping studies are currently in progress (Sandrin *et al.*, 1979a,b). (2) In a series of cocapping experiments, it could be shown that the specificities detected by the xenogeneic antiserum do not cocap with cell-surface Ig or with β_2-microglobulin, but that DRW and these specificities cocap (Sandrin *et al.*, 1979a,b); Sandrin, unpublished results). (3) In reciprocal blocking studies, it was found that DRW antisera could block the binding of rabbit anti-Ia sera and the xenogeneic antisera could block the binding of DRW antisera (Sandrin *et al.*, 1979a,b). Clearly, both antisera recognize similar structures on the cell surface, and the results are strikingly similar to those obtained in the murine system.

6.4. Polymorphism of Specificities Detected by Rabbit Anti-Ia Sera

When sera were raised to a number of different individuals, direct testing and absorption studies indicated that the sera were complex and contained multiple antibodies. At least ten different specificities have been identified thus far, but attempts to correlate these specificities with individual DRW specificities (DRW 1–8) have not met with great success either in family studies or from the typing of a limited panel. However, the complexities of the DRW system are still being defined, and at present we are typing limited panels provided by homozygous typing cells.

The results discussed above provide compelling evidence for the similarity of certain DRW specificities recognized by alloantisera and those detected by xenogeneic antisera. Their nature remains to be revealed, since chemical studies (including sugar inhibition tests) have only recently commenced. However, the detection of serum Ia antigens in man may have some practical value, as detailed below.

6.5. Functional Studies in Man

The content of Ia antigens in serum can readily be measured in man using a rosette inhibition technique. Several studies, analogous to those performed in the mouse, have now been attempted. In particular, the Ia antigen levels in serum have been assessed after *in vivo* antigenic stimulation, and also, a number of patients with tumors have been examined. After the injection of streptococcal, *Candida*, or mycobacterial antigens subcutaneously into sensitized individuals, there was a dramatic rise in serum Ia levels from 160–320 U/ml to more than 5000 inhibition U/ml of serum. This rise occurred before DTH skin reactivity was maximal and subsided before the skin induration had disappeared. Whether the Ia response in man is due to secretion of the antigen by T cells, as in the mouse, and is associated in some way with DTH responses is not known at present. In contrast to these findings was the uniform suppression of the level of Ia antigen in the sera of patients with different malignant tumors (Table 10). The level of suppression varied from 63 to 100% and

TABLE 10. Suppression of Serum Ia Levels in Patients with Tumors

Cancer	Cytostatic drugs	Ia inhibition titer[a]	Inhibition(%)
Nil (normals)[b]	–	320	—
Ovary	+	0	100
Colon	+	0	100
Colon	+	120	63
Colon	+	60	80
Disseminating	+	120	63
Breast	+	0	100
Pancreas	+	0	100
Lung	+	60	80
Hodgkin's disease	–	0	100
Acute lymphatic leukemia	–	0	100

[a]Results expressed as "inhibition units"/ml of serum (Parish *et al.*, 1976b).
[b]Based on data obtained from 30 individuals.

was independent of the presence of cytotoxic drugs (Sandrin *et al.*, 1979a). At present, the specificity of the suppression is being examined, but these two findings may have great value in determining an individual's T-cell status by a simple serum test. Furthermore, the testing, as yet in its early stages, may have value in monitoring therapy or as an aid to the diagnosis of the presence of malignant tumors.

7. Functional Significance of Carbohydrate-Defined Ia Antigens

The functional relevance of the carbohydrate-defined Ia antigens is still highly speculative. However, since virtually all functional studies of the *I* region have failed to differentiate between the protein-defined and carbohydrate-defined Ia antigens, all *I*-region phenomena now need to be reexamined and related to the two systems of antigens. For example, which family of antigens (if either) mediates the *Ir*-gene effects? Bearing these considerations in mind, three possible functions of the carbohydrate-defined Ia antigens are discussed below.

7.1. Surface-Membrane Receptors for Immunoregulatory Signals

There is now ample evidence from a wide range of biological systems that gangliosides can act as receptors on cells for regulatory molecules. The best-characterized receptor is the monosialoganglioside GM_1, which binds cholera toxin and subsequently results in adenylate cyclase activation (van Heyningen, 1974; Fishman and Brady, 1976). However, gangliosides have also been implicated in the cell-membrane receptors for tetanus toxin (van Heyningen, 1974), botulinum toxin (Simpson and Rapport, 1971), serotonin (van Heyningen, 1974), interferon (Vengris *et al.*, 1976), thyroid-stimulating hormone (Mullin *et al.*, 1978), and cell adhesion (Huang, 1978). At the immunological level, recent studies suggest that the receptor on macrophages for migration-inhibition factor is also a ganglioside (Higgins *et al.*, 1978). Similarly, since the carbohydrate-defined Ia antigens appear to be gangliosides, it seems likely that they may act as receptors for informational molecules between lymphoid cells. The observation that certain T-cell-derived gangliosides can inhibit *in vitro* antibody responses (Esselman and Miller, 1977) is consistent with this possibility.

At a more speculative level, if the *I* region codes for a family of glycosyltransferases and these enzymes are expressed at the cell surface (see Fig. 2), then interaction between the transferase and incompletely glycosylated carbohydrate Ia antigens on other cells or immunoregulatory factors could occur. Such a model has been proposed by Roseman (1970) to explain specific interaction between cells. In the case of the *I* region, the Ia antigens would represent a polymorphic system of recognition structures between cells. The selective advantage of this sort of polymorphism is that animal cell populations could resist infectious agents that attempted to resist the host's immune response by mimicry of the recognition structures.

7.2. Association with T-Cell-Derived Factors

There is now a large body of evidence that suggests that Ia antigenic specificities are associated with a range of immunoregulatory molecules or "factors" secreted by T cells. Both nonspecific (Armerding *et al.*, 1974) and antigen-specific (Munro and Taussig, 1975; Howie and Feldmann, 1977; McDougal *et al.*, 1977; Isac *et al.*, 1977; Tokuhisa *et al.*, 1978) helper factors of antibody formation have been shown to carry Ia antigens. Similarly, Ia antigens have been detected on antigen-specific suppressor factors of antibody formation (Tada *et al.*, 1976; Théze *et al.*, 1977), contact sensitivity (Greene *et al.*, 1977), and MLRs (Rich *et al.*, 1977). The *I* subregions controlling the antigens expressed by different factors vary somewhat. As a rule, factors that help antibody production carry *I-A*-subregion-defined Ia antigens, whereas suppressor factors of antibody formation and contact sensitivity bear *I-J*-subregion-controlled

TABLE 11. Ability of Rabbit Anti-Ia Serum Immunoabsorbents to Remove GAT-Specific and TGAL-Specific Helper Factors[a]

Spleen cells cultured with[b]:	Helper factor absorbed with:	IgM AFC/culture[c]	
		Filtrate	Eluate
GAT	—	10 ± 6	—
GAT-specific HF	—	17 ± 9	—
GAT + GAT-specific HF	—	257 ± 48	—
GAT + GAT-specific HF	Rabbit anti-Ia^k	60 ± 29	200 ± 12
GAT + GAT-specific HF	Rabbit anti-Ia^k control[d]	197 ± 7	7 ± 3
TGAL	—	23 ± 7	—
TGAL-specific HF	—	0	—
TGAL + TGAL-specific HF	—	293 ± 53	—
TGAL + TGAL-specific HF	Rabbit anti-Ia^k	3 ± 3	303 ± 70
TGAL + TGAL-specific HF	Rabbit anti-Ia^k control[d]	223 ± 46	17 ± 3

[a](HF) Helper factor; (AFC) antibody-forming cells.
[b]Each culture contained 3×10^6 unprimed B10 spleen cells, 5 μg/ml of antigen, and a 10^{-3} dilution of each helper-factor preparation. Helper factors were derived from CBA mice as previously described (Howie and Feldmann, 1977).
[c]Results represent either GAT AFC/culture in GAT experiment or TGAL AFC/culture in TGAL experiment ± standard errors of means.
[d]Rabbit anti-Ia^k from which all anti-Ia antibodies had been absorbed.

TABLE 12. Ability of Mouse and Rabbit Anti-Ia Sera to Block Absorption of GAT-Specific Helper Factor by Peritoneal Exudate Cells[a]

Antigen (GAT)	Helper factor	Absorption of HF by PEC[b]	Pretreatment of PEC[c]	IgM AFC to GAT/culture	
				Expt. 1	Expt. 2
+	−	—	—	20 ± 10	13 ± 13
−	+	No	—	13 ± 7	23 ± 15
+	+	No	—	190 ± 38	307 ± 26
+	+	Yes	Nil	60 ± 17	65 ± 19
+	+	Yes	A.TH NMS	40 ± 12	10 ± 10
+	+	Yes	A.TH anti-A.TL serum	143 ± 18	180 ± 35
+	+	Yes	Rabbit anti-Ia^k control	33 ± 15	17 ± 17
+	+	Yes	Rabbit anti-Ia^k	27 ± 5	37 ± 19

[a](HF) Helper factor; (PEC) peritoneal exudate cells; (AFC) antibody-forming cells; (NMS) normal mouse serum; (+ or −) presence in or absence of antigen or HF from culture. Culture conditions and rabbit antisera as in Table 11. Results include standard errors of means.
[b]0.5 ml of a 10^{-3} dilution of HF absorbed with 10^8 CBA PEC for 60 min at 37°C prior to addition to cultures.
[c]PEC (10^6/ml) pretreated with 1:20 dilution of mouse sera or 1:4 dilution of rabbit sera.

determinants. It was of interest, therefore, to determine whether carbohydrate-defined or protein-defined Ia antigens, or both, were associated with these immunoregulatory factors.

Recently, the nature of the Ia antigens carried by antigen-specific helper factors secreted by T cells was investigated (Howie *et al.*, 1979). It was found that both L-Glu^{60}-L-Ala^{30}-LTyr^{10} (GAT)-specific and poly-L(Tyr,Glu)-poly-DL-Ala-poly-L-Lys (TGAL)-specific helper factors from CBA/H (*H-2*^{k}) mice were retained and eluted from immunoabsorbent columns coupled with rabbit antibodies directed exclusively against the carbohydrate-defined Ia antigens (antiserum discussed in detail in Section 2.2) (Table 11). Mouse anti-Ia^k immunoabsorbents that carried antibodies against both the carbohydrate-defined and protein-defined Ia antigens also removed both helper factors (data not shown). However, these immunoabsorbants were unable to bind helper factor when they were pretreated with a dialyzable material in normal (*H-2*^{k}) mouse serum, which is known to neutralize antibodies against the carbohydrate-defined Ia antigens (Parish *et al.*, 1976c, 1977). In contrast, the binding of GAT-specific helper factor to *H-2*^{k} peritoneal exudate cells was significantly inhibited by mouse anti-Ia^k antibodies, but was not inhibited by rabbit anti-carbohydrate Ia antibodies (Table 12). Collectively, these results suggest that antigen-specific helper factors carry carbohydrate-defined Ia antigens, whereas the acceptor site for helper factor on peritoneal exudate cells (probably macrophages) consists of, or is closely associated with, the protein-defined Ia antigens. In fact, the ability of anti-Ia sera to block helper-factor uptake by peritoneal exudate cells is reminiscent of the masking of Fc receptors on lymphocytes by anti-Ia antibodies (Dickler, 1976; Stout *et al.*, 1977).

In another recent study (Liew *et al.*, 1980), a T-cell-derived factor that suppresses DTH to erythrocyte antigens (Liew and Chan-Liew, 1978) also appears to carry carbohydrate-defined Ia antigens. This conclusion was based on immunoabsorbent studies similar to the helper-factor experiments. It is also noteworthy that both the DTH suppressor factor (Liew *et al.*, 1980) and the GAT-specific helper factor carry *I-J*-subregion-controlled Ia antigens, whereas the TGAL-specific helper factor expresses *I-A*-subregion-defined determinants (Howie *et al.*, 1980), and yet all three of these factors appear to carry carbohydrate-defined Ia antigens (Table 13).

The functional significance of immunoregulatory factors carrying carbohydrate-defined Ia antigens is uncertain. The Ia antigens may be involved in the interaction of factors with target cells, analogous to the role of gangliosides as receptors on cells (see Section 7). In this context, it would be intriguing to know whether protein-defined Ia antigens on target cells recognize carbohydrate-defined Ia antigens on factors, as would be predicted from the hypothesis of Roseman (1970) (discussed in Section 7.1).

In a general sense, however, the presence of carbohydrate-defined Ia antigens on T-cell factors is compatible with the molecular weights of these glycoproteins. Most helper and suppressor factors have molecular weights of approximately 30,000–60,000 daltons (Munro and Taussig, 1975; Tokuhisa *et al.*, 1978; Takemori and Tada, 1975; Kapp *et al.*, 1976; Liew and Chan-Liew, 1978). Thus, it is difficult to envisage that such

TABLE 13. Summary of Ia Antigens Carried by Different Antigen-Specific T-Cell-Derived Factors

			Ia antigens on factor	
Factor	Response	Antigen specificity	Subregion origin	Carbohydrate Ia antigens?
Helper	Antibody	TGAL	*I-A*	Yes
Helper	Antibody	GAT	*I-J*	Yes
Suppressor	DTH	SRBC[a]	*I-J*	Yes

[a](SRBC) Sheep red blood cells.

factors could contain the complete protein-defined Ia antigens (molecular weight 58,000) or even the α(molecular weight 33,000) or β(molecular weight 25,000) chains, as well as possess antigen-binding capacity. A more tenable model for antigen-specific factors is that the polypeptide portion of the molecule specifies the antigen-binding site, whereas an oligosaccharide side chain attached either covalently by glycosylation or hydrophobically as a glycolipid carries Ia antigenicity.

7.3. Role as Antigen-Presenting Structures

It is now firmly established that self H-2K and H-2D antigens play a critical role in the recognition of foreign antigens by cytotoxic T cells (Doherty *et al.*, 1976; Shearer *et al.*, 1976). In a similar manner, it appears that self structures mapping to the *I* region are recognized in association with foreign antigen by the T cells that express helper activity (Katz and Benacerraf, 1975; Erb *et al.*, 1976), DTH (Miller *et al.*, 1976), and antigen-specific proliferation *in vitro* (Thomas *et al.*, 1977; R.H. Schwartz *et al.*, 1978).

It has been generally assumed that the protein-defined Ia antigens are probably associated with these *I*-region-restricted responses, although a formal demonstration of this association is difficult. However, our observation that the *I* region controls a second family of carbohydrate-defined antigens raises the possibility that for certain immune responses, the carbohydrate-defined antigens may mediate the restriction. For example, it could be envisaged that protein-defined Ia antigens may be involved in antigen presentation to T helper cells, whereas carbohydrate-defined Ia antigens could mediate antigen presentation to DTH T cells.

In fact, recent experiments (Basten *et al.*, 1980) suggest that the carbohydrate-defined Ia antigens may well be implicated in DTH induction. The experimental system was to immunize CBA ($H\text{-}2^k$) mice with dinitrofluorobenzene (DNFB), harvest spleen cells 36 hr later, and prepare an extract with a molecular weight of less than 14,000 from the cells. This extract, in the presence of additional DNFB, was capable of inducing naive CBA peritoneal exudate cells to express macrophage-migration inhibition, an *in vitro* correlate of DTH (J.R. David and Remold, 1976). The macrophage-migration inhibition was antigen-specific and was not induced by extracts from nonimmune mice. Thus, this spleen-cell extract from DNFB-treated mice appears to resemble transfer factor (TF) in its biological properties (Lawrence, 1974).

Immunochemically, the TF activity was removed by mouse anti-Ia^k sera and by a rabbit antiserum directed against the carbohydrate-defined Ia antigens. Furthermore, anti-dinitrophenyl (DNP) antibodies could absorb TF activity. Finally, the TF activity bound to concanavalin-A–Sepharose, a finding that further supports the notion that the TF molecule contains a carbohydrate portion.

Collectively, these results suggest that TF represents a complex between DNP (the immunogen) and the carbohydrate-defined Ia antigens. Presumably, this complex of immunogen and self Ia antigens is particularly potent at inducing DNP-specific DTH precursors, analogous to the role played by H-2K and H-2D antigens in the induction of cytotoxic T cells. Consistent with this interpretation are preliminary experiments that suggest that DNP-specific TF expresses some genetic restrictions in its action. Further experiments are required to establish that the carbohydrate-defined Ia antigens are implicated in DTH induction *in vivo.* It seems likely, however, that these antigens do play an important part in immune induction and regulation.

8. Conclusions

In this chapter, evidence is presented that suggests that a family of carbohydrate-defined Ia antigens exists in both mouse and man. These carbohydrate-defined antigens probably exist as glycolipids in serum and on cells and are distinct from the conventional glycoprotein Ia antigens. The level of these antigens in serum is under T-cell control, and in fact, serum levels can be used to assess general T-cell activity, particularly during different diseases. The functional significance of the carbohydrate Ia antigens is still uncertain, but they appear to be associated with certain immunoregulatory molecules and they may play a role in T-cell activation and in communication between lymphocytes.

ACKNOWLEDGMENTS. The original work reported in this review was supported by funds obtained from the NHMRC (Australia), the Australian Tobacco Research Foundation, and the National Institutes of Health (Grant No. CA21224). We also acknowledge the help of Terry Higgins and Mauro Sandrin in the preparation of this review.

References

Armerding, D., Sachs, D.H., and Katz, D.H., 1974, Activation of T and B lymphocytes *in vitro.* III. Presence of Ia determinants on allogeneic effect factor, *J. Exp. Med.* **140:**1717.

Basten, A., Croft, S., Parish, C.R., and McKenzie, I.F.C., 1981, Transfer of cell mediated immunity with cell free leukocyte extracts. III. Demonstration of Ia antigens in the specific component, *Cell Immunol.* (in press).

Callahan, G.N., Ferrone, S., Poulik, M.D., Reisfeld, R.A., and Klein, J., 1976, Characterization of Ia antigens in mouse serum, *J. Immunol.* **117:**1351.

Cantor, H., and Boyse, E.A., 1975, Functional classes of T lymphocytes bearing different Ly antigens. II. Cooperation between subclasses of Ly^+ cells in the generation of killer activity, *J. Exp. Med.* **141:**1390.

Cecka, M., McMillan, M., Murphy, D., Silver, J., McDevitt, H., and Hood, L., 1977, Partial amino acid sequence analyses of Ia molecules, in: *Ir Genes and Ia Antigens* (H.O. McDevitt, ed.), pp. 275–286, Academic Press, New York.

Cheers, C., and Pagram, F., 1979, Macrophage activation during experimental murine brucellosis: Basis for chronic infection, *Infect. Immunol.* **23:**197.

Cowing, C., Schwartz, B.D., and Dickler, H.B., 1978, Macrophage Ia antigens. I. Macrophage populations differ in their expression of Ia antigens, *J. Immunol.* **120:**378.

Cullen, S.E., Freed, J.H., Atkinson, P.H., and Nathenson, S.G., 1975, Evidence that protein determines Ia antigenic specificity, *Transplant, Proc.* **7:**237.

Cullen, S.E., Freed, J.H., and Nathenson, S.G., 1976, Structural and serological properties of murine Ia alloantigens, *Transplant, Rev.* **30:**236.

David, C.S., 1976, Serological and genetic aspects of murine Ia antigens, *Transplant. Rev.* **30:**229.

David, C.S., Neely, B.C., and Cullen, S.E., 1977, Inability to detect Ia antigens in mouse sera, in: *Ir Genes and Ia Antigens* (H.O. McDevitt, ed.), pp. 255–261, Academic Press, New York.

David J.R., and Remold, H.G., 1976, Macrophage activation by lymphocyte mediators and studies on the interaction of macrophage inhibitory factor (MIF) with its target cell, in: *Immunobiology of the Macrophage* (D.S. Nelson, ed.), pp. 401–450, Academic Press, New York.

Dickler, H.B., 1976, Lymphocyte receptors for immunoglobulin, *Adv. Immunol.* **24:**167.

Doherty, P.C., Blanden, R.V., and Zinkernagel, R.M., 1976, Specificity of virus-immune effector T cells for H-2K or H-2D compatible interactions: Implications for H-antigen diversity, *Transplant. Ref.* **29:**89.

Dresser, D.W., 1978, Most IgM-producing cells in the mouse secrete auto-antibodies (rheumatoid factor), *Nature (London)* **274:**480.

Dunlop, M.B.C., and Blanden, R.V., 1977, Mechanisms of suppression of cytotoxic T-cell responses in murine lymphocytic choriomeningitis virus infection, *J. Exp. Med.* **145:**1131.

Erb, P., Feldmann, M., and Hogg, N., 1976, Role of macrophages in the generation of T helper cells. IV. Nature of genetically related factor derived from macrophages incubated with soluble antigens, *Eur. J. Immunol.* **6:**365.

Esselman, W.J., and Miller, H.C., 1977, Modulation of B cell responses by glycolipid released from antigen-stimulated T cells, *J. Immunol.* **119:**1994.

Fishman, P.H., and Brady, R.O., 1976, Biosynthesis and function of gangliosides: Gangliosides appear to participate in the transmission of membrane-mediated information, *Science* **194:**906.

Freed, J.H., and Nathenson, S.G., 1977a, Antigenic structure of the Ia glycoprotein molecules, in: *Ir Genes and Ia Antigens* (H.O. McDevitt, ed.), pp. 263–273, Academic Press, New York.

Freed, J.H., and Nathenson, S.G., 1977b, Similarity of the carbohydrate structures of H-2 and Ia glycoproteins, *J. Immunol.* **119:**477.

Freed, J.H., David, C.S., Shreffler, D.C., and Nathenson, S.G., 1978, Structural studies of the protein portion of the H-2-linked Ia glycoprotein antigens of the mouse: Tryptic

peptide comparison of products from the *I-A* and *I-C* subregions of BIO.HTT, *J. Immunol.* **121**:91.
Freeman, R.R., and Parish, C.R., 1978, Spleen cell changes during fatal and self-limiting malarial infections of mice, *Immunology* **35**:479.
Friedberg, S.H., and Weissman, I.L., 1974, Lymphoid tissue architecture. II. Ontogeny of peripheral T and B cells in mice: Evidence against Peyer's patches as the site of generation of B cells, *J. Immunol.* **113**:1477.
Greene, M.I., Pierres, A., Dorf, M.E., and Benacerraf, B., 1977, The *I-J* subregion codes for determinants on suppressor factor(s) which limit the contact sensitivity response to picryl chloride, *J. Exp. Med.* **146**:293.
Hakomori, S-I., and Kobata, A., 1974, Blood group antigens, in: *The Antigens* (M. Sela, ed.), Vol. II, pp. 79–139, Academic Press, New York.
Hämmerling, G.J., 1976, Tissue distribution of Ia antigens and their expression on lymphocyte subpopulations, *Transplant. Rev.* **30**:64.
Hardy, B., Globerson, A., and Danon, D., 1973, Ontogenic development of the reactivity of macrophages to antigenic stimulation, *Cell. Immunol.* **9**:282.
Hardy, B., Mozes, E., and Danon, D., 1976, Comparison of the immune response potential of newborn mice to T-dependent and T-independent synthetic polypeptides, *Immunology* **30**:261.
Higgins, T.J., and Parish, C.R., 1980, Extraction of the carbohydrate-defined class of Ia antigens from murine spleen cells and serum, *Mol. Immunol.* **17**:1065.
Higgins, T.J., Sabatino, A.P., Remold, H.G., and David, J.R., 1978, Possible role of macrophage glycolipids as receptors for migration inhibition factor (MIF), *J. Immunol.* **121**:880.
Howie, S., and Feldmann, M., 1977, *In vitro* studies on H-2-linked unresponsiveness to synthetic polypeptides. III. Production of an antigen-specific T helper cell factor to (T,G)-A—L, *Eur. J. Immunol.* **7**:417.
Howie, S., Parish, C.R., David, C.S., McKenzie, I.F.C., Maurer, P.H., and Feldmann, M., 1979, Serological analysis of antigen specific helper factors specific for (T,G)-A—L and GAT, *Eur. J. Immunol.* **9**:501.
Huang, R.T., 1978, Cell adhesion mediated by glycolipids, *Nature (London)* **276**:624.
Isac, R., Dorf, M., and Mozes, E., 1977, The T-cell factor specific for poly (Tyr,Glu)-poly(Pro)-poly(Lys) is an *I*-region gene product, *Immunogenetics* **5**:467.
Jackson, D.C., Parish, C.R., and McKenzie, I.F.C., 1977, Detection and isolation of an Ia glycoprotein antigen from mouse serum, *Immunogenetics* **4**:267.
Jayawardena, A.N., Targett, G.A.T., Leuchars, E., Carter, R.L., Doenhoff, M.J., and Davies, A.J.S., 1975, T-cell activation in murine malaria, *Nature (London)* **258**:149.
Kapp, J.A., Pierce, C.W., De La Croix, F., and Benacerraf, B., 1976, Immunosuppressive factor(s) extracted from lymphoid cells of nonresponder mice primed with L-glutamic acid^{60}-L-alanine^{30}-L-tyrosine^{10} (GAT). I. Activity and antigenic specificity, *J. Immunol.* **116**:305.
Katz, D.H., and Benacerraf, B., 1975, The function and interrelationship of T cell receptors, *Ir* genes and other histocompatibility gene products, *Transplant. Rev.* **22**:175.
Kilburn, D.G., Smith, J.B., and Gorczynski, R.M., 1974, Nonspecific suppression of T lymphocyte responses in mice carrying progressively growing tumors, *Eur. J. Immunol.* **4**:784.
Lawrence, H.S., 1974, Transfer factor in cellular immunity, *Harvey Lect.* **68**:239.
Liew, F.Y., and Chan-Liew, W.L., 1978, Regulation of delayed-type hypersensitivity. II. Specific suppressor factor for delayed-type hypersensitivity to sheep erythrocytes in mice, *Eur. J. Immunol.* **8**:168.
Liew, F.Y., Sia, D.Y., Parish, C.R., and McKenzie, I.F.C., 1980, *MHC*-coded determi-

nants on antigen specific suppressor factor for delayed type hypersensitivity and surface phenotype of cells producing the factor, *Eur. J. Immunol.* **10**:305.

Marcus, D.M., and Cass, L.E., 1969, Glycosphingolipids with Lewis blood group activity: Uptake by human erythrocytes, *Science* **164**:553.

McDougal, J.S., Cort, S.P., and Gordon, D.S., 1977, Generation of T helper cells *in vitro*. III. Helper cell culture-derived factors are related to alloantigens coded for by the *I*-region of the *H-2* major histocompatibility complex, *J. Immunol.* **119**:1933.

McKenzie, I.F.C., and Parish, C.R., 1976, Secretion of Ia antigens by a subpopulation of T cells which are Ly-1$^+$, Ly-2$^-$ and Ia$^-$, *J. Exp. Med.* **144**:847.

McKenzie, I.F.C., Clarke, A.E., and Parish, C.R., 1977, Ia antigenic specificities are oligosaccharide in nature: Hapten inhibition studies, *J. Exp. Med.* **145**:1039.

McMillan, M., Cecka, J.M., Murphy, D.B., McDevitt, H.O., and Hood, L., 1977, Structure of murine Ia antigens: Partial NH_2-terminal amino acid sequences of products of the *I-E* or *I-C* subregion, *Proc. Natl. Acad. Sci. U.S.A.* **74**:5135.

Miller, J.F.A.P., Vadas, M.A., Whitelaw, A., and Gamble, J., 1976, Role of major histocompatibility complex gene products in delayed-type hypersensitivity, *Proc. Natl. Acad. Sci. U.S.A.* **73**:2486.

Mosier, D.E., Mathieson, B.J., and Campbell, P.S. 1977, Ly phenotype and mechanism of action of mouse neonatal suppressor T cells, *J. Exp. Med.* **146**:59.

Mullin, R.B., Pacuszka, T., Lee, G., Kohn, L.D., Brady, R.O., and Fishman, P.H., 1978, Thyroid gangliosides with high affinity for thyrotropin: Potential role in thyroid regulation, *Science* **199**:77.

Munro, A.J., and Taussig, M.J., 1975, Two genes in the major histocompatibility complex control immune response, *Nature (London)* **256**:103.

Okuda, K., and David, C.S., 1978, A new lymphocyte-activating determinant locus expressed on T cells, and mapping in *I-C* subregion, *J. Exp. Med.* **147**:1028.

Okuda, K., David, C.S., and Shreffler, D.C., 1977, The role of gene products of the *I-J* subregion in mixed lymphocyte reactions, *J. Exp. Med.* **146**:1561.

Parish, C.R., and McKenzie, I.F.C., 1977a, Mitogens and T-independent antigens stimulate T lymphocytes to secrete Ia antigens, *Cell. Immunol.* **33**:134.

Parish, C.R., and McKenzie, I.F.C., 1977b, Biosynthesis and antigenic nature of H-2K, H-2D and Ia antigens, in: *Progress in Immunology III* (T.E. Mandel, C. Cheers, C.S. Hosking, I.F.C. McKenzie, and G.J.V. Nossal, eds.), pp. 89–97, North-Holland, Amsterdam.

Parish, C.R., and McKenzie, I.F.C., 1978a, A detailed serological analysis of a xenogeneic anti-Ia serum, *Immunogenetics* **6**:183.

Parish, C.R., and McKenzie, I.F.C., 1978b, A sensitive rosetting method for detecting subpopulations of lymphocytes which react with alloantisera, *J. Immunol. Methods* **20**:173.

Parish, C.R., Chilcott, A.B., and McKenzie, I.F.C., 1976a, Low molecular-weight Ia antigens in normal mouse serum. I. Detection and production of a xenogeneic antiserum, *Immunogenetics* **3**:113.

Parish, C.R., Chilcott, A.B., and McKenzie, I.F.C., 1976b, Low molecular-weight Ia antigens in normal mouse serum. II. Demonstration of their T-cell origin, *Immunogenetics* **3**:129.

Parish, C.R., Jackson, D.C., and McKenzie, I.F.C., 1976c, Low molecular-weight Ia antigens in normal mouse serum. III. Isolation and partial chemical characterization, *Immunogenetics* **3**:455.

Parish, C.R., Jackson, D.C., and McKenzie, I.F.C., 1977, Evidence that Ia specificities are defined by carbohydrate, in: *Ir Genes and Ia Antigens* (H.O. McDevitt, ed.), pp. 243–253, Academic Press, New York.

Parish, C.R., Higgins, T.J., and McKenzie, I.F.C., 1978, Comparison of antigens recognized by xenogeneic and allogeneic anti-Ia antibodies: Evidence for two classes of Ia antigens, *Immunogenetics* **6**:343.
Parish, C.R., Freeman, R.R., McKenzie, I.F.C., Cheers, C., and Cole, G.A., 1979, Ia antigens in serum during different murine infections, *Infect. Immun.* **26**:422.
Parish, C.R., Higgins, T.J., and McKenzie, I.F.C., 1980, Lymphocytes express Ia antigens of foreign haplotype following treatment with neuroaminidase, *Immunogenetics* (in press).
Rabinowitz, S.G., 1976, Measurement and comparison of the proliferative and antibody responses of neonatal, immature and adult murine spleen cells to T-dependent and T-independent antigens, *Cell. Immunol.* **21**:201.
Rich, S.S., Orson, F.M., and Rich, R.R., 1977, *H-2* and non *H-2* gene control of T cell suppression of MLR, in: *Ir Genes and Ia Antigens* (H.O. McDevitt, ed.), pp. 559–565, Academic Press, New York.
Rogentine, G.N., and Plocinic, B.A., 1974, Carbohydrate inhibition studies of the naturally occurring human antibody to neuraminidase-treated human lymphocytes, *J. Immunol.* **113**:848.
Roseman, S., 1970, The synthesis of complex carbohydrates by multiglycosyl transferase systems and their potential function in intercellular adhesion, *Chem. Phys. Lipids* **5**:270.
Sandrin, M.S., Potter, T.A., Morgan, G.M., and McKenzie, I.F.C, 1978, Detection of mouse alloantibodies by rosetting with protein A coated sheep red cells, *Transplantation* **26**:126.
Sandrin, M.S., Vaughan, H.A., McKenzie, I.F.C., Tait, B.D., and Parish, C.R., 1979a, Ia antigenic specificities: Definition of human system and relevance to immune responses, *Transplant. Proc.* **XI**: 665.
Sandrin, M.S., Vaughan, H.A., McKenzie, I.F.C., Tait, B.D., and Parish, C.R., 1979b, The human Ia system: Definition and characterization by xenogeneic antisera, *Immunogenetics* **8**:185.
Schwartz, B.D., and Cullen, S.E., 1978, Chemical characteristics of Ia antigens, *Springer Semin. Immunopathol.* **1**:85.
Schwartz, R.H., Fathman, C.G., and Sachs, D.H., 1976a, Inhibition of stimulation in murine mixed lymphocyte cultures with an alloantiserum directed against a shared Ia determinant, *J. Immunol.* **116**:929.
Schwartz, R.H., David, C.S., Sachs, D.H., and Paul, W.E., 1976b, T-lymphocyte enriched murine peritoneal exudate cells. III. Inhibition of antigen-induced T lymphocyte proliferation with anti-Ia sera, *J. Immunol.* **117**:531.
Schwartz, R.H., Yano, A., and Paul, W.E., 1978, Interaction between antigen-presenting cells and primed T lymphocytes: An assessment of *Ir* gene expression in the antigen-presenting cell, *Immunol. Rev.* **40**:153.
Shearer, G.M., Rehn, T.G., and Schmitt-Verhulst, A.M., 1976, Role of the murine major histocompatibility complex in the specificity of *in vitro* T cells mediated lympholysis against chemically-modified autologous lymphocytes, *Transplant. Rev.* **29**:222.
Shreffler, D.C., and David, C.S., 1975, The *H-2* major histocompatibility complex and the *I* immune response region: Genetic variation, function and organization, *Adv. Immunol.* **20**:125.
Silver, J., 1977, Molecular structure of cell surface proteins determined by the murine MHC, in: *Progress in Immunology III* (T.E. Mandel, C. Cheers, C.S. Hosking, I.F.C. McKenzie, and G.J.V. Nossal, eds.), pp. 98–108, North-Holland, Amsterdam.
Silver, J., Russell, W.A., Reis, B.L., and Frelinger, J.A., 1977, Chemical characterization

of murine Ia alloantigens determined by the *I-E/I-C* subregions of the *H-2* complex, *Proc. Natl. Acad. Sci. U.S.A.* **74:**5131.

Simpson, L.L., and Rapport, M.M., 1971, The binding of botulinum toxin to membrane lipids: Sphingo-lipids, steroids and fatty acids, *J. Neurochem.* **18:**1751.

Spear, P.G., and Edelman, G.M., 1974, Maturation of the humoral immune response in mice, *J. Exp. Med.* **139:**249.

Springer, G.F., and Desai, P.R., 1977, Cross-reacting carcinoma-associated antigens with blood group and precursor specificities, *Transplant, Proc.* **9:**1105.

Steele, E.J., and Cunningham, A.J., 1978, High proportion of Ig-producing cells making autoantibody in normal mice, *Nature (London)* **274:**483.

Stout, R.B., Murphy, D.B., McDevitt, H.O., and Herzenberg, L.A., 1977, The Fc receptor on thymus-derived lymphocytes. IV. Inhibition of binding of antigen–antibody complexes to Fc-receptor-positive T cells by anti-Ia sera, *J. Exp. Med.* **145:**187.

Tada, T., Taniguchi, M., and David, C.S., 1976, Properties of antigen-specific suppressive T cell factor in the regulation of antibody response of mouse. IV. Special subregion assignment of the gene(s) that codes for the suppressive T-cell factor in the *H-2* histocompatibility complex, *J. Exp. Med.* **144:**713.

Takemori, T., and Tada, T., 1975, Properties of antigen-specific suppressive T-cell factor in the regulation of antibody response of the mouse. I. *In vivo* activity and immunochemical characterization, *J. Exp. Med.* **142:**1241.

Théze, J., Waltenbaugh, C., Dorf, M.E., and Benacerraf, B., 1977, Immunosuppressive factor(s) specific for L-glutamic acid^{50}-L-tyrosine^{50} (GT). II. Presence of *I-J* determinants on the GT-suppressive factor, *J. Exp. Med.* **146:**287.

Thomas, D.W., Yamashita, U., and Shevach, E.M., 1977, The role of Ia antigens in T cell activation, *Immunol. Rev.* **35:**97.

Tokuhisa, T., Taniguchi, M., Okumura, K., and Tada, T., 1978, An antigen-specific *I*-region gene product that augments the antibody response, *J. Immunol.* **120:**414.

Vadas, M.A., Miller, J.F.A.P., McKenzie, I.F.C., Chism, S.E., Shen, F.-W., Boyse, E.A., Gamble, J.R., and Whitelaw, A.M., 1976, Ly and Ia antigen phenotypes of T cells involved in delayed-type hypersensitivity and in suppression, *J. Exp. Med.* **144:**10.

van Heyningen, W.E., 1974, Gangliosides as membrane receptors for tetanus toxin, cholera toxin and serotonin, *Nature (London)* **249:**415.

Vengris, V.E., Reynolds, F.H., Hollenberg, M.D., and Pitha, P.M., 1976, Interferon action: Role of membrane gangliosides, *Virology* **72:**486.

12

Antigenic Products of the *HLA-D* Region

B.G. Solheim, D. Albrechtsen, and E. Thorsby

1. Introduction

A multitude of different cell-membrane alloantigens, complement factors, and components that may have important functions in the regulation of the immune response are controlled by the *HLA* genetic complex of chromosome 6 (W.F. Bodmer *et al.*, 1978). In this chapter, the identification, structure, tissue distribution, and clinical importance of the *HLA-D*-region antigens are discussed (see also Thorsby *et al.*, 1978). The HLA-D determinants are recognized by cellular techniques, while the HLA-D-related (DR) antigens are detected by serological methods. The relationship between the HLA-D determinants and HLA-DR antigens is also discussed.

The HLA-D determinants were first recognized by the mixed-lymphocyte culture (MLC) interaction (Yunis and Amos, 1971). These antigens induce the strongest stimulation in MLCs, and are detectable by HLA-D homozygous cell typing (HCT) (Thorsby and Piazza, 1975) or primed-lymphocyte typing (PLT) techniques (Sheehy *et al.*, 1975). Both HCT and PLT have, however, insufficient discriminative power and are time-consuming (120 and 40 hr, respectively).

Van Rood *et al.* (1975) were the first to describe serological detection of HLA-DR antigens on B cells and macrophages with platelet-absorbed pregnancy sera, and their findings have since been substantiated by a number of studies (see Kissmeyer-Nielsen, 1975). However, the serologi-

B.G. Solheim, D. Albrechtsen, and E. Thorsby • The Tissue Typing Laboratory, Rikshospitalet (The National Hospital), Oslo, Norway.

cal detection of HLA-DR antigens is also hampered by many practical problems. This was dramatically demonstrated in the 7th International Histocompatibility Workshop in 1977, where only 10 of 150 participating laboratories had an *r* value of 0.6 or better for two hidden duplicate sera (J.G. Bodmer *et al.*, 1978).

Finally, attention should be drawn to the close similarity between the Ia antigens in mice and the *HLA-D*-locus antigens in man. Both are responsible for the strongest stimulation in MLC tests, are involved in antigen presentation by macrophages, have a restricted tissue distribution, and are glycoproteins of comparable size (for further details, see Thorsby *et al.*, 1981).

2. Identification of *HLA-D*-Locus Products

2.1. Homozygous-Cell Typing

Modifications of the MLC reaction originally described by Bain *et al.* (1964) and Bach and Hirschhorn (1964) are the basis for HCT. The most important modification is the introduction of the "one-way" MLC in which lymphocytes from one person (A) are cocultured with lymphocytes from another person (B), the proliferative capacity of the latter lymphocytes being inhibited by radiation or mitomycin C, B*x*, where *x* indicates inhibition (Kasakura and Lovenstein, 1965; Bach and Voynow, 1966).

The test is generally performed in a micromethod, and proliferation peaks around day 5 and is assessed by radiolabeled thymidine incorporation (see, for example, Helgesen *et al.*, 1980). In the "one-way" MLC, AB*x*, the proliferative response is caused by antigenic differences between the lymphocytes, and the major stimulus for proliferation is incompatible HLA-D determinants on B*x* recognized by A (Yunis and Amos, 1971; Thorsby and Piazza, 1975).

In HCT, the stimulating lymphocytes are selected to be homozygous for their *HLA-D*-locus determinants. Thus, the responding lymphocytes will show strong proliferation when confronted with incompatible HLA-D determinants, while the response is low when the homozygous typing cell (HTC) shares the determinants with the responding one (Fig. 1) (Throsby *et al.*, 1978). A low response in HCT indicates the presence of an HLA-D determinant on the stimulated (responding) cell. Thus, the test is based on a "negative" MLC result, which requires great care in the interpretation of test results. A further problem is the number of factors that can induce lymphocyte proliferation and that when acting in concert possibly mask a typing response.

"Back-stimulation" is one of the problems in HCT. The irradiated

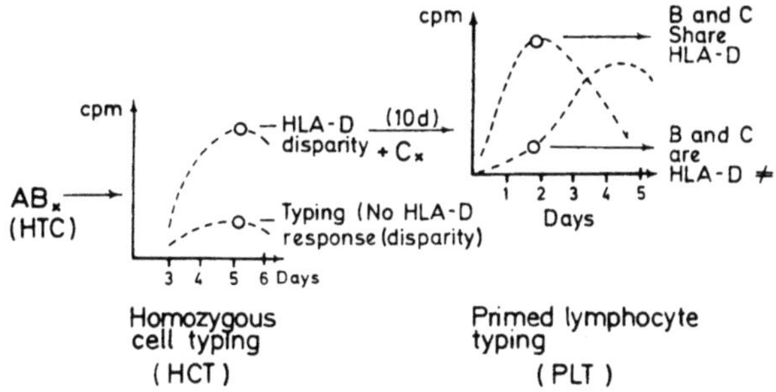

Figure 1. Homozygous-cell typing *(left)*: The top curve shows the MLC response (as incorporation of [^{3}H]thymidine) when A and B are disparate at HLA-D; the bottom curve shows the much weaker "typing" response observed when A shares the HLA-D determinants with B. Primed-lymphocyte typing *(right)*: After 10 days, stimulating cells from a third individual, C, are added. If B and C share HLA-D determinants, an early increased proliferation is observed. If B and C have no HLA-D determinants in common, no early increase is observed. From Thorsby *et al.* (1978).

HCT, on recognizing incompatibilities on the responder cells, may release blastogenic factors (Hirschberg *et al.*, 1974; Jörgensen *et al.*, 1974). In addition, HLA-non-D determinants can induce proliferation. This can be due to a second, weak, MLC-stimulating locus between *HLA-A* and *-B* (Eijsvoogel *et al.*, 1972; Thorsby *et al.*, 1973) and/or responses evoked by differences at *HLA-A and -B* (van Rood *et al.*, 1977; Albrechtsen *et al.*, 1978a; Suciu-Foca *et al.*, 1978). Due to these stimulating factors, clear-cut HCT is often difficult.

To improve the typing results, only those *HLA-D* homozygous cells that show good discrimination are used. In addition, all results (related to positive control cells) are doubly normalized by a special statistical approach (Ryder *et al.*, 1975). Nevertheless, a "gray area" of responses remains, wherein the presence or absence of a particular HLA-D determinant cannot be established. Retyping in some cases gives a clear-cut result, but often, doubtful responses are obtained once again. Of great value is the use of several HTC for each HLA-D determinant.

Table 1 shows the HLA-D determinants recognized and their approximate frequencies in a Norwegian population (Thorsby *et al.*, 1978). The frequencies differ among ethnic groups. Thus, for example, HLA-Dw3 is very rare in Japanese (Kashiwagi and Sasazuki, 1978).

Lymphoblastoid-cell lines homozygous for a given HLA-D determinant have been advocated as stimulating cells in HCT (Svedmyr *et al.*, 1975). The discriminative power has, however, proved inferior in these tests, and only very limited use is made of this approach.

HLA-D typing by sperm-lymphocyte culture also has its advocates (Festenstein and Halim, 1978). The method, however, has proved very

TABLE 1. HLA-D Determinants among Norwegians

Determinant	Number investigated	Antigen frequency	Gene frequency
HLA-Dw1	215	22.3	0.119
HLA-Dw2	215	30.2	0.165
HLA-Dw3	213	21.6	0.115
HLA-Dw4	181	22.2	0.124
HLA-Dw5	66	12.2	0.063
HLA-Dw6	215	10.7	0.055
HLA-Dw7	93	15.1	0.078
HLA-Dw8	209	8.6	0.044
HLA-Dw9	203	7.9	0.040
HLA-Dw10	Not tested		—
HLA-Dw11	Not tested		—
Blank	—	—	0.198

difficult to reproduce, and a recent paper by Law and Bodmer (1978) throws serious doubt as to the presence of HLA-A, -B, -C antigens, β_2-microglobulin, and HLA-DR antigens on sperm. These results have since been further substantiated with highly specific monoclonal antibodies from hybridomas (W.F. Bodmer, 1978, personal communication). The possibility that stimulation by sperm samples may be due to contaminating epithelial or macrophage cells must be borne in mind.

2.2. Primed-Lymphocyte Typing

This test relies on the specific clonal expansion by prior sensitization with a given HLA-D antigen in a one-way MLC (Sheehy *et al.*, 1975) and is derived from observation in mice (Andersson and Häyri, 1973). The priming can be performed between family members deviating by one haplotype or by HTC. When the primed cells are restimulated, an accelerated response is seen if the restimulating cells share the incompatible HLA-D antigen with the stimulating cell used for priming. Harvesting of the secondary MLC is usually after 24–48 hr (see Fig. 1).

The PLT was received with much enthusiasm, because it appeared to be a fast test for definition of HLA-D determinants. It has, however, proved technically difficult, and both HLA-non-D and non-HLA antigens have been reported to cause disturbing stimulation (Bardley *et al.*, 1978; Suciu-Foca *et al.*, 1977). In some of our studies of HLA-D determinants, the method has, however, proved valuable (Hirschberg *et al.*, 1977; Moen and Thorsby, 1978).

2.3. Serological Identification

A number of laboratories reported B-cell-specific antibodies in 1975 (Kissmeyer-Nielsen, 1975). Based on the findings by van Leuwen *et al.* (1973), van Rood *et al.* (1975) demonstrated the close relationship between B-cell-specific antibodies and HLA-D determinants. The designation HLA-DR (for D-related) was, however, first adopted in 1977. We could confirm this relationship with sera produced by planned immunization in HLA-D-incompatible, but HLA-A-, -B-, -C-compatible, combinations (Solheim *et al.*, 1975). A number of the B-cell-specific sera were also reported after screening against chronic lymphatic leukemia cells or B-cell lines, and antigenic systems based on these studies were postulated (e.g., Walford *et al.*, 1976). The relationship between the *HLA* system and B-cell antigens was generally accepted. However, many groups postulated that several loci within the *HLA* region coded for the antigens (Wernet, 1977).

In the 1977 Histocompatibility Workshop, 180 submitted antisera, representing previously published B-cell antisera and a number of new ones, were tested. The aims were (1) to compare the definition of antigens by different laboratories and adopt, if possible, a common standard nomenclature for generally recognized antigens; and (2) to test whether these antigens were identical to, or at least coded by, the same genes as the HLA-D determinants. Data from a set of B lymphocytes from healthy random Caucasoids reacting satisfactorily to control sera were tested by cluster analysis on all submitted B-cell antisera (J.G. Bodmer *et al.*, 1978). This resulted in the definition of the eight antigens DRw1–w7 and WIA8, which are closely associated with the corresponding HLA-D determinants. It could also be concluded that there is no evidence to define more than one locus currently. B-cell typing, however, has a number of pitfalls, which, as mentioned earlier, were clearly demonstrated by the 1977 Histocompatibility Workshop. In laboratories accustomed to B-cell typing, this has, however, proved to be the method of choice for the determination of *HLA-D*-locus antigens.

Optimal typing is generally performed with a two-stage technique at 20°C with T-cell-depleted peripheral-blood lymphocytes (Albrechtsen *et al.*, 1977a; J.G. Bodmer *et al.*, 1978). Depletion of T cells is simple and fast by rosetting with 2-aminoethylisothiouronium-bromide-treated sheep red blood cells (Pellegrino *et al.*, 1976) followed by Ficoll–Isopaque flotation (Böyum, 1968). Generally, cells are incubated with antiserum for 60 (or 30) min, rabbit complement is added, and the cells are incubated for 120 (or 60) min, followed by staining (of dead cells). In our experiments, the shorter incubation times are completely sufficient with good, strong antisera. Many typing reagents are, however, rather weak, and therefore the long method is often necessary.

HLA-DR typing can also be performed by a two-color fluorescence test for B cells that avoids enrichment of them (van Rood *et al.*, 1976). In this technique, B cells are stained with green fluorescein (FITC)-labeled anti-human IgG, and dead cells are stained with the red ethidium bromide. Antibody-dependent cell-mediated lympholysis has also been used for the detection of HLA-DR antigens (Dossetor *et al.*, 1975). In the screening of anti-HLA-A-, -B-, -C-contaminated anti-HLA-DR antisera, blocking of the former antigens by fowl anti-β_2-microglobulin has proved valuable (Bernoco *et al.*, 1976).

3. Production of HLA-DR Antisera

3.1. Alloantisera

Very many pregnancy sera must be screened before a good serum is found, and generally extensive platelet absorptions of HLA-A, -B, and -C antibodies have to be performed. We have produced very specific (non-absorbed) anti-HLA-DR sera by planned immunizations. In selected HLA-A, -B, -C-compatible HLA-D-deviating combinations, 3–6 × 10^7 peripheral-blood lymphocytes were injected intradermally (Albrechtsen *et al.*, 1977a). In five of eight cases (Table 2), antibodies specific for B cells (without prior absorptions) were produced. Three of these sera

TABLE 2. Effect of Planned Immunization in Eight HLA-A, -B, -C-Compatible, HLA-D-Disparate (MLC-Stimulating) Combinations.

Serum	HLA disparity[a]	Cytotoxicity of serum[b]	HLA-DR specificity	Association to:	DRw/Dw ++	+−	−+	−−	r^c
SOW	Dw2	100	DRw2	Dw2	31	4	0	85	0.92[d]
AH	Dw3	100	DRw3	Dw3	25	4	3	88	0.84[d]
SR	Dw4	70	DRw4	Dw4	14	2	11	93	0.64[d]
TL	Dw8	100	WIa8	Dw8	14	3	2	101	0.82[d]
TH	Dw6,[e]	100	DRw6+	Dw6+	15	46	0	59	0.31[d]
			DRw3	Dw3	28	33	0	59	0.56[d]
HB	Dw4	0	—	—	—	—	—	—	—
BB	Dw–[e]	0	—	—	—	—	—	—	—
EAH	Dw–[e]	0	—	—	—	—	—	—	—

[a]HLA disparity between immunizing cell donor and recipient.
[b]Percentage of Ig-positive cells from the immunizing donor killed by undiluted serum.
[c]Correlation coefficient ($r = \sqrt{x^2/n}$). [d]$n < 0.001$. [e]"Blank," unidentified HLA-D determinant.

TABLE 3. Detection of HLA-DR Alloantigenic Specificities with Unabsorbed Antisera from Rabbits Immunized with DR Antigens from HTC

Serum	Immunizing antigen	Serum specificity[a]	HLA-DR/serum reactivity				
			++	+−	−+	−−	*r*
IG2	DRw4	DRw4 (1:64)	19	0	14	13	0.48[b]
IG3	DRw4	DRw4 (1:8)	17	2	8	19	0.55[b]
IG4	DRw4	DRw4 (1:128)	19	0	15	12	0.45[b]
AE4	WIa8	WIa8 (1:8)	3	1	4	36	0.40[c]
BTB 1	WIa8	WIa8 (1:32)	4	0	7	32	0.45[c]

[a]At the dilution given in parentheses. [b]$p < 0.001$ (Fischer's exact test). [c]$p < 0.01$.

showed very high correlation to HLA-D determinants. Thus, planned immunization of human volunteers at present seems to represent the preferred method for raising DR antisera (see also Ferrara *et al.*, 1978).

By comparing different antisera, "heterogeneity" of some of the detectable HLA-DR antigens is apparent, indicating that the antigenic molecules may carry several separate ("private" and "public") determinants (Thorsby *et al.*, 1977; Albrechtsen *et al.*, 1978b). The HLA-DR antigens can be grouped after cross-reactivity, and the following patterns are most apparent: DR 1+2, 1+6, 2+6, 3+6, 4+5, 4+7, 4+8, and 5+8 (J.G. Bodmer *et al.*, 1978).

3.2. Xenoantisera

Highly specific anti-HLA-DR antibodies have been raised in rabbits (Humphreys *et al.*, 1976; Welsh and Turner, 1976; Ferrone *et al.*, 1977), and we have been able to demonstrate DR allospecificity in nonabsorbed rabbit antisera after immunization with purified HLA-DR antigen from *HLA-D*-homozygous cell lines (Table 3). The specificities are, however, detectable only at endpoint titration (Solheim *et al.*, 1978), and it has proved difficult to improve the specificity by absorptions.

A far more promising approach is the formation of DR-specific antibodies by hybrid myelomas (C.J. Barnstable *et al.*, 1978). Many centers are currently attempting this approach, and several antibodies recognizing public DR specificities have been produced. In the future, this approach may be the method of choice for raising antibodies; the possibility that the specificity might be too "high" for practical purposes (i.e., the antibody directed against a narrow "private" specificity) must, however, be borne in mind.

4. Structure of HLA-DR Antigens

Human Ia-like glycoprotein was first isolated from lymphoblastoid-cell lines by Snary *et al.* (1974) and Strominger *et al.* (1975). When prepared by detergent extraction, it is composed of two subunits, 29,000 and 34,000 daltons (p 29,34), respectively, whereas the papain-solubilized analogue has subunits of 23,000 and 30,000 daltons (Springer *et al.*, 1978; Humphreys *et al.*, 1976). This molecular complex demonstrates structural similarity with murine Ia antigens and can be used to raise xenoantisera with many of the functional properties of murine Ia and human B-cell-specific alloantisera (Cresswell and Geier, 1975; Möller, 1976). We have been able to demonstrate (Kaufman *et al.*, 1978; Giphart *et al.*, 1977) that anti-HLA-DR alloantisera are directed against the p 29, 34 complex, thus proving that this complex carries the antigenic site for these antibodies. This observation has been extended by Klareskog *et al.* (1978), who demonstrated that the DR alloantigenic specificity is localized to the 34,000-dalton subunit of the complex. By a somatic-cell-hybridization technique, B.A. Barnstable and Jones (1978) also provided evidence that the 34,000-dalton chain carries the HLA-DR alloantigenic specificity. Thus, it is now firmly established that p 29, 34, and most probably its 34,000-dalton subunit, carries the human HLA-DR alloantigens.

In the cell membrane, the different HLA-DR antigens are independent of each other (Albrechtsen *et al.*, 1978b), but closely associated with the Fc receptor of B lymphocytes (e.g., Solheim *et al.*, 1976).

5. Tissue Distribution

Unlike the classic transplantation antigens HLA-A, -B, and -C, the *HLA-D*-locus antigens have a restricted tissue distribution. By cellular techniques, HLA-D determinants have been clearly demonstrated on B lymphocytes, macrophages, endothelial cells, and skin cells (for references, see Thorsby *et al.*, 1977). Their presence on sperm is more controversial.

By serology, HLA-DR antigens have in general been found on the same tissues (Wernet, 1976). In the case of epidermis, it has been demonstrated that the antigens reside in the Langerhans cells and not in the epithelial cells (Rowden *et al.*, 1977; Klareskog *et al.*, 1977). The presence of HLA-DR antigens on endothelial cells has been further substantiated by Hirschberg *et al.* (1979). Recently, immunoabsorbent-purified rabbit anti-human-HLA-DR antisera were used in the demonstration of Ia antigens in a wide range of guinea pig tissues (Wiman *et al.*, 1978). Thus, epithelial cells in the bronchi, intestine, gallbladder, kidney pelvis, and urinary bladder are positive. In addition, Ia antigens were detected on salivary glandular epithelium, lactating mammary epithelial cells, and Kupfer cells of the liver. It is striking that the epithelium of these tissues is specially characterized by an abundance of IgA-secreting cells. Due to the extensive similarity between Ia antigens in different species, the tissue distribution in guinea pigs is also highly relevant for human studies. In humans, we have been able to demonstrate HLA-DR antigens in the epithelium of small-intestine biopsies (Scott *et al.*, 1980).

In addition, HLA-DR antigens have been reported on human null cells (Wernet, 1976). This finding still needs confirmation. In resting T cells, however, less than 10% express DR antigens detectable by DR alloantisera (Albrechtsen *et al.*, 1977c) or xenoantisera specific for p 29,34 (Fu *et al.*, 1978). By treatment of T cells with HLA-DR alloantisera and subsequent incubation with complement, the responsiveness to the mitogen concanavalin A (Con A) is almost abolished, while no or only weak inhibition of the responsiveness to phytohemagglutinin (PHA), antigens such as purified protein derivative PPD), or allogeneic cells is observed (see Tables 4 and 8) (Albrechtsen *et al.*, 1977c). Furthermore, using similar pretreatment, the activity of the nonspecific suppressor cells generated in human MLC tests is also strongly inhibited (Hirschberg and Thorsby, 1977). Preliminary studies indicate that the HLA-DR antigenic determinants present on B cells may be different from those present on the subpopulation of T cells responsible for generation of the Con A response (Albrechtsen *et al.*, 1977c). By treatment of T cells with xeno-anti-DR sera and complement, the generation of helper activity as assayed by generation of plaque-forming cells is also impeded (Fu *et al.*, 1978). DR antigens also seem to be present on transformed MLC-activated T cells; furthermore, they appear to be present on activated cyto-

TABLE 4. Inhibition of Mitogen- and Antigen-Reactive Lymphocytes by Pretreatment with Anti-HLA-DRw2 Antiserum and Complement[a]

Pretreatment[b]	Cell donor[c]	Control	PHA (1:100[d])	Con A (1 mg/ml[d])	PPD
NS	A	327 ± 56	33,194 ± 831	21,592 ± 1,448	4249 ± 309
Anti-DRw2		224 ± 62	22,111 ± 3,746	3,285 ± 466	4701 ± 401
NS	B	300 ± 91	20,746 ± 954	12,157 ± 1,285	1214 ± 54
Anti-DRw2		438 ± 64	19,483 ± 1,079	14,147 ± 1,830	1561 ± 135

[a] For further details, see Albrechtsen *et al.* (1977b). Results are mean cpm ± S.E.
[b] Normal serum (NS) or antiserum + rabbit complement, 60 min at 37°C.
[c] HLA-DRw type: (A) DRw2; (B) DRw1. [d] Optimal mitogen concentration.

TABLE 5. Tissue Distribution of HLA-D Determinants and HLA-DR Antigens

Tissue	HLA-D	HLA-DR[a]
B lymphocytes	+	+
Null cells		+?
Macrophages	+	+
T lymphocytes		
T helper		
Resting		−
Activated		+(?)
T killer		
Resting		−
Activated		+(?)
T suppressor		
Resting		−
Activated		+
T Con-A-responsive		+
T MLC-responsive		−
Epidermal cells (Langerhans cells)	+	+
Endothelial cells	+	+
Intestinal epithelium (small intestine)		+
Sperm	+?	+?

[a](?) Detected only by xenoantisera.

toxic T cells responsible for cell-mediated lympholysis (Evans *et al.*, 1978).

In leukemias, HLA-DR-positive leukemic cells have been found to form E-rosettes (Fu *et al.*, 1978). In one case of Sezary's syndrome, we have observed a patient with HLA-DR antigens on the malignant T cells (Solheim *et al.*, 1979b).

Thus, the majority of resting T cells do not express HLA-DR antigens detectable by currently applied methods. On activated T cells, however, and in some leukemic cases, the majority of the T cells may express HLA-DR antigens. The tissue distribution of HLA-DR antigens is summarized in Table 5.

6. Relationship between HLA-D Determinants and HLA-DR Antigens

The HLA-DR antigens and HLA-D determinants are closely associated on a population level, they are almost always inherited together in families, and they have a similar tissue distribution, and anti-HLA-DR antisera will specifically cause stimulator-cell inhibition of MLC.

The high association between HLA-DR antigens and HLA-D determinants in the Norwegian population is demonstrated in Table 6 (see Albrechtsen *et al.*, 1978a). The associations are seen to be very high except for the antigens HLA-Dw4/DRw4 and Dw6/DRw6. Both HLA-Dw4 and -Dw6 are rather difficult specificities (Thorsby and Piazza, 1975; Festenstein *et al.*, 1978). This and the fact that there are no monospecific HLA-DRw4 and -Dw6 antisera explain the discrepancies. Very similar associations were obtained at the 7th International Histocompatibility Workshop (J.G. Bodmer *et al.*, 1978a). The association is also demonstrated by the circumstance that the strength of MLC stimulation in unrelated combinations is significantly influenced by the degree of HLA-DR incompatibility between stimulating and responding cells (Fig. 2). Virtually no stimulation is seen in HLA-identical sibs, and the modest stimulation observed in HLA-DR-compatible combinations can be explained by HLA-non-D antigens.

The correlation between HLA-D determinants and HLA-DR antigens has not been extensively studied in disease states, but some data have been published on dermatitis herpetiformis and gluten-sensitive enteropathy (Solheim *et al.*, 1977; Keuning *et al.*, 1976; Ek *et al.*, 1978). We found the association between HLA-Dw3 and HLA-DRw3 less pronounced, and in particular there were a number of cases with relative responses around 60–80% with HLA-Dw3 HTC and positive reaction with anti-HLA-DRw3 antisera. In a recent study, we looked at the distribution of HLA-Dw3 determinants and HLA-DRw3 antigens in 37 children with gluten-sensitive enteropathy. HLA-D typing for Dw1–Dw10 was performed with 20 HTC; two Dw3 HTC were used, and this was the only antigen demonstrating increased frequency. HLA-DRw3 typing was performed with 36 anti-HLA-DR alloantisera, covering the specificities

TABLE 6. Association between HLA-D Determinants and HLA-DR Antigens in Unrelated Norwegians

HLA-D	HLA-DR	Number investigated	++	+−	−+	−−	*r*
Dw1	DRw1	119	18	1	0	100	0.94[a]
Dw2	DRw2	119	30	1	2	86	0.91[a]
Dw3	DRw3	118	25	3	0	90	0.91[a]
Dw4	DRw4	116	17	1	14	83	0.63[a]
Dw5	DRw5	95	6	1	0	88	0.84[a]
Dw6	DRw6	118	13	6	14	85	0.65[a]
Dw7	DRw7	115	15	0	1	99	0.93[a]
Dw8	DRw8	118	12	1	1	104	0.87[a]

[a] $p < 0.001$.

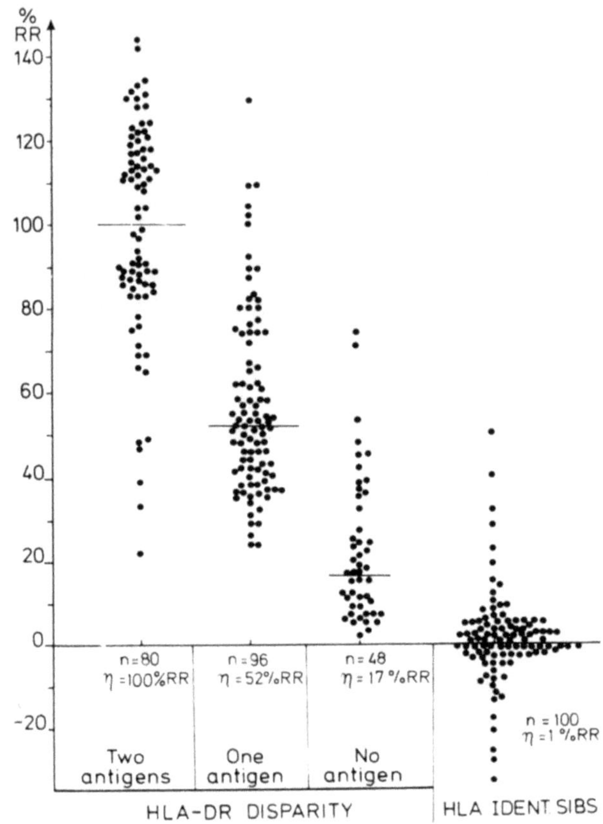

Figure 2. Relative responses (RR) in MLCs between unrelated cell donors disparate for two, one, and zero HLA-DR specificities, and between HLA-identical siblings. From Albrechtsen *et al.* (1978a).

DRw1–7 and WIA8. As can be seen in Table 7, more patients were HLA-DRw3 than HLA-Dw3. Of the nine patients who were HLA-Dw3-negative but HLA-DRw3-positive, six had relative responses below 80% with both HTC. In three patients in whom the HLA-Dw3 typing was found to be doubtful, one HTC gave typing response, the other did not. On the other hand, Keuning *et al.* (1976) found good correlation between HLA-D and DR typing in patients with gluten-sensitive enteropathy. They, however, repeated HCT several times and used a larger number of Dw3 HTC. Non-HLA, B-cell-associated antigens have been suggested in gluten-sensitive enteropathy Mann *et al.*, 1976; Pena *et al.*, 1978), but the methods applied for their detection are rather special, and the results not confirmed by other groups. We are therefore prone to suggest abnormal activity against weak MLC-stimulating antigens in some patients with celiac disease. In addition, possible stimulation by traces of glutten derivatives in serum added to culture media might be an explanation. However, the possibility that HLA-D determinants and HLA-DR antigens are products of two different but closely linked loci must also be considered.

Another argument for two different loci defining HLA-D and HLA-DR comes from studies of different ethnic groups that seem to show some clear-cut discrepancies (W.F. Bodmer *et al.* 1978). Nonrandom association has been reported for a number of HLA antigens. Thus, linkage disequilibrium exists between some HLA-A and -B, between many -B and -C, and most pronounced between some -B and D/DR antigens (Kissmeyer-Nielsen, 1975; W.F. Bodmer *et al.*, 1978). However, none of these associations can be compared in strength to the one between HLA-D determinants and HLA-DR antigens. Differences in associations between HLA-D determinants and HLA-non-D MLC-stimulating determi-

TABLE 7. Association between HLA-Dw3 and HLA-DRw3 in 37 Children with Gluten-Sensitive Enteropathy

HLA-Dw3/HLA-DRw3				
++	+−	−+	−−	*r*
20	0	9	5	0.41 ($p < 0.025$)

RR[a] in HTC for three patients with doubtful HLA-Dw3 typing and nine patients with discrepant results:

Doubtful	Discrepant
22.65	43.68
27.68	49.61
20.98	51.65
	54.75
	57.67
	66.70
	76.103
	82.85
	97.149

[a](RR) Relative response.

HLA-Dw3 was defined as follows:
Present: (a) RR < 40% for both HTC.
(b) RR < 40% for one and 40% < RR < 60% for the other HTC.
Doubtful: (a) RR < 40% for one and > 60% for the other HTC.
(b) 40% < RR < 60% for both HTC.
Absent: All other RR values.

HLA-DwR3 was defined as follows:
Present: Positive reaction with at least two out of three typing sera.
Doubtful: Positive with only one out of three typing sera.

nants in different races can be an explanation for some of the discrepancies observed.

Of seven HLA recombinant families studied in Oslo, five included HLA-A/B-D and two HLA-A-B/D recombinant children. In these families, the HLA-DR specificities always traveled with the *HLA-B-D* or *HLA-D* chromosomal region. In 23 families with 79 children (N = 127), no triplets for HLA-DR have been observed. However, HLA-D/DR recombinations have been suggested (Festenstein, 1978, personal communication.) The observations have not yet been confirmed by others, and technical problems especially involved with HCT suggest caution in the interpretations. The analogy of human HLA-D determinants and HLA-DR antigens to mice Ia antigens (for discussion, see Thorsby *et al.*, 1980), however, makes it tempting to assume more than one locus in man also.

A striking argument not only for a close genetic association, but also for a close association of HLA-D/DR in the cell membrane, is given by MLC-inhibition experiments (Jonker *et al.*, 1975; Lawler *et al.*, 1977; Albrechtsen *et al.*, 1977b, 1978b). The presence of anti-HLA-DR antisera in MLCs results in specific inhibition of stimulating cells carrying the relevant HLA-DR antigen, while responder cells are not significantly affected (Table 8). Also, stimulation in PLT is inhibited by anti-HLA-DR antisera (Hirschberg *et al.*, 1977). Finally, some very interesting findings by Bergholtz and Thorsby (for references, see Thorsby *et al.*, 1980) should be mentioned. They demonstrate that immune T cells recognize

TABLE 8. Inhibition of Stimulating Cells, but Not Responding Cells, by Anti-HLA-DRw2 Antiserum[a]

Cell type[b]	Normal serum	Anti-DRw2 serum
Stimulating cell[c]		
A	7,710 ± 584	1,855 ± 151
B	13,350 ± 891	10,219 ± 1,268
Autologue	587 ± 73	425 ± 43
Responding cell[d]		
A	9,441 ± 862	6,186 ± 341
Autologue	768 ± 36	367 ± 23
B	7,897 ± 534	8,260 ± 791
Autologue	889 ± 51	634 ± 8

[a]The MLC tests were performed with either 20% normal serum (NS) or 10% NS + 10% (inactivated) immune serum present throughout the culture period. For further details, see Albrechtsen *et al.* (1977b). Results are mean cpm ± S.E.

[b]HLA-DRw type: (A) DRw2, 3; (B) DRw5,6.

[c]Serum donor used as responding cell.

[d]Serum donor used as stimulating cell.

PPD optimally only when PPD is presented by macrophages carrying *HLA-D/DR* gene products present during priming. Also, this response is specifically inhibited by monospecific anti-HLA-DR alloantisera, which further underlines the central role of the HLA-DR antigens.

Taken together, available data indicate that HLA-DR antigens are identical or very closely linked, both genetically and in the cell membrane, to the HLA-D determinants. If they are identical, it remains to be seen whether the determinants triggering B cells for alloantibody production are the same as those that stimulate T cells in MLC or are part of the signal for T-cell activation by protein antigens. The answers to these questions must await better biochemical characterization of the gene products. In any case, the close association has made HLA-DR typing very useful for the identification of HLA-D determinants, although some care should be exercised in disease studies and different ethnic groups.

Finally, it should be mentioned that recent studies have indicated the existence of other "DR-like" antigenic molecules coded for by the *HLA* region (Abelson and Mann, 1977; Tosi *et al.*, 1978). The influence of these products on MLC and the precise localization of the loci are not defined.

7. Clinical and Biological Importance

7.1. Transplantation

In renal transplantation, the results indicate that HLA-D determinants (Sachs *et al.*, 1977; Solheim *et al.*, 1979a) and HLA-DR antigens (Albrechtsen *et al.*, 1978c; Ting and Morris, 1978; Persijn *et al.*, 1978; Martins Da Silva, *et al.*, 1978) have a significant influence on the fate of the grafts. HLA-DR matching results in good kidney graft survival irrespective of matching for HLA-A and -B antigens (Albrechtsen *et al.*, 1978c), and in bone-marrow transplantation, HLA-D compatibility appears to be more important than compatibility for HLA-A, -B, and -C antigens (Copenhagen Study Group of Immunodeficiencies, 1973; Horowitz *et al.*, 1975; Goldman, 1977). These findings have important practical implications because the polymorphism of the *HLA-D/DR* gene products is restricted compared to that of the *HLA-A, -B,* and *-C* gene products. The chance of finding a compatible unrelated combination for the former antigens is thus rather good.

In vitro studies, and analogy with murine data, suggest that the HLA-D determinants play the greatest role in the initial triggering of an immune response toward allogeneic tissue, and that the HLA-A, -B, and -C antigens are the major targets of the humoral and cellular effector phase (van Rood, 1973; Thorsby, 1974; Bach *et al.*, 1976). However, HLA-D determinants are apparently able to induce production of anti-HLA-DR antibodies, and also in T-cell-mediated lympholysis, the HLA-DR antigens can be target antigens (Albrechtsen *et al.*, 1979).

In mice, antibodies directed against the Ia antigens, particularly those coded for by *I-A*, may cause enhancement of H-2-disparate grafts (McKenzie and Henning, 1977; Staines *et al.*, 1977). One explanation put forward is that anti-Ia antibodies might inhibit sensitization of T helper cells. For this reason, one has looked for a possible beneficial effect on clinical kidney transplantation of recipient antibodies reacting with B cells of the kidney donor. A positive cross-match with only donor B cells is generally not associated with hyperacute rejection (Ting and Morris, 1978; Soullillou *et al.*, 1978; Albrechtsen *et al.*, 1978c; Iwaki *et al.*, 1979), in contrast to a positive cross-match involving anti-HLA-A, -B, and -C antibodies (Kissmeyer-Nielsen and Kjerbye, 1967). An enhancing effect of anti-HLA-DR antibodies has, however, not been demonstrated. In contrast, a trend toward inferior graft survival has even been reported (Albrechtsen *et al.*, 1978c; Iwaki *et al.*, 1979).

7.2. Disease Associations

Several studies have demonstrated that there exists a similar or stronger association between some of the HLA-DR antigens (HLA-D determinants) and certain diseases than for the corresponding HLA-B antigens (Dausset and Svejgaard, 1977). This is most pronounced for gluten-sensitive enteropathy and dermatitis herpetiformis (Ek *et al.*, 1978; Keuning *et al.*, 1976; Solheim *et al.*, 1977), where over 90% of affected individuals have the DRw3 antigen. Associations are also seen in multiple sclerosis, and some organ-specific autoimmune diseases such as Addison's disease, thyrotoxicosis, insulin-dependent diabetes, chronic active hepatitis, myasthenia gravis, and Goodpasture's syndrome (Table 9). Rheumatoid arthritis, especially of progressive type (Roitt *et al.*, 1978) and being seropositive (Dobloug *et al.*, 1979), is associated with HLA-DRw4. It is interesting to note that the disease associations in Caucasians are mostly to HLA-DRw3, but that some associations also exist to DRw2 and DRw4. The negative association between insulin-dependent diabetes and DRw2 is very interesting, and might indicate a protective effect of this gene product. It should further be pointed out that HLA-DRw2 and Drw3 are the DR antigens showing most significant nonrandom associations to certain HLA-B (and -A) antigens: DRw2 to HLA-B7 (and -A3) and DRw3 to HLA-B8 (and -A1).

One explanation for these associations may be that the molecules carrying these specificities have important functions in the regulation of specific immune responsiveness. Data from different studies in animals

TABLE 9. Associations between HLA-D/DR and Certain Diseases[a]

Disease	Antigen	Frequency (%) Patients	Controls	Relative risk
Gluten-sensitive enteropathy	DRw3	97	24	56.4
Dermatitis Herpetiformis	DRw3	96	24	48.1
Organ-specific autoimmune diseases				
Multiple sclerosis	DRw2	40–70	18–29	4.8
	DRw3	35–37	14–24	6.7
Addison's disease	Dw3	70	26	6.3
Grave's disease	Dw3	50–54	24–26	3.7
Insulin-dependent diabetes	DRw2	0–7	22–29	0.24
	DRw3	36–59	11–24	5.7
	DRw4	32–58	16–28	2.8
Chronic active hepatitis	DRw3	68	24	6.6
Myasthenia gravis	DRw3	44	21	2.9
Goodpasture's disease	DRw2	88	32	13.1
Rheumatoid arthritis	DRw4	70	28	5.8

[a]For further details, see Ryder *et al.* (1978).

(Miller and Vadas, 1977; Doherty *et al.*, 1976) and humans (see Thorsby *et al.*, 1980) suggest that the major histocompatibility antigens play an important role in T-cell activation by different antigens. For example, recognition of the HLA-DR antigens of macrophages is part of the signal for T-helper-cell activation by protein antigens.

The *HLA-D*-locus antigens may thus be part of a network through which cell–cell signals are conveyed in the immunological system, and recognition of "self" HLA-D/DR may be of paramount importance for activation of T cells. The involvement of HLA-D/DR in macrophage–T cell collaboration may explain the association between certain HLA-D/DR determinants and some diseases in that the HLA-D/DR molecules themselves may be directly involved by differing in their ability to display antigenic determinants in an immunogenic way to T cells (see Thorsby *et al.*, 1980). Other possible mechanisms, such as *Ir* genes in linkage disequilibrium with HLA-D/DR, must, however, also be considered, and of course it must be stressed that HLA is not the only factor determining disease susceptibility.

8. Conclusion

Both our studies and those of others have demonstrated that the antigenic products of the *HLA-D* region, the HLA-D determinants and the HLA-DR antigens, are very closely associated both on a population level and in the cell membrane. No firm evidence has yet been presented that demonstrates that more than one locus codes for HLA-D/DR. However, an extremely high linkage disequilibrium could explain the HLA-D/DR associations. Further biochemical and population studies in different races must be performed to solve the question of one or several loci coding for HLA-D/DR. Meanwhile, the close association has made HLA-DR typing a most convenient tool for the determination of the *HLA-D* region. By HLA-DR typing, *HLA-D*-region antigenic products can be taken into account in clinical medicine.

The restricted tissue distribution and probable central role of the HLA-D/DR antigens in cell collaboration in the immune system open a new perspective for the *HLA-D*-region products in general and clinical immunology.

ACKNOWLEDGMENTS. The Norwegian Council for Science and the Humanities, the Norwegian Cancer Society, and Mr. Anders Jahre's Fund for the Promotion of Science have supported our studies. The secretarial help of Mrs. E. Garmann, K. Goyer, and L. Berger is gratefully acknowledged.

References

Abelson, L.D., and Mann, D.L., 1978, Genetic control of B-cell alloantigens: Evidence for gene(s) linked to the HLA-A locus, *Tissue Antigens* **11**:101.

Albrechtsen, D., Solheim, B.G., and Thorsby, E., 1977a, Serological identification of five HLA-D associated (Ia-like) determinants, *Tissue Antigens* **9**:153.

Albrechtsen, D., Solheim, B.G., and Thorsby, E., 1977b, Antiserum inhibition of the mixed lymphocyte culture (MLC) interaction: Inhibitory effect of antibodies reactive with HLA-D associated determinants, *Cell. Immunol.* **28**:258.

Albrechtsen, D., Solheim, B.G., and Thorsby, E., 1977c, The presence of Ia-like determinants on a subpopulation of human T lymphocytes, *Immunogenetics* **5**:149.

Albrechtsen, D., Bratlie, A., Nousiainen, H., Solheim, B.G., Winther, N., and Thorsby, E., 1978a, Serological typing of HLA-D: Predictive value in mixed lymphocyte cultures (MLC), *Immunogenetics* **6**:91.

Albrechtsen, D., Solheim, B.G., and Thorsby, E., 1978b, Relationship of HLA-D associated B lymphocyte (Ia-like) antigens in the cell membrane, *Tissue Antigens* **11**:372.

Albrechtsen, D., Flatmark, A., Jervell, J., Halvorsen, S., Solheim, B.G., and Thorsby, E., 1978c, Significance of HLA-D/DR matching in renal transplantation, *Lancet* **2**:1126.

Albrechtsen, D., Arnesen, E., Solheim, B.G., and Thorsby, E., 1979, Significance of HLA-D matching and of B cell cross-match tests, *Transplant. Proc.* **11**:743.

Andersson, L., and Häyry, P., 1973, Specific priming of mouse thymus dependent lymphocytes to allogeneic cells *in vitro*, *Eur. J. Immunol.* **3**:595.

Bach, F.H., and Hirschhorn, K., 1964, Lymphocyte interaction: A potential histocompatibility test *in vitro*, *Science* **143**:813.

Bach, F.H., and Voynow, N.K., 1966, 1-Way stimulation in mixed leukocyte cultures, *Science* **153:**545.

Bach, F.H., Bach, M.L., and Sondel, P., 1976, Differential function of major histocompatibility complex antigens in T lymphocyte activation, *Nature (London)* **259:**273.

Bain, B., Vas, M.R., and Lowenstain, L., 1964, The development of large immature mononuclear cells in mixed leukocyte cultures, *Blood* **23:**108.

Barnstable, B.A., and Jones, E.A., 1978, Isolation, structure and genetics of HLA-A, -B, -C and -DRw (IA) antigens, *Br. Med. Bull.* **34:**241.

Barnstable, C.J., Bodmer, W.F., Brown, G., Galfre, G., Milstein, C., Williams, A.F., and Ziegler, A., 1978, Production of monoclonal antibodies to group A erythrocytes, HLA and other human cell surface antigens—new tools for genetic analysis, *Cell* **14:**9.

Bernoco, D., Bernoco, M., Ceppelini, R., Poulik, M.D., van Leeuwen, A., and van Rood, J.J., 1976, Cell antigens of the HLA system: A simple serotyping technique based on non-cytotoxic anti-β-2-microglobulin, *Tissue Antigens* **8:**253.

Bodmer, J.G., Pickbourne, P., and Richards, S., 1978, Ia serology, in: *Histocompatibility Testing 1977,* (W.F. Bodmer, J.R. Batchelor, J.G. Bodmer, H. Festenstein, and P.J. Morris, eds.), pp. 35–82, Munksgaard, Copenhagen.

Bodmer, W.F., Batchelor, J.R., Bodmer, J.G., Festenstein, H., and Morris, P.J. (eds.), 1978, *Histocompatibility Testing 1977,* Munksgaard, Copenhagen.

Böyum, A., 1968, Separation of leucocytes from blood and bone marrow, *Scand. J. Clin. Lab. Invest.* **21,** Suppl. 97.

Bradley, B., Oliver, R.T.D., Mendell, N., and Stevens, A., 1978, The primed lymphocyte (PL) exchange, in: *Histocompatibility Testing 1977* (W.F. Bodmer, J.R. Batchelor, J.G. Bodmer, H. Festenstein, P.L. Morris, eds.), pp. 142–152, Munksgaard, Copenhagen.

Copenhagen Study Group of Immunodeficiencies, 1973, Bone-marrow transplantation from an HL-A non-identical but mixed lymphocyte culture identical donor, *Lancet* **1:**1146.

Cresswell, P., and Geier, S.S., 1975, Antisera to human B-lymphocyte membrane glycoproteins block stimulation in mixed lymphocyte culture, *Nature (London)* **237:**147.

Dausset, J., and Svejgaard, A. (eds.), 1977, *HLA and Disease,* Munksgaard, Copenhagen.

Dobloug, J., Førre, Ø., and Thorsby, E., 1979, HLA-DRw4 and rheumatoid arthritis, *Lancet* **1:**549.

Doherty, P.C., Götze, D., Trinchieri, G., and Zinkernagel, M., 1976, Models for recognition of virally modified cells by immune thymus-derived lymphocytes, *Immunogenetics* **3:**517.

Dossetor, J.B., Kovithavongs, T., Marchuk, L., Butcher, D., St. Louis, G.T., and Schlaut, J., 1975, A caucasoid isolate: Hutterites; Correlation between ABCIL reactivity of a serum and stimulation by a typing cell, in: *Histocompatibility Testing 1975* (F. Kissmeyer-Nielson, ed.), pp. 620–624, Munksgaard, Copenhagen.

Eijsvoogel, V.P., van Rood, J.J., Toit, E.D., and Schellekens, P.T.A., 1972, Position of a locus determining mixed lymphocyte reactions distinct from the known HL-A loci, *Eur. J. Immunol.* **2:**413.

Ek, J., Albrechtsen, D., Solheim, B.G., and Thorsby, E., 1978, Strong association between an HLA-Dw3 associated B cell alloantigen and coeliac disease, *Scand. J. Gastroenterol.* **13:**229.

Evans, R.L., Faldetta, T.J., Humphreys, R.E., Pratt, D.M., Yunis, E.J., and Schlossman, S.F., 1978, Peripheral human T cells sensitized in mixed leucocyte culture synthesize and express Ia-like antigens, *J. Exp. Med.* **148:**1440.

Ferrara, G.B., Tosi, R., Longo, A., Castellani, A., Viviani, C., and Carminati, G., 1978, A safe blood transfusion procedure for immunization against major histocompatibility complex determinants in man, *Transplantation* **26:**150.

Ferrone, S., Pellegrino, M.A., and Reisfeld, R.A., 1977, Immunogenicity of human B cell antigens solubilized from cultured human lymphoid cells, *J. Immunol.* **118:**1036.

Festenstein, H., and Halim, K., 1978, Sperm lymphocyte culture (SLC), in: *Histocompatibility Testing 1977*, (W.F. Bodmer, J.R. Batchelor, J.G. Bodmer, H. Festenstein, and P.J. Morris, eds.), pp. 153–154, Munksgaard, Copenhagen.

Festenstein, H., Oliver, R.T.D., Sachs, J.A., McMichael, A.J., Bodmer, W.F., and Mendell, N.R., 1978, Overall analysis of the HTC data based on clusters, patterns and antigen reports, in: *Histocompatibility Testing 1977* (W.F. Bodmer, J.R. Batchelor, J.G. Bodmer, H. Festenstein, and P.J. Morris, eds.), pp. 115–134, Munksgaard, Copenhagen.

Fu, S.M., Chiorazzi, N., Wang, C.Y., Montazeri, G., Kunkel, H.G., Ko, H.S., and Gottlieb, A.B., 1978, Ia-bearing T lymphocytes in man: Their identification and role in the generation of allogeneic helper activity, *J. Exp. Med.* **148:**1423.

Giphart, M.J., Kaufman, J.F., Fuks, A., Albrechtsen, D., Solheim, B.G., Bruning, J.W., and Strominger, J.L., 1977, HLA-D associated alloantisera react with molecules similar to Ia antigens, *Proc. Natl. Acad. Sci. U.S.A.* **74:**3533.

Goldman, S.F., 1977, Selection of related and unrelated bone marrow donors, *Transplant. Proc.* **9:**507.

Helgesen, A., Hirschberg, H., and Thorsby, E., 1980, Mixed lymphocyte culture microtechnique, in: NIAID Manual of Tissue Typing Techniques, DHEW Publication No. (NIH) 80 545:148.

Hirschberg, H., and Thorsby, E., 1977, Activation of human suppressor cells in mixed lymphocyte cultures, *Scand. J. Immunol.* **6:**809.

Hirschberg, H., Rankin, B., and Thorsby, E., 1974, Production of blastogenic factor by mitomycin-treated cells in mixed lymphocyte cultures, *Transplantation* **17:**323.

Hirschberg, H., Albrechtsen, D., Solheim, B.G., and Thorsby, E., 1977, Inhibition of human mixed lymphocyte culture stimulation by anti-HLA-D associated antisera: Studies with primed responding cells, *Eur. J. Immunol.* **7:**26.

Hirschberg, H., Moen, T., and Thorsby, E., 1979, Specific destruction of human endothelial cell monolayers by anti DRw antisera, *Transplantation* **28:**116.

Horowitz, S.D., Groshong, T., Bach, F.H., Hong, R., and Yunis, E.J., 1975, Treatment of severe combined immunodeficiency with bone marrow from unrelated, mixed lymphocyte culture nonreactive donor, *Lancet* **2:**431.

Humphreys, R.E., McCune, J.M., Chess, L., Herrman, H.C., Malenka, D.J., Mann, D.L., Parham, P., Schlossman, S.F., and Strominger, J.L., 1976, Isolation and immunological characterization of a human, B-lymphocyte-specific, cell surface antigen, *J. Exp. Med.* **144:**98.

Iwaki, Y., Terasaki, P.I., Weil, R., Koon, L., and Starzl, T. 1979, Retrospective tests of B-cold lymphocytotoxins and transplant survival at a single center, *Transplant. Proc.* **11:**941.

Jonker, M., Persijn, G.G., and van Rood, J.J., 1975, MLC inhibition studies with sera from multiparous women, in: *Histocompatibility Testing 1975* (F. Kissmeyer-Nielson, ed.), pp. 594–603, Munksgaard, Copenhagen.

Jörgensen, F., Lamm, L.U., and Kissmeyer-Nielsen, F., 1974, MLC typing and blastogenic factor, *Tissue Antigens* **4:**404.

Kasakura, S., and Lowenstein, L., 1965, The effect of irradiation *in vitro* on mixed leukocyte cultures and on leukocyte cultures with phytohaemagglutinin, in: *Histocompatibility Testing 1965* (D.B. Amos and J.J. van Rood, eds.), pp. 211–212, Munksgaard, Copenhagen.

Kashiwagi, N., and Sasazuki, T., 1978, HLA-D in Japanese, in: *Histocompatibility Testing 1977* (W.F. Bodmer, J.R. Batchelor, J.G. Bodmer, H. Festenstein, and P.J. Morris, eds.), p. 135, Munksgaard, Copenhagen.

Kaufman, J., Fuks, A., Giphart, M., Solheim, B., and Strominger, J.L., 1978, Immunological studies of human Ia-like antigens, in: *Ir Genes and Ia Antigens* (H. McDevitt, ed.), pp. 235–242, Academic Press, New York.

Keuning, J.J., Pena, A.S., van Leeuwen, A., van Hoff, J.P., and van Rood, J.J., 1976, HLA-Dw3 associated with coeliac disease, *Lancet* **1:**506.

Kissmeyer-Nielsen, F., (ed.), 1975, *Histocompatibility Testing 1975,* Munksgaard, Copenhagen.

Kissmeyer-Nielsen, F., and Kjerbye, K.E., 1967, Lymphocytotoxic microtechnique: Purification of lymphocytes by flotation, in: *Histocompatibility Testing 1967* (E.S. Curtoni, P.L. Mattiuz, and R.M. Tosi, eds.), pp. 381–383, Munksgaard, Copenhagen.

Klareskog, L., Malmnäs-Tjernlund, U., Forsum, U., and Peterson, P.A., 1977, Epidermal Langerhans cells express Ia antigens, *Nature (London)* **268:**248.

Klareskog, L., Rask, L., Fohlman, J., and Peterson, P.A., 1978, Heavy HLA-DR (Ia) antigen chain is controlled by the MHC region, *Nature (London)* **275:**762.

Law, H.Y., and Bodmer, W.F., 1978, Use of microimmobilization and microagglutination assays for attempted detection of HLA antigens and β_2-microglobulin on human sperm, *Tissue Antigens* **12:**249.

Lawler, S.D., Hockley, A.B., Jones, E.H., Mrazek, I., and Dewar, P.J., 1977, Inhibition of mixed lymphocyte cultures by Ia antibodies, *Tissue Antigens* **10:**140.

Mann, D.L., Katz, S.I., Nelson, D.L., Abelson, L.D., and Strober, W., 1976, Specific B cell antigens associated with gluten-sensitive enteropathy and dermatitis herpetiformis, *Lancet* **1:**110.

Martins Da Silva, B., Jeannet, M., and Vassalli, M., 1978, Matching renal grafts (letter), *Lancet* **1:**1047.

McKenzie, I.F.C., and Henning, M.M., 1977, Studies of immunogenicity and enhancement of alloantigens of the various regions of the H-2 complex, *Transplant. Proc.* **9:**609.

Miller, J.F.A.P., and Vadas, M.A., 1977, The major histocompatibility complex: Influence on immune reactivity and T-lymphocyte activation, *Scand. J. Immunol.* **6:**771.

Moen, T., and Thorsby, E., 1978, Specificity of human lymphocytes primed against allogeneic cells *in vitro.* I. Optimalization of culture conditions for detection of HLA-D specificity, *Tissue Antigens* **12:**367.

Möller, G. (ed.), 1976, *Transplantation Reviews,* Vol. 30, Munksgaard, Copenhagen.

Pellegrino, M.A., Ferrone, S., and Theofilopoulos, A.N., 1976, Isolation of human T and B lymphocytes by rosette formation with 2-aminoethylisothiouronium bromide (AET)-treated sheep red blood cells and with monkey red blood cells, *J. Immunol. Methods* **11:**273.

Pena, A.S., Mann, D.L., Hague, N.E., Heck, J.A., van Leeuwen, A., van Rood, J.J., and Strober, W., 1978, Genetic basis of gluten-sensitive enteropathy, *Gastroenterology* **75:**230.

Persijn, G.G., Gabb, B.W., van Leeuwen, A., Nagtegaal, A., Hogeboom, J., and van Rood, J.J., 1978, Matching for HLA antigens of A, B, and DR loci in renal transplantation by Eurotransplant, *Lancet* **1:**1278.

Roitt, I.M., Corbett, M., Festenstein, H., Jaraquemada, D., Papasteriadis, C., Hay, F.C., and Nineham, L.J., 1978, HLA-DRw4 and prognosis in rheumatoid arthritis, *Lancet* **1:**990.

Rowden, G., Lewis, M.G., and Sullivan, A.K., 1977, Ia antigen expression on human epidermal Langerhans cells, *Nature (London)* **268:**247.

Ryder, L.P., Thomsen, M., Platz, P., and Svejgaard, A., 1975, Data reduction in LD typing, in: *Histocompatibility Testing 1975* (F. Kissmeyer-Nielsen, ed.), pp. 557–562, Munksgaard, Copenhagen.

Ryder, L.P., Andersen, E., and Svejgaard, A., 1978, HLA and disease, Third report from the HLA and disease registry.

Sachs, J.A., Festenstein, H., Tuffnel, V.A., and Paris, A.M.I., 1977, Collaborative scheme for tissue typing and matching in renal transplantation. IX. Effect of HLA-A, -B and -D locus matching, pretransplant transfusion and other factors on 612 cadaver renal grafts, *Transplant. Proc.* **9:**483.

Scott, H., Solheim, B.G., Brandtzaeg, P., and Thorsby, E., 1980, HLA-DR-like antigens in the epithelium of the human small intestine, *Scand. J. Immunol.* **12:**77.

Sheehy, M.J., Sondel, P.M., Bach, M.L., Wank, R., and Bach, F.H., 1975, A rapid assay using primed lymphocytes, *Science* **188:**1308.

Snary, D., Goodfellow, P., Hayman, M.J., Bodmer, W.F., and Crumpton, M.J., 1974, Subcellular separation and molecular nature of human histocompatibility antigens (HL-A), *Nature (London)* **247:**457.

Solheim, B.G., Bratlie, A., Winther, N., and Thorsby, E., 1975, LD typing with antisera produced by planned immunization, in: *Histocompatibility Testing 1975* (F. Kissmeyer-Nielsen, ed.), pp. 713–718, Munksgaard, Copenhagen.

Solheim, B.G., Thorsby, E., and Möller, E., 1976, Inhibition of the Fc receptor of human lymphoid cells by antisera recognizing determinants of the HLA system, *J. Exp. Med.* **143:**1568.

Solheim, B.G., Albrechtsen, D., Thorsby, E., and Thune, E., 1977, Strong association between an HLA-Dw3 associated B cell alloantigen and dermatitis herpetiformis, *Tissue Antigens* **10:**114.

Solheim, B.G., Fuks, A., Smith, L., Strominger, J.L., and Thorsby, E., 1978, Possible detection of HLA-DR alloantigenic specificities in man with unabsorbed rabbit antisera, *Scand. J. Immunol.* **8:**15.

Solheim, B.G., Flatmark, A., Halvorsen, S., Jervell, J., and Thorsby, E., 1979a, The influence of HLA-A, -B, -C and -D matching and pretransplant blood transfusions on kidney graft survival, *Transplant. Proc.* **11:**748.

Solheim, B.G., Braathen, L.R., Hovig, T., and Strominger, J.L., 1979b, Evidence for the presence of human Ia-like (HLA-DR) and T-cell specific antigens on Sezary cells, *Scand. J. Immunol.* **10:**381.

Soullillou, J.P., Peyrat, M.A., and Guenel, J., 1978, Association between treatment-resistant kidney allograft rejection and post-transplant appearance of antibodies to donor B lymphocyte alloantigens, *Lancet* **1:**354.

Springer, T., Kaufman, J., Terhorst, G., and Strominger, J.L., 1978, Studies of the structure of the human Ia-like antigen, in: *Ir Genes and Ia Antigens* (H.O. McDevitt, ed.), pp. 229–234, Academic Press, New York.

Staines, N.A., Guy, K., Fish, F., Sworn, J.L., Davies, D.A.L., and Festenstein, H., 1977, Passive enhancement and antigens of different regions of the mouse H-2 complex, *Transplant. Proc.* **9:**941.

Strominger, J.L., Chess, L., Herrmann, H.C., Humphreys, R.E., Malenka, D., Mann, D., McCune, J.M., Parham, P., Robb, R., Springer, T.A., and Terhorst, C., 1975, Isolation of histocompatibility antigens and of several B cell specific proteins from cultured human lymphocytes, in: *Histocompatibility Testing 1975* (F. Kissmeyer-Nielsen, ed.), pp. 719–730, Munksgaard, Copenhagen.

Suciu-Foca, N., Susinno, E., Nicholson, J., Fotino, M., Molinaro, A.P., and Rubinstein, P., 1977, Complete typing of the HLA region in families. IV. The genetics of HLA-D as seen by the HTC and PLT methods, *Transplant. Proc.* **9:**1751.

Suciu-Foca, N., Rubinstein, P., Susinno, E., Broell, J., Weiner, J., and Reemtsma, K., 1978, Quantitation of HLA-D differences, *Tissue Antigens* **12:**94.

Svedmyr, E.A.J., Leibold, W., and Gatti, R.A., 1975, Possible use of established cell lines for MLR locus typing, *Tissue Antigens* **5:**186.

Thorsby, E., 1974, The human major histocompatibility system, *Transplant. Rev.* **18:**51.

Thorsby, E., and Piazza, A., 1975, Typing for HLA-D (LD1 or MLC) determinants, in: *Histocompatibility Testing 1975* (F. Kissmeyer-Nielsen, ed.), pp. 414–458, Munksgaard, Copenhagen.

Thorsby, E., Hirschberg, H., and Helgesen, A., 1973, A second locus determining human

MLC response: Separate lymphocyte populations recognize the products of each different MLC locus allele in allogeneic combinations, *Transplant. Proc.* **5:**1523.

Thorsby, E., Albrechtsen, D., Hirschberg, H., Kaakinen, A., and Solheim, B.G., 1977, MLC-activating HLA-D determinants: Identification, tissue distribution and significance, *Transplant. Proc.* **9:**393.

Thorsby, E., Albrechtsen, D., Bergholtz, B.O., Hirschberg, H., and Solheim, B.G., 1978, Identification and significance of products of the HLA-D region, *Transplant. Proc.* **10:**313.

Thorsby, E., Bergholtz, B., and Nousiainen, H., 1981, Self *HLA-D* region products restrict human T-lymphocyte activation by antigen, in : *Current Trends in Histocompatibility,* Vol. 2 (R.A. Reisfeld and S. Ferrone, eds.), Plenum Press, New York.

Ting, A., and Morris, P., 1978, Matching for B cell antigens of the HLA-DR series in cadaver renal transplantation, *Lancet* **1:**575.

Tosi, R., Tanigaki, N., Centis, D., Ferrara, G.B., and Pressman, D., 1978, Immunological dissection of human Ia molecules, *J. Exp. Med.* **148:**1592.

van Leeuwen, A., Schuit, H.R.E., and van Rood, J.J., 1973, Typing for MLC (LD). II. The selection of nonstimulator cells by MLC inhibition tests using SD identification stimulator cells (MISIS) and fluorescence antibody studies, *Transplant. Proc.* **5:**1539.

van Rood, J.J., 1973, LD–SD interaction *in vivo* and the allograft reaction, *Transplant. Proc.* **5:**1747.

van Rood, J.J., van Leeuwen, A., Parlevliet, J., Termijtelen, A., and Keuning, J.J., 1975, LD typing by serology. IV. Description of a new locus with three alleles, in: *Histocompatibility Testing 1975* (F. Kissmeyer-Nielsen, ed.), pp. 629–636, Munksgaard, Copenhagen.

van Rood, J.J., van Leeuwen, A., and Ploem, J.S., 1976, Simultaneous detection of two cell populations by two-colour fluorescence and application to the recognition of B cell determinants, *Nature (London)* **262:**795.

van Rood, J.J., van Leeuwen, A., Termijtelen, A., and Bradley, B., 1977, The predictive value of HLA-D matching for the outcome of the MLC test, *Tissue Antigens* **10:**148.

Walford, R.L., Gossett, T., Troup, G.M., Gatti, R.A., Mittal, K.K., Robins, A., Ferrara, G.B., and Zeller, E., 1976, The Merrit alloantigenic system of human B lymphocytes: Evidence for thirteen possible factors including one six-member segregant series, *J. Immunol.* **116:**1704.

Welsh, K.I., and Turner, M.J., 1976, Preparation of antisera specific for human B cells by immunization of rabbits with immune complexes, *Tissue Antigens* **8:**197.

Wernet, P., 1976, Human Ia type alloantigens: Methods of detection, aspects of chemistry and biology, markers for disease states, *Transplant. Rev.* **30:**271.

Wernet, P. (ed.), 1977, Human Ia type and PLT antigens: Genetic aspects and correlation to other histocompatibility determinants, *Scand. J. Immunol.* **6:**367.

Wiman, K., Curman, B., Forsum, U., Klareskog, L., Malmnäs-Tjernlund, U., Rask, L., Trägardh, L., and Peterson, P.A., 1978, Occurrence of Ia antigens on tissues of non-lymphoid origin, *Nature (London)* **276:**711.

Yunis, E.J., and Amos, D.B., 1971, Three closely linked genetic systems relevant to transplantation, *Proc. Natl. Acad. Sci., U.S.A.* **68:**3031.

13

The Polymorphism of *I*-Region-Encoded Antigens among Wild Mice

Edward K. Wakeland and Jan Klein

1. Introduction

Genes in the major histocompatibility complex (MHC) have been shown to control the expression of several cell-surface antigens that are involved in the differentiation and activation of cells of the immune system. These antigens can be divided into two classes on the basis of functional and structural criteria (Klein, 1977). The class I antigens are the targets of the transplantation reaction, are involved in the recognition of virus-infected cells, have a molecular weight of about 44,000 daltons, and are nonconvalently associated with β_2-microglobulin. The class II antigens are involved in the regulation of the antibody response to soluble antigens and mediate many of the interactions of immunocompetent cells. Those class II antigens that have been structurally characterized consist of two polypeptide chains and are not associated with β_2-microglobulin.

The class I genes of most mammalian species are highly polymorphic. Previous studies from this laboratory have revealed that murine class I antigens encoded by the *H-2K* and *H-2D* genes are extremely polymorphic in wild-mouse populations (Klein, 1970; Klein *et al.*, 1978a). Serological typing of wild mice with alloantisera specific for known H-2 antigens suggests that more than 60 alleles of the class I genes in the *H-2K* and *H-2D* regions are present in *Mus musculus* (Duncan *et al.*, 1979). Although many other genes are polymorphic in wild mice (Berry and Peters, 1977), the polymorphism of the class I H-2 antigens is unparalleled

Edward K. Wakeland and Jan Klein • Department of Immunogenetics, Max-Planck-Institute for Biology, Tübingen, West Germany.

among the currently known genetic systems in the mouse. What selective forces, if any, are operating to maintain this polymorphism is not known.

The serologically detected polymorphism of class I antigens reflects the extensive structural variations in the protein products of the class I alleles. Recent technical developments have allowed direct structural comparisons of the class I antigens produced among inbred lines of mice (Brown *et al.*, 1974; Vitetta *et al.*, 1976; Henning *et al.*, 1976; Silver and Hood, 1976; Ewenstein *et al.*, 1976). Data obtained with both peptide mapping and microsequencing techniques demonstrate considerable structural variations in the primary structure of the class I antigens. Peptide-mapping data indicate that the structural polymorphism is distributed throughout the molecule and not localized in any single region (Brown *et al.*, 1974). Microsequencing data indicate that allelic class I products of the inbred lines may vary in from 10 to 30% of their primary structure (Maizels *et al.*, 1978). This amount of variation has prompted some investigators to suggest that the currently recognized class I alleles actually represent separate genes that are inherited as a "gene family" the expression of which is controlled by a regulatory mechanism (Bodmer, 1972).

The murine class II genes in the *I* region of the *H-2* complex were originally defined by their influence on the magnitude of the humoral immune response of certain inbred mice to synthetic polypeptide antigens (Benacerraf and McDevitt, 1972). The products of most of the class II genes in the *I* region are cell-surface antigens (denoted Ia antigens) that can be detected with specific alloantisera (David, 1977). The products of only two genes, *Ia-1* of the *IA* subregion and *Ia-5* of the *IE* subregion, can be assayed by a standard antibody-mediated cytotoxicity test with normal spleen cells, or immunoprecipitated from radiolabeled spleen-cell extracts. These Ia antigens are present on the majority of B cells and on macrophages of spleen and lymph nodes. The analysis of antisera prepared against Ia antigens of inbred mice indicates that they are complex and polymorphic.

Structural studies of the Ia antigens indicate that both *Ia-1* and *Ia-5* code for molecules that consist of two polypeptide chains, designated alpha (α) and beta (β), with molecular weights of approximately 30,000–35,000 and 25,000–30,000 daltons, respectively (Cullen *et al.*, 1976). The isolated α and β chains of the *Ia-1* and *Ia-5* products can be distinguished by their amino-terminal amino acid sequences, indicating that none of the subunits is shared between the two products (Cook *et al.*, 1977; McMillan *et al.*, 1978a; Silver *et al.*, 1976; Cecka *et al.*, 1978). Data obtained with both microsequencing and tryptic-peptide-mapping techniques demonstrate considerable structural variations among inbred alleles of the β chains from both *Ia-1* and *Ia-5* products (Freed 1978; Cook *et al.*, 1979). In contrast, little or no structural variations have been detected among inbred line alleles of either Ia antigen's α chains (Cook *et al.*, 1979; Freed, 1978; McMillan *et al.*, 1978b).

We are studying the polymorphism of the Ia antigens in wild mice. Because of the complexity of these antigens, we are using two approaches. First, we are analyzing the Ia antigens of a collection of cogenic lines carrying wild-derived *H-2* haplotypes on a C57BL/10 Sn background. In addition, we use these lines to refine the specificity of our typing reagents. Second, we trap and serologically type wild mice in the field.

2. Serological Analyses of the *I*-Region Antigens Present in a Collection of Wild-Derived *H-2* Haplotypes

2.1. Origin of the B10.W Lines

Cogenic lines carrying wild-derived *H-2* haplotypes on a C57BL/10Sn (B10) background have been produced. The development of these B10.W (where "W" stands for "wild") lines has been described elsewhere (Klein, 1973, 1975). Briefly, the progeny of wild male mice with an Ss^h phenotype were repeatedly backcrossed to an Ss^l B10.Br (*H-2*^{k}) strain. In each backcross generation, the progeny carrying the wild-derived *H-2* haplotype were detected by their Ss^h phenotypes. The lines were established as homozygous for wild-derived *H-2* haplotypes by intercrossing the Ss^h progeny of the final backcross generation and selecting among the *H-2*^{k}-negative progeny for the founding stock. At present, 29 B10.W lines have been completed. Table 1 lists these lines with their respective numbers of generations at the time of testing and the origins of their wild-mouse ancestors.

Two features of the production of these lines are relevant to the interpretation of data obtained through their analysis. All but three of these lines (B10.MOL1, B10.CAS2, B10.CAA2) were derived from male wild mice that were trapped in or near Ann Arbor, Michigan. Thus, the *H-2* haplotypes of these mice are representative of the trappable population of wild mice in a restricted geographical area and are not necessarily representative of wild mice in general. Consequently, estimates of the polymorphism of *H-2* genes based solely on an analysis of the B10.W lines are *minimum* estimates of the polymorphism present in the entire wild-mouse population. As with any *H-2* cogenic line, a variable amount of the chromosome 17 bordering on either side of the selected *H-2* complex is also present in each B10.W line. What effect (if any) these additional wild-derived loci may have on the H-2 antigens of the B10.W lines is not known.

TABLE 1. List of B10.W Congenic Lines Used in the Present Study

Line	Generation	Wild-mouse origin
B10.BUA1	N12F4	Butcher farm, 1651 Knight Rd., Ann Arbor, Mich. (barn)
B10.BUA16	N17F3	Butcher farm, 1651 Knight Rd., Ann Arbor,Mich. (barn)
B10.BUA19	N13F6	Butcher farm, 1651 Knight Rd., Ann Arbor, Mich. (barn)
B10.CAA2	N10F3	Ribblet House, Menco Park, Calif. (garage)
B10.CAS2	N10F4	*Mus castaneus* from Dr. M. Potter
B10.CHA2	N12F5	CH farm on Scio-Church Rd., Ann Arbor, Mich. (corncrib)
B10.CHR51	N12F4	CH farm, Wagner Rd., Ann Arbor, Mich. (granary)
B10.DRB62	N13F5	DR farm, 6350 Waters Rd., Ann Arbor, Mich. (barn)
B10.GA20	N13F6	Geigen farm, 5540 Five Mile Rd., Ann Arbor, Mich. (barn)
B10.GA37	N13F6	Geigen farm, 5540 Five Mile Rd., Ann Arbor, Mich. (barn)
B10KEA2	N13F5	King farm, 10075 North Territorial Rd., Ann Arbor, Mich. (barn)
B10.KPA42	N9F7	Kapp farm, 4330 Nixon Rd., Ann Arbor, Mich. (granary)
B10.KPA132	N8F5	Kapp farm, 4330 Nixon Rd., Ann Arbor, Mich. (granary)
B10.KPB128	N9F4	Kapp farm, 4330 Nixon Rd., Ann Arbor, Mich. (corncrib)
B10.LIB18	N8F4	Ks farm, Liberty Road, Ann Arbor, Mich. (granary)
B10.LIB55	N10F4	Ks farm, Liberty Road, Ann Arbor, Mich. (granary)
B10.MOL1	N10F2	*Mus molossinus* from Dr. M. Potter
B10.SAA48	N11F5	NB farm, Austin Rd., Saline, Mich. (granary)
B10.SNA57	N8F5	SN farm, Liberty Rd., Ann Arbor, Mich. (corncrib)
B10.SNA70	N9F5	SN farm, Liberty Rd., Ann Arbor, Mich. (corncrib)
B10.STA10	N8F4	Stein farm, 4200 Liberty Rd., Ann Arbor, Mich. (barn)
B10.STA12	N7F5	Stein farm, 4200 Liberty Rd., Ann Arbor, Mich. (barn)
B10.STA39	N11F7	Stein farm, 4200 Liberty Rd., Ann Arbor, Mich. (barn)
B10.STA62	N10F4	Stein farm, 4200 Liberty Rd., Ann Arbor, Mich. (barn)

TABLE 1. *(continued)*

Line	Generation	Wild-mouse origin
B10.STC77	N9F6	Stein farm, 4200 Liberty Rd., Ann Arbor, Mich. (corncrib)
B10.STC90	N8F6	Stein farm, 4200 Liberty Rd., Ann Arbor, Mich. (corncrib)
B10.WOA105	N12F4	Wolf farm, 2801 Tessmer Rd., Ann Arbor, Mich. (granary)

2.2. Typing of the B10.W lines with Reagents Specific for Ia Antigens of the Inbred Lines

The B10.W lines were typed with alloantisera detecting Ia antigens of inbred lines. A total of 34 Ia antigens have been described thus far by the various laboratories working on Ia serology with inbred mice (listed in Klein *et al.*, 1978b). Almost all these antigens have been mapped to either the *Ia-1* or the *Ia-5* gene by analysis with inbred *H-2* recombinant lines or coprecipitation and cocapping techniques.

The Ia alloantisera used in our study were selected from a panel of about 50 antisera produced in the authors' laboratory. The prime factor for the selection of typing reagents was a high specific cytotoxic titer against the appropriate target cells. The selected antisera detected 17 Ia antigens among the inbred lines, 5 of which had not been previously reported (Wakeland and Klein, 1979). The strain combinations used to produce these allo-antisera, the absorptions required to make them oligospecific, the appropriate target cells, and any additional antibody activities present in the sera after absorption are listed in Table 2.

The B10.W lines were tested for the presence of inbred Ia antigens with these alloantisera by direct cytotoxicity and absorption analyses. In each instance, an inbred antigen was assigned only to those B10.W lines that fully absorbed the reactivity of the anti-serum for the appropriate inbred target cells. In several instances, lymphocytes from individual B10.W lines that reacted with these typing reagents by direct cytotoxicity were unable to absorb all their reactivity against the inbred target cells. For example, lymphocytes from line B10.STC90 were lysed to a high titer by anti Ia.2 antiserum (K464 in Table 2). However, absorption of K464 with B10.STC90 lymphocytes would not remove all the reactivity of this reagent for B10.BR target cells. These results indicate that B10.STC90 contains an antigen that cross-reacts with Ia.2. Similar cross-reactions were observed with antisera to antigens Ia.5, Ia.11, Ia.12, Ia.15, Ia.24, and Ia.31. The Ia antigens assigned to the B10.W lines are listed in Table 3.

TABLE 2. Alloantisera Used for Detection of Ia Specificities

Code No.	Antigen detected	Recipient	Donor	Absorption	Target	Other antibodies
K593	1	(A.BY × B10..HTT)F_1	A.TL	—	B10.M	Ia.2,Ia.19
K464	2	(LP.RIII × B10.T (6R)F_1	AQR	B10.PL	B10.BR	—
K228	4	(B10 × A.TL)F_1	B10.HTT	B10.RIII	B10.S	—
K212	5	(A.TL × B10)F_1	B10.HTT	—	B10.P	Ia.4,Ia.24
K595	7	(B10 × R107)F_1	B10.A(5R)	—	B10.D2	—
NIH8+	8	(A × B10.A)F_1	B10.A(5R)	—	B10.D2	H-2.33,Ia.20,+
K548	11	(B10.A × A)F_1	B10.D2	B10.STC77[a]	B10.D2	—
K228	12	(B10 × A.TL)F_1	B10.HTT	B10.PL	B10.RIII	—
K594	15	(A.TH × B10.HTT)F_1	A.TL	B10.RIII	B10	—
K499	17	(B10.Q × DBA/2)F_1	AQR	B10.A(5R) B10.WB	B10.S	Ia.2, Ia.19
K417	19	(B10.HTT × A.SW)F_1	A.TL	B10.PL	B10.RIII	Ia.2
K30	20	(B10.D2 × A)F_1	HTI	EL4, B10.RIII	B10	—
K228	24	(B10 × A.TL)F_1	B10.HTT	—	B10.PL	Ia.4, Ia.12
K464	31	(LP.RIII × B10.T (6R)F_1	AQR	—	B10.PL	Ia.2
K499	32	(B10.Q × DBA/2)F_1	AQR	B10.A (4R)	B10.P	Ia.34
K499	33	(B10.Q × DBA/2)F_1	AQR	B10.A (5R)	B10.WB	Ia.2, Ia.17, Ia.19, Ia.31
K499	34	(B10.Q × DBA/2)F_1	AQR	B10.A(4R), B10.P	B10.A(5R)	—

[a] Absorption with B10.STC77 removes antibodies to the *H-2K*^{d} allele.

TABLE 3. Distribution of Ia Specificities among B10.W Lines

	Ia specificity																
Line	1	2	4	5	7	8	11	12	15	17	19	20	24	31	32	33	34
SNA57	—	—	—	—	7	8	—	—	15	—	—	—	—	—	32	—	34
SNA70	1	2	—	—	7	—	—	—	15	17	19	—	—	31	32	33	34
STA10	—	—	—	—	7	—	—	—	15	—	—	—	—	—	32	—	—
STA12	—	—	—	—	7	—	—	—	15	—	—	—	—	—	32	—	—
STA39	—	—	—	—	7[a]	—	—	—	15	—	—	—	—	—	32	—	34
STA62	—	—	—	—	7	8	—	—	15	—	—	20	—	—	32	—	34
STC77	—	—	—	5	7[a]	—	—	—	—	—	—	—	—	—	32	—	—
STC90	1	—	—	—	7	—	—	—	15	17	19	—	—	31	32	33	34
BUA1	—	—	—	5	7	—	—	12	—	17	—	—	24	—	32	33	34
BUA16	—	—	—	5	7	—	—	12	—	17	—	—	24	—	32	33	34
BUA19	—	—	—	5	7	—	—	12	—	17	—	—	24	—	32	33	34
KPA42	—	—	—	—	7	8	—	—	15	—	—	—	—	—	32	—	—
KPA44	—	—	—	5	7	—	—	12	—	17	—	—	24	—	32	33	34
KPA132	—	—	—	—	7	8	—	—	15	—	—	—	—	—	32	—	—
KPB128	—	—	4	5	7	—	—	12	—	17	—	—	24	—	32	33	34
LIB18	—	—	—	5	7	—	—	12	—	17	—	—	24	—	32	33	34
LIB55	—	—	—	—	7	—	—	—	15	—	—	—	—	—	32	—	—
GA20	—	—	—	—	7	—	—	—	—	17	—	—	—	—	32	33	—
GA37	—	—	4	5	7	—	—	12	—	17	—	—	24	—	32	33	34
KEA2	—	—	—	—	7[a]	—	—	—	—	—	—	—	—	—	—	—	—
KEA5	—	—	—	—	7	—	—	—	—	—	—	—	—	—	32	—	—
MOL1	1	2	—	—	7	—	—	—	15	17	19	—	—	31	32	33	34
CAS2	—	—	—	—	—	—	—	—	—	—	—	—	—	—	—	—	—
CHR51	—	—	—	5	7	—	—	—	—	—	—	—	—	—	32	—	—
CHA2	1	2	—	—	7	—	—	—	15	17	19	—	—	31	32	33	34
WOA105	—	—	—	—	7	8	—	—	15	—	—	—	—	—	32	—	—
SAA48	—	—	—	—	7	—	—	—	—	—	—	—	—	32	—	—	
DRB62	—	—	—	—	7	8	—	—	15	—	—	—	—	—	32	—	34
CAA2	—	—	—	5	7	—	—	—	—	—	—	—	—	32	—	—	

[a]These lines have lower levels of Ia.7 when measured by absorptive capacity.

2.3. Estimates of *I*-Region Polymorphism of Inbred and B10.W Lines

The inbred and B10.W lines can be organized into groups on the basis of their Ia phenotypes. Antigens encoded by the *Ia-1* and *Ia-5* genes can be analyzed separately to determine the minimum number of alleles of each gene, and then together to estimate the minimum number of *I*-region haplotypes present within the 40 inbred and B10.W strains.

The phenogroups formed by Ia antigens encoded by *Ia-1* are listed in Table 4. Fourteen Ia antigens were found in 15 different combinations among the inbred and B10.W lines. Thus, a minimum estimate of 15 *Ia-1*

TABLE 4. Phenogroups Formed by Antigens Localized to *Ia-1* Products

Prototype line	H-2	Characteristic phenogroup	Other lines
B10	b	8, 15, 20	STA62
B10.D2	d	8, 11, 15	—
B10.M	f	1, 5, 17, 33	—
B10.WB	j	5, 15, 33	—
B10.BR	k	1, 2, 15, 17, 19, 31, 33	MOL1, CHA 2, SNA 70
B10.P	p	5	STC77, CHR51, CAA2
B10.RIII	r	1, 5, 12, 17, 19, 24, 33	—
B10.S	s	4, 5, 12, 17, 24, 33	KPB128, GA37
B10.PL	u	1, 5, 15, 17, 24, 31, 33	—
B10.SM	v	8, 15	KPA42, SNA57, KPA132, WOA105, DRB62
B10.STA10	w 13	15	STA12, LIB55, STA39
B10.STC90	w 15	1, 15, 17, 19, 31, 33	—
B10.BUA1	w 16	5, 12, 17, 24, 33	BUA16, BUA19, LIB18, KPA44
B10.GA20	w 23	17, 33	—
B10.KEA2	w 24	—	KEA5, CAS2, SAA48

alleles is necessary to explain these data. Some of the B10.W lines, such as B10.STA10 and B10.CAS2, have alleles that code for few or none of these antigens. This observation suggests that the *Ia-1* alleles of these strains code for antigens that are quite different from those of inbred lines. Fourteen of the B10.W lines have *Ia-1* alleles the products of which are serologically indistinguishable from those of either $Ia\text{-}1^b$, $Ia\text{-}1^k$, $Ia\text{-}1^p$, $Ia\text{-}1^s$, or $Ia\text{-}1^u$ (Table 4). Whether the products of these wild-

TABLE 5. Phenogroups Formed by Antigens Localized to *Ia-5* Products

Prototype line	H-2	Characteristic phenogroup	Other lines
B10	b	—	B10.M, B10.Q, B10.S, CAS2
B10.D2	d	7	KEA2
B10.P	p	7, 32	B10.WB, B10.PL, STA10 STA12, STC77, KPA42 KPA132, GA20, KEA5, CHR51,WOA105, SAA48, CAA2, LIB55
B10.BR	k	7, 32, 34	B10.RIII, B10.SM, SNA57, SNA70, STA39, STA62, STC90, BUA1, BUA19, BUA16,KPA44, KPB128, LIB18,GA37, MOL1, DRB62, CHA2

derived *Ia-1* alleles are structurally identical to their inbred counterparts remains to be determined. However, recent data obtained with antisera prepared against these particular B10.W lines indicate that in some instances their *Ia-1* products can be distinguished serologically from those of the prototype inbred lines (Wakeland and Klein, unpublished observations). Comparative tryptic peptide mapping of the products of the serologically indistinguishable *Ia-1* alleles will establish whether they represent closely related or identical alleles.

The phenogroups formed by antigens encoded by *Ia-5* are presented in Table 5. The three Ia antigens encoded by *Ia-5* were found in four different combinations. In contrast to the results obtained with antisera to *Ia-1*-encoded antigens, no new *Ia-5* alleles were detected among the B10.W lines with the reagents used. These results place a minimum estimate of the polymorphism of *Ia-5* at four alleles.

The phenogroups obtained by combining all the *I*-region antigens are presented in Table 6. A total of 21 different *I*-region haplotypes were detected. Several of the B10.W lines, such as B10.CAS2, B10.SAA48, and B10.KEA2, are negative for most or all of the inbred Ia antigens. Other lines have *I*-region haplotypes the products of which are serologi-

TABLE 6. Phenogroups Formed by Antigens of *Ia-1* and *Ia-5* Products

Prototype line	H-2	Characteristic phenogroups	Other lines
B10	b	8, 15, 20	—
B10.D2	d	7, 8, 11, 15	—
B10.M	f	1, 5, 17	—
B10.WB	j	5, 7, 15, 32, 33	—
B10.BR	k	1, 2, 7, 15, 17, 19, 31, 32, 33, 34	SNA70, MOL1, CHA2
B10.P	p	5, 7, 32	STC77, CHR51, CAA2
B10.Q	q	5	—
B10.RIII	r	1, 5, 7, 12, 17, 19, 24, 32, 33, 34	—
B10.S	s	4, 5, 12, 17, 24, 33	—
B10.PL	u	1, 7, 15, 17, 24, 31, 32, 33	—
B10.SM	v	7, 8, 15, 32, 34	SNA57, DRB62
B10.STA10	w13	7, 15, 32	STA12, LIB55
B10.STA62	w23	7, 15, 20, 32	—
B10.STC90	w15	1, 7, 15, 17, 19, 31, 32, 33, 34	—
B10.BUA1	w16	5, 7, 12, 17, 24, 32, 33, 34	BUA16, BUA19, LIB18, KPA44
B10.KPA132	w1	7, 8, 15, 32	KPA42, WOA105
B10.KPB128	w19	4, 5, 7, 12, 17, 24, 32, 33, 34	GA37
B10.GA20	w24	7, 17, 32, 33	KEA5
B10.KEA2	w25	7	—
B10.CAS2	w17	—	—
B10.SAA48	w3	7, 32	—

cally indistinguishable from those encoded by *H-2*^{k}, *H-2*^{p}, or *H-2*^{v}. These results suggest that some of the *I*-region haplotypes of inbred mice may be present in wild-mouse populations, but that most wild mice have haplotypes not found among the inbred *H-2* haplotypes of independent origin.

Several interesting features of the polymorphism of *Ia-1* are apparent from the typing of the B10.W lines. The frequencies of *Ia-1*-encoded antigens ranged from 0.0 (Ia.11) to 0.41 (Ia.15,17) among the B10.W lines. In addition, several of the typing reagents that were monospecific when tested on inbred lines were split by the B10.W lines into multiple reactivities. All these properties are the expected characteristics of a highly polymorphic gene.

Results obtained with antisera to the *Ia-5*-encoded antigens contrasted sharply with those of the *Ia-1* products. Only four *Ia-5* alleles were detected in our survey, and all these were present among the inbred lines. None of the typing reagents for *Ia-5* products was split into component antibodies by the B10.W lines, and the frequencies of their respective antigens ranged from 0.52 (Ia.34) to 0.97 (Ia.7). These results demonstrate a distinct difference in the serologically detected polymorphism of the *Ia-1* and *Ia-5* genes. Our data suggest that *Ia-1* is nearly as polymorphic as the class I *H-2K* and *H-2D* genes, while *Ia-5* is considerably less polymorphic than either. However, the possibility that *Ia-5* controls antigens the polymorphism of which is not readily detected with the available antisera cannot be ruled out. A structural comparison of the *Ia-5* products from appropriate B10.W lines will resolve this question.

The recent findings of Jones *et al.* (1978) may be relevant to our results concerning the polymorphism of *Ia-5*. These authors have demonstrated that the lighter polypeptide chain (presumably the β chain) of the *Ia-5* product is encoded in the *IA* subregion, while the heavier chain (presumably the α chain) is encoded in the *IE* subregion. Since all the antigens of *Ia-5* products are encoded by the *IE* subregion, these results indicate that alloantisera specific for *Ia-5* products are interacting only with the α chain. This would suggest that the four *Ia-5* alleles that we have detected in our survey represent variations in the α chain of the *Ia-5* product and do not represent the polymorphism of the β chain.

2.4. Detection of Natural Recombinants among the B10.W Lines

Many of the B10.W lines have inbred-like *H-2* alleles in combinations that are absent in the standard inbred recombinant panel. By combining the class I antigen typing results (Zaleska-Rutczynska and Klein, 1977; Duncan and Klein, unpublished results) with the class II antigen typing data, a table of "natural" recombinant B10.W lines can be compiled

TABLE 7. List of B10.W Lines Representing Natural Recombinations of Inbred *H-2* Alleles

Line	H-2 haplotype	H-2 regions[a] *K*	*A,B*	*E,C*	*S*	*D*
KEA5	*w5*	*d*	*w*	*w*	*w*	*w*
SNA70	*w8*	*k*	*k*		*w*	*w*
BUA19	*w22*	*w*	*w*	*w*	*w*	*k*
MOL1	*w12*	*k*	*k*		*w*	*w*
STC77	*w14*	*d*	*w*	*w*	*w*	*w*
CHR51	*w18*	*d*	*w*	*w*	*w*	*w*
KPB128	*w19*	*s*	*s*	*w*	*w*	*b*
GA37	*w21*	*s*	*s*	*w*	*w*	*w*
CAA2	*w11*	*f*	*w*	*w*	*w*	*w*
CHA2	*w26*	*q*	*k*		*w*	*w*
STA62	*w27*	*w*	*b*	*w*	*w*	*w*

[a]Vertical lines denote points of recombination relative to the inbred *H-2* alleles. A "*w*" indicates that the marker gene for this region does not resemble an inbred allele.

(Table 7). As Table 7 shows, 11 of the B10.W lines are natural recombinants containing one or more of the inbred class I or class II alleles. These results suggest that intra-*H-2* recombination is a common event among wild mice and that the wild-mouse population represents a large reservoir of potentially useful *H-2* recombinants.

3. Serological Typing of the Ia Antigens of Wild Mice from Texas

3.1. Trapping and Typing Wild Mice in Texas

Wild mice were trapped in seven different geographical areas of Texas during the summer and fall of 1977. About 50% of the mice were trapped at five different localities within a 150-km radius of Dallas, Texas. The remainder were trapped at several locations in southern Texas near the town of Harlington (about 500 km from Dallas). Most of the mice were trapped in or near farm buildings where grain or food was being stored. In one instance (Cross Creek ranch, Table 10), all the mice trapped probably came from a single nest that we located in an unused grain silo. The exact distribution of the mice trapped in other farm buildings is unknown and thus could represent multiple breeding units. Over 100 mice were trapped during the survey, and 88 of these were successfully brought to the laboratory and typed for Ia antigens.

The typing reagents used for our survey are listed and described in Table 8. All these reagents were specific for their antigens in direct cytotoxicity testing of the inbred and B10.W lines. Splenic lymphocytes were typed with these reagents for Ia antigens using a standard two-stage microcytotoxicity test. About 5% of the wild mice had spleen cells that were nonspecifically lysed (>25% dead cells) by normal mouse serum plus complement (our standard control). These mice could not be typed for Ia antigens and were excluded from the survey. Also, occasional weak cross-reactions (titer 1:4) were noted with some of the reagents. These reactions were not designated as positives when assigning antigens. All our reagents had a titer of 1:16 or more when tested on appropriate target cells from homozygous or heterozygous animals.

3.2. Frequency and Distribution of Ia Antigens in Texas Wild Mice

The phenotypic frequencies of ten Ia antigens among Texas wild mice are presented in Table 9. The frequencies of *Ia-1*-encoded antigens ranged from 0.034 (Ia-1.4) to 0.450 (Ia-1.1). The three private antigens of this group (2, 4, 11) had the lowest frequencies of all the antigens tested. The two *Ia-5*-encoded antigens surveyed had frequencies of 0.77 (Ia-5.7) and 0.324 (Ia-5.32). The higher frequencies of the *Ia-5*-encoded antigens are consistent with our previous results with the B10.W lines and suggest that this gene is less polymorphic among Texas wild mice than *Ia-1*.

The organization of wild-mouse populations into closed breeding

TABLE 8. Alloantisera Used for the Detection of Ia Antigens among Trapped Wild Mice

Code No.	Antigen detected	Recipient	Donor	Absorption	Other antibody
K593	2	(A.BY × B10.HTT)F_1	A.TL	B10.RIII, B10.STC90	—
K593	19	(A.BY × B10.HTT)F_1	A.TL	B10.M	Ia.2
K593	1	(A.BY × B10.HTT)F_1	A.TL	—	Ia.2, Ia.19
K464	2	[LP.RIII × B10.T (6R)]F_1	AQR	B10.PL, B10.STC90	—
K464	31	[LP.RIII × B10.T (6R)]F_1	AQR	—	Ia.2
K228	4	(B10 × A.TL)F_1	B10.HTT	B10.RIII	—
K228	12	(B10 × A.TL)F_1	B10.HTT	B10.PL	Ia.4
K228	24	(B10 × A.TL)F_1	B10.HTT	—	Ia.4, Ia.12
K595	7	(B10 × R107)F_1	B10.A (5R)	—	—
K509	7	[B10.A (4R) × 129]F_1	B10.A (2R)	—	—
K548	11	(B10.A × A)F_1	B10.D2	B10.STC77	—
K499	32	(B10.Q × DBA/2)F_1	AQR	B10.A (4R)	—

TABLE 9. Phenotypic Frequencies of Ia Antigens among Wild Mice Trapped in Texas

Specificity	*H-2* subregion	Fraction of positive wild mice	Phenotypic frequency
1	*IA*	18/40	0.450
2	*IA*	12/88	0.136
4	*IA*	3/88	0.034
11	*IA*	9/88	0.102
12	*IA*	15/88	0.170
19	*IA*	6/40	0.150
24	*IA*	31/88	0.352
31	*IA*	34/88	0.386
7	*IE*	68/88	0.772
32	*IE*	12/37	0.324

units called "demes" had been recognized for some time (for references, see Klein, 1975). This type of breeding structure results in localized inbreeding and predicts that mice from one locality will be genetically homogeneous. Table 10 presents the Ia phenotypes of mice trapped at 12 different geographic locations. Of the 26 phenotypes detected, as many as 5 were found at a single location. These results indicate that although mice from the same locality tend to have similar Ia phenotypes, 2 or more *I*-region haplotypes are often present in the local populations. A larger survey will be necessary to determine the relationship of the demic population structure and the distribution of Ia phenotypes among wild mice.

3.3. An Estimate of *I*-Region Heterozygosity among Wild Mice

An estimation of the *I*-region heterozygosity of wild mice was obtained by breeding trapped wild males with *H-2*-homozygous inbred stocks and testing the progeny for segregating Ia antigens. If a wild male was heterozygous for *I*-region genes, then his Ia phenotype would segregate as two distinct phenotypes among the progeny. By typing the wild male and his progeny for Ia antigens, a minimum estimate of the frequency of *I*-region-heterozygous mice could be obtained.

The fraction of mice heterozygous for *IA*- and *IE*-encoded antigens is summarized in Table 11. Nine male mice from five different localties had *IA*-encoded antigens detected by our typing reagents, and seven of these mice (78%) were heterozygous. Nineteen male mice from nine localities could be typed for *IE*-encoded antigens, and nine of these (47%) were heterozygotes. A total of eight mice could be tested for both *IA*- and *IE*-encoded antigens, and seven of these (87.5%) were heterozygotes.

These results indicate that most wild mice are heterozygous for *I*-region genes.

The high degree of *I*-region heterozygosity detected in our study is unprecedented in comparison to other genetic systems in the mouse. Recently, Berry and Peters (1977) estimate the overall mean heterozygosity of enzymatic loci in wild mice at 6%. The *I*-region heterozygosity detected in our survey is an order of magnitude higher than this value.

TABLE 10. Geographic Distributions of Ia Phenotypes among Texas Wild Mice

Location	Number of mice	Phenotype
Cross Creek ranch,	2	Ia-1.2, Ia-1.31, Ia-5.7
Grapevine	2	Ia-1.24, Ia-1.31, Ia-5.7
	5	Ia-1.31, Ia-5.7
	5	Ia-1.24, Ia-5.7
Airport barn, Grapevine	4	Ia-5.7
Wolf farm,	3	Ia-1.24, Ia-5.7
Valley View	3	—
	2	Ia-1.1, Ia-1.31, Ia-5.7
	1	Ia-1.1, Ia-1.2, Ia-1.19, Ia-1.31, Ia-5.7
	1	Ia-1.11, Ia-1.2, Ia-1.24, Ia-5.7
Pesche farm,	1	Ia-1.12, Ia-1.24, Ia-5.7
Valley View	1	Ia-1.1, Ia-1.2, Ia-1.11, Ia-1.19, Ia-1.31, Ia-5.7
	1	Ia-1.1, Ia-1.31, Ia-5.7
	2	Ia-1.1, Ia-1.2, Ia-1.4, Ia-1.12, Ia-1.19, Ia-1.24, Ia-1.31, Ia-5.7
Miller dairy, McKinney	4	Ia-1.1, Ia-1.2[a], Ia-1.19, Ia-1.31, Ia-5.7
Oakbrook stables,	3	Ia-1.2, Ia-1.24, Ia-1.31, Ia-5.7
Dallas	1	Ia-1.31, Ia-5.7
Duncan farm barns,	3	Ia-1.31, Ia-5.7
Harlington	3	Ia-1.11, Ia-5.7
	3	—
Duncan farm fields,	7	Ia-5.7
Harlington	5	Ia-1.24, Ia-5.7
Harlington grain elevator, Harlington	2	Ia-1.11, Ia-5.7
Knight farm,	2	Ia-1.4, Ia-1.12, Ia-1.24
Harlington	1	Ia-1.11, Ia-2.24, Ia-1.31, Ia-5.7
CF farm,	1	Ia-1.24[a]
Denision	2	Ia-1.24[a], Ia-1.1, Ia-1.31
Sulfur Springs	3	Ia-1.1, Ia-1.31, Ia-5.7

[a]Probably a cross-reacting antigen.

TABLE 11. *I*-Region Heterozygosity among Texas Wild Mice

Geographic location	Fraction of mice heterozygous	
	IA subregion	*IE* subregion
Duncan farm, Harlington	2/3	5/9
Oakbrook stables, Dallas	1/2	0/1
Cross Creek ranch, Grapevine	2/2	0/1
Miller dairy, McKinney	—	0/1
Airport barn, Grapevine	—	1/1
Wolf dairy, Valley View	1/1	1/1
Au garage, Austin	—	1/1
Grain elevator, Harlington	—	0/1
Pesche dairy, Valley View	1/1	1/1

4. Conclusions

These studies indicate that *Ia-1* of the *IA* subregion is a highly polymorphic gene with a minimum of 15 alleles among the inbred and B10.W lines. The low frequencies of *Ia-1*-encoded private specificities in Texas wild mice suggest that many more alleles remain to be discovered. Currently, we can estimate that the *Ia-1*-encoded private specificities of inbred lines occur with frequencies of 0.05 to 0.10 in wild-mouse populations. These are higher frequencies than are observed with class I private specificities (Duncan *et al.*, 1979) and suggest that *Ia-1* may be slightly less polymorphic than *H-2K* and *H-2D*.

In contrast, *Ia-5* of the *IE* subregion has considerably less serologically detectable polymorphism than *H-2K, H-2D*, or *Ia-1*. If this result is confirmed by structural comparisons of allelic *Ia-5*-encoded products, then it suggests that *Ia-5* may be subject to different selective pressures than *Ia-1, H-2K,* and *H-2D*. The currently detectable polymorphism of *Ia-5* is comparable to that observed among enzymatic loci.

An analysis of the geographical distribution and heterozygosity of *I*-region alleles among wild-mouse populations will yield valuable information concerning the selective pressures affecting the evolution of these genes. The data we have obtained in our Texas survey indicate that wild mice can be typed for Ia antigens by serological methods with existing reagents. Although the sample size is small, some tentative conclusions about the Ia antigens of wild mice can be made. The high frequency of *I*-region heterozygotes and the multiple *I*-region phenotypes of mice from single localities are characteristics that would not be expected in a population organized as tightly closed breeding units. If Texas wild mice do form demes—and there is no reason to assume that they do not—then our results suggest that other factors such as selective pressure may be influencing the allelic distribution and heterozygosity of *I*-region genes. A larger survey with more typing reagents will allow an analysis of the factors responsible for the maintainance of *I*-region polymorphism in wild-mouse populations.

References

Benacerraf, B., and McDevitt, H.O., 1972, Histocompatibility-linked immune response genes, *Science* **175**:273.

Berry, R.J., and Peters, J., 1977, Heterogeneous heterozygosities in *Mus musculus* populations, *Proc. R. Soc. London Ser. B.* **197**:485.

Bodmer, W.F., 1972, Evolutionary significance of the HL-A system, *Nature* (*London*) **237**:139.

Brown, J.L., Kato, K., Silver, J., and Nathenson, S.G., 1974, Notable diversity in peptide composition of murine *H-2K* and *H-2D* alloantigens, *Biochemistry* **13**:3174.

Cecka, M., McMillan, M., Murphy, D., Silver, J., McDevitt, H., and Hood, L., 1978, Partial amino acid sequence analyses of Ia antigens, in: *Ir Genes and Ia Antigens* (H.O. McDevitt, ed.), pp. 275–286, Academic Press, New York and London.

Cook, R., Vitteta, E.S., Capra, J.D., and Uhr, J.W., 1977, The partial amino acid sequence of murine Ia molecules: Lack of homology between murine I-C^d and human P29, *Immunogenetics* **5**:437.

Cook, R., Uhr, J.W., Vitetta, E.S., and Capra, J.D., 1979, Structural studies on the murine Ia alloantigens. III. Tryptic peptide comparisons of allelic products of the *I-E/C* subregion, *Mol. Immunol.* **16**:29.

Cullen, S.E., Freed, J.H., and Nathenson, S.G., 1976, Structural and serological properties of murine Ia alloantigens, *Transplant. Rev.* **30**:236.

David, C.S., 1977, The major histocompatibility system of the mouse, in: *The Major Histocompatibility System in Man and Animals* (D. Gotze, ed.), pp. 255–290, Springer-Verlag, Berlin, Heidelberg, New York.

Duncan, W.R., Wakeland, E.K., and Klein, J., 1979, Histocompatibility-2 system in wild mice. VIII. Determination of the frequencies of *H-2K, H-2D,* and *I* region encoded antigens in populations of wild mice, *Immunogenetics* **9**:261.

Ewenstein, B.M., Freed, J.H., Mole, L.E., and Nathenson, S.G., 1976, Localization of the papain cleavage site of H-2 glycoproteins, *Proc. Natl. Acad. Sci. U.S.A.* **73**:915.

Freed, J.H., 1978, Comparison of primary structures of Ia products from the I-A and I-E/C subregion, *J. Immunol.* **121**:1609.

Henning, R., Milner, R.J., Reske, K., Cunningham, B.A., and Edelman, G.M., 1976, Subunit structure, cell surface orientation and partial amino acid sequences of murine histocompatibility antigens, *Proc. Natl. Acad. Sci. U.S.A.* **73**:118.

Jones, P.P., Murphy, D.B., and McDevitt, H.O., 1978, Two-gene control of the expression of a murine Ia antigen, *J. Exp. Med.* **148**:925.

Klein, J., 1970, Histocompatibility-2 (H-2) polymorphism in wild mice, *Science* **168**:1362.

Klein, J., 1973, Polymorphism of the H-2 loci in wild mice, in *International Symposium on Standardization of HL-A Reagents* (R.H. Regamey and J.V. Sparck, eds.), pp. 251–256, S. Karger, Basal.

Klein, J., 1975, *The Biology of the Mouse Histocompatibility-2 Complex,* Springer-Verlag, New York.

Klein, J., 1977, Evolution and function of the MHS: Facts and speculations, in *The Major Histocompatibility System in Man and Animals* (D. Gotze, ed.), pp. 339–378, Springer-Verlag, Berlin, Heidelberg, New York.

Klein, J., Duncan, W.R., Wakeland, E.K., Zaleska-Rutczynska, Z., Huang, H.J., and Hsu, E., 1978a, Characterization of the H-2 haplotypes in wild mice, in: *Workshop of the Origin of Inbred Strains of Mice* (H.C. Morse, ed.), pp. 667–687, Academic Press, New York.

Klein, J. Flaherty, L., Vandeberg, J.L., and Shreffler, D.C., 1978b, H-2 haplotypes, genes, regions, and antigens: First listing, IMmunogenetics **6**:489.

Maizels, R.M., Frelinger, J.A., and Hood, L., 1978, Partial amino acid sequences of mouse transplantation antigens, *Immunogenetics* **7**:428.

McMillan, M., Cecka, J.M., Murphy, D.B., McDevitt, H.O., and Hood, L., 1978a, Partial amino acid sequences of murine Ia antigens of the I-EC^{d} subregion, *Immunogenetics* **6**:137.

McMillan, M., Cecka, J.M., Frelinger, J.G., Murphy, D., Frelinger, J.A., McDevitt, H.O., and Hood, L., 1978b, Chemical characterization of murine Ia antigens, *J. Immunol.* **121**:1608.

Silver, J., and Hood, L., 1976, Preliminary amino acid sequences of transplantation antigens: Genetic and evolutionary implications, in: *Contemporary Topics in Molecular Immunology* (H.M. Eisen and R.A. Reisfeld, eds.), pp. 221–229, Plenum Press, New York.

Silver, J., Cecka, J.M., McMillan, M., and Hood, L., 1976, Chemical characterization of products of the H-2 complex, XLI, *Cold Spring Harbor Symp. Quant. Biol.* **41**:477.

Vitetta, E.S., Capra, J.D., Klapper, D.G., Klein, J., and Uhr, J., 1976, The partial amino-acid sequence of an *H-2K* molecule, *Proc. Natl. Acad. Sci. U.S.A.* **73**:905.

Wakeland, E.K., and Klein, J., 1979, Histocompatibility-2 system in wild mice. VII. Serological analysis of 29 wild-derived *H-2* haplotypes with antisera to inbred *I* region antigens, *Immunogenetics* **8**:27.

Zaleska-Rutczynska, Z., and Klein, J., 1977, Histocompatibility-2 system in wild mice. V. Serological analysis of sixteen B10.W congenic lines, *J. Immunol.* **119**:1903.

14

HLA Polyclonal and Monoclonal Xenoantibodies

Production, Characterization, and Application to the Study of HLA Antigens

Barry S. Wilson, Ah-Kau Ng, Vito Quaranta, and Soldano Ferrone

1. Introduction

A myriad of cellular functions are mediated through cell–cell interactions and are a result of communication by surface-membrane structures; therefore, these structures, particularly human histocompatibility (HLA) antigens and their functions, are the subjects of intense analysis. The characterization of these membrane components would be quite difficult were it not that most of these molecules are antigenic and elicit the production of specific antibodies through allo- or xenoimmunization. Alloimmunization produces antibodies to antigenic determinants that are polymorphic within a species (alloantigens); the latter method produces antibodies to these determinants as well as to species-specific determinants. Virtually all allo- and xenoantisera contain multiple populations of antibodies that differ in affinity, specificity, and titer, and are the products of distinct clones of cells. These conventional allo- and xenoantisera will be referred to as polyclonal antisera.

The use of polyclonal antibodies has enabled investigators to (1) identify the complexity of cell-surface structures expressed by different

Barry S. Wilson, Ah-Kau Ng, Vito Quaranta, and Soldano Ferrone • Department of Immunology, Scripps Clinic and Research Foundation, La Jolla, California 92037.

cells; (2) enumerate and isolate different cell populations; (3) determine the physical relationships among various antigenic structures on the cell membrane; (4) detect and quantitate cell-membrane antigens shed into body fluids; and (5) isolate antigens for the purposes of determining their molecular structures and analyzing their primary amino acid sequences. Specificity, affinity, and availability are the critical factors that determine the successful application of antibody reagents in these investigations.

The specificity of polyclonal antisera can be controlled by reducing the antigenic dissimilarities between donor and recipient through an appropriate selection, by using purified antigens as immunogens, or by appropriately absorbing unwanted antibodies from the antisera. Nevertheless, small amounts of unwanted contaminating antibodies may remain in the antisera and cause the spurious effects that have been occasionally observed. For instance, one published example that is pertinent to the field of HLA antigens indicated that the inhibitory effects of HLA-A,B alloantisera on mixed lymphocyte reactions, originally attributed to HLA-A,B alloantibodies (Ceppellini *et al.*, 1971), were actually caused by contaminating antibodies to antigenic structures controlling this reaction.

The recent development of the hybridoma technique for producing monoclonal antibodies (Köhler and Milstein, 1975) began an era of new antibody reagents. With this technique, antibody-secreting cells are fused with myeloma cells to form a hybridoma that can be isolated as a single cell-derived clone and grown indefinitely by tissue culturing. The culture medium of the growing hybridoma contains the secreted homogeneous antibodies. In contrast to polyclonal xenoantisera, specific monoclonal antibodies can be developed through immunization with antigenically complex immunogens (e.g., cells) because cell-culturing techniques enable the isolation of a single antibody-secreting cell for clonal development. In addition, monoclonal antibodies are homogeneous in their affinity and specificty for the single determinant to which they are directed. Conceivably, this hybridoma technique can be used to dissect the humoral immune response into its component antibodies to yield a library of antibodies specific for various determinants of virtually any antigen.

Antibodies to HLA antigens have detected two major types of molecules: One type, the classic HLA-A,B,C antigens, is expressed on all nucleated cells and consists of a 43,000-molecular-weight glycopeptide, noncovalently associated with β_2 microglobulin (β_2-μ) (Grey *et al.*, 1973; Nakamuro *et al.*, 1973; Peterson *et al.*, 1974). The HLA-A,B,C alloantigenic determinants are located on the 43,000-molecular-weight component (Nakamuro *et al.*, 1975). The other molecular type, the recently identified HLA-DR antigens, has a restricted tissue distribution, is serologically polymorphic, and consists of two noncovalently associated subunits of approximately 34,000 (α chain) and 29,000 molecular weight (β

chain) (Ferrone *et al.*, 1978a). Whether the HLA-DR allo-antigenic determinant is associated with the α or the β chain or both is at present a matter of controversy. Peptide mapping, somatic cell hybridization, and/or binding studies of alloantisera with isolated α and β chains have been used to determine the source of the structural polymorphism. Some investigators claim that HLA-DR polymorphism resides in the α chain (Snary *et al.*, 1977; Ikeman *et al.*, 1978; Klareskog *et al.*, 1978a), and others have implicated the β chain (Tosi *et al.*, 1978; Silver and Ferrone, 1979; Walker *et al.*, this volume).

The studies of HLA antigens generally have used alloantisera from pregnant women or from recipients of blood transfusions or allografts or both. These alloantisera have been invaluable for defining the genetic organization of the *HLA* region and the serological polymorphism of its gene products. However, because alloantisera are generally low in titer and affinity and are difficult to obtain in large amounts, they are of limited value in immunochemical studies of HLA antigens. These limitations prompted production of HLA xenoantisera, which offer the advantages of vigorous immunization methods and large-volume production of antisera at the peak of the immune response. Such antisera contain high-titer and high-affinity antibodies that are invaluable for analyzing the molecular profiles of HLA antigens.

In this chapter, we will first conduct a historical survey of the literature that pertains to the production of polyclonal and monoclonal xenoantibodies to HLA antigens. In the next three sections, we will describe our current methods for preparing and characterizing these HLA xenoantibodies, as well as their applications to the study of HLA antigens. The last section compares our results to the published results of other investigators, and it also contains some speculation on the mechanisms that control the production of xenoantibodies to HLA antigenic determinants.

2. Historical Review

2.1. Polyclonal Xenoantisera to HLA-A,B,C Allospecificities

The history of xenoantisera production to HLA-A,B,C allotypic specifities can be divided into two distinct segments depending on which form of the antigen is used for immunization: the early studies used intact human cells as immunogens; later studies used semipurified antigens. In 1964, Shulman *et al.* (1964) immunized animals phylogenetically distant from humans (rabbits, guinea pigs, rats, and dogs) with whole human blood cells or buffy coat leukocytes. The resulting xenoantisera contained high-titer antibodies to human leukocytes, but unfortunately, none of these antisera recognized HLA-A,B,C, alloantigens. Attempts to make these antisera specific were unsuccessful, since absorption with any one platelet or leukocyte preparation removed all the antibodies that reacted with cells from other donors. Chimpanzees were also investigated for their responses to HLA-A,B,C allospecificities because serological assays with both human and chimpanzee alloantisera showed a cross-reactivity between certain HLA-A,B allospecificities and chimpanzee alloantigens (Shulman *et al.*, 1964, 1965; Metzger *et al.*, 1965; Metzger and Zmijewski, 1966; Balner *et al.*, 1967). Antisera were produced that, after the appropriate absorptions with human cells, detected polymorphic specificities expressed on human leukocytes (Shulman *et al.*, 1965; Metzger *et al.*, 1965); however, these antigens correlated poorly with the specificities defined by HLA-A,B,C alloantisera. Thus, the investigators concluded that chimpanzee antisera would not be useful for large-scale production because of the low specificity and affinity of the antisera as compared with conventional human alloantisera. The failure of these initial studies, together with the prevailing dogma that xenoimmunization elicits antibodies only to common and not to allotypic determinants, caused most investigators to give up all hope of producing xenoantisera to the HLA-A,B,C allospecificities.

Eventually, purified preparations of HLA antigens became available through research about the chemical nature of these antigens and brought new interest for producing xenoantisera. In contrast to the earlier studies, some of the animals immunized with purified soluble antigens produced xenoantisera that, when appropriately diluted or adsorbed or both, were highly specific for certain HLA-A,B,C alloantigens (Table 1). In these studies, most of these xenoantisera were directed to either HLA-A1, A2, A9, or B7, which were the predominant allospecificities in the immunogen. The question of whether rabbits can produce xenoantibodies to other alloantigens (not listed in Table 1) will require further study. Despite these successful reports, further development of xenoantisera to HLA-A,B,C allospecificities did not ensue because of a general skepticism about the appropriateness of the antisera for tissue typing. Nonetheless, these studies had definitely established that xenoimmunization of species phylogenetically distant from humans can elicit xenoantisera that define the serological polymorphism of the HLA-A,B,C antigens.

2.2. Polyclonal Xenoantisera to Common Determinants of HLA-A,B,C Antigens

The existence of common antigenic determinants among HLA-A,B,C molecules that bear different allospecificities was not apparent until the molecule was structurally characterized. Previous to that time,

TABLE 1. Polyclonal Xenoantisera to the Heavy Chains of the HLA-A,B,C Molecular Complex

Immunogen	Antibody source	Specificity	Reference
Papain-solubilized leukemia-cell antigens	Rabbit	Common	Batchelor (1969)
Papain-solubilized RPMI-4265-cell antigens (A2, A9, B7, B12)	Rabbit	A2, B7, A9, B12	Einstein *et al.* (1971)
3-M-KCl-solubilized lymphoid-cell antigens	Rabbit	Allospecific	Ferrone *et al.* (1972)
Papain-solubilized spleen-cell antigens (A1, B7)	Monkey	A1, B7 Common	Metzgar and Miller (1972, 1973); Sanderson and Welsh (1973)
3-M-KCl-solubilized lymphoid-cell antigens	Chicken	Common	David *et al.* (1973)
Serum A9 antigens	Rabbit	A9	Billing and Terasaki (1974)
Serum A9 antigens	Rabbit	A24	Ferrone *et al.* (1975)
Papain-solubilized RPMI-1788-cell antigens	Rabbit	Common	Nakamuro *et al.* (1975)
Papain-solubilized A2 antigens purified from RPMI 4265 cells	Rabbit	A2	Robb *et al.* (1975)
Purified *A*-locus and *B*-locus antigens from RPMI 4265 cells	Rabbit	*HLA-A* locus *HLA-B* locus	Cresswell and Ayres (1976)
Papain-solubilized HLA antigens from spleen cells	Rabbit	Common	Rask *et al.* (1976)
Serum A9 antigens	Rabbit	A9	Ferrone *et al.* (1977a)
Man–mouse hybrid cells containing chromosome 6	Mouse	Common	Aden *et al.* (1978)
Immune-absorbed HLA-A, B, and C	Rabbit	Common	B.S. Wilson *et al.* (1978)
Papain-solubilized spleen cells	Rabbit	Common	L.A. Wilson and Gallaspy (1978)
Serum and cellular high-density lipproteins	Goat and rabbits	A2, A9, B15, B44	Richierdi *et al.* (1979)

xenoantibodies that reacted with cells expressing different HLA-A,B,C alloantigens were thought to be detecting a species-specific antigen (Bachvaroff and Rapaport, 1973) rather than common determinants of the HLA-A,B,C molecules. Later, amino acid analysis (Mann *et al.*, 1970) and peptide mapping (Reisfeld *et al.*, 1973) of purified HLA-A,B,C antigens revealed their homogeneous natures and indicated that the alloantigenic sites were located in a small portion of the molecules (Reisfeld *et al.*, 1973); thus, the molecule could bear multiple common determinants. These determinants were later shown to be located on both the heavy chain and β_2-μ of each of the HLA-A,B,C molecular complexes. Xenoantisera to β_2-μ have been produced against the free β_2-μ molecule isolated from the urine of patients with renal tubular diseases (Berggard and Bearn, 1968) or against the complete HLA-A,B,C molecular complexes (Sanderson, 1977).

Xenoantisera to common determinants of the HLA-A,B,C heavy chains were produced using a variety of methods and are listed in Table 1. The first report of a xenoantiserum specific for common determinants of the HLA-A,B,C molecules was by Batchelor (1969), who immunized rabbits with partially purified HLA-A2 substances. One of his xenoantisera seemed to react with common determinants, since it reacted with all human lymphocytes, regardless of their HLA-A,B,C phenotypes. In addition, Fab and Fab_2 fragments prepared from this xenoantiserum could competitively block the binding of HLA-A2 alloantibodies to lymphocyte targets. From these experiments, Batchelor concluded that the xenoantiserum reacted with a species-specific antigen that either was part of the HLA-A2 determinant or was in close proximity to this determinant on the same molecule. This antiserum most likely was directed to the heavy chain or to β_2-μ or to both. Similarly, Metzger and Miller (1973) described a monkey xenoantiserum that precipitated HLA antigens expressing various allospecificities. In still another study, a rabbit antiserum produced against rhesus donkey cell-membrane antigens cross-reacted with the HLA-A,B,C heavy chains (Katagari *et al.*, 1974). Thus, common determinants for HLA-A,B,C heavy chains are shared among different species, a finding confirmed more recently with monoclonal antibodies (Parham *et al.*, 1979).

Xenoantisera, especially those directed to β_2-μ, have greatly assisted the study of HLA-A,B,C antigens in the following ways: (1) The molecular characterizations and partial amino acid sequences of HLA-A,B,C antigens have been determined by using molecules purified by affinity chromatography on xenoantibody adsorbents (Ballou *et al.*, 1976; Allison *et al.*, 1978b). (2) By using the allo- and xenoantisera to study the serological expression of HLA-A,B,C antigens in human–murine hybrid cells, it was found that the gene coding for the HLA-A,B,C heavy chains is located at chromosome 6 (Van Someren *et al.*, 1974) and the gene coding for β_2-μ at chromosome 15 (Goodfellow *et al.*, 1975). (3) Serological tests designed to screen human sera for allo-antibodies to HLA-DR antigens involve cells with HLA-A,B,C antigens that were blocked by prior treatment with xenoantibodies to β_2-μ or by prior treatment with xenoantibodies to common determinants of the HLA-A,B,C heavy chains (Indiveri *et al.*, 1979a,c; 1980b.). (4) Evolutionary relationships between *HLA-A,B* loci and murine *H-2K,D* loci were defined by the serological cross-reactivity of xenoantisera to HLA-A,B molecules (Götze *et al.*, 1972; David *et al.*, 1973), a finding confirmed by the high degree of homology in the partial amino acid sequence of murine H-2K,D and human HLA-A,B antigens (Silver and Hood, 1977).

Xenoantisera that detect determinants expressed exclusively by products of only one of the three *HLA-A,B,C* loci have been produced. One such xenoantiserum was described by Cresswell and Ayres (1976), who immunized rabbits with either a purified *HLA-A*-locus product (A2) or *HLA-B*-locus products (B7, B12). These structures were separated from each other by subjecting purified HLA-A,B,C substances from cultured B-lymphoid cells (RPMI 4265) to ion-exchange chromatography. The resulting xenoantisera cross-reacted weakly with molecules of the nonimmunizing locus; cross-reactivity could be eliminated by specific absorption with these molecules, indicating that in addition to determinants specific for particular loci, there are some determinants shared between the HLA-A,B series molecules. This finding was extended by Rask *et al.* (1976) to include the *C*-locus molecules, and suggests that the *HLA-A,B,C* loci arose through gene duplication and subsequently diversified to acquire their individual determinants.

Rabbits immunized with isolated HLA-A,B,C heavy chains denatured by treatment with heat, acids, or guanidine-HCl can elicit antisera that react very strongly with the denatured molecules, yet these antisera essentially do not react with the native structures (Tanigaki and Nakamuro, 1974; Ploegh *et al.*, 1979). It has recently been reported that such antisera to cryptic or denatured HLA-A,B,C determinants are able to react with newly synthesized HLA-A,B,C heavy chains translated from cell-free messenger RNA (Ploegh *et al.*, 1979). The *de novo* synthesized HLA-A,B,C heavy chains seem to lack all other native antigenic determinants, as evidenced by their lack of reaction with HLA-A,B, alloantisera or a monoclonal xenoantibody to HLA-A,B,C common determinants.

2.3. Monoclonal Xenoantibodies to HLA-A,B,C Antigens

A summary of the monoclonal antibodies produced against HLA-A,B,C heavy chains is shown in Table 2. Lampson *et. al.* (1978) were the

TABLE 2. Monoclonal Xenoantibodies to the Heavy Chain of the HLA-A,B,C Molecular Complex

Immunogen	Antibody source	Specificity	Reference
Cell membranes of tonsil lymphocytes	Mouse hybridoma	Common	Barnstable *et al.* (1978)
Human lymphocytes	Mouse-spleen fragment	A2	Lampson *et al.* (1978)
Papain-solubilized A2 antigens purified from RPMI 4265 cells	Mouse hybridoma	A2, common	Parham and Bodmer (1978)
Cultured human cells	Mouse hybridoma	Bw4	Indiveri *et al.* (1980a)

first to attempt production of monoclonal antibodies to HLA-A,B,C antigens by using the splenic focus assay (Klinman, 1969), originally employed for studying the developmental aspects of the humoral immune response at the level of individual clones. In this assay, splenocytes from a mouse immunized with human lymphoid cells were used to repopulate the spleen of an X-irradiated recipient mouse with limited numbers of immune B lymphocytes. The recipient spleen was then sliced into small fragments, with each containing a single clone derived from the transferred cells, and cultured *in vitro*. Unfortunately, the splenocytes were short-lived, and although there were some that secreted antibody to HLA-A,B,C antigens, there was barely enough material for analytical purposes. This problem was overcome when Köhler and Milstein (1975) developed the hybridoma technique, in which an antibody-secreting cell achieves long-lasting life after being fused with a myeloma tumor cell. After monoclonal alloantibodies were generated to the major histocompatibility antigen of rats (Williams *et al.*, 1977) and mice (Lemke *et al.*, 1978), Barnstable *et al.* (1978) applied the hybridoma technique to produce monoclonal antibodies to HLA-A,B,C antigens. These hybridomas were derived from murine splenocytes immunized with a membrane preparation of human tonsil lymphocytes. Most of the resultant monoclonal antibodies were directed to cell-membrane antigens of wide tissue distribution; however, one of these, termed W6/32, reacted with the 43,000-molecular-weight and 12,000-molecular-weight molecules of the HLA-A,B,C complexes. Subsequent serological studies with somatic cell hybrids and blocking of immunoprecipitation by soluble β_2-μ indicated that W6/32 was specific for determinants located on most if not all of the 43,000-molecular-weight HLA-A,B,C heavy chains. In other experiments, Trucco *et al.* (1978) fused myeloma cells with splenocytes from mice immunized with human lymphoblastoid cells. The investigators isolated several hybridomas that secreted monoclonal antibodies to β_2-μ and thus concluded that β_2-μ is more immunogenic than the HLA-A,B,C heavy chains, a finding that contrasts to our results. Parham and Bodmer (1978) produced hybridoma lines derived from splenocytes of mice immunized with chemically purified HLA-A2 antigens. Of 14 hybridoma clones that secreted monoclonal antibodies to HLA-A,B,C antigens, 10 seemed to recognize common determinants of the HLA-A,B,C heavy chains, while the other 4 hybridomas detected allospecific determinants. Thus, the goal of pioneer research to provide an unlimited supply of xenoantisera to detect HLA allospecificities is becoming a reality. Our own research on developing monoclonal xenoantibodies to HLA antigens will be discussed later in this review.

2.4. Xenoantibodies to HLA-DR Antigens

The development of xenoantisera to HLA-DR antigens has progressed quite rapidly as a result of the experience gained with HLA-A,B,C antigens and because of the strong immunogenicity of HLA-DR molecules in animals of several species. A large majority of the polyclonal HLA-DR xenoantisera that have been produced to date react with common structures of the HLA-DR molecule. A list of the HLA-DR xenoantisera to common or to allotypic determinants appears in Table 3. This list excludes xenoantisera first claimed to be specific for leukemia antigens, then reinterpreted, but not formally proven as specific for HLA-DR antigens. In contrast to the HLA-A,B,C xenoantisera, there have been only a few reports of xenoantisera reactive with HLA-DR allospecificities (Solheim *et al.*, 1978; Ferrone *et al.*, 1977b, 1978b). These reports are not as well documented as are the allospecific xenoantisera to the HLA-A,B,C molecule, mainly because the gene products of the *HLA-DR* loci are still incompletely identified.

3. Polyclonal Xenoantisera to HLA Allospecificities

3.1. Introduction

Initially, we developed polyclonal xenoantisera to HLA-A,B,C allospecificities to determine the immunogenicity of HLA-A,B,C alloantigens subjected to conventional biochemical purification procedures. Ultimately, locating the positions of alloantigenic determinants on the HLA-A,B,C molecules and identifying the smallest molecular fragments that

TABLE 3. Polyclonal Xenoantisera and Monoclonal Xenoantibodies to HLA-DR Antigens

Immunogen	Antibody source	Specificity of antiserum	Reference
Papain-solubilized RPMI-4265-cell antigens	Rabbit	Common	Cresswell and Geier (1975)
Papain-solubilized leukemia-cell antigens	Rabbit	Common	Billing *et al.* (1976)
Detergent-solubilized membrane and submembrane glycoproteins of BR 18 cells	Mice/rabbit	Common	Goodfellow *et al.* (1976)
Papain-solubilized HLA-DR antigens from 1M-1 cells	Rabbit	Common	Humphreys *et al.* (1976)
Antibody-precipitated HLA-DR antigens isolated from spleen cells solubilized by detergent	Rabbit	Common	Welsh and Turner (1976)
Lipid-associated HLA antigens from lymphoblastoid cells	Rabbit	Allospecific	Ferrone *et al.* (1977b)
Detergent-solubilzied HLA-DR antigens from BR 18 cells	Rabbit	Common	Snary *et al.* (1977)
Papain-solubilized HLA-DR antigens from from RPMI 4265 cells	Rabbit	Common	Springer *et al.* (1977)
Lipid-associated HLA antigens from lymphoblastoid cells and cultured human lymphoid cells mixed with anti-T-cell xenoantisera	Goats/rabbits	Allospecific Common	Ferrone *et al.* (1978b)
HLA-DR antigens from leukemia cells	Rabbit	Common	Klareskog *et al.* (1978b)
Antibody-precipitated HLA-DR antigens isolated from RPMI 1640 cells solubilized with detergent	Rabbit	Allospecific	Solheim *et al.* (1978)
Lipid-associated HLA antigens from lymphoblastoid cells and cultured human lymphoid cells mixed with anti-T-cell xenoantisera	Goats/rabbits	Allospecific	Belvedere *et al.* (1980a)
Cultured human cells	Mice (monoclonal)	Common	Molinaro *et al.* (1980)
Immune-adsorbed HLA-DR antigens from lymphoblastoid cells	Rabbits	Common	B.S. Wilson *et al.* (1979b)

still retain immunogenic activity via such purification procedures should enable correlation of the structures of the molecules with their biological functions. Later on, we abandoned the classic biochemical approach and structurally analyzed HLA-A,B,C antigens with a more rapid and simple immunochemical isolation method that entails using specific antisera to these radiolabeled antigens. The first few experiments demonstrated that alloantisera would be of little value in this approach, since they seemed to have insufficient amounts of high-affinity antibodies. Attempts to concentrate high-affinity alloantibodies by adsorption and subsequent elution from lymphoid cells, although occasionally yielding a useful reagent, failed to provide enough antibody reagents for routine investigation. Thus, we focused on the development of high-titer and high-affinity xenoantisera that would isolate HLA-A,B,C alloantigens, and we decided to use microsequencing techniques (Silver and Hood, 1977) for determining the primary amino acid sequences of individual HLA-A,B,C allospecificities isolated by specific xenoantibodies. To avoid mixed sequences at the residues coding for the allospecificities, xenoantisera to HLA-A,B,C allospecificities were chosen rather than xenoantisera to β_2-μ (Ballou *et al.*, 1976). Having produced xenoantisera to HLA-A,B,C allospecificities, we found these antisera useful in other areas of HLA investigation. For example, xenoantisera could be used to define cross-reactions on subsets of HLA-A,B,C antigens that are poorly immunogenic or non-immunogenic in allogeneic combinations. Such cross-reactions may be envisioned as common portions of different allospecificities, much like the public specificities of the murine *H-2* system. In addition, the knowledge we gained in developing and analyzing xenoantisera to HLA-A,B,C allospecificities has been applied to developing xenoantisera to HLA-DR allospecificities. Finally, we hypothesized that xenoantisera to HLA allospecificities could define the way rabbit complement functions in the lymphocytotoxic test for HLA typing. It is our contention that rabbit complement is more efficient than human complement in lysing lymphocytes coated with HLA antibody, possibly because the rabbit complement contains natural antibodies (Ferrone *et al.*, 1971) directed to polymorphic human lymphocytic antigens (Mittal *et al.*, 1973a,b). Thus, effective lysis of target cells by HLA alloantibodies requires additional interactions on the cell surface by antigen–antibody complexes with the antibodies provided by the natural lymphocytotoxic antibodies in rabbit complement. Support for this theory is that appropriate adsorption of rabbit complement with human lymphocytes results in both the loss of natural antibodies and increased lytic efficiency over human complement, but does not affect the level of complement activity measured by a standard hemolytic assay with antibody-coated sheep erythrocytes. Nonetheless, the decrease in lytic efficiency may still be due to adsorption of certain rabbit-complement components that are undetected by a standard hemolytic assay. Therefore, we used xenoantisera to HLA antigens to further validate our theory about the mechanism of action of rabbit complement. The rationale was as follows: If additional anti-human lymphocytic antibodies are required from rabbit complement for the effective lysis of target cells by HLA antibodies, then xenoantisera containing antibodies to HLA as well as to other lymphocytic-membrane structures may be able to lyse lyphocytes with the appropriate HLA phenotypes in conjunction with human complement. Removal of contaminating antibodies by appropriate adsorptions should cause the antisera to lose their cytotoxicity with human complement and exhibit a reaction characteristic of allospecificity in conjunction with rabbit complement. This approach does not involve any adsorption of the complement source, and therefore rules out the argument that adsorption may be affecting the levels of certain complement components in rabbit serum.

3.2. Xenoantisera to Cellular HLA-A,B,C Antigens

To produce xenoantisera specific for HLA-A,B,C alloantigens, we (Ferrone *et al.*, 1972) injected rabbits with HLA antigens solubilized from cultured B-lymphoid cells by hypertonic salt extraction; the resulting antisera required extensive adsorptions with lymphoid cells to remove contaminating antibodies to non-HLA-A,B,C structures. A few of these xenoantisera did show specificity for some HLA-A,B alloantigens (Ferrone *et al.*, 1972, 1973); however, the correlation coefficients with HLA-A,B,C alloantisera in cytotoxicity tests were far too low for a tissue-typing reagent. Also, the difficulty encountered in reproducing the large-scale adsorptions with different batches of antisera and the low affinity of the antibodies that remained after adsorption made this approach both expensive and impractical for large-scale production.

Although the adsorbed xenoantisera were neither discriminatory enough for tissue typing nor of high enough affinity for immunochemical studies, in their unadsorbed forms, they were useful for assessing the serological cross-reactivity between murine H-2 and human HLA-A,B,C alloantigens (Götze *et al.*, 1972). The unadsorbed xenoantisera reacted differently with lymphocytes from separate strains of mice. After a preparation of soluble H-2 antigens inhibited the cytotoxicity of the cross-reactive xenoantisera, it was evident that H-2 antigens were involved in this reaction. Furthermore, when the mice that did not express cross-reactivity for HLA-A,B,C antigens were sensitized to soluble HLA-A,B,C antigens, they rejected skin grafts from the cross-reactive strains at an accelerated rate in contrast to their comparatively well tolerated skin grafts from unreactive strains (Götze *et al.*, 1973). This phenomenon indicates that the murine major histocompatibility loci, *H-2K* and *D* are the targets of the cross-reaction with the HLA-A,B,C xenoantisera.

3.3. Xenoantisera to Serum HLA-A,B,C Antigens

The discovery of soluble HLA-A,B antigens in serum (Charlton and Zmijewski, 1970; Billing *et al.*, 1973; Miyakawa *et al.*, 1973; Oh *et al.*, 1975; Pellegrino *et al.*, 1974) provided investigators with an unusual source of immunogens, which did not have to undergo harsh solubilization procedures required for extraction of cellular antigens; therefore, it seemed plausible that these serum antigens might retain more of their native configurations and be better sources of immunogens than the cellular molecules. Since soluble HLA-A9 antigens were present in the serum in greater amounts than were the other allospecificities (Pellegrino *et al.*, 1974; Belvedere *et al.*, 1979a), our efforts focused on this specificity. The following methods were used to purify HLA-A,B antigens from serum (Ferrone *et al.*, 1977a): (1) affinity chromatography on β_2-μ immunoadsorbents; (2) ammonium sulfate precipitation followed by gel filtration, ion-exchange chromatography, and polyacrylamide gel electrophoresis; and (3) ultracentrifugation in a KBr density gradient (density = 1.23). The latter method, which isolates HLA-A,B,C antigens because of their high-density lipoprotein (HDL) character (Allison *et al.*, 1977a), provided the most effective immunogen as evidenced by the early appearance of high-titer rabbit antibodies that persisted for months after boostering.

Antisera from rabbits immunized with serum HLA-A,B antigens showed no specificity for any HLA-A,B,C alloantigens in cytotoxicity tests; however, after removal of unwanted antibodies by either of several methods—(1) dilution with medium or serum from an HLA-A9 negative donor; (2) adsorption with serum proteins coupled to immunoadsorbents; (3) adsorption with cells lacking HLA-A,B,C antigens, such as erythrocytes (Harris and Zervas, 1969) or Daudi cells (Reisfeld *et al.*, 1975); or (4) adsorption with cells of the appropriate HLA-A,B,C allospecificities—many antisera exhibited high correlation coefficients with HLA alloantisera. Those instances where specificity for HLA-A9 was achieved by adsorption with cells lacking detectable HLA-A,B,C antigens (erythrocytes and Daudi cells) indicates that some rabbits produced few if any antibodies to HLA-A,B,C common determinants.

Because many tissue-typing experts are skeptical about whether xenoantisera specific for HLA-A,B allospecificities can be produced, we sent our HLA-A9 xenoantisera to several HLA typing laboratories for independent confirmation of the specificity of the xenoantisera. The results from these laboratories unanimously confirmed the specificity of the HLA-A9 xenoantisera (Ferrone *et al.*, 1975, 1977a). Genetic studies performed with a limited number of families with particular HLA types indicated that one of our HLA-A9 xenoantisera (No. 1828) reacted with antigenic structures segregating with HLA-A9 antigens (Albert, personal communication); this finding and the results from other immunochemical and serological analyses provided additional evidence for the HLA-A9 specificity of our xenoantisera (Allison *et al.*, 1978a; Belvedere *et al.*, 1979a). In lysostrip tests, HLA-A9 allo- or xenoantisera treatment of human lymphoid cells subsequently treated with appropriate antiglobulin antiserum resulted in a specific loss of susceptibility to lysis mediated by either reagent. Similarly, human cells coated with Fab_2 antibody fragments from HLA-A9 allo- or xenoantisera acquired specific resistance to the cytotoxic effects of either reagent. Sodium dodecyl sulfate–polyacrylamide gel electrophoresis analysis of sequential immunodepletion experiments indicated that HLA-A9 allo- and xenoantisera both reacted with 43,000-molecular-weight and 12,000-molecular-weight components that corresponded with, respectively, the heavy and light chains of HLA-A9. Taken together, these data clearly show that HLA-A9 xenoantisera react specifically with the HLA-A9 molecule detected by HLA-A9 alloantisera.

An immunoadsorption assay was developed to determine whether the HLA-A9 xenoantisera react with the same antigenic determinant(s) recognized by HLA-A9 alloantisera (Allison *et al.*, 1977b). In this assay, soluble HLA-A9 antigens adsorbed to an HLA-A9 xenoantibody coupled to a Sepharose column were tested for their capacity to adsorb antibody from HLA-A9 alloantisera. Adsorption indicates that the antigen has bound to the xenoantibody adsorbent through determinant(s) separate from those recognized by the alloantisera. On the other hand, lack of adsorption indicates that the xenoantibody adsorbent binds the same or closely associated determinants recognized by the alloantisera. At least one of several HLA-A9 xenoantisera screened in this assay (no. 2958) reacted with the same or closely associated determinants recognized by the alloantisera. Recent studies in collaboration with Dr. P. Richiardi (Institute of Medical Genetics, Turin, Italy) suggest that goat or rabbit antisera to serum HDL shows specificity for HLA-A,B alloantigens other than A9 when adsorbed with platelets or leukocytes (Richiardi *et al.*, 1979). This study suggests that the HDL method may be successfully applied for generating xenoantisera to a variety of HLA-A,B allospecificities.

3.4. Xenoantisera to Cellular HLA-DR Antigens

The development of xenoantibodies to HLA-DR alloantigens involved immunizing rabbits and goats with a suspension of cultured human

B-lymphoid cells precoated with a xenoantiserum to a human T-cell line (Molt-4) or with HLA antigens solubilized from cultured human B-lymphoid cells by 3 M KCl and partially purified by flotation in a KBr gradient (density = 1.23) (Ferrone *et al.*, 1977b, 1978b; Belvedere *et al.*, 1980a.) Antibodies to non-HLA-DR structures in the immunogen have been used in other systems to suppress the immune response to these determinants (Cerottini *et al.*, 1969; Greaves and Brown, 1975). Xenoantisera to the B-cell lines were serologically and immunochemically analyzed for HLA-DR antibodies. These xenoantisera or Fab_2 fragments from them were tested by the lysostrip or Fab_2 blocking test, respectively, for their abilities to induce cultured B-lymphoid cells to resist complement-dependent lysis mediated by HLA-DR alloantisera. In indirect immunoprecipitation and subsequent sodium dodecyl sulfate–polyacrylamide gel electrophoresis, the xenoantisera reacted with two components having the characteristic molecular weights of the HLA-DR α (34,000 molecular weight) and α (29,000 molecular weight) chains. Xenoantisera containing HLA-DR antibodies were adsorbed with erythrocytes, human T-lymphoid cell lines (Molt 4, 1301), or cultured human B-lymphoid cells of the appropriate HLA-DR phenotype. The specificities of the adsorbed xenoantisera were assessed by cytotoxicity testing on a panel of B lymphocytes typed with HLA-DR alloantisera submitted to the 7th International Histocompatibility Workshop. Our results, which were later confirmed by other laboratories, indicate the nine xenoantisera showed a significant, albeit low, correlation with DR alloantisera (Ferrone *et al.*, 1977b, 1978b; Belvedere *et al.*, 1979c). The inability to achieve higher correlation coefficients might result from (1) incomplete characterization of HLA-DR allospecificities, (2) inability of xenoantisera to recognize the same determinants reacting with alloantisera, (3) contaminating antibodies to non-HLA-DR structures or to HLA-DR common determinants, and/or (4) technical artifacts with alloantisera in the cytotoxicity test. Nevertheless, the correlation coefficient does indicate that some xenoantisera can recognize HLA-DR allospecificities after adsorption with human cells lacking HLA-DR antigens [e.g., erythrocytes (Ferrone *et al.*, 1978a)]. A similar finding with some xenoantisera to serum HLA-A9 antigens (Allison *et al.*, 1978a) suggests that certain animals produce more antibodies to HLA allospecificities than to HLA common determinants.

3.5. Application for Biological and Structural Studies of HLA Antigens

An HLA-A9 xenoantiserum (No. 2958) was used to purify intrinsically labeled HLA-A9 antigens from Victor cells for determining their partial N-terminal primary amino acid sequence (Allison *et al.*, 1978b). The amino acid sequence of the first 20 residues at the amino terminus of

TABLE 4. Cross-Reactivity of HLA-A9 Xenoantisera with HLA-A,B Alloantigens in a Fab_2 Blocking Assay[a]

	HLA alloantigens[b]									
	A locus					*B* locus				
Fab_2 preparation	1	2	3	9	32	5	8	14	18	w4
1417 D	+	ND	+	+	ND	–	ND	ND	ND	+
1418 D	+	+	+	+	–	–	–	–	–	+
1419 D	–	–	ND	+	ND	–	ND	–	–	–

[a]Peripheral-blood lymphocytes from at least five donors were treated with Fab_2 fragments for 60 min at 25°C. The cells were then tested for susceptibility to complement-dependent cytotoxicity mediated by at least three HLA-A and -B alloantisera.
[b](+) Positive or (–) negative for blocking; (ND) not done.

the molecule had a high degree of homology with other allospecificities coded for by the *HLA-A,B* loci, indicating that the HLA-A9 alloantigen is not located in the first 20 amino-terminal residues of the molecule.

The patterns of cross-reactivities of xenoantisera to HLA-A,B,C allospecificities are generally similar to the patterns of cross-reactivities of alloantisera (Richiardi *et al.*, 1979); however, the following three differences were noted: (1) The cross-reaction of HLA-A9 antibodies with Bw4 occurred for 6 of 12 xenoantisera (Table 4), although there are only two published reports of this alloantisera cross-reaction (Legrand and Dausset, 1975; Scalamogna *et al.*, 1976), suggesting that HLA-A9 and Bw4 share a common portion, which is either poorly immunogenic or rarely occurs as a histoincompatibility in allogeneic combinations. (2) Some xenoantisera may mediate the cytotoxicity of lymphocytes that express a cross-reactive alloantigen. For example, some HLA-A9 xenoantisera mediate lysis of lymphocytes that lack HLA-A9 antigens, but express the cross-reactive HLA-A2 specificity (Ferrone and Mittal, unpublished observations). This finding may reflect a higher affinity of xenoantibodies than of alloantibodies for the cross-reactive antigen or may reflect increased sensitivity of the lymphocytotoxicity test performed without human serum components that block the effect of rabbit complement (Ferrone *et al.*, 1979). (3) Xenoantisera may detect cross-reactions among certain HLA-A,B,C alloantigens that had not previously been discovered with alloantisera (Belvedere *et al.*, 1980b). This could conceivably occur if certain determinants shared among various alloantigens are more immunogenic in xenogeneic than in allogeneic combinations.

The mechanism by which rabbit complement functions with HLA antibodies in the lymphocytotoxicity test was determined by studying the cytotoxicity of HLA xenoantisera after adsorption with leukocytes and platelets (Richiardi *et al.*, 1979). The unadsorbed xenoantiserum (Table 5) reacted to a similar extent with lymphocytes from donors with different HLA-A,B,C alloantigens. After adsorption with a pool of platelets, the xenoantiserum showed no differential cytotoxic reactivity in conjunction with rabbit complement, although in conjunction with human complement, a pattern of reactivity compatible with the recognition of certain HLA-A,B,C specificities was observed. In contrast, after the appropriate adsorptions with leukocytes, the xenoantiserum exhibited a loss of cytotoxicity in conjunction with human complement, whereas allospecificity was observed in conjunction with rabbit complement. Similar results were obtained with HLA-DR xenoantisera: limited adsorption with erythrocytes and T-lymphoid cells resulted in reagents that in conjunction with rabbit complement were cytotoxic to both B- and T-lymphoid cells, whereas in conjunction with human complement, they were specific for certain HLA-DR alloantigens (Belvedere *et al.*, 1979b, 1980a). Further adsorption of the HLA-DR xenoantisera resulted in a lack of cytotoxicity in conjunction with human complement, although in conjunction with rabbit complement, specific cytotoxicity for B lymphocytes was observed. Since complement-dependent lysis of target cells requires a minimum density of antigen–antibody interactions on the cell membrane (Linscott, 1970), we contend that the inability of alloantisera to lyse target cells in conjunction with human complement reflects a low density of individual alloantigens expressed by the cells. However, human complement can affect cytotoxicity if antisera contain additional antibodies to determinants other than the allospecificity, as has been observed with the HLA-A,B,C xenoantisera after adsorption with platelets, and with the HLA-DR xenoantisera after limited adsorption with human erythrocytes and cultured human T-lymphoid cells. Therefore, the ability of rabbit complement to affect cytotoxicity in conjunction with HLA allospecific antibodies most likely results from sublytic amounts of natural antibodies

TABLE 5. Cytotoxic Activity of HLA-A,B,C Xenoantisera in Conjunction with Human and Rabbit Complement[a]

HLA-A,B,C xenoantiserum No.	Adsorption	Complement source	Xenoantiserum titer (reciprocal)[b]	Positive reaction (%)	Allospecificity
65-R63	None	Human/rabbit	32/256	100/100	—/—
	Platelets	Human/rabbit	ND	40/100	A2/—
	Leukocytes	Human/rabbit	ND	0/29	—/A2 and A28
167	None	Human/rabbit	64/1000	100/100	—/—
	Platelets	Human/rabbit	ND	20/100	A9/—
	Leukocytes	Human/rabbit	ND	0/35	—/A9

[a] Each antiserum was tested with peripheral-blood lymphocytes from at least 40 HLA-typed donors.
[b] (ND) Not done.

in rabbit sera that increase antigen–antibody interactions on the target cells sensitized with HLA antibodies to levels sufficient for complement lysis.

4. Polyclonal Xenoantisera to Common Determinants of HLA Antigens

4.1. Introduction

Our interest in producing xenoantibodies to common determinants of HLA antigens was to have a reagent that detected these molecules on cells and in body fluids and isolated these antigens for structural analyses previous to knowledge of the alloantigenic makeup of the sample. We also felt that these xenoantisera would facilitate the screening of undefined allo- and xenoantisera for antibodies to HLA and would increase the accuracy of HLA typing. For example, inhibition of antibody binding to target cells coated with HLA xenoantibodies provides a rapid assay for obtaining presumptive evidence that the antibodies are directed to HLA antigens. In addition, the lack of accuracy due to contaminating antibodies in some alloantisera used for HLA typing may be eliminated by coating the target cells with Fab_2 fragments from xenoantisera to the contaminant antigens (e.g., block HLA-DR when testing for HLA-A,B,C antigens). Finally, cross-reactivity studies performed with xenoantisera to HLA common determinants and cells from various species along the phylogenetic tree may provide useful information on the evolutionary development of gene products of the major histocompatibility complex.

We have produced xenoantisera to common structures of HLA-A,B,C antigens by using two immunization methods that efficiently limit the contaminant antigens from the immunogen and thus obviate the need for laborious biochemical purifications or extensive antiserum adsorptions. In one method, the immunogens were man–mouse hybrid cells that contain a limited number of human chromosomes but nevertheless express HLA antigens. With the other method, the immunogens were HLA antigens adsorbed from detergent-solubilized preparations of human cells on HLA-antibody-loaded *Staphylococcus aureus* Cowan I strain (SACI) bacteria.

4.2. Xenoantisera to HLA Antigens Expressed on Man–Mouse Somatic-Cell Hybrids

Hybrids between human and murine somatic cells undergo a random loss of human chromosomes that enables the chromosomal localization of genes responsible for human cell functions (McKusick and Ruddle, 1977). Thus, hybrid cells expressing HLA antigens, but with limited expression of other surface antigens due to the reduction of human genetic material, may represent a functionally purified HLA immunogen. This method is depicted schematically in Fig. 1.

Of 12 xenoantisera to human melanoma–murine fibroblast hybrid cells, 2 contained antibodies to common determinants of HLA-A,B,C antigens (Pellegrino *et al.*, 1979). The xenoantisera (1) maintained their cytotoxicity for HLA-A,B,C antigens after adsorptions with Daudi cells lacking HLA-A,B,C antigens (Reisfeld *et al.*, 1975); (2) were not cytotoxic for cells the HLA-A,B,C antigens of which were blocked from reaction with Fab_2 fragments of xenoantisera to human β_2-μ, (3) could precipitate the classic HLA-A,B,C bimolecular complexes from lymphoid cells with different HLA phenotypes; (4) did not react with ^{125}I-labeled β_2-μ; and (5) lost their cytotoxic activity to peripheral lymphocytes from five unrelated subjects after the antisera were absorbed with any of five different cultured human B-lymphoid cell lines.

As yet, we are unable to elicit xenoantibodies to HLA-DR antigens by using hybrids produced by fusing murine fibroblasts with human melanoma or B-lymphoid cells. Although these hybrids contain chromosome 6, which carries the genes coding for HLA-DR allospecificity, they still fail to elicit xenoantibodies in rabbits (Glassy *et al.*, 1979). Since HLA-DR antigens are considered differentiation antigens, fusion of HLA-DR-bearing cells with cells that do not express these antigens may preclude expression of HLA-DR antigens. Support for this possibility is the lack of expression of HLA-DR antigens on hybrids derived from the fusion of

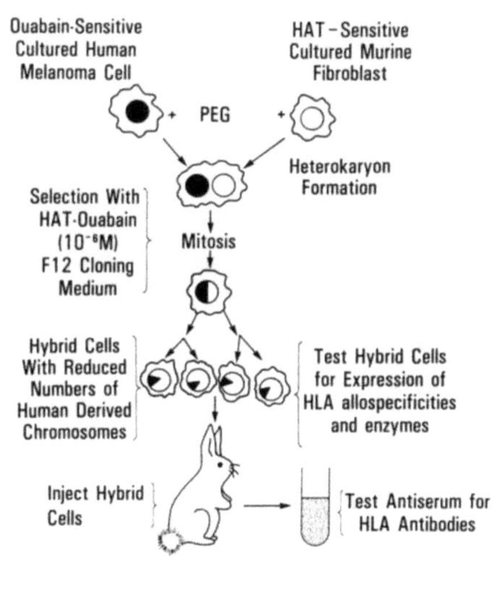

Figure 1. Production and selection of human–murine hybrids used for eliciting HLA xenoantibodies. A human melanoma cell line is fused with a TK− murine fibroblast with the aid of polyethylene glycol (PEG). The parental cells are killed by HAT–ouabain selective medium, and the surviving hybrid cells are then isolated and tested for expression of HLA alloantigens and isoenzymes. Those hybrids expressing HLA alloantigens are used as immunogens in xenogeneic combinations.

Daudi cells with HeLa cells (Indiveri and Ferrone, unpublished observations). However, if this is not the case, then our hybrids could possibly lack a chromosome coding for one of the two HLA-DR polypeptide chains, so that the molecule either is not synthesized, is not inserted into the cell membrane, or is not antigenic. A situation where the expression of a two-chain structure requires the genetic information for both polypeptide chains occurs with Daudi cells that lack the genetic information for β_2-μ (Zeuthen *et al.*, 1977) but contain the genetic information for the HLA-A,B,C heavy chains (Fellous *et al.*, 1977). Daudi cells do not express any HLA-A,B,C heavy-chain structures on the cell surface (Reisfeld *et al.*, 1975) and do not elicit xenoantibodies to HLA-A,B,C antigens (unpublished observations).

4.3. Xenoantisera to HLA Antigens Bound to *Staphylococcus aureus* Cowan I Strain Immunoadsorbents

The SACI–antigen–antibody technique was designed as a fast and simple method for producing HLA xenoantisera. According to the protocol for this technique (Fig. 2), the IgG antibodies from a specific antiserum are immobilized by binding to SACI through a cell-wall component known as protein A (Forsgren and Sjoquist, 1966). The antibody-loaded SACI can then bind their corresponding antigens from a detergent-solubilized preparation of a human cell line. Once the SACI–antigen–antibody complexes have been washed free of unbound antigens, they are injected into rabbits to elicit xenoantisera. We used SACI coated with antibodies from an anti-human β_2-μ xenoantiserum to bind HLA-A,B,C antigens from a detergent preparation of either cultured B-cell lines (B.S. Wilson *et al.*, 1978), T-cell lines, or melanoma-cell lines. The specificities of the xenoantisera produced against antigens from these three types of

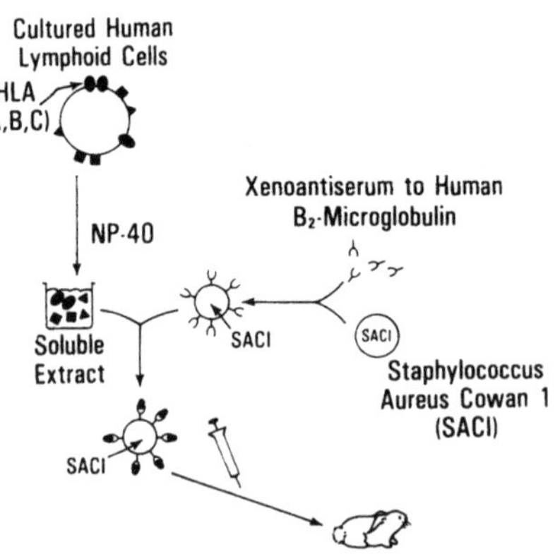

Figure 2. Production of xenoantibodies to HLA-A,B,C antigens by using the *Staphylococcus aureus* Cowan I strain (SACI) antigen–antibody technique. The IgG fraction of a xenoantiserum to human β_2-μ was bound to SACI through reaction with protein A. The SACI–Ig complexes are mixed with a NP-40 detergent preparation of a lymphoid-cell line in order to bind HLA-A,B,C antigens. The unbound cellular antigens are removed by washing, and the SACI–HLA-A,B,C complexes are then injected into rabbits to elicit xenoantibodies.

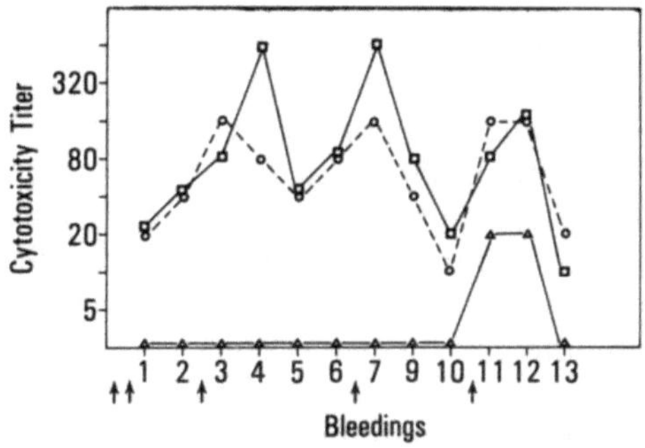

Figure 3. Cytotoxic antibody production to HLA-A,B,C antigens following immunization using the SACI–antigen–antibody technique. Rabbit No. 9698 was injected with HLA-A,B,C antigens from the cultured human T-cell line 1301. These antigens were bound to SACI via anti-human β_2-μ xenoantibodies. Arrows indicate when injections were made. Multiple bleedings were performed to test the xenoantiserum for cytotoxicity to HLA-A,B,C-bearing cells [WI-L2 cultured lymphoid cells (□) and human peripheral-blood lymphocytes (○)] and with cells lacking HLA-A,B,C antigens [Daudi cells (Δ)].

cultured cells were similar, so the following discussion applies to all three cell types.

Cytotoxic xenoantisera were produced after three to five injections of the SACI–HLA-A,B,C complexes (Fig. 3). In complement-dependent cytotoxicity tests, as well as in indirect rosette assays, the unadsorbed xenoantisera had high titers to cells expressing HLA-A,B,C antigens. On the other hand, the xenoantisera reacted poorly with Daudi cells that lack HLA-A,B,C antigens (Reisfeld *et al.*, 1975) and with cells having HLA-

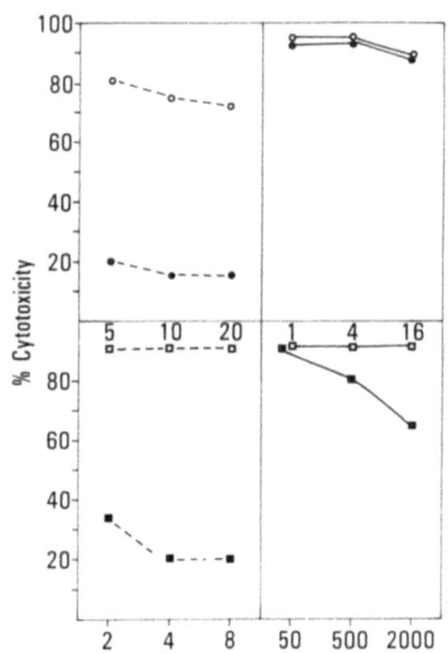

Figure 4. Serological specificity of xenoantisera to HLA-A,B,C antigens prepared by the SACI–antigen–antibody technique. Cultured human B-lymphoid cells (WI-L2) coated with Fab_2 fragments from either a xenoantiserum to human β_2-μ (top panels, ●) or from a normal rabbit serum (top panels, ○) were tested for their susceptibility to lysis by a xenoantiserum (No. 8492) to HLA-A,B,C antigens (top left panel) and an HLA-DRw4 alloantiserum (top right panel). Fab_2 fragments from an HLA-A,B,C xenoantiserum (No. 8826, bottom panels, ■) and Fab_2 fragments from normal rabbit serum (bottom panels, □) were tested for their abilities to block the lysis of WI-L2 cells by an anti HLA-A1 alloantiserum (bottom left panel) and a xenoantiserum to human β_2 (bottom right panel).

A,B,C antigens blocked by Fab_2 fragments from a xenoantiserum to β_2-μ. Both inhibition of a rosette assay and Fab_2 blocking studies indicated that the xenoantisera were reacting exclusively with HLA-A,B,C antigens. An example of Fab_2 blocking is shown in Fig. 4. It is interesting to note that Fab_2 fragments from the xenoantisera induced resistance to lysis by HLA-A,B alloantisera, and to a partial extent by a xenoantiserum to β_2-μ. The partial blocking may be explained by the possible presence of free β_2-μ antigen sites on the cell surface (Poulik *et al.*, 1973) or by a displacement of the Fab_2 fragments. Further analyses of the xenoantisera implied that they were reacting with common determinants located exclusively on the heavy chain(s) because: (1) they were unable to bind significant amounts of purified ^{125}I-labeled human β_2-μ; (2) they maintained their reactivity with HLA-A,B,C molecules in the presence of free β_2-μ (Fig. 5); and (3) after adsorption with a panel of HLA-A,B,C lymphocytes, they lost their cytotoxic activity to five HLA-typed cultured human lymphoid-cell lines expressing different HLA phenotypes.

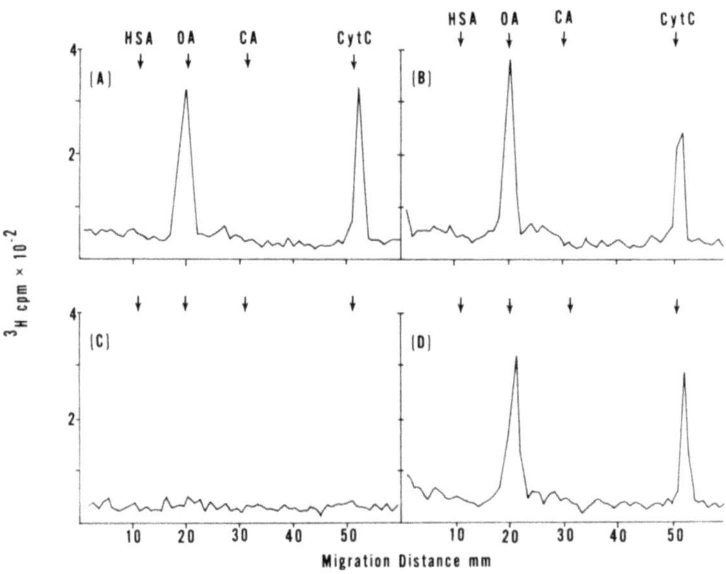

Figure 5. Immunoprecipitation of HLA-A,B,C molecules by xenoantiserum 8492 in the presence of purified human β_2-μ. Immunoprecipitation of [^{3}H]leucine-labeled RPMI 1788 glycoprotein with a xenoantiserum to human β_2-μ (A,C) and by the xenoantiserum 8492 (B,D,) was performed in the presence (C,D) or the absence (A,B,) of 10 μg purified-free human β_2-μ. Immunoprecipitates were analyzed by electrophoresis on 12.5% polyacrylamide gels containing 0.1% sodium dodecyl sulfate. The molecular-weight standards human serum albumin (HSA), 68,000; ovalbumin (OV), 44,000; carbonic acid anhydrase (CA), 29,000; and cytochrome *c* (CytC), 13,000, were electrophoresed on a companion gel.

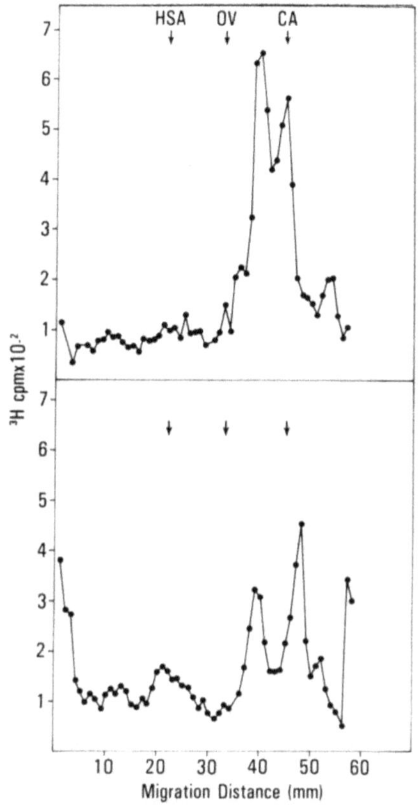

Figure 6. Mobility of HLA-DR α and β chains on sodium dodecyl sulfate–polyacrylamide gels under reducing and nonreducing conditions. HLA-DR antigens were immunoprecipitated from a [^{3}H]leucine-labeled RPMI 1788 glycoprotein preparation using a xenoantiserum prepared by injection of RPMI 4098 HLA-DR antigens bound to SACI strain bacteria (8612). The immunoprecipitates were boiled in 2% sodium dodecyl sulfate in the presence (top graph) and absence (bottom graph) of 2% 2-mercaptoethanol and then electrophoresed on 8% polyacrylamide gels containing 0.1% sodium dodecyl sulfate. The molecular-weight standards human serum albumin (HSA), 68,000; ovalbumin (OV), 44,000; and carbonic acid anhydrase (CA), 29,000, were electrophoresed on a companion gel.

Although the various cell types used as sources of HLA-A,B,C antigens had little effect on the quality of antibodies produced to these structures, they generated contaminant antibodies that reacted with other cellular antigens that were detectable in the later bleedings. Those contaminant antibodies directed to HLA-DR are avoidable when cell lines lacking HLA-DR antigens (i.e., T-lymphoid cells) are used as sources of HLA-A,B,C antigens. The antibodies to other contaminant antigens can be eliminated by predepleting the detergent preparation used as a source of HLA-A,B,C antigens with appropriate antibodies bound to SACI.

Xenoantisera to HLA-DR antigens were prepared by the SACI–antigen–antibody technique and subsequent characterization of these xenoantisera was performed in a manner similar to the preparation and characterization of xenoantisera to HLA-A,B,C antigens except that anti-HLA-DR xenoantibodies were bound to SACI and detergent extracts of cultured B-lymphoid cells served as sources of HLA-DR antigens (Wilson *et al.*, 1979b). Rabbits injected with HLA-DR antigens bound to SACI usually produced cytotoxic xenoantisera after the third immunization. The resulting unadsorbed xenoantisera reacted preferentially with B-lymphoid cells rather than with T-lymphoid cells in both cytotoxicity and rosetting assays, suggesting specificity for HLA-DR antigens. Lysostrip analysis, Fab_2 blocking, and rosette inhibition indicated that these putative HLA-DR xenoantisera were reacting with the molecules detected by HLA-DR alloantisera, but not with those detected by HLA-A,B alloantisera. In immunoprecipitation, the xenoantisera reacted with two chains of approximately 34,000 and 29,000 molecular weight. The increased mobility of the lighter component under nonreducing conditions identified it as the β chain and consequently the heavier component as the α chain of the HLA-DR molecule (Fig. 6) (Ferrone *et al.*, 1978a).

Two of the xenoantisera were analyzed in adsorption studies to determine whether they were reacting with either common determinants or allospecific determinants of the HLA-DR molecule. Adsorption of the antiserum with five different cell lines failed to result in differential cytotoxicity when tested against a panel of five cultured B-lymphoid-cell lines. Thus, these xenoantisera were specific for common determinants of the HLA-DR molecule. Whether these determinants are expressed on both chains or only on one chain of the HLA-DR complex is unknown.

Initially, these HLA-DR xenoantisera were highly specific for the HLA-DR molecule; however, in some cases, contaminant antibodies to the HLA-A,B,C antigens were detectable in the later bleedings. The generation of these contaminants could be eliminated by predepleting the detergent preparation, used as a source of HLA-DR antigens, with anti-human β_2-μ antibodies bound to SACI. In addition, the choice of cell lines used as sources of HLA-DR immunogens is also important in maintaining the selectivity of the xenoantisera for HLA-DR antigens (e.g., contaminant antibodies to an antigen of approximately 80,000 molecular weight were observed in a xenoantiserum prepared to HLA-DR from RPMI 4098 cells, but were absent from a xenoantiserum prepared to HLA-DR from Raji cells).

4.4. Application for Biological and Structural Studies of HLA Antigens

HLA antigens have been successfully detected by xenoantisera to common determinants of these antigens. Thus, primary structural analysis of HLA-DR antigens such as peptide mapping (Silver and Ferrone, 1979) and N-terminal amino acid sequence (Allison *et al.*, 1978c) has relied on the immunochemical purification of HLA-DR antigens by high-affinity xenoantibodies to common determinants. The results of these studies indicated that the smaller polypeptide chain of the HLA-DR molecule (the β chain) exhibits extensive structural polymorphism and thus should contain the amino acid residues involved in the HLA-DR alloantigenic moiety (Silver and Ferrone, 1979).

The HLA-DR xenoantisera have also been used to detect, on tumor cells, the presence of histocompatibility antigens that are expressed as a result of malignant transformation. Screening human tumor cells of nonlymphoid origin in serological and immunochemical tests demonstrated that cultured melanoma cells expressed HLA-DR antigens (B.S. Wilson *et al.*, 1979a, 1980), in contrast to their nonmalignant counterparts (melanocytes) (Klareskog *et al.*, 1977; Rowden *et al.*, 1977). The cultured melanoma cells expressed lower amounts of HLA-DR antigens than did cultured B-lymphoid-cell lines, resulting apparently from a decreased synthesis of these antigens. However, the molecular structures of the melanoma-derived DR antigens were similar to those of HLA-DR antigens from human B-lymphoid cells.

Another use of xenoantisera to HLA-DR has been to detect the level of these antigens in body fluids of normal individuals and patients with various diseases (B.S. Wilson *et al.*, 1979b; Indiveri *et al.*, 1980a). Inhibition of rosette assays between HLA-DR xenoantisera and B-lymphoid cells has been used to demonstrate that a large percentage of patients with chronic lymphocytic leukemia have elevated levels of HLA-DR serum antigens. This assay also detected HLA-DR antigens in the urine of normal individuals and patients with chronic lymphocytic leukemia.

Xenoantisera to common structures of HLA antigens and their Fab_2 fragments can be used as blocking reagents in screening human sera for alloantibodies to these antigens (Indiveri *et al.*, 1979a,b). Antibodies elicited in chickens against HLA-DR antigens bound to SACI are currently being investigated for their use in screening human sera for alloantibodies because fowl antibodies are unable to fix mammalian complement components (Rice, 1948), and thus can be used to block cytotoxicity of human alloantibodies without having to prepare them as Fab_2 fragments.

Cross-reactivity analyses with xenoantisera to HLA common determinants have revealed some evolutionary relationships between human HLA antigens and murine H-2 antigens at the molecular level. Antibodies isolated from HLA xenoantisera through adsorption–elution from murine cells were shown by both serological (direct cytotoxicity and Fab_2 blocking assays) and immunochemical tests (indirect immunoprecipitation and sequential immunodepletions) to cross-react with human and murine histocompatibility antigens (Callahan *et al.*, 1979, 1980; Ferrone, unpublished results). This immunological cross-reactivity is in agreement with the high degree of homology in the primary amino acid sequence of HLA-A,B,C and H-2 antigens (Silver and Hood, 1977) and HLA-DR and Ia antigens (Allison *et al.*, 1978c) and strongly suggests that these antigens have similarities in their tertiary structures.

5. Monoclonal Xenoantibodies to HLA Antigens

5.1. Introduction

Although the availability of antibodies with well-defined specificity was an obvious advantage and constituted sufficient motivation for producing monoclonal antibodies, the possibility that the hybridoma technique could generate a library of antibodies specific for the various antigenic determinants of the HLA molecules provided additional impetus. These antibodies may potentially identify new relationships such as cross-reactivity among various HLA allelic products, which are not detectable with conventional alloantisera, as well as new cross-reactivities among a multiplicity of other immune molecules. Furthermore, monoclonal xenoantibodies produced against certain cells might detect HLA alloantigens mutated by malignant transformation of cells. Finally, the isolation of enzymatic fragments of HLA antigens for further biochemical analysis may be facilitated by affinity chromatography with monoclonal antibodies. Most of these studies would be quite difficult, if not impossible, with polyclonal xenoantisera, since such antisera react with multiple determinants of each immunogen.

5.2. Production and Screening of Antibodies

We originally attempted monoclonal antibody production by fusing murine myeloma cells with splenocytes from rabbits immunized to HLA antigens, since rabbits produce antibodies that react with HLA allotypic specificities. However, we abandoned this approach because of a low fusion efficiency and because of poor stability of the rabbit–murine hybridomas. We then switched to murine–murine hybridomas and used an experimental design similar to the method published by Gefter *et al.* (1977). Briefly, mice were immunized with Victor cells (B-lymphoid), BwV cells (melanoma), or purified HLA antigens. The immune splenocytes were fused with myeloma lines P3-X63-Ag8 or P3-NS1-1-Ag4-1 aided by the addition of polyethylene glycol. After overnight culturing, the cells were placed in microtiter wells (2×10^5 cells/well) and grown in a selective medium containing hypoxanthine, aminopterin, and thymidine (HAT medium). Two weeks later, virtually all the parental myeloma cells were killed by the selective medium and all the unfused splenocytes died, leaving cultures of growing somatic-cell hybrids.

This protocol required screening of the supernatant fluids from developing clones for antibody activity to the immunizing cells either with a radioimmunometric binding assay using ^{125}I-labeled rabbit anti-mouse Ig or with an indirect rosette microassay using erythrocytes coated with rabbit anti-mouse Ig antibodies. The clonal supernatants possessing antibody activity were studied further to determine whether they reacted with HLA antigens. Presumptive evidence of specificity for certain HLA antigens was obtained when the clonal supernatants showed differential reactivity with cells expressing or lacking the appropriate antigens. Daudi cells, erythrocytes, or cells the HLA-A,B,C antigens of which were blocked from reaction by xenoantisera to β_2-μ or to common determinants of the heavy chains of HLA-A,B,C antigens were used as target cells lacking HLA-A,B,C antigens. On the other hand, T-lymphoid cells, erythrocytes, or cells the HLA-DR antigens of which were blocked by treatment by antisera to common structures of these antigens were used as cells lacking HLA-DR antigens. The hybridoma supernatants, presumed to contain antibodies to HLA antigens, were tested by the microcytotoxicity assay for their abilities to mediate complement-dependent lysis of lymphocytes. This characteristic is a requirement for these antibodies that will be tested for allospecificity, since the microcytotoxicity test is the established method for tissue typing. Subsequently, all the cytotoxic antibodies were tested for allospecificity against a large panel of HLA-typed cells in the microcytotoxicity test. Finally, both the cytotoxic and the other noncytotoxic antibodies were assessed for their reactivity with the classic molecular structures comprising the HLA antigens by indirect immunoprecipitation and sodium dodecyl sulfate–polyacrylamide gel electrophoresis. Those antibodies that reacted with polymorphic HLA determinants other than the known alloantigens were tested in sequential immunodepletion experiments vs. xenoantisera either to β_2-μ or to common structures of the HLA molecules to assess whether these determinants are expressed on all HLA-A,B,C or HLA-DR molecules or on specific subsets of these antigens.

5.3. Characterization of a Monoclonal Xenoantibody to HLA-A,B,C Antigens

Myeloma cell P3-X63-Ag8 was fused with splenocytes from a mouse immunized with cultured Victor cells. The resulting hybrid produced monoclonal antibody No. 28, which reacted in both the cytotoxicity and the ^{125}I-radioimmunometric assay with Victor cells, but not with Daudi cells or with Victor cells treated with Fab_2 fragments derived from a xenoantiserum to HLA-A,B,C common determinants, leading us to conclude that this antibody reacted with HLA-A,B,C antigens. This conclusion was confirmed by immunochemical evidence demonstrating that antibody No. 28 detected the same 43,000-molecular-weight and 12,000-molecular-weight structures that were detected with a xenoantiserum to common determinants of the HLA-A,B,C heavy chain. The

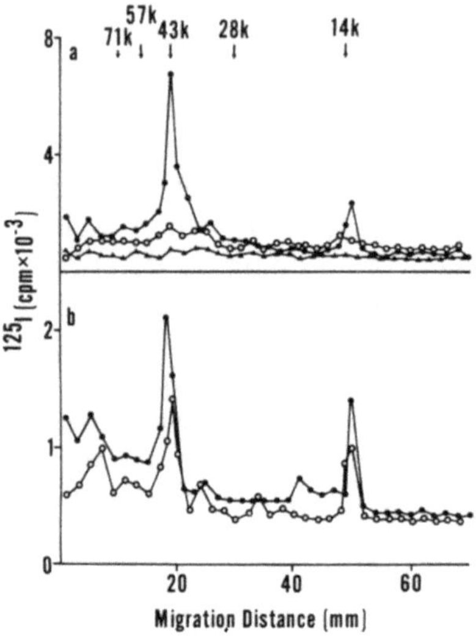

Figure 7. Reactivity of monoclonal xenoantibody No. 28 with HLA-A,B,C antigens from a cultured B-lymphoid-cell line. ^{125}I-labeled glycoprotein from cultured B-lymphoid Victor cells was first cleared of material that reacted with normal rabbit serum (●). The glycoprotein was also further depleted either once (▲) or twice (○) with monoclonal antibody No. 28. All three depleted fractions were then reacted in immunoprecipitation with either antibody No. 28 (top graph) or with a xenoantiserum (No. 9698) to common determinants of the HLA-A,B,C heavy chain (bottom graph). The immunoprecipitates were electrophoresed on 12.5% polyacrylamide tube gels containing 0.1% sodium dodecyl sulfate. The position of molecular-weight markers is shown at the top of the figure.

previous results, together with the lack of reactivity with β_2-μ, indicate that antibody No. 28 detects a determinant on the heavy chains of the HLA-A,B,C molecular complex. Sequential immunodepletion experiments indicated that antibody No. 28 cannot deplete all the Victor cell HLA-A,B,C molecules that were detected with a xenoantiserum (No. 9698) to common structures of these antigens (Fig. 7).

5.4. Characterization of a Monoclonal Xenoantibody to HLA-DR Antigens

Monoclonal antibody No. 80, derived from the same fusion as antibody No. 28, reacted with B-lymphoid cells, but not T-lymphoid cells, in the ^{125}I-radioimmunometric binding assay. This antibody was presumed specific for HLA-DR antigens after it could not mediate cytotoxicity of B-lymphoid cells pretreated with Fab$_2$ fragments from a xenoantiserum to the HLA-DR antigens. Antibody No. 80 was confirmed specific for HLA-DR antigens by several independent HLA-typing laboratories (Molinaro *et al.*, 1980). Although antibody No. 80 did not show specificity for any known HLA-DR alloantigens, the determinants detected by antibody No. 80 are apparently expressed by a subpopulation of the HLA-DR molecules. This conclusion was obtained from immunodepletion experiments in which a xenoantiserum to common structures of HLA-DR antigens depleted all molecules detected by antibody No. 80, whereas antibody No. 80 was unable to deplete all the molecules detected by the xenoantiserum (Fig. 8). We have not yet determined which of the HLA-DR polypeptide chains carries the determinant detected by antibody No. 80; however, we do know that this determinant is different from the one recognized by another monoclonal antibody, No. 70, since lymphoid cells coated with antibody No. 70, which is an IgG1 and does not bind complement, are still susceptible to the cytotoxic effects of antibody No. 80 (Molinaro *et al.*, 1980).

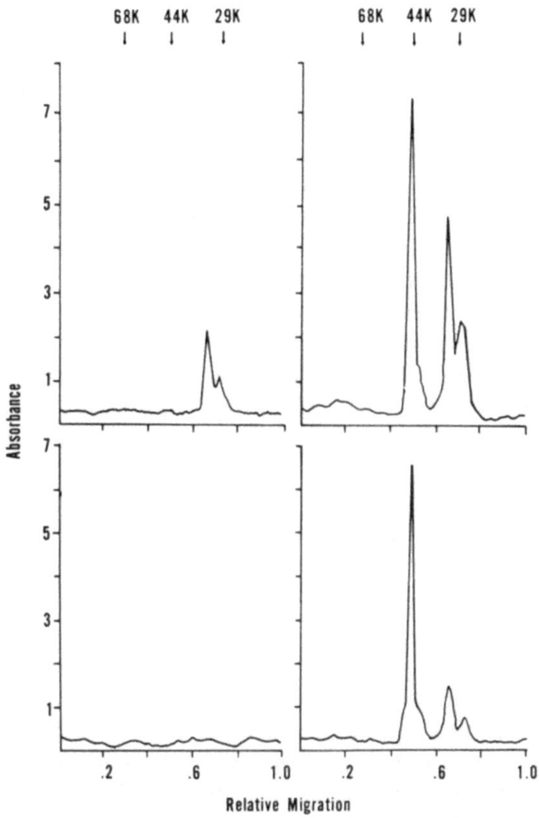

Figure 8. Reactivity of monoclonal antibody No. 80 in indirect immunoprecipitation with B-lymphoid cell HLA-DR antigens. A [^{35}S]methionine-labeled glycoprotein preparation of the Victor B-lymphoid-cell line was first cleared of material reactive with normal rabbit serum (top panels) or with monoclonal antibody No. 80 (bottom panels). The remaining glycoproteins were then reacted in immunoprecipitation either with monoclonal antibody No. 80 (left-hand panels) or with a xenoantiserum (No. 3634) to common determinants of HLA-DR antigens (right-hand panels). The immunoprecipitates were electrophoresed on 10% polyacrylamide slab gels containing 0.1% sodium dodecyl sulfate. Autoradiographs were scanned at 550 mm and the absorbance was plotted vs. relative migration. The positions of molecular-weight markers are shown at the top of the figure. Left to right: bovine serum albumin, ovalbumin, carbonic anhydrase.

5.5. Application for Biological and Structural Studies of HLA Antigens

Because of their unquestionable specificity, monoclonal xenoantibodies to HLA antigens should allow us to verify some of the results obtained with polyclonal xenoantisera. One such study deals with the expression of HLA-DR antigens on stem cells. Evidence in the murine system that Ia antigens (the analogue of HLA-DR antigens) are lacking on mouse stem cells (Basch *et al.*, 1977) raises doubts about the conclusion that human stem cells express HLA-DR antigens, since the latter studies have used polyclonal allo- and xenoantisera that may contain contaminating antibodies reacting with the stem cells. Through the use of monoclonal antibodies that eliminate any concern for contaminant antibodies, we demonstrated conclusively that human stem cells do indeed express HLA-DR antigens (Fitchen *et al.*, 1980). The difference between the human and murine stem cells, if not technical in nature, suggests the development of divergent regulatory mechanisms in hemopoietic stem cells after speciation. Another controversy is the relationship between the HLA-Bw4 alloantigens and the receptor for the third component of human complement (C3). Using monoclonal antibodies and polyclonal xenoantisera to the HLA-A,B,C molecular complexes, we showed that HLA-A,B,C antigens are both spatially and structurally unrelated to the C3 receptor (Indiveri *et al.*, 1980a).

Monoclonal antibodies are being used to isolate and characterize specific subpopulations of cells (Indiveri *et al.*, unpublished).

6. Conclusion

The data summarized in the previous sections clearly indicate that two types of antibodies can be produced to HLA antigens through cross-species immunization, paralleling observations with xenoantisera to the MHC antigens of mice (Sachs *et al.*, 1971, 1973; Staines *et al.*, 1973; Parish *et al.*, 1976; Morello *et al.*, 1978; Kvist *et al.*, 1978a,b; Hoffman-Fezer *et al.*, 1978), rats (Poloskey *et al.*, 1975; Edwards *et al.*, 1977), and guinea pigs (Clement *et al.*, 1979). One type of antibody directed to determinants common to all molecules of a single group (e.g., HLA-A,B,C), is referred to as an anti-common HLA antibody. The other type reacts with the allotypic determinants that define serological polymorphism of HLA antigens. The former type of antibody has been generally accepted by the scientific community; however, the latter type is regarded with skepticism exemplified by a recent quotation from Sanderson and Thorsby (1977), who concluded that HLA allospecificity "has only been established unequivocally for serological reagents raised within a species."

It is not absolutely clear which factors control the immune responses of rabbits such that in some cases certain antisera react preferentially with common determinants in contrast to other cases when these antisera react preferentially with alloantigenic determinants. One factor may be the inheritance of immune-response genes enabling rabbits to respond to common or to allotypic determinants. Another factor may be the antigenic makeup of the individual rabbit. Thus, xenoantibody responses directed predominantly to alloytpic rather than common determinants may occur when the antigenic dissimilarity between rabbits and humans approaches that of an allogeneic combination. Support for this notion comes from the fact that the primary structures of histocompatibility antigens have been highly conserved through evolution as evidenced by (1) the high degree of amino acid sequence homology among histocompatibility antigens from various species and (2) the detection of shared alloantigens between rabbits and humans (Schulman *et al.*, 1964; Albert *et al.*, 1969). A third factor may be the immunogen source (i.e., serum or cellular). Fourth, purification methods may have different effects on the expression of certain alloantigenic determinants. In our experience, lipid-associated materials from either cells or serum elicit xenoantibodies to HLA allospecificities most successfully. The high lipid content of this preparation may in some way simulate conditions at the cell membrane and thus help to maintain the active conformation of the alloantigenic determinants. Support for this hypothesis comes from studies in which removal of lipid by digestion with papain destroys the immunogenicity of the HLA molecule without having any apparent effect on antigenicity (unpublished observations). Alternatively, the situation wherein the SACI–antigen–antibody immunization technique elicits antibodies to common rather than to allotypic determinants may result from blocking or denaturing of the allotypic determinants when the antigen is presented in combination with antibody. The SACI bacteria might also effect the response to common rather than to allotypic determinants.

There are several reports in the literature that claim that β_2-μ is more immunogenic than the HLA-A,B,C heavy chains when the complete bimolecular complex is injected into either mice (Trucco *et al.*, 1978) or rabbits (Sanderson, 1977). Our results contrast to these reports. Chiefly, we have used the HDL fraction of serum or cells and the SACI–antigen–antibody technique to immunize rabbits, whereas the other investigators have used either whole cells (Trucco *et al.*, 1978) or papain-digested and biochemically purified HLA-A,B,C antigens (Sanderson, 1977).

Xenoantisera have been most useful for characterizing HLA antigens: xenoantibodies to β_2-μ, HLA-A,B,C heavy chain, and HLA-DR have been successfully used to isolate HLA antigens for analyzing their molecular profiles and their chemical structures via peptide mapping and primary amino acid sequencing. These studies would not have been feasible with alloantisera because of the difficulty in obtaining sufficient amounts and because their antibodies are low in affinity and titer. Paradoxically, the xenoantisera are not accepted as an alternative to alloantisera for tissue typing, although the specificity of HLA-A9 xenoantisera has been verified by independent laboratories and the xenoantisera are being distributed by the National Institute of Health, leading us to conclude that the lack of acceptance is unfounded. Monoclonal xenoantibodies should not suffer the same prejudice as did polyclonal xenoantisera, since these antibodies are homogeneous and therefore specificity is certain. We are unable to predict whether murine monoclonal xenoantibodies can be prepared to all the HLA allospecificities or whether those antibodies that react with each allospecificity can function in the cytotoxicity tests and are therefore useful.

Aside from the practical applications of monoclonal xenoantibodies, there is the exciting possibility that these reagents may detect all the various determinants of the HLA molecules, running the gamut from common to public specificities, all the way to private specificities. When antibodies to such determinants become available, cross-reactivity studies will reveal evolutionary relationships among various HLA alloantigens and among these antigens and their analogues in other species.

ACKNOWLEDGMENTS. This work was supported by grants from the National Institutes of Health, a special fellowship of the Leukemia Society of America (B.W. and A.N.), a fellowship of the Leukemia Society of America (V.Q.), and an American Heart Association Established Investigatorship Award (S.F.). The authors wish to acknowledge the secretarial assistance of Mr. D. Trinko and the editorial assistance of Mrs. P. Minick. This is publication number 2017 from Scripps Clinic and Research Foundation.

References

Aden, D.P., Mausner, R., and Knowles, B.B., 1978, Production of HLA antibody in mice immunized with syngeneic mouse–human hybrid cells containing human chromosome 6, *Nature (London)* **271**:375.

Albert, E., Kano, K., Abeyounis, C.J., and Milgrom, F., 1969, Detection of human lymphocyte isoantigens by rabbit homotransplantation sera, *Transplantation* **5**:466.

Allison, J.P., Pellegrino, M.A., Ferrone, S., Callahan, G.N., and Reisfeld, R.A., 1977a, Biologic and chemical characterization of HLA antigens in human serum, *J. Immunol.* **118**:1004.

Allison, J.P., Pellegrino, M.A., Reisfeld, R.A., and Ferrone, S., 1977b, An immunadsorption technique for analysis of antigenic determinants reacting with HLA xenoantisera, *Transplant. Proc.* **9**:1691.

Allison, J.P., Belvedere, M., Reisfeld, R.A., Pellegrino, M.A., and Ferrone, S., 1978a,

Serological and immunochemical characterization of HLA-A9 xenoantisera, *J. Immunol.* **121**:579.

Allison, J.P., Ferrone, S., Walker, L.E., Pellegrino, M.A., Silver, J., and Reisfeld, R.A., 1978b, The partial amino acid sequence of HLA-A9 antigen purified with a specific xenoantiserum, *Transplantation* **26**:451.

Allison, J.P., Walker, L.E., Pellegrino, M.A., Ferrone, S., Reisfeld, R.A., Frelinger, J.A., and Silver, J., 1978c, Murine Ia and human DR antigens: Homology of amino terminal sequences, *Proc. Natl. Acad. Sci. U.S.A.* **75**:3953.

Bachvaroff, R., and Rapaport, F.T., 1973, Immunological studies of the relationship between HL-A and species specific antigenic sites on the human lymphocyte surface, *Transplantation* **15**:586.

Ballou, B., McKean, D.J., Freedlander, E.F., and Smithies, O., 1976, HLA membrane antigens: Sequencing by intrinsic radioactivity, *Proc. Natl. Acad. Sci. U.S.A.* **73**:4487.

Balner, H., VanLeeuwen, A. Dersjant, H., and van Rood, J.J., 1967, Defined leukocyte antigens of chimpanzees: Use of chimpanzee isoantisera for leukocyte typing in man, *Transplantation* **5**:624.

Barnstable, C.J., Bodmer, W.F., Brown, G., Galfre, G., Milstein, C., Williams, A.F., and Ziegler, A., 1978, Production of monoclonal antibodies to Group A erythrocytes, HLA and other human cell surface antigens—New tools for genetic analysis, *Cells* **14**:9.

Basch, R.S., Janossy, G., and Greans, M.F., 1977, Murine pluripotential stem cells lack Ia antigen, *Nature* (*London*) **270**:520.

Batchelor, J.R., 1969, The relationship between HLA specificity and a human species antigen, *Transplantation* **7**:554.

Belvedere, M., Allison, J.P., Reisfeld, R.A., Pellegrino, M.A., and Ferrone, S., 1979a, Serum HLA antigens: Serological and immunogenic properties, in: *HLA Antigens in Clinical Medicine and Biology* (S. Ferrone, E.S. Curtoni, and S. Gorni, eds.) p. 19, Garland STPM Press, New York.

Belvedere, M., Olivetti, E., Pelligrino, M.A., and Ferrone, S., 1979b, Reactivity of DR xenoantisera in a cytotoxic test with human complement, *Transplant. Proc.* **11**:1327.

Belvedere, M., Pellegrino, M.A., and Ferrone, S., 1980a, Xenoantisera to DRw allospecificities, *J. Immunogenet.* **7**:167.

Belvedere, M., Richardi, P., Pellegrino, M.A., and Ferrone, S., 1980b, Fab_2 fragments from HLA xenoantigens specifically block cytolosis mediated by HLA-A,B alloantisera, *J. Immunogenet.* **7**:215.

Berggard, I., and Bearn, A.G., 1968, Isolation and properties of a low molecular weight β_2-globulin occurring in human biological fluids, *J. Biol. Chem.* **243**:4095.

Billing, R.J., and Terasaki, P.I., 1974, Rabbit antisera to HL-A9 isolated from normal serum, *Transplantation* **17**:231.

Billing, R., Mittal, K.K., and Terasaki, P.I., 1973, Isolation of soluble molecule HL-A antigens from normal human sera by ion exchange chromatography, *Tissue Antigens* **3**:251.

Billing, R., Rafizadeh, B., Drew, I., Hartman, G., Gale, R., and Terasaki, P., 1976, Human B-lymphocyte antigens expressed by lymphocytic and myelocytic leukemia cells. 1. Detection by rabbit antisera, *J. Exp. Med.* **144**:167.

Callahan, G.N., Ng, A., Pellegrino, M.A., and Ferrone, S., 1979, Cross reacting xenoantibodies to human and murine β_2-microglobulin, *Transplant. Proc.* **11**:1739.

Callahan, G.N., Pellegrino, M.A., and Ferrone, S., 1980, Cross reacting xenoantibodies to the heavy chain of HLA-A, B and H-2 antigens: Preparation and serological and immunochemical characterization, *Scand. J. Immunol.* **12**:297.

Ceppellini, R., Bonnard, G.P., Coppo, F., Miggiano, V.C., Pospisil, M., Curtoni, E.S., and Pellegrino, M.A., 1971, Mixed leukocyte cultures and HL-A antigens. I. Reactivity of young fetuses, newborns and mothers at delivery, *Transplant. Proc.* **3**:58.

Cerottini, J.P., McConahey, P.J., and Dixon, F.J., 1969, Specificity of the immunosuppression caused by passive administration of antibody, *J. Immunol.* **103:**268.

Charlton, R.K., and Zmijewski, C.M., 1970, Soluble HL-HA antigen: Localization in the β-lipoprotein fraction of human serum, *Science* **170:**636.

Clement, L.T., Kask, A.M., Schwartz, B.D., and Shevach, E.M., 1979, Analysis of guinea pig membrane proteins recognized by heterologous antilymphocite sera, *Transplantation* **27:**397.

Cresswell, P., and Ayres, J.L., 1976, HLA antigens: Rabbit antisera reacting with all A series or all B series specificities, *Eur. J. Immunol.* **6:**82.

Cresswell, P., and Geier, S.S., 1975, Antisera to human B-lymphocyte membrane glycoproteins block stimulation in mixed lymphocyte culture, *Nature* (*London*) **257:**147.

David, C.S., Klein, J., and Shreffler, D.C., 1973, Serologic homology between H-2 and HL-A system, *Transplant. Proc.* **5:**461.

Edwards, P.A., Kunz, H.W., and Gill, T.J., 1977, Genetic studies in inbred rats. VIII. The production of xenoantisera against Ag-B histocompatibility antigens, *J. Immunogenet.* **4:**53.

Einstein, A.B., Mann, D.L., Gordon, H.G., Trapani, R.J., and Fahey, J., 1971, Heterologous antisera against specific HL-A antigens, *Transplantation* **12:**299.

Fellous, M., Kamoun, M., Wiels, J., Dousset, J., Clements, G., Zeuthen, J., and Klein, G., 1977, Induction of HLA expression in Daudi cells after cell fusion, *Immunogenetics* **5:**423.

Ferrone, S., Cooper, N.R., Pellegrino, M.A., and Reisfeld, R.A., 1971, The lymphocytotoxic reaction: The mechanism of rabbit complement action, *J. Immunol.* **107:**939.

Ferrone, S., Natali, P.G., Hunter, M., Terasaki, P.I., and Reisfeld, R.A., 1972, Immunogenicity of soluble HL-A alloantigens, *J. Immunol.* **108:**1718.

Ferrone, S., Pellegrino, M.A., Götze, D., Mittal, K.K., Terasaki, P.I., and Reisfeld, R.A., 1973, Cytotoxic heteroantisera against soluble HL-A antigens, in: *International Symposium on Standardization of HLA Reagents,* Copenhagen, 1972, *Symp. Ser. Immunobiol.,* Vol. 18, p. 218, S. Karger, Basel.

Ferrone, S., Pellegrino, M.A., Billing, R., Terasaki, P.I., and Reisfeld, R.A., 1975, Production of anti-W24 xenoantisera in rabbits, *Tissue Antigens* **5:**41.

Ferrone, S., Mittal, K.K., Pellegrino, M.A., Allison, J.P., and Reisfeld, R.A., 1977a, Immunogenicity of HLA antigens purified from serum, *Transplantation* **23:**7.

Ferrone, S., Pellegrino, M.A., and Reisfeld, R.A., 1977b, Immunogenicity of human B cell antigens solubilized from cultured human lymphoid cells, *J. Immunol.* **118:**1036.

Ferrone, S., Allison, J.P., and Pellegrino, M.A., 1978a, Human DR (Ia-like) antigens: Biological and molecular profile, in: *Contemporary Topics in Molecular Immunology* (H.N. Eisen and R.A. Reisfeld, eds.), p. 239, Plenum Press, New York.

Ferrone, S., Naeim, F., Indireri, F., Walker, L.E., and Pellegrino, M.A., 1978b, Xenoantisera to human DR antigens: Serological and immunochemical characterization, *Immunogenetics* **7:**349.

Ferrone, S., Pellegrino, M.A., and Allison, J.P., 1979, Rabbit complement in the cytotoxic test with antibody-coated nucleated cells: Properties and role of human antigens reactive with rabbit natural antibodies, in: *HLA Antigens in Clinical Medicine and Biology* (S. Ferrone, E.S. Curtoni, and S. Gorni, eds.), p. 58, Garland STPM Press, New York.

Fitchen, J.H., Ferrone, S., Quarranta, V., Molinaro, G.A., and Cline, M., 1980, Monoclonal antibodies to HLA-A, B and DR antigen inhibit colony formation by human myeloid progenitor cells, *J. Immunol.* **125:**2004.

Forsgren, A., and Sjoquist, J., 1966, "Protein A" from *S. aureus.* I. Pseudo-immune reaction with human globulin, *J. Immunol.* **97:**882.

Gefter, M.L., Margulies, D.H., and Scharff, M.D., 1977, A simple method for polyethylene glycol-promoted hybridization of mouse myeloma cells, *Somat. Cell Genet.* **3:**231.

Glassy, M.C., Pellegrino, M.A., Quaranta, V., Molinaro, G.A., and Ferrone, S., 1979, Lack of DR antigens on human B lymphocyte–mouse fibroblast hybrids that express HLA-A, B antigens, *Transplant. Proc.* **11**:1719.

Goodfellow, P.N., Jones, E.A., van Heyningen, V., Solomon, E., Bobrow, M., Miggiano, V., and Bodmer, V.F., 1975, The β_2-microglobulin gene is on chromosome 15 and not in the HL-A region, *Nature (London)* **254**:267.

Goodfellow, P., Barnstable, C., Jones, E., Bodmer, W.F., Crumpton, M.J., and Snary, D., 1976, Production of specific antisera to human B lymphocytes, *Tissue Antigens* **7**:105.

Götze, D., Ferrone, S., and Reisfeld, R.A., 1972, Serologic cross-reactivity between H-2 and HL-A antigens. I. Specific reactivity of rabbit anti-HL-A sera against murine cells, *J. Immunol.* **109**:439.

Götze, D., Lee, S., Ferrone, S., Pellegrino, M.A., and Reisfeld, R.A., 1973, Cross-reactivity between HL-A and H-2 antigens. II. Allogeneic sensitization by xenogeneic soluble lymphocyte antigens (HL-A), *Transplant Proc.* **5**:467.

Greaves, M.F., and Brown, B., 1975, Antisera to acute lymphoblastic leukemia cells, *Clin. Immunol. Immunopathol.* **4**:67.

Grey, H.M., Kubo, R.T., Colon, S.M., Poulik, M.D., Cresswell, P., Springer, T., Turner, M., and Strominger, J.C., 1973, The small subunit of HL-A antigens is β_2-microglobulin, *J. Exp. Med.* **138**:1608.

Harris, R., and Zervas, J.D., 1969, Reticulocyte HL-A Antigens, *Nature (London)* **221**:1062.

Hoffmann-Fezer, G., Götze, D., Rodt, H., and Theirfelder, S., 1978, Immunohistochemical localization of xenogenic antibodies against Ia^K lymphocytes on B cells and reticular cells, *Immunogenetics* **6**:367.

Humphreys, R.E., McCune, J.M., Chess, L., Herrman, H.C., Malenka, D.J., Mann, D.L., Parham, P., Schlossman, S.F., and Strominger, J.L., 1976, Isolation and immunologic characterization of a human, B-lymphocyte-specific, cell surface antigen, *J. Exp. Med.* **144**:98.

Ikeman, R.L., Sullivan, A.K., Kositsky, R., Bartok, K., and Jerry, L.M., 1978, Molecular variants of human Ia-like antigens, *Nature (London)* **272**:267.

Indiveri, F., Fagiolo, U., Pellegrino, M.A., and Ferrone, S., 1979a, Uremic patients immunized with planned blood transfusions: Detection of HLA antibodies with the cytotoxic test and an indirect rosette microassay, *Transplant. Proc.* **11**:167.

Indiveri, F., Wilson, B.S., Pellegrino, M.A., and Ferrone, S., 1979b, Detection of human histocompatibility antigens with an indirect rosette microassay. *J. Immunol. Methods* **29**:101.

Indiveri, F., Pellegrino, M.A., Quaranta, V., Molinaro, G.A., and Ferrone, S., 1980a, Monoclonal and polyclonal xenoantibodies to the HLA-A,B,C antigenic molecular complex do not affect the functional activity of C3 receptors, *Z. Immunitätsforsch. Immunobiol.* (in press).

Indiveri, F., Wilson, B.S., Natali, P.G., Pellegrino, M.A., and Ferrone, S., 1980b, Immunogenicity of DR antigens isolated from body fluids, *Transplant Proc.* **12**:121.

Katagari, M., Tanigaki, N., Kreifter, V.P., and Pressman, D., 1974, "Common" antigenic structures of HL-A antigens. III. An HL-A common antigenic marker closely associated with HL-A alloantigenic activity and detected by the use of rabbit anti-rhesus monkey cell membrane antibodies, *Immunology* **27**:487.

Klareskog, L., Tjernlund, U.M., Forsum, U., and Peterson, P.A., 1977, Epidermal Langerhans cells express Ia antigens, *Nature (London)* **268**:248.

Klareskog, L., Rask, L., Fohlman, J., and Peterson, P.A., 1978a, Heavy HLA-DR (Ia) antigen chain is controlled by the MHC region, *Nature (London)* **275**:762.

Klareskog, L., Tragardh, L., Lindblom, J.B., and Peterson, P.A., 1978b, Reactivity of a rabbit antiserum against highly purified HLA-DR antigens, *Scand. J. Immunol.* **7**:199.

Klinman, N.R., 1969, Antibody with homogenous antigen binding produced by spleen foci in organ culture, *Immunochemistry* **6**:757.
Köhler, G., and Milstein, C., 1975, Continuous cultures of fused cells secreting antibody of predefined specificity, *Nature (London)* **256**:495.
Kvist, S., Klareskog, L., and Peterson, P.A., 1978a, Identification of H-2 and Ia-antigen analogues in several species by immunological cross-reactions of xenoantisera, *Scand. J. Immunol.* **7**:447.
Kvist, S., Osterberg, L., and Peterson, P.A., 1978b, Reactions and cross-reactions of a rabbit anti-H2 antigen serum, *Scand. J. Immunol.* **7**:265.
Lampson, L.A., Levy, R., Crumet, F.C., Ness, D., and Pious, D., 1978, Production *in vitro* of murine antibody to a human histocompatibility alloantigen, *Nature (London)* **271**:461.
Legrand, L., and Dausset, J., 1975, The complexity of the HL-A gene product. II. Possible evidence for a "public" determinent common to the first and second HL-A series, *Transplantation* **19**:177.
Lemke, H., Hammerline, G., Hohmann, C., and Rajewsky, K., 1978, Hybrid cell lines secreting monoclonal antibody specific for major histocompatibility antigens of the mouse, *Nature (London)* **271**:249.
Linscott, W.D., 1970, An antigen density effect on the hemolytic efficiency of complement, *J. Immunol.* **104**:1307.
Mann, D.L., Fahey, J.L., and Nathenson, S.G., 1970, Molecular comparisons of papain solubilized H-2 and HL-A alloantigens, in: *Histocompatibility Testing* (P.I. Terasaki, ed.), p. 461, Munksgaard, Copenhagen.
McKusick, V.A., and Ruddle, F.H., 1977, The status of the gene map of the human chromosomes, *Science* **196**:390.
Metzgar, R.S., and Miller, J.L., 1972, Production of HL-A specific antibodies in monkeys by immunization with soluble HL-A antigen, *Transplantation* **13**:467.
Metzgar, R.S., and Miller, J.L., 1973, Production of precipitating primate antibodies to human membrane antigen(s) with HL-A activity by immunization with soluble HL-A antigens, *J. Immunol.* **110**:1097.
Metzgar, R.S., and Zmijewski, C.M., 1966, Species distribution of human tissue isoantigens. I. Detection of human tissue isoantigens in chimpanzees, *Transplantation* **4**:84.
Metzgar, R.A., Zmijewski, C.M., and Amos, D.B., 1965, Serological activity of human and chimpanzee antisera to human leukocyte isoantigens, in: *Histocompatibility Testing* (P.S. Russel and H.J. Winn, eds.), Publ. No. 1129, National Academy of Science Research Councils, p. 45.
Mittal, K.K., Ferrone, S., Mickey, R.M., Pellegrino, M.A., Reisfeld, R.A., and Terasaki, P.I., 1973a, Serological characterization of natural anti-human lymphocytotoxic antibodies in mammalian sera, *Transplantation* **16**:287.
Mittal, K.K., Ferrone, S., Mickey, M.R., Pellegrino, M.A., Reisfeld, R.A., and Terasaki, P.I., 1973b, Specificity of lymphocytotoxic anti-human antibodies in normal rabbit sera, *Tissue Antigens* **3**:**88**.
Miyakawa, Y., Tanigaki, N., Kreiter, V.P., Moore, G.E., and Pressman, D., 1973, Characterization of soluble substances in the plasma carrying HL-A alloantigenic activity and HL-A common antigenic activity, *Transplantation* **15**:312.
Molinaro, G.A., Quaranta, V., and Ferrone, S., 1980, Characterization of the specificity of DR monoclonal antibodies. *Transplant Proc.* **11**:1748.
Morello, D., Gachelin, G., Dubois, P.L., Tanigaki, N., Pressman, D., and Jacob, F., 1978, Absence of reaction of a xenogenic anti-H-2 serum with mouse embryonal carcinoma cells, *Transplantation* **26**:119.

Nakamuro, K., Tanigaki, N., and Pressman, D., 1973, Multiple common properties of human β_2-microglobulin and the common portion fragment derived from HL-A antigen molecules, *Proc. Natl. Acad. Scie. U.S.A.* **70:**2863.

Nakamuro, K., Tanigaki, N., and Pressman, D., 1975, Common antigenic structures of HL-A antigens. VI. Common antigenic determinants located on the 33,000-dalton alloantigenic fragment portion of papain-solubilized HL-A antigens, *J. Immunol.* **29:**1119.

Oh, S.K., Pellegrino, M.A., Ferrone, S., Sevier, E.D., and Reisfeld, R.A., 1975, Soluble HL-A antigens in serum. I. Isolation and purification, *Eur. J. Immunol.* **5:**161.

Parham, P., and Bodmer, W.F., 1978, Monoclonal antibody to a human histocompatibility alloantigen HLA-A2, *Nature (London)* **276:**397.

Parham, P., Sehgal, P.K., and Brodsky, F.M., 1979, Anti-HLA-A,B,C monoclonal antibodies with no alloantigenic specificity in humans define polymorphisms in other primate species, *Nature (London)* **279:**639.

Parish, C.R., Chilcott, A.B., and McKenzie, I.F.C., 1976, Low molecular weight Ia antigens in normal mouse serum. I. Detection and production of a xenogeneic antiserum, *Immunogenetics* **3:**113.

Pellegrino, M.A., Ferrone, S., Pellegrino, A., Oh, S.K., and Reisfeld, R.A., 1974, Evaluation of two sources of soluble HL-A antigens: Platelets and serum, *Eur. J. Immunol.* **4:**250.

Pellegrino, M.A., Wilson, B.S., and Ferrone, S., 1979, Immunogenicity of HLA-A,B antigens expressed by human melanoma–murine fibroblast cell hybrids, *Transplant. Proc.* **11:**1706.

Peterson, P.A., Rask, L., and Lindblom, J.B., 1974, Highly purified papain-solubilized HL-A antigens contain β_2-microglobulin, *Proc. Natl. Acad. Sci. U.S.A.* **71:**35.

Ploegh, H.L., Cannon, O.E., and Strominger, J.L., 1979, Cell-free translation of the mRNAs for the heavy and light chains of HLA-A and HLA-B antigens, *Proc. Natl. Acad. Sci. U.S.A.* **76:**2273.

Poloskey, P.E., Kunz, H.W., and Gill, T.J., 1975, Genetic studies in inbred rats. V. Xenoantisera against two major histocompatability antigens raised by immunization with red cells, *J. Immunogenet.* **2:**189.

Poulik, M.D., Bernoco, M., Bernoco, D., and Ceppellini, R., 1973, Aggregation of HL-A antigens at the lymphocyte surface induced by an anti-serum to β_2-microglobulin, *Science* **182:**1352.

Rask, L., Lindblom, J.B., and Peterson, P.A., 1976, Structural and immunological similarities between HLA antigens from three loci, *Eur. J. Immunol.* **6:**93.

Reisfeld, R.A., Pellegrino, M.A., Ferrone, S., and Kahan, B.D., 1973, Chemical and molecular nature of HL-A antigen, *Transplant. Proc.* **5:**447.

Reisfeld, R.A., Sevier, E.D., Pellegrino, M.A., Ferrone, S., and Poulik, M.D., 1975, Association of HL-A antigen and β_2-microglobulin at the cellular and molecular level, *Immunogenetics* **2:**183.

Rice, C.E., 1948, Inhibitory effects of certain avian and mammalian antisera in specific complement-fixation systems, *J. Immunol.* **59:**365.

Richiardi, P., Pellegrino, M.A., and Ferrone, S., 1979, Xenoantisera to allotypic specificities of HLA-A and -B antigens: Serologic characterization, *Transplantation* **28:**333.

Sachs, D.H., Winn, H.J., and Russell, P.S., 1971, The immunologic response to xenografts, *J. Immunol.* **107:**481.

Sachs, D.H., McKenzie, I.F.C., Winn, H.J., and Russell, P.S., 1973, Serologic distinction between soluble species-specific and strain-specific transplantation antigens, *Transplant. Proc.* **5:**477.

Sanderson, A.R., 1977, HLA "help" for human β_2-microglobulin across species barriers, *Nature (London)* **269:**414.

Sanderson, A.R., and Thorsby, E., 1977, Anti-MHC xenoantisera and alloterminology, *Transplantation* **23:**525.

Sanderson, A.R., and Welsh, K.I., 1973, HL-A specific antibodies by immunization of *Macaca irus* (Cynomologus) monkeys with purified HL-A substances, *Transplant. Proc.* **5:**471.

Scalamogna, M., Mercuriali, F., Pizzi, G., and Sirchia, G., 1976, Cross-reactivity between the first and second segregant series of the HLA system, *Tissue Antigens* **7:**125.

Shulman, N.R., Marder, V.J., Hiller, M.C., and Collier, E.M., 1964, Platelet and leukocyte isoantigens and their antibodies: Serologic, physiologic and clinical studies, *Prog. Hematol.* **4:**222.

Shulman, N.R., Moor-Jankowski, J., and Hiller, M.C., 1965, Platelet and leukocyte isoantigens common to man and other animals, in: *Histocompatibility Testing 1965* (H. Balner, F.J. Cleton, and J.G. Fernisee, eds.), p. 113, Munksgaard, Copenhagen.

Silver, J., and Ferrone, S., 1979, Structural polymorphism of human DR antigens, *Nature (London)* **279:**436.

Silver, J., and Hood, L., 1977, Preliminary amino acid sequences of transplantation antigens: Genetic and evolutionary implications, in: *Contemporary Topics in Molecular Immunology* (H.N. Eisen and R.A. Reisfeld, eds.), p. 35, Plenum Press, New York.

Snary, D., Barnstable, C.J., Bodmer, W.F., Goodfellow, P.N., and Crumpton, M.J., 1977, Cellular distribution, purification, and molecular nature of human Ia antigens, *Scand. J. Immunol.* **6:**441.

Solheim, B.G., Fuks, A., Smith, L., Strominger, J.L., and Thorsby, E., 1978, Possible detection of HLA-DR alloantigenic specificities in man with unadsorbed rabbit antisera, *Scand. J. Immunol.* **8:**15.

Springer, T.A., Kaufman, J.F., Siddoway, L.A., Giphart, M., Mann, D.L., Terhorst, C., and Strominger, J.L., 1976, Chemical and immunological characterization of HL-A linked B lymphocyte alloantigens, *Cold Spring Harber Symp. Quant. Biol.* **41:**387.

Staines, N.A., O'Neill, G.J., Guy, K., and Davies, D.A.L., 1973, Xenoantisera against lymphoid cells: Specificity and use in monitoring purification of mouse and human histocompatibility antigens, *Tissue Antigens* **3:**1.

Tanigaki, N., and Nakamuro, K., 1974, Common antigenic structures of HL-A antigens. V. An antigenic determinant characteristic of a 33,000 dalton fragment of HLA molecules, *Transplantation* **18:**74.

Tosi, R., Tanigaki, N., Centis, D., Ferrara, G.B., and Pressman, D., 1978, Immunological dissection of human Ia molecules, *J. Exp. Med.* **148:**1592.

Trucco, M.M., Stocker, J.W., and Ceppellini, R., 1978, Monoclonal antibodies against human lymphocyte antigens, *Nature (London)* **273:**666.

van Someren, H., Westerveld, A., Hagemeirjer, A., Mees, J.R., Meera Khan, P., and Zaalberg, O.B., 1974, Human antigen and enzyme markers in man–Chinese hamster somatic cell hybrids: Evidence for synteny between the HL-A, PGM_3, ME_1 and IPO-B loci, *Proc. Natl. Acad. Sci. U.S.A.* **71:**962.

Welsh, K.I., and Turner, M.J., 1976, Preparation of antisera specific for human B cells by immunization of rabbits with immune complexes, *Tissue Antigens* **8:**197.

Williams, A.F., Galfre, G., and Milstein, C., 1977, Analysis of cell surfaces by xenogeneic myeloma-hybrid antibodies: Differentiation antigens of rat lymphocytes, *Cell* **12:**683.

Wilson, B.S., Pellegrino, M.A., Reisfeld, R.A., and Ferrone, S., 1978, A simple method for production of specific xenoantisera to human histocompatibility (HLA-A, -B,-C) antigens, *Transplant. Proc.* **10:**741.

Wilson, B.S., Indiveri, F., Pellegrino, M.A., and Ferrone, S., 1979a, DR (Ia-like) antigens on human melanoma cells: Serological detection and immunochemical characterization, *J. Exp. Med.* **149:**658.

Wilson, B.S., Indiveri, F., Pellegrino, M.A., and Ferrone, S., 1979b, Production and characterization of DR xenoantisera: Use for detection of serum DR antigens, *J. Immunol.* **122:**1967.

Wilson, B.S., Indiveri, F., Molinaro, G.A., Quaranta, V., and Ferrone, S., 1980, Characterization of DR antigens on cultured melanoma cells by using monoclonal antibodies, *Transplant. Proc.* **12:**125.

Wilson, L.A., and Gallaspy, G.T., 1978, Xenoantibody directed against molecular components of the HLA system, *Transplantation* **26:**35.

Zeuthen, J., Friedrich, U., Rosen, A., and Klein, I., 1977, Structural abnormalities in chromosome 15 in cell lines with reduced expression of β_2-microglobulin, *Immunogenetics* **4:**567.

II

CHEMISTRY

15

Structural Studies of the Murine Ia Alloantigens

Richard G. Cook, J. Donald Capra, Jonathan W. Uhr, and Ellen S. Vitetta

1. Introduction

The *I* region of the murine major histocompatibility complex (MHC) regulates a variety of immune functions through the control of cellular interactions and antigen responsiveness (Benacerraf and McDevitt, 1972; reviewed in Klein, 1975; Shreffler and David, 1975; Katz, 1977). The gene products thus far demonstrated for the *I* locus are cell-surface glycoproteins, designated as the Ia (immune-associated) antigens (Shreffler *et al.*, 1974). Numerous studies have demonstrated that anti-Ia alloantisera inhibit many *I*-region-controlled immune responses. These include the induction of both T-lymphocyte proliferation (R.H. Schwartz *et al.*, 1976a, 1978a) and antibody synthesis (J.A. Frelinger *et al.*, 1975; Niederhuber and Frelinger, 1976) by certain antigens, successful collaboration among immunocompetent cells (Katz *et al.*, 1974; Pierce *et al.*, 1976; Kappler and Marrack, 1976), immune suppression (Murphy *et al.*, 1976; Tada *et al.*, 1976; Pierres *et al.*, 1978), and the induction of mixed-lymphocyte reactions (MLR) (Meo *et al.*, 1975). Thus, the Ia antigens may function as recognition units that mediate interactions among cells and/or between cells and antigen.

Functional, serological, and biochemical analyses have discriminated five *I* subregions: *I-A*, *-B*, *-J*, *-E*, and *-C* (Fig. 1) (Shreffler and David, 1975;

Richard G. Cook, J. Donald Capra, Jonathan W. Uhr, and Ellen S. Vitetta • Department of Microbiology, University of Texas Southwestern Medical School, Dallas, Texas 75235.

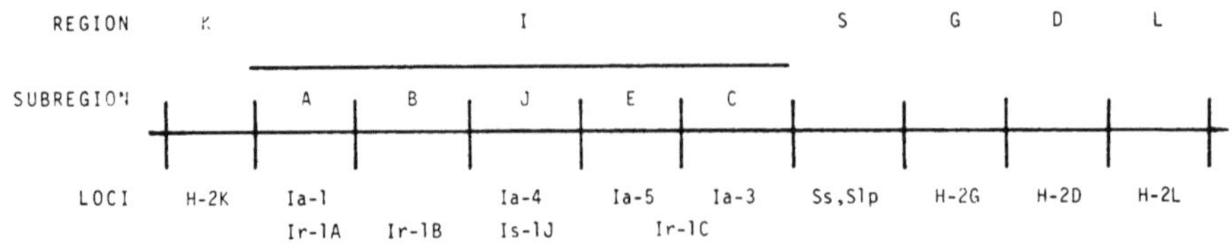

Figure 1. Genetic map of the *H-2* complex.

Shreffler *et al.*, 1976). The *I-A* subregion controls several phenotypic traits including immune-response (*Ir*) genes, determinants (Lad-1) that elicit mixed-lymphocyte reactivity (MLR) (Klein, 1975), and Ia alloantigens (Cullen *et al.*, 1976). The *I-B* subregion is defined only by *Ir* genes (Lieberman *et al.*, 1972; Sachs *et al.*, 1978); no Ia antigens have been detected for this subregion. The *Ia-4* locus (*I-J* subregion) controls surface determinants found on several subpopulations of T lymphocytes (reviewed in Murphy, 1978). These include suppressor, helper, Con-A-promoter, and MLR-stimulator T cells. Several suppressor factors also carry I-J determinants. To date, there has been no biochemical characterization of the molecule(s) carrying these determinants.

The two loci between *I-J* and *S* are designated *I-E* and *I-C*; due to the recent difficulty in distinguishing between these two loci, the terminology *I-E/C* has frequently been used. The *I-C* subregion was originally defined by *Ir* genes (Merryman and Maurer, 1974) and also by Ia serological specificities Ia.6 and 7 (David, 1976). The *I-E* subregion was defined serologically (Ia.22) by Shreffler *et al.* (1976). However, recent data from David and Cullen (1978) suggest that Ia.7 be reassigned to the *I-E* subregion, since it coprecipitates with I-E specificity 23. There has been great difficulty in detecting an I-C specific alloantigen (Ia.6); however, Delovitch *et al.* (1977) have detected two distinct molecules controlled by the I-E–I-C loci. It was not determined whether one of the antigens was encoded by *I-C*. The problems in defining an I-C alloantigen may be explained by recent data that suggest that I-C determinants are found on T cells (Okuda and David, 1978). Rich *et al.* (1978) have also found I-C determinants (Ia.6) on an MLR-suppressor factor. Alloantigens expressing Ia.7 can be immunoprecipitated independently of the I-A alloantigens (Cullen *et al.*, 1976; Delovitch *et al.*, 1977) and represent the second class of readily immunoprecipitable Ia antigens. Since the issue may not be completely resolved, for simpicity we shall consider the Ia.7-positive alloantigens as I-E/C molecules.

Thus, the *I-A* and *I-E/C* subregions encode the two predominant (at least biochemically detectable) species of Ia antigens; these molecules are found predominantly on B lymphocytes (Cullen *et al.*, 1976; Delovitch and McDevitt, 1975; Vitetta and Cook, 1979). No alloantigens have as yet been characterized for *I-J* and *I-C*, although these loci do appear to control surface determinants found on subsets of T lymphocytes.

Over the past two years, the primary structural analysis of the Ia alloantigens has been a major focus of our laboratories. The primary aim of these studies is to biochemically characterize the Ia antigens in an effort to gain insight into the molecular mechanisms through which these putative receptor molecules might function. Following a brief section on procedures utilized for isolation of Ia antigens, this chapter will present our findings on: (1) the expression of A and E/C alloantigens predominantly on B cells; (2) the primary structural characterization of the A and E/C antigens; and (3) the genetic and functional implications suggested by these studies and those of others.

2. Isolation of Ia Antigens

2.1. Radiolabeling and Sodium Dodecyl Sulfate–Polyacrylamide Gel Electrophoresis

In all our studies, the Ia antigens were isolated from radiolabeled (^{3}H, ^{14}C, or ^{125}I) splenic lysates by immunoprecipitation and sodium dodecyl sulfate–polyacrylamide gel electrophoresis (SDS-PAGE). Briefly, 2–4 × 10^{8} splenocytes from various congenic strains (Table 1) were radiolabeled for 6–8 hr with either ^{3}H (100–200 μCi/ml) or ^{14}C (10–20 μCi/ml) amino acids (Vitetta *et al.*, 1976a; Cook *et al.*, 1978a). For surface-labeling experiments, the cells were labeled with ^{125}I at 1 × 10^{8} cells/ml using

TABLE 1. Haplotypes of Mouse Strains Utilized

	H-2 haplotypes								
		I							
Strain	*K*	*A*	*B*	*J*	*E*	*C*	*S*	*G*	*D*
B10 or C57BL/6	*b*	*b*	*b*	*b*	*b*	*b*	*b*	*b*	*b*
B10.BR	*k*	*k*	*k*	*k*	*k*	*k*	*k*	*k*	*k*
B10.D2	*d*	*d*	*d*	*d*	*d*	*d*	*d*	*d*	*d*
B10.RIII	*r*	*r*	*r*	*r*	*r*	*r*	*r*	*r*	*r*
B10.P	*p*	*p*	*p*	*p*	*p*	*p*	*p*	*p*	*p*
B10.AQR	*q*	*k*	*k*	*k*	*k*	*d*	*d*	*d*	*d*
B10.A or A/J	*k*	*k*	*k*	*k*	*k*	*d*	*d*	*d*	*d*
B10.A(3R)	*b*	*b*	*b*	*b*	*k*	*d*	*d*	*d*	*d*
B10.A(5R)	*b*	*b*	*b*	*k*	*k*	*d*	*d*	*d*	*d*
B10.A(4R)	*k*	*k*	*b*	*b*	*b*	*b*	*b*	*b*	*b*
B10.HTT	*s*	*s*	*s*	*s*	*k*	*k*	*k*	*k*	*k*

the lactoperoxidase-catalyzed procedure as described (Vitetta *et al.*, 1971). Cells were centrifuged from the labeling medium, washed in Tris-buffered saline (TBS), and lysed with Nonidet P-40 (NP-40) (Cook *et al.*, 1978a). Lysates were centrifuged to remove nuclei, debris, and aggregates and either dialyzed against TBS or chromatographed on lentil lectin [*Lens culinaris* hemagglutinin (LcH)]–sepharose (Cook *et al.*, 1978b). The lysates or LcH-adherent material was cleared of Ig and nonspecific material with rabbit anti-mouse Ig (RAMIg) (Vitetta *et al.*, 1976a) and the protein-A-bearing Cowan I strain of *Staphylococcus aureus* (Kessler, 1975; Cullen and Schwartz, 1976). The I-A and I-E/C alloantigens were subsequently immunoprecipitated with alloantisera (100 μl/10^8 cell equivalents) and *S. aureus*. The alloantisera and the subregions and specificities that they detect are summarized in Table 2. Immune complexes were

TABLE 2. Description of Alloantisera

Antiserum		H-2 haplotypes[a]									I-regions detected by immunoprecipitation
			I								
Designation	Combination	*K*	*A*	*B*	*J*	*E*	*C*	*S*	*G*	*D*	
D2αA	Recipient: B10.D2	*d*	*d*	*d*	*d*	*d*	*d*	*d*	*d*	*d*	
	Donor: B10.A	*k*	*k*	*k*	*k*	*k*	*d*	*d*	*d*	*d*	*A*
HTIα5R	Recipient: (B10 ×	*b*	*b*	*b*	*b*	*b*	*b*	*b*	*b*	*b*	
	HTI)F_1	*b*	*b*	*b*	*b*	*b*	*b*	*b*	?	*d*	
	Donor: B10.A(5R)	*b*	*b*	*b*	*k*	*k*	*d*	*d*	*d*	*d*	*E*
Aα5R	Recipient: (A ×	*k*	*k*	*k*	*k*	*k*	*d*	*d*	*d*	*d*	
	B10.A)F_1	*k*	*k*	*k*	*k*	*k*	*d*	*d*	*d*	*d*	
	Donor: B10.A(5R)	*b*	*b*	*b*	*k*	*k*	*d*	*d*	*d*	*d*	*A*
A.THαA.TL	Recipient: A.TH	*s*	*s*	*s*	*s*	*s*	*s*	*s*	*s*	*s*	
	Donor: A.TL	*s*	*k*	*k*	*k*	*k*	*k*	*k*	*k*	*d*	*A,E*
HTTαA.TL	Recipient: (A.BY ×	*b*	*b*	*b*	*b*	*b*	*b*	*b*	*b*	*b*	
	B10.HTT)F_1	*s*	*s*	*s*	*s*	*k*	*k*	*k*	*k*	*d*	
	Donor: A.TL	*s*	*k*	*k*	*k*	*k*	*k*	*k*	*k*	*d*	*A*
B6αCBA	Recipient: C57BL/6	*b*	*b*	*b*	*b*	*b*	*b*	*b*	*b*	*b*	
	Donor: CBA	*k*	*k*	*k*	*k*	*k*	*k*	*k*	*k*	*k*	*E*

[a]Potential reactivities are boxed.

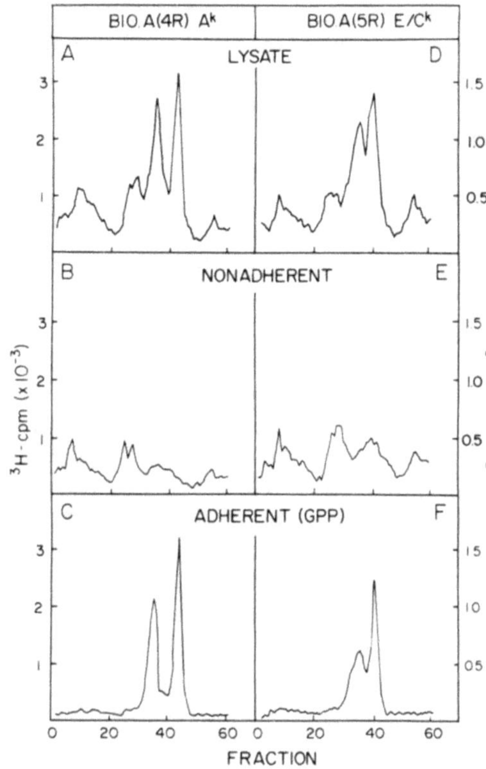

Figure 2. Comparison of Ia antigens precipitated from lysates, Lc-H-Non-adherent material, and Lc-H-adherent material. B10.A(5R) and B10.A(4R) splenocytes were labeled with [^{3}H]-Leu; one half of each lysate was chromatographed on LcH–sepharose. Equal aliquots (cell equivalents) of the lysates, nonadherent, and glycoprotein pools (GPP) were reacted with A.THαA.TL to isolate the A^k (A–C) and E/C^k (D–F) alloantigens.

eluted from the *S. aureus* with SDS solubilizing buffer and electrophoresed in the Laemmli discontinuous gel system (Laemmli, 1970; Cullen *et al.*, 1976) to resolve the α and β subunits.

2.2. Lentil Lectin Affinity Chromatography

The lentil lectin affinity chromatography step provides a simple and efficient procedure for enriching for Ia antigens, as demonstrated previously by Cullen *et al.* (1976). Approximately 5–10% of the acid-insoluble radioactive proteins adhere to the lectin column. Recoveries of the A and E/C alloantigens from the lysate and the LcH-adherent and nonadherent fractions are shown in Fig. 2 (Cook *et al.*, 1978b). B10.A(4R) and B10.A(5R) splenocytes were labeled with [^{3}H]leucine. Half of each lysate was chromatographed on LcH–sepharose; nonadherent and adherent pools were collected, concentrated, and dialyzed. After removal of Ig and nonspecific material, 100 μl A.TH anti-A.TL was added to each sample and immune complexes were removed with *S. aureus;* A.TH anti-A.TL reacts with A^k of B10.A(4R) and E/C^k of B10.A(5R). Figures 2A and

2D demonstrate that both the A and E/C products are readily precipitated from lysates. Note that the α and β chains of A separate better than those of E/C; molecular-weight markers were not coelectrophoresed in these gels, but were in subsequent experiments presented in the following sections. Ia antigens of either subregion *were not* detected in the LcH-nonadherent pools (Figs. 2-B and 2-E). It is of interest that the 45,000-dalton "nonspecific" peak observed in lysates appears to be present in the LcH-nonadherent pool. In contrast, the adherent fraction does contain α and β chains of Ia molecules (Figs. 2-C and 2-F). The background observed in the glycoprotein pool (GPP) is greatly reduced compared to that seen in the lysates.

The recoveries of Ia antigens from lysates and GPP are approximately equal. However, the decrease in the size of the α-chain peaks in the GPP may be due to the removal of nonspecific material that coelectrophoreses with the α chains. Thus, the A and E/C alloantigens (*k* haplotype) adhere to LcH; other data (not presented) revealed that all the Ia antigens analyzed in these studies adhere to lentil lectin.

2.3. Molecular-Weight Comparisons

For molecular-weight comparisons of the A and E/C antigens from different haplotypes, ^{3}H and ^{14}C double-label techniques were used to allow unambiguous detection of electrophoretic variations. In these experiments, the ^{3}H- and ^{14}C-labeled samples were mixed prior to elution from *S. aureus.* All gels were fractionated and then counted in Beckman EP cocktail in a liquid scintillation counter; using a $^{3}H/^{14}C$ ratio of 4:1 and appropriate channel discriminators, the ^{14}C cpm crossover to the ^{3}H cpm channel was negligible (<10%). [^{3}H]-IgG used as a molecular-weight marker for PAGE was prepared from secretions of P3 myeloma cells.

2.4. NH_2-Terminal Sequence Analysis

For structural analysis of these antigens, the α and β subunits were located by counting a small aliquot of each gel fraction and then extracted from the gel matrix with .05% SDS and lyophilized. For amino acid sequence analysis, the α and β subunits were dialyzed against distilled H_2O and loaded in a Beckman 890 sequencer as described (Vitetta *et al.*, 1976a; Capra *et al.*, 1976; Cook *et al.*, 1978a). The thiazolinone derivatives from samples labeled with a single amino acid were lyophilized and then counted in a liquid scintillation counter. In multiple amino acid labeling experiments, the thiazolinone derivatives from each sequencer step were converted to phenylthiohydantoin (PTH) amino acids by aqueous HCl and evaporated to dryness. These PTH amino acids were dissolved in methanol along with a standard PTH amino acid mixture and identified by high-pressure liquid chromatography (Cook *et al.*, 1978a).

2.5. Comparative Tryptic Peptide Mapping

We have also examined the A and E/C antigens for primary structural variation by comparative tryptic peptide mapping techniques (Cook *et al.*, 1979a). In these experiments, the samples were solubilized with 1–2 ml H_2O containing 1 mg human gamma-globulin (HGG) as carrier and dialyzed for 6–12 hr against 0.1 M NH_4HCO_3, pH 8.0. The molecules to be compared (e.g., [^{3}H]-E/C$^k\alpha$ and [^{14}C]-E/C$^p\alpha$) were then mixed at a ^{3}H/^{14}C cpm ratio of 3–4:1. Tos-Phe-CH_2-CL-trypsin was added in 0.001 N HCl at a ratio of 1:10 the amount of HGG. After a 1-hr incubation at 37°C, additional trypsin at a ratio of 1:20 was added and the digestion continued at 37°C for 12–16 hr. The pH was then lowered to approximately 3.0 with glacial acetic acid and the samples lyophilized. Before chromatography, peptides were solubilized in 0.05 M pyridine acetate (PA), pH 3.13, and centrifuged at 3000 rpm to remove acid-insoluble material. From 70 to 90% of the input counts per minute was recovered as acid-soluble. Tryptic peptides were separated by cation-exchange chromatography on Technicon Chromobeads Type P using a microbore column (3 mm × 150 mm) maintained at 54°C by a water jacket. Soluble peptides (1–2 ml) were loaded onto the column in 0.05 M PA, pH 3.13. After the column was washed with 5–6 ml starting buffer, a pH–ionic strength gradient was applied using a Varigard gradient maker. Forty milliters of each of the following PA buffers was used: 0.05 M, pH 3.13; 0.1 M, pH 3.54; 0.2 M, pH 4.02; 0.5 M, pH 4.50; and 2.0 M, pH 5.0 (Brown *et al.*, 1974). Twenty-drop fractions were collected into scintillation vials and the contents evaporated. Water (0.5 ml) was added to each vial for solubilization and the samples counted in a scintillation counter. The ^{3}H and ^{14}C cpm were normalized and corrected for channel spillover.

3. Surface Expression of I-A- and I-E/C-Encoded Molecules by B Lymphocytes

Unlike Ig receptors, which are confined to B cells, Ia antigens are found on numerous cell types, including sperm (Hammerling *et al.*, 1975; Delovitch *et al.*, 1978), epidermal cells (Delovitch and McDevitt, 1975; J.G. Frelinger *et al.*, 1978), macrophages (Delovitch and McDevitt, 1975; R.H. Schwartz *et al.*, 1976b), and subsets of both T (Fathman *et al.*, 1975; B.D. Schwartz *et al.*, 1977; Goding *et al.*, 1975) and B (Sachs and Cone, 1973; David *et al.*, 1973; Götze *et al.*, 1973; Press *et al.*, 1976) lymphocytes. However, like the Ig receptors, the Ia antigens have been implicated as important molecules in B-cell triggering. Thus, anti-Ia sera have been shown to block responses to TI and TD antigens and to mitogens (Marrack and Kappler, 1977; Henry and Chan, 1977; J.A. Frelinger *et al.*, 1978; Neiderhuber *et al.*, 1975). In addition, such sera can block B-cell colony formation (Kincade and Ralph, 1976), the mixed-lymphocyte culture (MLC)-stimulating activity of B cells (Meo *et al.*, 1975), and the ability of B cells to be stimulated by nonspecific T-cell factors (Marrack and Kappler, 1977).

To date, few attempts have been made to relate the distribution of Ig to antigens encoded by different *I* subregions, although recent studies by J.A. Frelinger *et al.* (1978) suggest that the majority of I-A- and I-E/C-encoded molecules are coexpressed on immunocompetent B cells. We have extended these studies by comparing the expression of surface IgM and IgD molecules to the presence of the I-A and I-E/C antigens on normal spleen cells (Vitetta and Cook, 1979). In these experiments, enzymatically radioiodinated spleen cells were treated with complement (C′) and antisera directed against I-A, I-E/C, or Ig. The dead cells were removed by sedimentation on 1*g* fetal calf serum (FCS) gradients (Goodman *et al.*, 1975; Vitetta *et al.*, 1976b). The viable small lymphocytes were recovered and lysed, and the lysates were treated with antisera directed against Ig or Ia; the complexes were absorbed to *S. aureus* (Cowan I). The supernatants of these precipitates were then treated with antisera directed against I-A, I-E/C, and H-2 and the complexes bound to *S. aureus*. Radioactivity was eluted in SDS, reduced, and electrophoresed on SDS gels by the procedures of either Maizel (1966) or Laemmli (1970). By comparing the areas under μ, δ, or Ia (α and β) peaks in the lysates of the killed vs. the control population, we were able to assess the effect of deleting a population bearing one specific marker on the recovery of molecules from the remaining viable cells. These studies were confined to small lymphocytes and did not take into account either large lymphocytes, plasma cells, or macrophages, all of which sediment with the dead cells in the 1 *g* gradients.

3.1. Effect of Anti-Ig + C′ on the Recovery of Cells Bearing IgM and IgD

The first series of experiments determined whether the anti-Ig sera were effective in deleting Ig^+ (B) cells. In these experiments, we examined the surface Ig's on small lymphocytes that survived treatment with anti-Ig + C′. In seven experiments, anti-Ig + C′ killed 36–63% of the radioiodinated cells. As described previously (Vitetta *et al.*, 1976b), and as shown in Fig. 3, no Ig could be precipitated from lysates of the surviv-

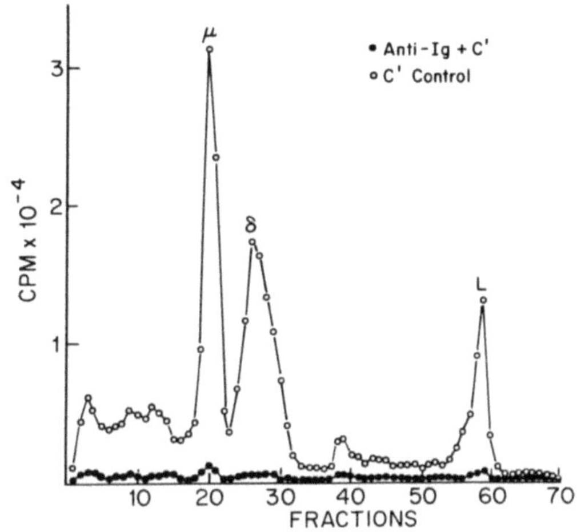

Figure 3. Effect of eliminating Ig⁺ cells on the recovery of cell-surface Ig (IgM and IgD) from surviving small lymphocytes. Radio-iodinated B10.A(5R) spleen cells were treated with anti-Ig + C′ and the dead cells were eliminated on 1*g* gradients. The viable small lymphocytes were lysed and the lysates precipitated with anti-Ig and *S. aureus*. Immune complexes were eluted, reduced, mixed with [^{3}H]-μ and L chains, and electrophoresed on 7.5% gels.

ing cells. These experiments suggest that virtually all Ig-bearing cells can be eliminated by treatment with anti-Ig + C′.

3.2. Effect of Anti-Ig + C′ on the Recovery of Cells Bearing I-A and I-E/C Antigens

To determine whether the elimination of Ig^+ cells resulted in the loss of I-A and I-E/C molecules, radioiodinated 4R or 5R spleen cells were treated with anti-Ig + C′, and the lysates of the viable small lymphocytes were examined by immunoprecipitation for I-A and I-E/C molecules. It should be noted that enzymatic radioiodination of intact cells labels only the β chains of Ia molecules, whereas biosynthetic labeling labels both α and β chains (B.D. Schwartz *et al.*, 1978). As indicated in Fig. 4, there was a 95% reduction in radioactive I-A and I-E/C in the lysates of the surviving cells. These results confirm previous studies showing that the majority of Ia antigens are expressed on B cells and indicate that the I-A- and I-E/C-encoded molecules are present almost exclusively on Ig^+ cells. These studies did not, however, indicate whether some Ig^+ cells bear I-A and others bear I-E/C or whether both Ia antigens are present on the same Ig^+ cells.

3.3. Effect of Anti-I-A or Anti-I-E/C + C′ on the Recovery of Cells Bearing IgM and IgD

In experiments described above, we had demonstrated that the elimination of Ig^+ cells resulted in the loss of cells bearing I-A and I-E/C. The reverse experiments were performed to determine whether elimination of

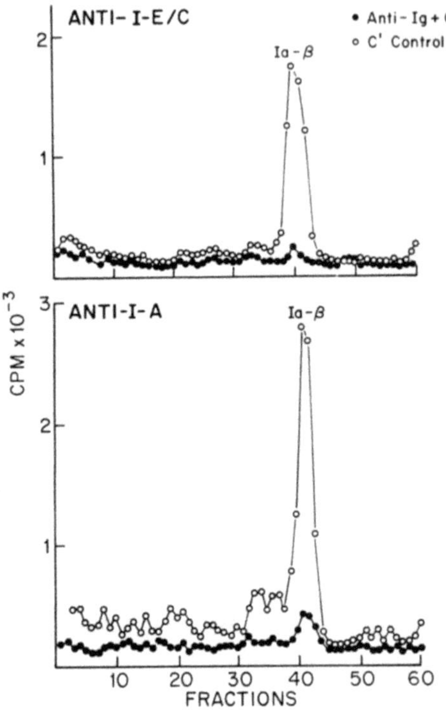

Figure 4. Effect of eliminating Ig$^+$ cells on the recovery of cell-surface I-E/C (top panel) and I-A (bottom panel) molecules from surviving small lymphocytes. The experiment in the top panel was performed with 5R cells, the experiment in the bottom panel with 4R cells. Both lysates were precleared with RAMIg and *S. aureus*. I-E/C and I-A molecules were precipitated with A.THαA.TL and *S. aureus* and electrophoresed on 7.5% gels.

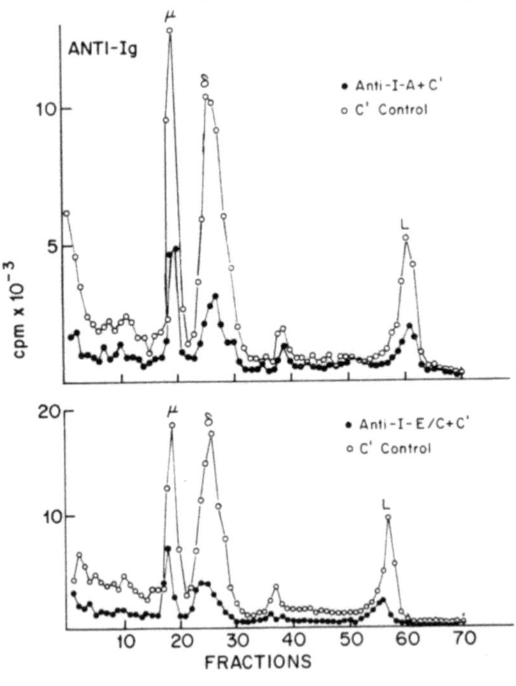

Figure 5. Effect of eliminating I-A$^+$ cells (top panel) or I-E/C$^+$ cells (bottom panel) on the recovery of cell-surface Ig from surviving small lymphocytes. The experiments in the top panel were performed with B10.BR cells and HTTαATL serum, the experiments in the bottom panel with 5R cells and HTIα5R serum. Both lysates were treated with anti-Ig and *S. aureus* and the immunoprecipitates electrophoresed on 7.5% gels.

cells bearing I-A or I-E/C resulted in a parallel loss of Ig+ cells. When radioiodinated 5R and B10.BR cells were treated with either anti-I-A or anti-I-E/C + C′, radioactive IgM and IgD were reduced by approximately 65% (Fig. 5), indicating that some of the Ig+ cells (bearing IgM and IgD) lack sufficient quantities of I-A or I-E/C to be deleted by the anti-Ia sera + C′.

3.4. Effect of Anti-I-A or Anti-I-E/C + C′ on the Recovery of I-A or I-E/C Antigens from Surviving Cells

To determine whether I-A and I-E/C molecules are on the same cell, radioiodinated B10.BR splenocytes were treated with anti-I-A + C′. The surviving small lymphocytes were lysed and treated with antisera directed against H-2K and I-A or H-2K and I-E/C. The use of an antiserum con-

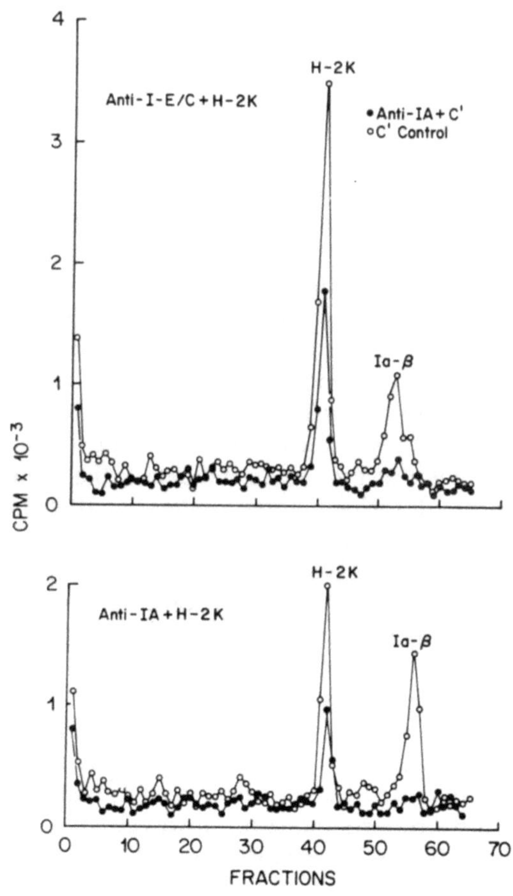

Figure 6. Effect of eliminating I-A+ cells on the recovery of cell-surface I-E/C and H-2K (top panel) and I-A and H-2K (bottom panel) from surviving cells. B10.BR cells were treated with HTTαA.TL + C′. Lysates were precleared with RAMIg, and the supernatant was precipitated with B6αCBA (top panel) or D2αA (bottom panel) and *S. aureus* and the immunoprecipitate electrophoresed on 7.5% gels.

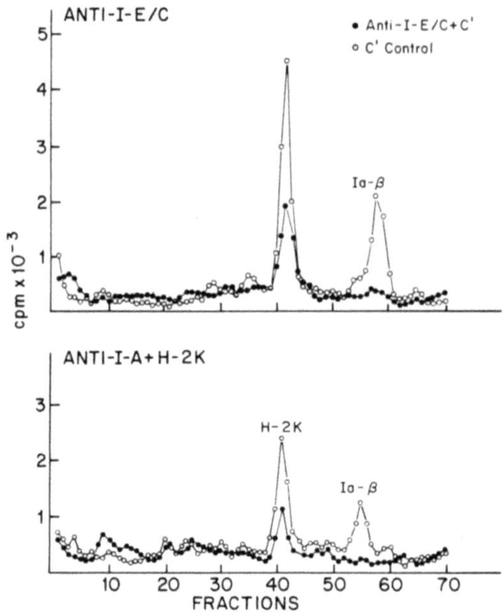

Figure 7. Effect of eliminating I-E/C$^+$ cells on the recovery of cell-surface I-E/C (top panel) and I-A and H-2K (bottom panel) from surviving cells. B10.A(5R) cells were treated with HTIα5R + C′. The lysate was precleared with RAMIg and *S. aureus*; the supernatant was precipitated with A.THαA.TL (top panel) or Aα5R (bottom panel) and the immunoprecipitate electrophoresed on 7.5% gels. The nature of the 44K material in the top panel is unclear.

taining anti-H-2K as well as anti-Ia activity represented a quantitative control in that approximately 50% of the H-2K molecules should be present on T cells and not eliminated by the anti-Ia + C′. As can be seen in Fig. 6, the elimination of I-A$^+$ cells resulted in a greater than 95% loss of I-E/C molecules, clearly demonstrating that the two *I*-subregion-encoded molecules are expressed on the *same* cells. In both instances, the H-2 peak was reduced by approximately 50%, reflecting the molecules present on the surviving T cells.

The reverse experiment, using anti-I-E/C + C′ on ^{125}I-labeled cells, is shown in Fig. 7. As indicated, the results are analogous to the experiments described above, indicating that the majority of I-A and I-E/C are expressed on the same cells.

The observation that the majority of Ia antigens are expressed and synthesized by B cells is consistent with many previous reports. In addition, our findings are also consistent with studies that have shown that some Ig$^+$ cells either lack Ia antigens or express very low densities of Ia molecules (Press *et al.*, 1976).

Our results suggest that all I-A and I-E/C molecules are expressed exclusively by Ig$^+$ cells. However, a number of published reports have documented the expression of Ia antigens on T cells and macrophages. Those reports indicate, however, that the subpopulations of T cells that bear Ia can be minor ones and that both the Ia$^+$ T cells and Ia$^+$ macrophages bear low densities of I-A, I-E/C, or I-J antigens. It is therefore possible that the amounts of Ia on these subsets would not be detected in our assay. Moreover, although some of our sera could have anti-I-J activity, I-J antigens have not yet been detected by immunoprecipitation.

Our studies do not address the question of the function of I-A and I-E/C molecules on B cells. Nevertheless, the expression of both subregion molecules on the same cells raises provocative questions concerning their function. Thus, there is considerable evidence, particularly at the T cell–macrophage level, that Ia antigens are the products of *Ir* genes and that Ia molecules play a major role in cell–cell recognition and, possibly, antigen presentation (Katz and Benacerraf, 1975; R.H. Schwartz *et al.*, 1978b; Rosenthal, 1978). However, at present, the relationship between *Ir* genes and Ia antigens in the B cell is unclear. It is puzzling that most examples of *Ir* gene control appear to be at the macrophage–T cell level, whereas I-A and I-E/C antigens are expressed almost exclusively on B cells. Further functional and biochemical studies will be required to resolve this paradox.

4. Structural Analysis of the I-A Alloantigens

Most of the serological polymorphism detected for the *I*-region alloantigens can be mapped to the *A* subregion; at least 11 of the 23 defined Ia specificities are controlled by this subregion (Shreffler and David, 1975; Klein *et al.*, 1978; B.D. Schwartz and Cullen, 1978). Most of the standard *H-2* haplotypes express an I-A alloantigen, and like the H-2 K and D alloantigens, both public and private specificities have been demonstrated.

4.1. General Structural Features

We have examined the A^k, A^b, and A^d alloantigens for electrophoretic variation by SDS-PAGE using sensitive double-label (^3H and ^{14}C) techniques (Cook *et al.*, 1978b). Under reducing conditions, the α- and β-subunit apparent molecular weights for all three of these products are 34,000 and 26,000 daltons, respectively. The α and β chains of A^k coelectrophorese with those of A^b (Fig. 8A) and A^d (not shown). Identical patterns have been observed for A alloantigens immunoprecipitated from both lysates and LcH-adherent material. These molecular weights are consistent with the molecular-weight ranges for Ia antigens reported by others (Cullen *et al.*, 1976; Silver *et al.*, 1976; Jones, 1977).

Analysis of these *A*-subregion products on SDS-PAGE under nonreducing conditions revealed a dominant peak (~80%) at 65,000 daltons

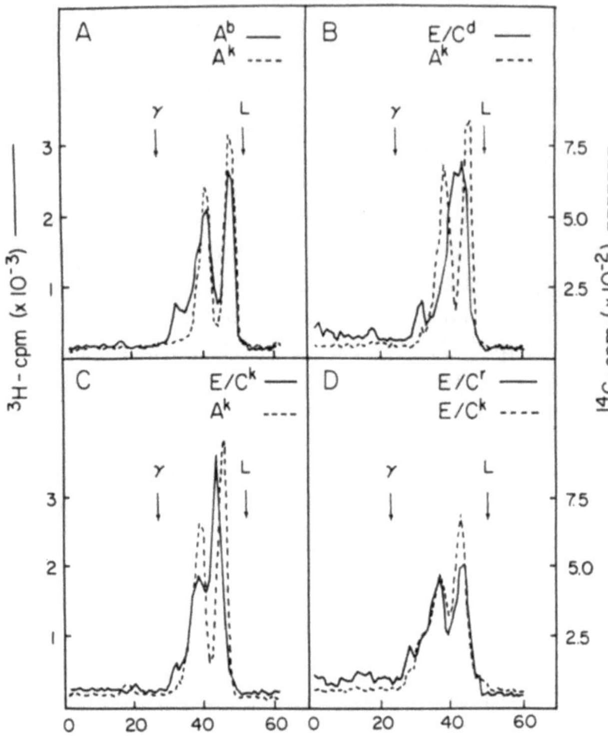

Figure 8. SDS-PAGE analysis of *A*- and *E/C*-subregion products precipitated from glycoprotein pools. Appropriate ^3H (——) and ^{14}C (----) immunoprecipitates from designated strains were mixed, solubilized in the presence of 2-ME, and electrophoresed on 12.5% gels. ^{14}C-labeled B10.A(4R) precipitated with A.THαA.TL is compared to [^3H]-B10.A(5R) precipitated with Aα5R (Fig. 8A, A^b vs. A^k); [^3H]-B10.D2 precipitated with HTIα5R (Fig. 8B, E/C^d vs. A^k); [^3H]-B10.BR precipitated with HTIα5R (Fig. 8C, E/C^k v. A^k). In Fig. 8D, [^{14}C]-B10.BR precipitated with HTIα5R is compared to ^3H-RIII/2J precipitated with HTIα5R (E/C^r vs. E/C^k).

and minor peaks (~ 20%) at 34,000 (α) and 26,000 (β) daltons. A similar finding has been reported by Cullen *et al.* (1976). However, the possibility exists that the disulfide bonding of the α and β chains of I-A was an artifact generated during detergent lysis, as has been described for the apparent dimerization of the murine H-2 alloantigen (Henning *et al.*, 1976). To test this possibility, B10.A(4R) splenocytes were labeled with [^3H]leucine, centrifuged from the labeling medium, and divided into equal aliquots. One aliquot was suspended in TBS (control) and the other in TBS containing 10 mM iodoacetamide to alkylate free sulfhydryl groups. After 15 min at 4°C, both cell suspensions were centrifuged and lysed in TBS–NP-40 (control) or TBS–NP-40 containing 100 mM iodoacetamide.

Glycoprotein pools were then prepared from each by LcH affinity chromatography, and the I-A^k alloantigens were immunoprecipitated and analyzed by SDS-PAGE under reducing and nonreducing conditions. Results are shown in Fig. 9; Figs. 9A and 9C show that under normal lysing conditions, the α and β chains are disulfide-bonded (mol. wt. 65,000 daltons) and that reduction generates α and β polypeptides. Under nonreducing conditions, a small proportion (~20%) of the molecules are not disulfide-bonded. However, as shown in Fig. 9-B, lysis in the presence of an alkylating agent and electrophoresis in the absence of 2-mercaptoethanol (2-ME) results in the total disappearance of the $\alpha-\beta$ dimer and the appearance of only α and β chains; electrophoresis in the presence of reducing agent yields a similar profile (Fig. 9D).

Therefore, the disulfide-bonded $\alpha-\beta$ dimer appears to be an artifact generated during detergent lysis. A similar finding has been reported by B.D. Schwartz and Cullen (1978). That the 65,000-dalton peak indeed consists of α and β chains is shown in Fig. 10. The 65,000-dalton peak (Fig. 9A) was eluted from the gel matrix, lyophilized, solubilized in sample buffer with or without 2-ME, and electrophoresed on 12.5% gels. In the absence of reducing agent, the 65,000-dalton peak remains intact (Fig. 10A), and reduction generates α and β chains (Fig. 10B). The $\alpha-\beta$ dimerization of the A^b and A^d products can also be prevented by pretreatment and lysis in the presence of alkylating agents (not shown). Thus, the allelic A^k, A^b, and A^d alloantigens appear identical with respect to subunit molecular weight and the tendency of the α and β chains to form disulfide-bonded dimers.

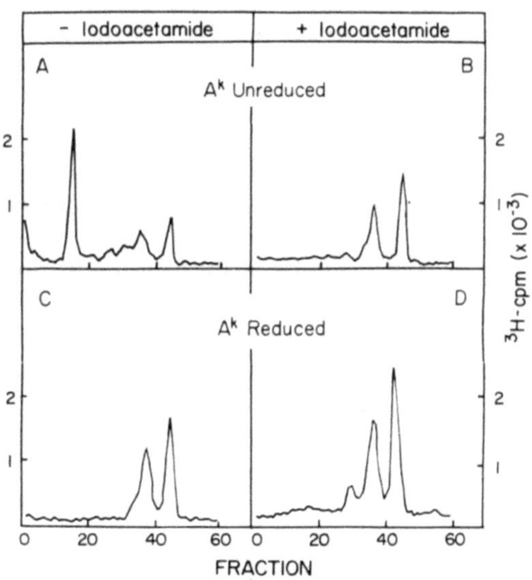

Figure 9. Effect of iodoacetamide in the lysis buffer on the molecular association of I-A^k molecules. B10.A(4R) splenocytes were radiolabeled and lysed with or without iodoacetamide. Glycoprotein pools were prepared by LcH affinity chromatography. Equal aliquots (cell equivalents) of each were precipitated with A.THαA.TL and the precipitates solubilized with or without 2-ME and analyzed on SDS-PAGE (12.5% gels).

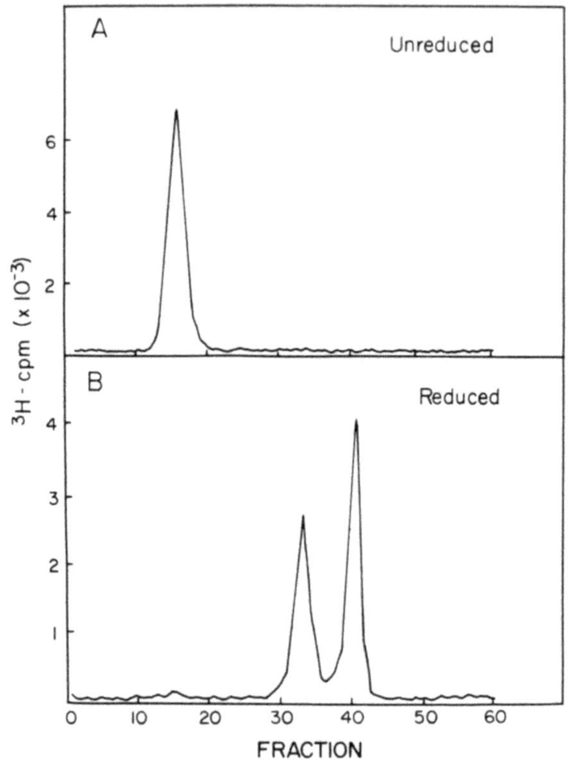

Figure 10. Generation of α and *β* chains by reduction of the 65,000-dalton I-A product. B10.A(4R) splenocytes were radiolabeled, lysed without iodoacetamide, and chromatographed on LcH–sepharose. The *A*-subregion product was precipitated with A.THαA.TL and electrophoresed without reduction on 12.5% gels. The 65,000-dalton peak was collected, lyophilized, resuspended in sample buffer with or without 2-ME, and electrophoresed on 12.5% gels.

4.2. NH_2-Terminal Sequence Analysis

At the primary structural level, the I-A (also I-E/C) allelic products are currently being analyzed by comparative tryptic peptide mapping and by NH_2-terminal sequence analysis. It is hoped that with the use of these procedures, the extent and nature of allelic variation that exists in these molecules can be deduced.

We have examined the α and β subunits of the A^k and A^b alleles by NH_2-terminal sequencing (Cook *et al.*, 1978c, 1979b). As shown in Table 3, there is no detectable allelic variation between the *k* and *b* α polypeptides, although only 6 assignments could be made in the first 20 residues of these molecules. The other positions are apparently occupied

TABLE 3. Partial NH_2-Terminal Amino Acid Sequences of I-A Alloantigens[a]

	1	2	3	4	5	6	7	8	9	10	11	12	13	14	15	16	17	18	19	20
A^b_α				ILE		ALA			VAL			TYR				VAL	TYR			
A^k_α				ILE		ALA			VAL			TYR				VAL	TYR			
A^b_β			SER		ARG	HIS	PHE	VAL	TYR		PHE	—	—	—		TYR	PHE			
A^k_β			SER		ARG	HIS	PHE	VAL	—		PHE	PRO	PRO	PHE		TYR	PHE			

[a]Dashes at positions 9, 12, 13, and 14 of the β polypeptides indicate sequence differences between A^k and A^b. These haplotype-associated differences are also boxed.

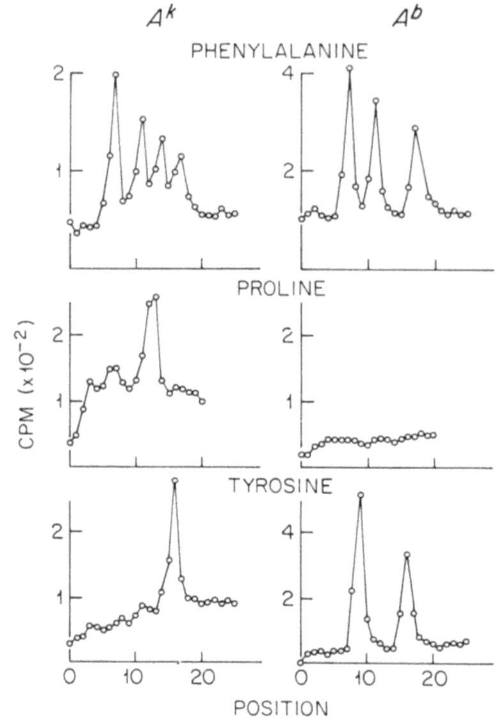

Figure 11. Sequence analysis of the β polypeptides of A^k and A^b. Profiles are presented only for those amino acids that differ between *k* and *b* haplotypes.

by those amino acids (glycine, glutamic, and aspartic acids and glutamine and asparagine) that cannot be adequately incorporated into normal splenocytes. Signficant allelic variation was, however, demonstrated in the β polypeptides at positions 9, 12, 13, and 14; sequencer profiles showing these allelic differences are depicted in Fig. 11. McMillan *et al.* (1978) have also examined the A^k and A^b antigens for NH_2-terminal sequence, and although their data are less complete, the results are completely consistent with ours—NH_2-terminal sequence differences are evident only in the β subunits.

4.3. Comparative Tryptic Peptide Mapping

The A^k and A^b alloantigens have also been compared by tryptic peptide mapping, which is a powerful tool for gaining insight into the structural relatedness among proteins. While allelic variation was shown only for the A β subunits by NH_2-terminal sequencing, peptide mapping of these molecules demonstrates allelic structural variation for both the α and β polypeptides (Fig. 12). As shown in the top panel, the A^k and A^b α subunits differ significantly; only 55% of their tryptic peptides coelute.

The β chains (bottom panel) also show considerable allelic variation, having only 40% coelution of tryptic peptides. Preliminary data comparing the A^k and A^d alloantigens indicate that a similar degree of variation also exists in the α and β subunits of these allelic products. It must be pointed out that this technique does tend to overestimate the degree of structural variation between molecules. For example, a single amino acid substitution in a peptide could alter its charge such that it elutes from the ion-exchange column at a different position. Generally, a 40–50% homology by peptide mapping techniques represents an 80–90% homology by amino acid sequence.

Since allelic variation can be demonstrated by peptide mapping for both the α and β subunits of the A alloantigens (*k* and *b* haplotypes), it appears that both subunits are encoded by or at least controlled by the MHC. The use of congenic strains of mice having the same "background genes" and differing only at their MHC allows one to dismiss non-MHC genes as being the reason for these allelic differences. NH_2-terminal se-

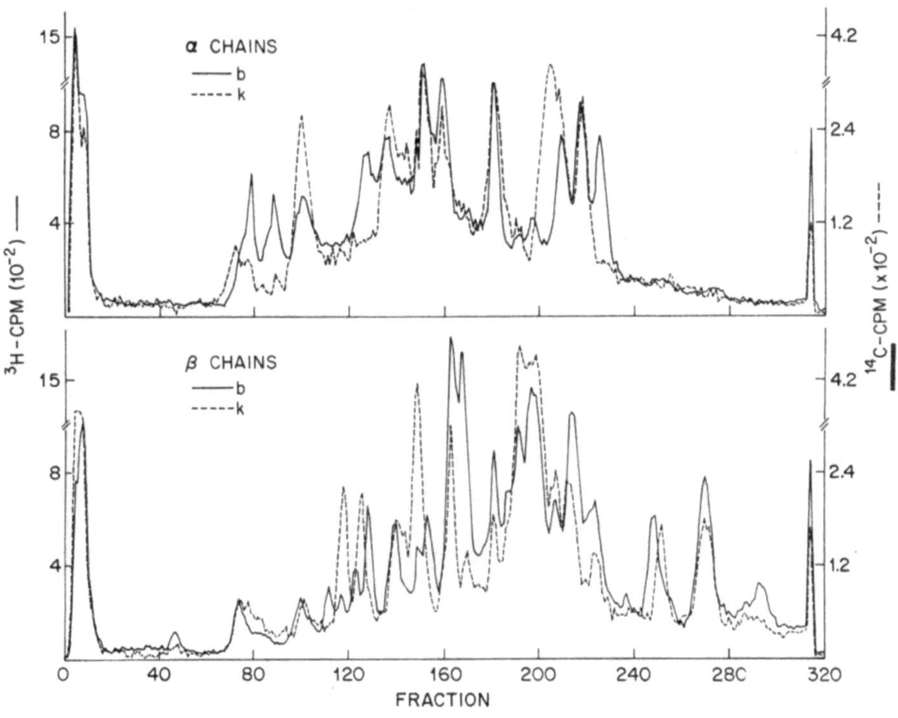

Figure 12. Ion-exchange chromatography of tryptic digests of the α (top panel) and β (bottom panel) subunits of the A^k and A^b alloantigens. ^{3}H-labeled A^b α and β subunits are compared with ^{14}C-labeled A^k α and β subunits.

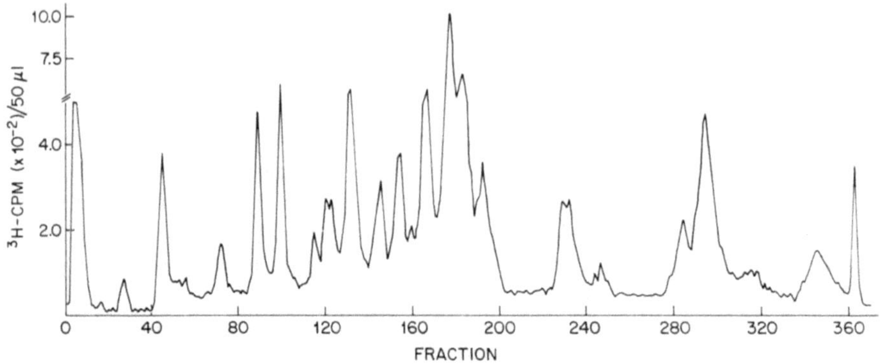

Figure 13. Representative tryptic peptide map utilized for the isolation of peptides for sequencing. The AK β chain was isolated from B10.A(4R) splenocytes labeled with [^{3}H]-Arg, Lys, Phe, Leu, His, and Val.

quence analysis has thus far detected differences only in the β subunits. Preliminary experiments utilizing peptide analysis of the A alloantigens from appropriate intra-*I*-region recombinants indicate that both the α and β subunits are controlled or encoded by the *I-A* subregion (data not presented).

A current project in our laboratories is the determination of the complete amino acid sequence of the A^k β subunit. Even though technical limitations of radioisotopic labeling will probably not allow the assignment of all residues, we feel that enough of the sequence can be ascertained to allow meaningful comparisons with allelic products that will subsequently be examined. It is hoped that this type of comparison will elucidate the extent and nature of primary structural variation that exists in these polypeptides. By radiolabeling with a mixture of amino acids, sufficient radioactivity can be recovered in peptides, generated by enzymatic cleavage, to allow an accurate amino acid sequence determination. Figure 13 shows a representative tryptic peptide map utilized for the isolation of peptides for sequencing. Unfortunately, at present, the amino acid assignments in these peptides are too sparse to merit inclusion in this chapter; however, the data derived by these techniques are thus far entirely reproducible and should in the near future be informative.

5. Structural Analysis of the I-E/C Alloantigens

In contrast to the *I-A* subregion, only four serological specificities have been defined for the *I-E/C* subregion (Shreffler *et al.*, 1976; David and Cullen, 1978; Klein *et al.*, 1978). These include a public specificity,

Ia.7, that is carried by all serologically detectable E/C alloantigens, and three private specificities, Ia.21, 22, and 23, found on the *p, k,* and *d* allelic products, respectively. No I-E/C alloantigens have been detected for the *b, f, q,* and *s* haplotypes.

5.1. General Structural Features

We have characterized four allelic E/C alloantigens (*k, r, p,* and *d*) with respect to the apparent molecular weights of their α and β subunits (Cook *et al.*, 1978b). As shown in Fig. 8, there are differences in the molecular weights of the α and β polypeptides of the E/C antigens (reducing conditions). The A^k subunits are compared with those of E/C^d in Fig. 8B and with those of E/C^k in Fig. 8C. The E/C^d and also E/C^p (not shown) α and β subunits do not coelectrophorese with those of A^k and have apparent molecular weights of 31,000 and 29,000 daltons. The other two E/C antigens analyzed, E/C^k and E/C^r, have similar subunit molecular weights of 34,000 and 28,000 daltons (Fig. 8D). A summary of the apparent molecular weights of the E/C and also the A alloantigens is shown in Table 4. Thus, quite surprisingly, there appears to be allelic or haplotype-associated molecular-weight variation in the E/C α and β subunits. These molecular-weight differences among the E/C antigens may be due to primary structural variation within the polypeptide portions of the molecules, differing degrees of glycosylation, or postsynthetic processing of precursor forms.

To test the latter possibility, mixing experiments were performed in an effort to detect postsynthetic events that might be limited to a particular subregion or haplotype (data not shown). A glycoprotein pool containing $[^3H]$-E/C^k (or E/C^r) was mixed with an *unlabeled* lysate containing E/C^p (or E/C^d). The E/C molecules were then immunoprecipitated and analyzed by SDS-PAGE. If post synthetic processing was responsible for the haplotype-associated molecular-weight variation, the α and β chains of E/C^k (34,000 and 28,000) should be converted to molecular weights of 31,000 and 29,000 daltons observed for E/C^p molecules. However, the

TABLE 4. Summary of Ia Molecular Weights

I-subregion product	Haplotypes	Molecular weights (daltons) α Chain	β Chain
A	*k, b, d*	34,000	26,000
E/C	*k, r*	34,000	28,000
E/C	*p, d*	31,000	29,000

E/C^k and E/C^r α and β chains retained molecular weights of 34,000 and 28,000, respectively. The reciprocal experiment ([^{3}H]-E/C^p mixed with unlabeled E/C^k) also revealed no molecular-weight discrepancies—E/C^p (and E/C^d) α and β chains remained poorly separated with molecular weights of 31,000 and 29,000 daltons. These experiments are by no means rigorous and conclusive, but suggest that the differences are not explicable by proteolytic processing.

We examined the possibility that carbohydrate may be influencing apparent molecular weight by electrophoresis of radiolabeled I-E/C antigens on gels of different percentage acrylamide. Varying degrees of glycosylation among the α and β subunits should be reflected by changes in apparent molecular weight. Electrophoresis on 10, 12.5, and 15% gels revealed no detectable molecular-weight shifts in either the α or β subunits. However, these experiments are not sufficient evidence to rule out a carbohydrate influence. A definitive answer as to whether varying degrees of glycosylation or differences within the polypeptide portions of the molecule are responsible for the molecular-weight shifts must ultimately await amino acid sequence analysis.

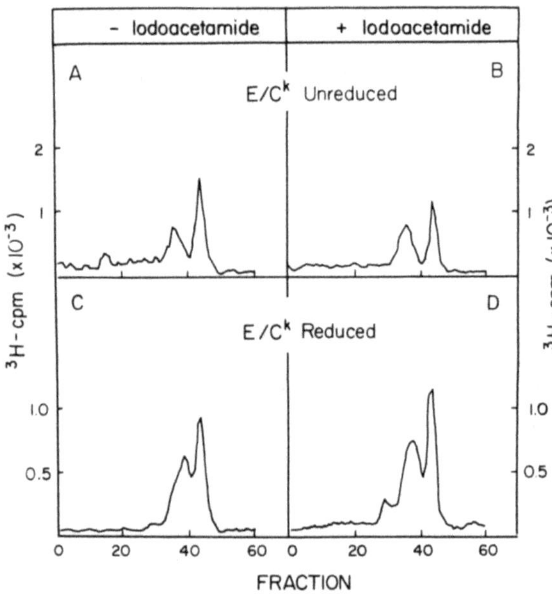

Figure 14. Effect of iodoacetamide in the lysis buffer on the molecular association of I-E/C^k molecules. B10.A(5R) splenocytes were radiolabeled and lysed with or without iodoacetamide. Glycoprotein pools were prepared by LcH affinity chromatography. Equal aliquots (cell equivalents) of each were precipitated with A.THαA.TL and the precipitates solubilized with or without 2-ME and analyzed on SDS-PAGE (12.5% gels).

TABLE 5. Partial NH_2-Terminal Amino Acid Sequences of I-E/C Alloantigens[a]

	1	2	3	4	5	6	7	8	9	10	11	12	13	14	15	16	17	18	19	20	21	22
E/C^k_α	ILE	LYS			HIS	THR	ILE	ILE		ALA		PHE	TYR	LEU	LEU	PRO			ARG			PHE
E/C^r_α	ILE	LYS			HIS	*	ILE	ILE		*		PHE	TYR	LEU	LEU	*			ARG			PHE
E/C^k_β	VAL	ARG		SER	ARG	PRO		PHE	LEU		TYR	—	LYS	SER				PHE	TYR			
E/C^r_β	VAL	ARG		SER	ARG	PRO		PHE	LEU		TYR	SER	THR	SER				PHE	TYR			

[a]The asterisks at positions 6, 10, and 16 of the E/C^r α polypeptide indicate that THR, ALA, and PRO were not tested. The dash at position 12 of the E/C^k β polypeptide indicates that SER is not present. Haplotype-associated differences between the β polypeptides of E/C^k and E/C^r are boxed.

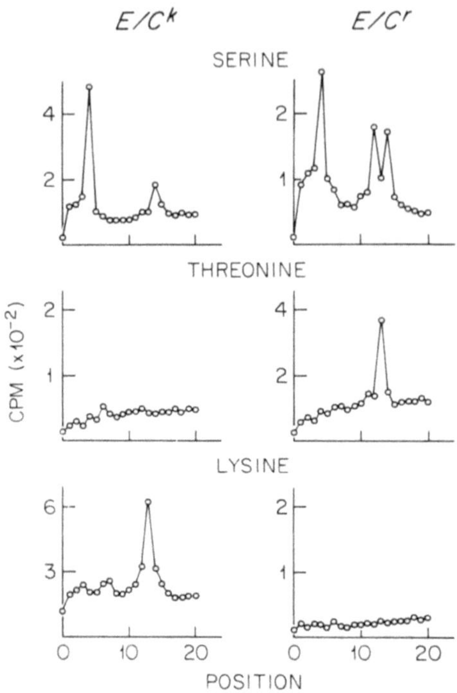

Figure 15. Sequence analysis of the β polypeptides of E/C^k and E/C^r. Profiles only are presented for those amino acids that differ between *k* and *r* haplotypes.

Unlike the A alloantigens, the E/C α and β subunits do not disulfide bond to form dimers under normal detergent lysing conditions (Cook *et al.*, 1978b; B.D. Schwartz and Cullen, 1978). As shown in Fig. 14, the E/C^k [also E/C^p, E/C^d, and E/C^r (not shown)] alloantigens migrate as free α and β chains under nonreducing conditions, in the presence and in the absence of iodoacetamide. In the unreduced form, the α and β subunits of the E/C antigens appear to resolve better; this has also been observed by Silver *et al.* (1979), who found the molecular weight of the unreduced β chain to be 24,000 daltons. This is probably due to an intrachain disulfide bond in the β chain that in the unreduced state gives the molecule a more compact conformation and thus a lower apparent molecular weight. Structural variations such as this could also explain the molecular-weight differences observed between the E/C allelic products.

5.2. NH_2-Terminal Sequence Analysis

The NH_2-terminal sequences of the α and β subunits of the E/C^k and E/C^r alloantigens are shown in Table 5 (Cook *et al.*, 1979b). No differences were detected between the α polypeptides, although we were unable to sufficiently incorporate threonine, alanine, and proline into the E/C^r α subunits. The β subunits of *r* and *k* show haplotype-associated variation at positions 12 and 13 (Fig. 15). McMillan *et al.* (1978) and

Allison *et al.* (1978) have examined the E/C^k and E/C^d antigens and found no variation between the α chains, but did find a difference in the β polypeptides—E/C^d β has a valine at position 12 while E/C^k β does not. Our analysis of the E/C^r β subunit demonstrates a serine at position 12; therefore, the chains of E/C^k, E/C^d, and E/C^r all differ at this position. Thus, as with the *A*-subregion alloantigens, NH_2-terminal sequence variation between the E/C allelic products can be detected only in the β subunits.

5.3. Comparative Tryptic Peptide Mapping

The E/C alloantigens from *k, r, p,* and *d* haplotypes have also been examined structurally by comparative peptide mapping of tryptic peptides (Cook *et al.*, 1979a). Antisera against Ia.7 (HTIα5R) were used to immunoprecipitate all these E/C products. SDS-PAGE gel profiles shown in Fig. 16 demonstrate that the α and β subunits from all four haplotypes are well resolved; E/C^p and E/C^d were electrophoresed on 10% gels,

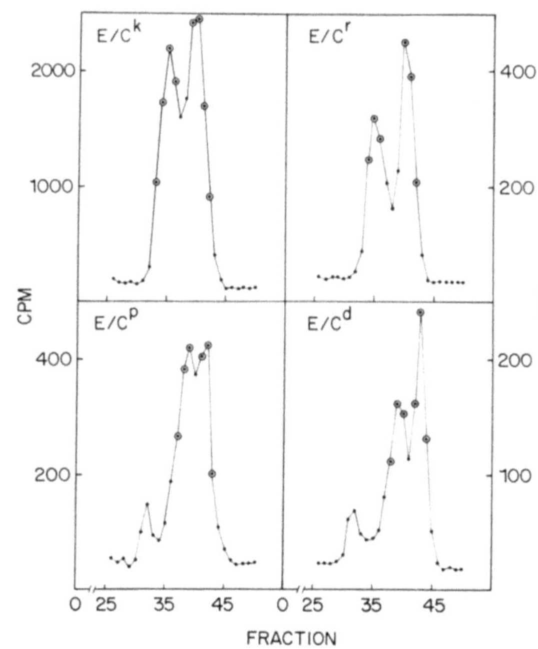

Figure 16. SDS-PAGE analysis of *E/C*-subregion products precipitated from glycoprotein pools with HTIα5R, B10.BR splenocytes (E/C^k) were labeled with [^{3}H]-L,Y,K,R; B10.RIII (E/C^r), B10.P (E/C^p), and B10.D2 (E/C^d) splenocytes were labeled with [^{14}C]-L,Y,K,R. E/C^k and E/C^r subunits were separated on 12.5% gels, and E/C^p and E/C^d on 10% gels. Points for the fractions pooled for α and β subunits are circled.

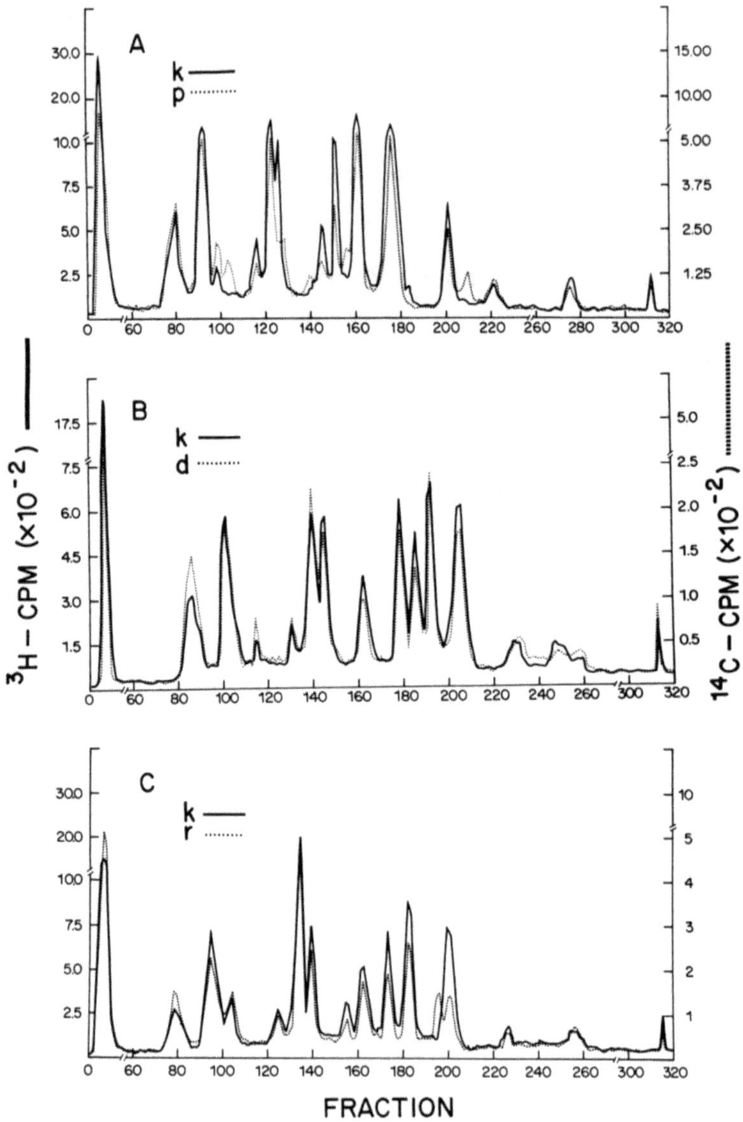

Figure 17. Ion-exchange chromatography of tryptic digests of E/C α polypeptides. ^{3}H-labeled E/C^{k} α chains are compared with ^{14}C-labeled E/C^{p} (A), E/C^{d} (B), and E/C^{r} (C) α chains.

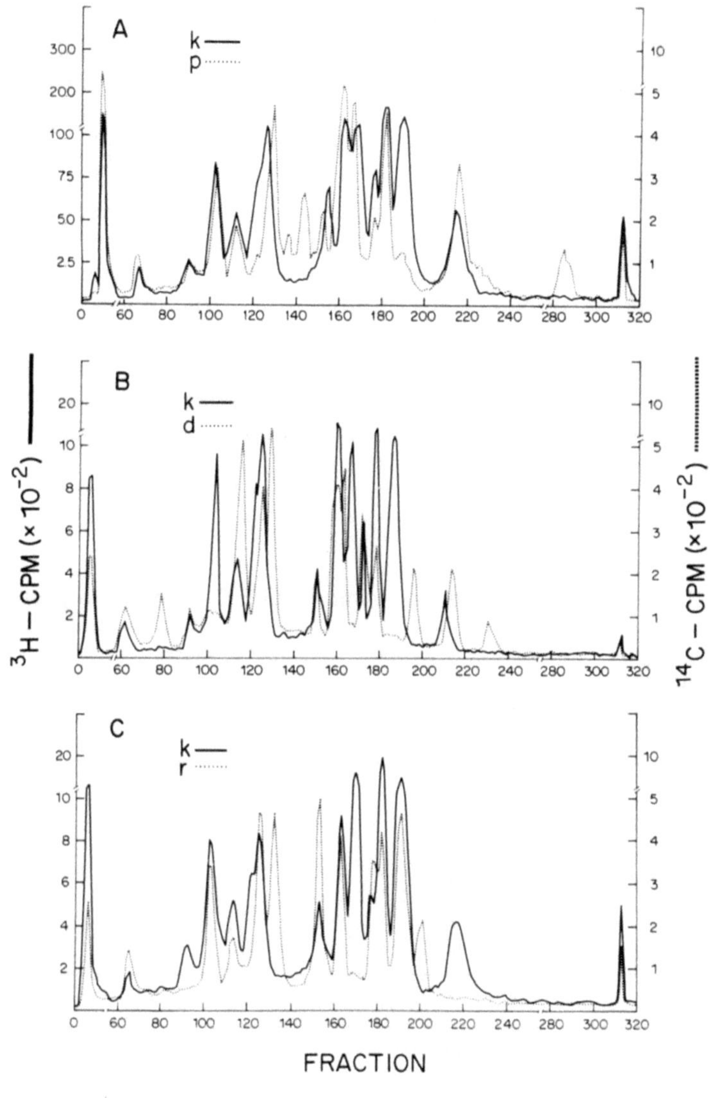

Figure 18. Ion-exchange chromatography of tryptic digests of E/C β polypeptides. ^{3}H-labeled E/C^k β chains are compared with ^{14}C-labeled E/C^p (A), E/C^d (B), and E/C^r (C) β chains.

which seem to yield a better resolution of the α and β subunits. In Figs. 17 and 18, the α and β subunits of ^{3}H-labeled E/C^k are compared with those of ^{14}C-labeled E/C^p, E/C^d, and E/C^r. Little variation was detected in the α chains—E/C^k α tryptic peptides showed approximately 84, 93, and 97% coincidence of elution with E/C^p, E/C^d, and E/C^r. In contrast, the E/C β-chain peptide comparisons showed a remarkable degree of allelic variation (Fig. 18). The β-chain tryptic peptides from E/C^k displayed only 48% coelution with E/C^p and E/C^d, and 69% coelution with E/C^r (Table 6). Utilizing isoelectric focusing to separate tryptic peptides, Silver *et al.* (1979) have reported similar findings. These authors examined E/C^k and E/C^d and could detect peptide variation only in the β subunits. Thus, by this technique, the α polypeptides exhibit little structural variation, as is observed for classic allelic products; the β chains, on the other hand, are quite dissimilar and contain structural variation not typically found for most alleles. This same degree of variation between alleles was observed for the *A* subregion α *and* β chains (*k* and *b* haplotypes) and also for the H-2 K and D alloantigens (Brown *et al.*, 1974).

TABLE 6. Tryptic Peptide Comparisons of E/C α and β Polypeptides

E/C-subregion haplotype	Number of tryptic peptides	Number of shared peptides	Percentage coincidence[a]
	α Chains		
k *p*	14 17	13	84
k *d*	14 14	13	93
k *r*	14 15	14	97
	β Chains		
k *p*	14 15	7	48
k *d*	14 15	7	48
d *r*	14 12	9	69

[a]Percentage coincidence was determined by the following formula: (number of shared peptides/average number of peptides) × 100.

5.4. Genetic Control of the E/C Alloantigens

The apparent allelic variation in the E/C α and β subunits detected by peptide mapping, and the haplotype-associated NH_2-terminal sequence variation in the β chains, suggest that both the E/C alloantigen subunits are encoded within the MHC. Recent data by Jones *et al.* (1978) have demonstrated that the E/C alloantigens are indeed controlled by two different *I*-region loci—one in *A* and the other in *E/C*. Specific anti-I-E/C immunoprecipitates were examined by two-dimensional gel analysis; by this technique, proteins are separated in the first dimension by their charge (isoelectric focusing) and in the second dimension by apparent molecular weight (SDS-PAGE). When analyzed in the two-dimensional gel system, the E/C alloantigens consist of two electrophoretically distinct species of polypeptides. Subsequent analysis of the anti-E/C immunoprecipitates and whole splenic lysates from intra-*I*-region recombinants and F_1 hybrids demonstrated that the two E/C polypeptides were controlled by different genes. A locus in *E/C* encoded one polypeptide; the other polypeptide, designated as Ae, was controlled by the *A* subregion. Thus, strains with the same haplotype in *E/C*, but different haplotypes, in *A*, expressed E/C alloantigens with electrophoretically distinct Ae polypeptides. By this technique of two-dimensional gel analysis, it was not possible to ascertain whether the variation in Ae was due to posttranslational modification or primary structural differences. In an effort to confirm and extend these observations to the more conventional $\alpha-\beta$ subunit nomenclature, and also to determine the possible nature of the observed electrophoretic variation, we have compared the E/C α and β subunits from appropriate *I*-region recombinants by peptide mappings (Cook *et al.*, 1979c).

The strains we have analyzed are shown in Table 7; all are *k* haplotype in *E/C*, but vary in *A* (*k*, *b*, or *s*). The E/C α chains from B10.A, B10.A(3R), and B10.A(5R) showed coelution of all tryptic peptides (Fig. 19). Also, no differences were detected between B10.HTT and B10.A α chains (not shown). However, there were notable differences among the β subunits of B10.A(3R) or (5R) and B10.HTT. Figure 20 demonstrates that there are distinct tryptic peptide differences between the β subunits of B10.A and 3R or 5R; these differences are denoted by arrows. The bottom panel is a control showing the reproducibility of the system. Both 3R and 5R are *b* haplotype for the *A* subregion, and thus the E/C β polypeptides from these two strains should be identical; this is shown in Fig. 21. We have examined another intra-*I*-region recombinant, B10.HTT, which is *s* haplotype in the *A* subregion. As would be predicted, the E/C β chains from HTT are different from those of both B10.A and B10.A(3R) (Fig. 22).

TABLE 7. Summary of Peptide Mapping Data on the E/C Antigens from Recombinant Strains[a]

Strains	*H-2* haplotypes									Percentage of coelution of tryptic peptides with B10.A E/C subunits	
		I									
	K	*A*	*B*	*J*	*E*	*C*	*S*	*G*	*D*	α	β
B10.A	*k*	*k*	*k*	*k*	*k*	*d*	*d*	*d*	*d*	100	100
B10.AQR	*q* ↳	*k*	*k*	*k*	*k*	*d*	*d*	*d*	*d*	ND	100
B10.A(5R)	*b*	*b*	*b* ←|	*k*	*k*	*d*	*d*	*d*	*d*	100	60
B10.A(3R)	*b*	*b*	*b*	*b* ←|	*k*	*d*	*d*	*d*	*d*	100	60
B10.HTT	*s*	*s*	*s*	*s* ←|	*k*	*k*	*k*	*k*	*d*	100	56

[a]The arrows indicate that the β chain must be encoded to the right (→) or left (←) of that locus.

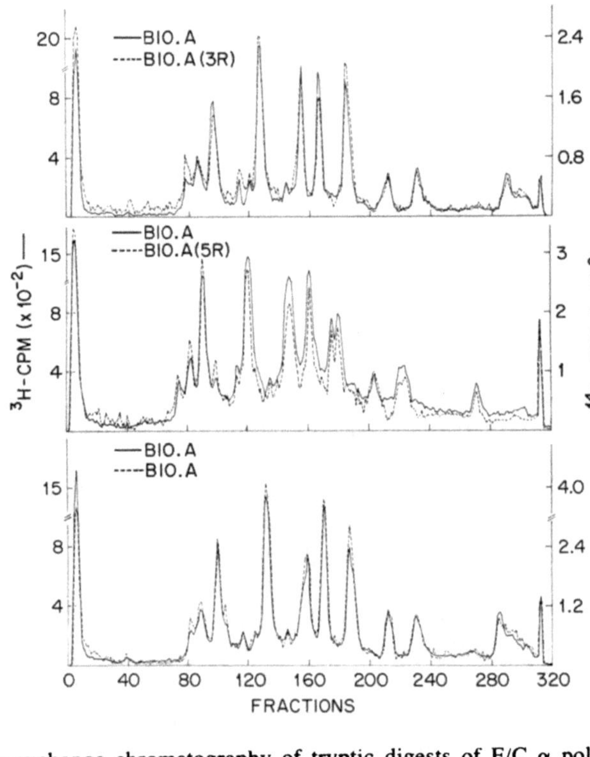

Figure 19. Ion-exchange chromatography of tryptic digests of E/C α polypeptides. ^{3}H-labeled E/C^k α chains from B10.A are compared with ^{14}C-labeled E/C^k α chains from B10.A(3R) (A), B10.A(5R) (B), B10.A (C).

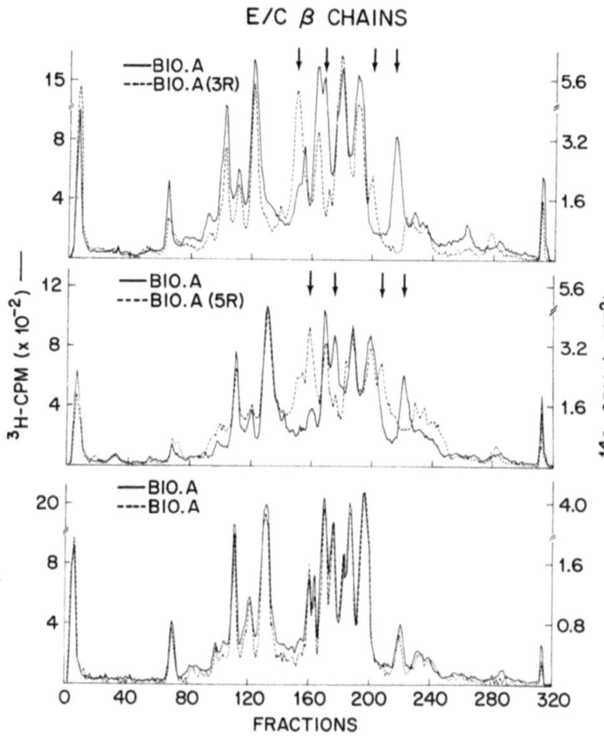

Figure 20. Ion-exchange chromatography of tryptic digests of E/C β polypeptides. ^{3}H-labeled E/C^k β chains from B10.A are compared with ^{14}C-labeled E/C^k β chains from B10.A(3R) (A), B10.A(5R) (B), and B10.A (C). Major peptide differences are denoted by arrows.

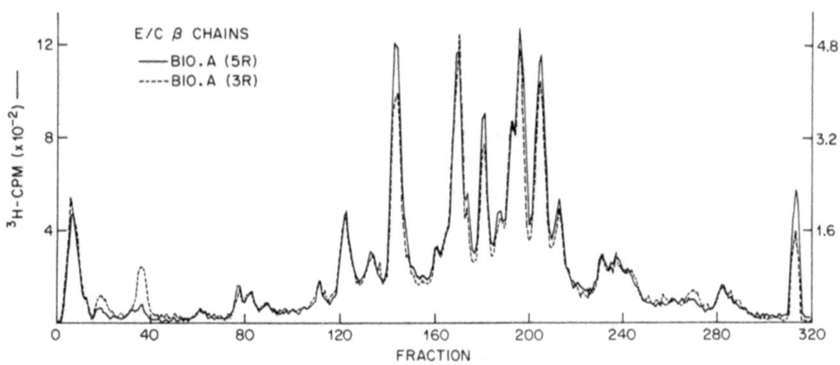

Figure 21. Ion-exchange chromatography of tryptic digests of E/C β polypeptides. ^{3}H-labeled E/C^k βchains from B10.A(5R) and B10.A(3R) are compared.

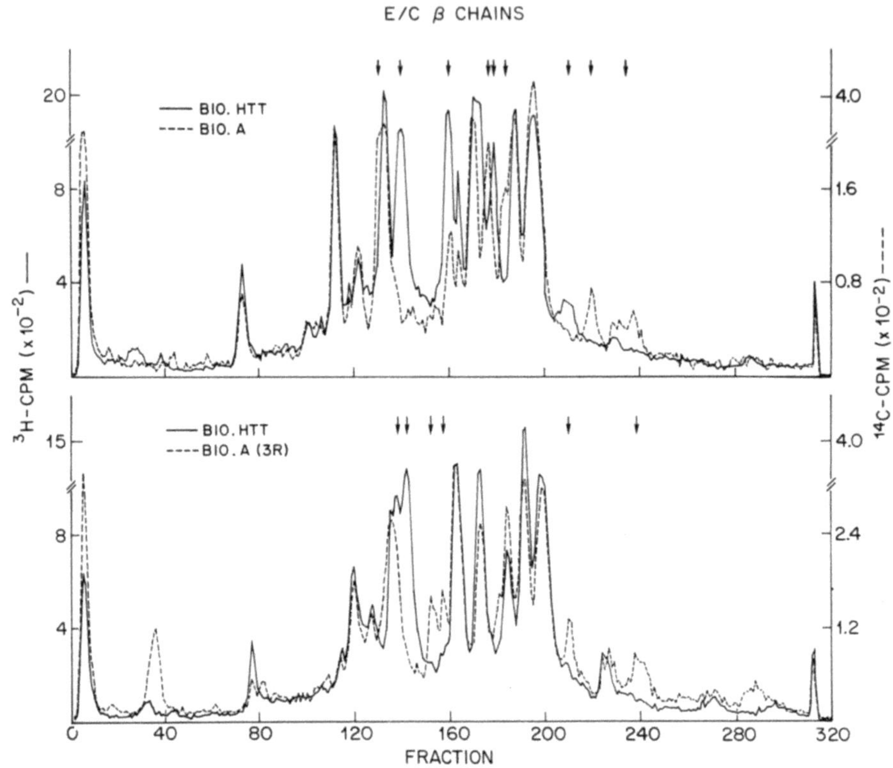

Figure 22. Ion-exchange chromatography of tryptic digests of E/C β polypeptides. ^{3}H-labeled E/C^k β chains from B10.HTT are compared with ^{14}C-labeled E/C^k β chains from B10.A (top panel) and B10.A(3R) (bottom panel). Major peptide differences are denoted by arrows.

Thus, while all four strains possess the *k* allele in the *E/C* subregion, the E/C β subunits from B10.A(3R) or (5R) and B10.HTT show approximately 40% variation by peptide mapping. Posttransitional modification (e.g., glycosylation) could not account for such extensive structural variation, and in addition, tryptic Ia glycopeptides have been detected only in the first (fall-through) peptide peak from the ion-exchange column (R.G. Cook and E.S. Vitetta, unpublished observations). These data demonstrate that the structural gene for the E/C β subunit lies outside *E/C* and to the left of *I-J* (see Table 7). A comparison of the β subunits from B10.A and B10.AQR revealed no peptide differences (not shown); this maps the E/C β-chain structural gene to the right of *H-2K* and into *A* or *B*.

That the E/C^k α subunits from all strains analyzed by peptide mapping appear identical implies that the α subunit is encoded by *E/C* and that the allospecificity Ia.7 is a determinant(s) controlled by this chain. The β polypeptide may exert a conformational influence on this allodeterminant, but cannot contain the determinant(s), since serological ambiguities would have been observed in the assignment of Ia.7 to *E/C*.

6. Conclusions and Implications

6.1. The A and E/C Alloantigens Are Coexpressed on Ig^+ (B) Lymphocytes

Subpopulations of lymphocytes were killed with cytotoxic antisera to I-A, I-E/C, or Ig determinants and the surviving cells examined for each of these molecules by immunoprecipitation. By this technique, the A and E/C alloantigens can be detected only on Ig^+ lymphocytes and are coexpressed on the same cell.

6.2. Primary Structural Differences Exist between the A and E/C Alloantigens

Although both the A and E/C antigens consist of two polypeptide chains, α and β, they can be differentiated by their apparent subunit molecular weights and by their capacities to form disulfide-bonded α–β dimers during detergent lysis. By NH_2-terminal sequence analysis, there is no apparent homology between the A and E/C α chains or between the β chains. There are limited tryptic peptide mapping comparisons between the *A*- and *E/C*-subregion products, but the data suggest that there is little structural relatedness (Freed *et al.*, 1978).

6.3. Allelic Variation Is Detected in the α and β Subunits of Both the A and E/C Alloantigens

There are multiple amino acid sequence differences between allelic α chains of the A and E/C molecules; thus far, no allelic variation in the α subunits has been detected by sequence analysis. Comparative tryptic peptide analysis has demonstrated marked allelic variation (~40–50%) in the Aα, A β, and E/C β chains and detectable (~10%) variation in E/C α allelic products. Since congenic mouse strains, which differ only at the MHC, have been utilized, the allelic variation observed indicates that all four subunits (A α and β, E/C α and β) are encoded within the MHC.

6.4. The I-E/C Alloantigen α and β Subunits Are Both Encoded within the *I* Region

The evidence previously reported by Jones *et al.* (1978) indicated that the E/C alloantigens were controlled by two *I*-region loci—*A* and *E/C*. We have confirmed and extended this observation, demonstrating by comparative peptide analysis that the *structural genes* for the E/C α and β subunits are encoded within the *E/C* and *A* or *B* subregions, respectively. To our knowledge, there is no biological precedent, for a two-chained molecule, which is not synthesized as a polyprotein, to contain subunits that are genetically linked; the significance of this observation for the E/C alloantigens is not clear at present. The finding that this two-chain Ia alloantigen is encoded by separate genes is further evidence that the E/C α polypeptide (only minor allelic variation by peptide mapping) is encoded within the MHC—the antisera used to isolate the E/C molecules detect Ia specifcity 7, which unequivocally maps to the *right* of *I-J,* and the β chain of E/C antigens is unequivocally encoded to the *left* of *I-J*. This requires that specificity 7 be associated with the α polypeptide and therefore be *I*-region (*I-E/C*)- controlled. Preliminary experiments indicate that both subunits of the I-A alloantigen are *I*-region-encoded. Figure 23 presents our current interpretation of the genetic organization and expression of the A and E/C alloantigens.

6.5. The Murine E/C Alloantigens and the Human DR Alloantigens are Homologous by NH_2-Terminal Sequence

Although there are limited sequence data available for any of these molecules, there is striking homology between the human DR antigens and the murine E/C, but not A, alloantigens (see Tables 8 and 9). The

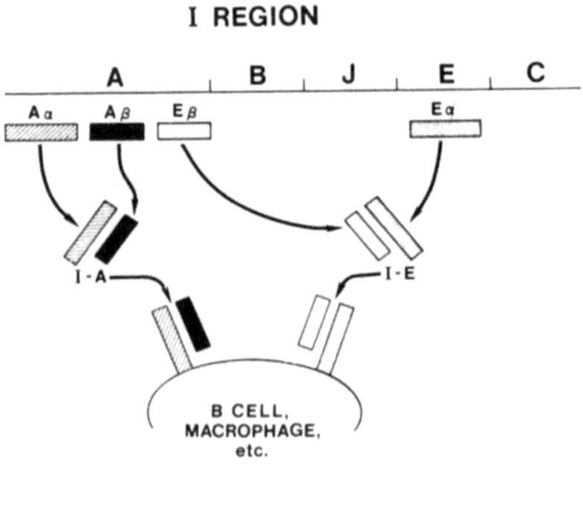

Figure 23. Interpretive model of the genetic organization and expression of the A and E/C alloantigens. The order of the Aα, Aβ, and Eβ "genes" in the *A* subregion is not known; also, our results have not eliminated the *B* subregion as the locus that encodes Eβ. For simplicity, E is used instead of E/C.

TABLE 8. NH_2-Terminal Sequence Comparisons between Murine and Human Ia α Subunits[a]

	1	2	3	4	5	6	7	8	9	10	11	12	13	14	15	16	17	18	19	20	21	22
A α				ILE		ALA			VAL			TYR				VAL	TYR					
E/C α	ILE	LYS			HIS	THR	ILE	ILE		ALA		PHE	TYR	LEU	LEU	PRO			ARG			PHE
DR α					HIS	VAL						PHE	TYR	LEU		PRO						PHE
P34	ILE	LYS	GLU	GLU(ARG)		VAL	ILE		GLN	ALA	GLU	PHE	TYR	LEU	ASN							

[a]The A and E/C α-chain sequence data are from Cook *et al*. (1979b). The human DR α and P34 sequences are from Silver *et al*. (1979) and Springer *et al*. (1977), respectively. A box indicates sequence identities between the human and murine E/C molecules.

TABLE 9. NH_2-Terminal Sequence Comparisons between Murine and Human Ia β Subunits[a]

	1	2	3	4	5	6	7	8	9	10	11	12	13	14	15	16	17	18	19	20
A β			SER		ARG	HIS	PHE	VAL	TYR		PHE	PRO	PRO	PHE		TYR	PHE			
E/C β	VAL	ARG		SER	ARG	PRO		PHE	LEU		TYR	SER VAL	LYS THR	SER				PHE	TYR	
DR β	[ ]					PRO		PHE	LEU	TYR	TYR	VAL						PHE	TYR	
P29	[ ]	GLY	ASP	VAL	PRO			PHE	LEU	GLU	GLN	VAL								

[a]The prototypic A and E/C β-chain sequence data are from Cook *et al*. (1979b) with the exception of VAL at position 12 in E/C, which is from McMillan *et al*. (1978). The DR β and P29 sequences are from Silver *et al*. (1979) and Springer *et al*. (1977), respectively. The DRβ and P29 sequences have been shifted by one residue to maximize homology with E/C β (denoted by brackets). Sequence identification between E/C β and the human products is denoted with boxes.

human β-chain sequences must be shifted to the right by one amino acid to attain homology with the E/C β chains. Whether or not both subunits of the human alloantigens are MHC-encoded is not clear. Two groups (Barnstable *et al.*, 1978; Klareskog *et al.*, 1978) have presented evidence that the α polypeptides are encoded within the MHC, while a recent report by Tosi *et al.* (1978) suggests that only the β subunit is controlled by the *HLA* region. Due to the sequence homology between the human and murine E/C antigens, and the evidence demonstrating that both E/C subunits are *I*-region-encoded, it is possible that both the α and β subunits of the human DR antigens are controlled by *HLA*-linked loci. An *I-A*-subregion homologue has not been demonstrated in man, although there is evidence for additional DR specificities (Tosi *et al.*, 1978).

6.6. The Two-Gene Control of the E/C Alloantigens May Help to Explain Gene Complementation

Several synthetic polypeptides (Dorf *et al.*, 1975; Munro and Taussig, 1975) and protein antigens (Sachs *et al.*, 1978; Berzofsky, 1978), which are under *Ir* gene control, require the presence of responder alleles at two distinct *I*-region loci. In most instances, the two loci have been mapped to *A* and *E/C*. Due to the complexities inherent in each system that displays dual *Ir* gene control, it is not possible to generalize whether each of the controlling *Ir* loci recognize the same or different antigenic determinants. For the myoglobin (Berzofsky, 1978) and nuclease (Sachs *et al.*, 1978) responses, it appears that different *Ir* loci control responsiveness to different antigenic determinants. Thus, these two antigens do not appear to require *complementation* between two genes for the generation of a response. Responsiveness to GLΦ, on the other hand, does require gene complementation (responder alleles at two loci) for the generation of both antibody synthesis (Dorf *et al.*, 1975) and T-lymphocyte proliferation (R.H. Schwartz *et al.*, 1976c). The two genes determining responsiveness to GLΦ have been designated as α, which maps in *E/C*, and β, which maps in *A*. The demonstration that the E/C alloantigen is controlled by both the *E/C* (α-chain) and *A* (β-chain) loci offers a molecular mechanism whereby both subregions might control the response to GLΦ. Thus, the E/C alloantigen alone would designate responsiveness to GLΦ. An alternative explanation is that both the A and E/C antigens are needed, and that the complementation observed is a requirement for the expression of two responder alloantigens and not just a "hybrid" E/C alloantigen. R.H. Schwartz *et al.* (1978a) have demonstrated that anti-A *and* anti-E/C alloantisera inhibit T-cell proliferation to GLΦ, suggesting that both alloantigens may be required. However, as mentioned by the authors, there were inconsistencies observed for anti-I-A alloantisera inhibition experiments (R.H. Schwartz *et al.*, 1978a,c), and therefore caution should be observed in the final interpretation of these results. Both models are consistent with the requirement for the coexpression of the GLΦ responder α and β genes on the same antigen-presenting cell (R.H. Schwartz *et al.*, 1978c). Obviously, further studies are needed to clarify the mechanism by which dual *Ir* genes control immune responsiveness.

ACKNOWLEDGMENTS. We wish to thank Susan Kourvelas, Mary Bagby, Pam Liu, Yuh-Minh Tseng, Sam Lin, Becky Himmel, Sam Chinn, Terri Wallis, Beth Tierney, Donna Atherton, and Peggy Frank for excellent technical assistance during various phases of this work, and Judy Hahn and Daisi Margoulides for careful and patient preparation of this manuscript. We also thank Mark Siegelman for his contributions to the E/C^r sequence data. This work was supported in part by generous grants from the National Institutes of Health, American Cancer Society, and National Science Foundation.

References

Allison, J.P., Walker, L.E., Russell, W.A., Pellegrino, M.A., Ferrone, S., Reisfeld, R.A., Frelinger, J.A., and Silver, J., 1978, Murine Ia and human DR antigens: Homology and amino terminal sequences, *Proc. Natl. Acad. Sci. U.S.A.* **75**:3953.

Barnstable, C.J., Jones, E.A., Bodmer, W.F., Bodmer, J.G., Arce-Gomez, B., Snary, D., and Crumpton, M.J., 1978, Genetics and serology of HL-A-linked human Ia antigens, *Cold Spring Harbor Symp. Quant. Biol.* **41**:443.

Benacerraf, B., and McDevitt, H.O., 1972, Histocompatibility-linked immune response genes, *Science* **175**:273.

Berzofsky, J.A., 1978, Genetic control of the immune response to mammalian myoglobins in mice. I. More than one I-region gene in H-2 controls the antibody response, *J. Immunol.* **120**:360.

Brown, J.L., Kato, K., Silver, J., and Nathenson, S.G., 1974, Notable diversity in peptide compostion of murine H-2K and H-2D alloantigens, *Biochemistry* **13**:3174.

Capra, J.D., Vitetta, E.S., Klapper, D.G., Uhr, J.W., and Klein, J., 1976, Structural studies on protein products of murine chromosome 17: Partial amino acid sequence of an $H\text{-}2K^b$ molecule, *Proc. Natl. Acad. Sci. U.S.A.* **73**:3661.

Cook, R., Vitetta, E.S., Capra, J.D., and Uhr, J.W., 1977, The partial amino acid sequence of a murine Ia molecule: Lack of homology between murine $I\text{-}C^d$ β and human P29, *Immunogenetics* **5**:437.

Cook, R.G., Vitetta, E.S., Uhr, J.W., Klein, J., Wilde, C.E., III, and Capra, J.D., 1978a, Structural studies on protein products of murine chromosome 17. III. Partial amino acid sequence of an $H\text{-}2K^q$ molecule, *J. Immunol.* **121**:1015.

Cook, R.G., Uhr, J.W., Capra, J.D., and Vitetta, E.S., 1978b, Structural studies on the murine Ia alloantigens. II. Molecular weight characterization of the I-A and I-E/C subregions, *J. Immunol.* **121**:2205.

Cook, R.G., Carroll, M.C., Uhr, J.W., Vitetta, E.S., and Capra, J.D., 1978c, Studies on the protein products of murine chromosome 17: A status report, *Transplant. Proc.* **10**:695.

Cook, R.G., Vitetta, E.S., Uhr, J.W., and Capra, J.D., 1979a, Structural studies on the murine Ia alloantigens. III. Tryptic peptide comparisons of allelic products of the *I-E/C* subregion, *Mol. Immunol.* **16**:29.

Cook, R.G., Siegelman, M.H., Capra, J.D., Uhr, J.W., and Vitetta, E.S., 1979b, Structural studies on murine Ia alloantigens. IV. Partial NH_2-terminal sequences of the I-A and I-E/C subregion products, *J. Immunol.* **122**:2232.

Cook, R.G., Vitetta, E.S., Uhr, J.W., and Capra, J.D., 1979c, Structural studies on the murine Ia alloantigens. V. Evidence that the structural gene for the I-E/C beta polypeptide is encoded within the *I-A* subregion, *J. Exp. Med.* **144**:981.

Cullen, S.E., and Schwartz, B.D., 1976, An improved method for isolation of H-2 and Ia alloantigens using immunoprecipitation induced by protein A-bearing staphylococci, *J. Immunol.* **117**:136.

Cullen, S.E., Freed, J.H., and Nathenson, S.G., 1976, Structural and serological properties of murine Ia alloantigens, *Transplant. Rev.* **30**:236.

David, C.S., 1976, Serologic and genetic aspects of murine Ia antigens, *Transplant. Rev.* **30**:299.

David, C.S., and Cullen, S.E., 1978, Murine Ia antigens: Identification and mapping of Ia.23 and further definition of the *I-E* subregion, *J. Immunol.* **120**:1659.

David, C.S., Shreffler, D.C., and Frelinger, J.A., 1973, New lymphocyte antigen system (Lna) controlled by the Ir region of the mouse H-2 complex, *Proc. Natl. Acad. Sci. U.S.A.* **70**:2509.

Delovitch, T.L., and McDevitt, H.O., 1975, Isolation and characterization of murine Ia antigens, *Immunogenetics* **2**:39.

Delovitch, T.L., Murphy, D.B., and McDevitt, H.O., 1977, Immunochemical evidence for three Ia loci in the *I*-region of the *H-2* complex, *J. Exp. Med.* **146**:1549.

Delovitch, T.L., Press, J.L., and McDevitt, H.O., 1978, Expression of murine Ia antigens during embryonic development, *J. Immunol.* **120**:818.

Dorf, M.E., Stimpfling, J.H., and Benacerraf, B., 1975, Requirement for two H-2 complex Ir genes for the immune response to the L-Glu, L-Llys, L-Phe terpolymer, *J. Exp. Med.* **141**:1459.

Fathman, C.G., Cone, J.L., Sharrow, S.O., Tyrer, H., and Sachs, D.H., 1975, Ia alloantigen(s) detected on thymocytes by use of a fluorescence-activated cell sorter, *J. Immunol.* **115**:584.

Freed, J.H., David, C.S., Shreffler, D.C., and Nathenson, S.G., 1978, Structural studies of the protein portion of the H-2-linked Ia glycoprotein antigens of the mouse: Tryptic peptide comparison of products from the I-A and I-C subregions of B10.HTT, *J. Immunol.* **121**:91.

Frelinger, J.A., Neiderhuber, J.E., and Shreffler, D.C., 1975, Inhibition of immune responses *in vitro* by specific antiserums to Ia antigens, *Science* **188**:268.

Frelinger, J.A., Hibbler, F.J., and Hill, S.W., 1978, Expression of *I-A* and *I-E,C* region-coded Ia antigens on functional B cell subpopulations, *J. Immunol.* **121**:2376.

Frelinger, J.G., Wettstein, P.J., Frelinger, J.A., and Hood, L., 1978, Epidermal Ia molecules from the I-A and I-EC subregions of the mouse H-2 complex, *Immunogenetics* **6**:125.

Goding, J.W., White, E., and Marchalonis, J.J., 1975, Partial characterization of Ia antigens on murine thymocytes, *Nature* (*London*) **257**:230.

Goodman, S.A., Vitetta, E.S., Melcher, U., and Uhr, J.W., 1975, Cell surface Ig. XIII. Distribution of IgM and IgD-like molecules on small and large cells of mouse spleen, *J. Immunol.* **114**:1646.

Götze, D., Reisfeld, R.A., and Klein, J., 1973, Serologic evidence for antigens controlled by the Ir region in mice, *J. Exp. Med.* **138**:1003.

Hammerling, G.J., Mauve, G., Goldberg, E., and McDevitt, H.O., 1975, Tissue distribution of Ia antigens: Evidence for Ia antigens on sperm cells and macrophages, *Immunogenetics* **1:**428.

Henning, R., Milner, R.J., Reske, K., Cunningham, B.A., and Edelman, G.M., 1976, Subunit structure, cell surface orientation and partial amino-acid sequences of murine histocompatibility antigens, *Proc. Natl. Acad. Sci. U.S.A.* **73:**118.

Henry, C., and Chan, E.L., 1977, Expression and function of I-region determinants on immunocompetent cells. I. Selective expression of I-C region determinants on immune cells, *J. Immunol.* **119:**737.

Jones, P.P., 1977, Analysis of H-2 and Ia molecules by two-dimensional gel electrophoresis, *J. Exp. Med.* **146:**1261.

Jones, P.P., Murphy, D.B., and McDevitt, H.O., 1978, Two-gene control of the expression of a murine Ia antigen, *J. Exp. Med.* **148:**925.

Kappler, J.W., and Marrack, P.C., 1976, Helper T cells recognize antigen and macrophage surface components simultaneously, *Nature (London)* **262:**797.

Katz, D.H., 1977, Genetic control of immune responses and cellular interactions, in: *Lymphocyte Differtiation, Recognition, and Regulation,* pp. 530–597, Academic Press, New York.

Katz, D.H., and Benacerraf, B., 1975, The function and interrelationships of T-cell receptors, Ir genes and other histocompatibility gene products, *Transplant. Rev.* **22:**175.

Katz, D.H., Graves, M., Dorf, M.E., DiMuzio, H., and Benacerraf, B., 1974, Cell interactions between histoincompatible T and B lymphocytes. VII. Cooperative responses between lymphocytes are controlled by genes in the I region of the H-2 complex, *J. Exp. Med.* **141:**263.

Kessler, S.W., 1975, Rapid isolation of antigens, from cells with a staphylococcal protein A-antibody adsorbent: Parameters of the interaction of antigen–antigen complexes with protein A, *J. Immunol.* **115:**1617.

Kincade, P.W., and Ralph, P., 1976, Regulation of clonal B lymphocyte proliferation by anti-immunoglobulin or anti-Ia antibodies, *Cold Spring Harbor Symp. Quant. Biol.* **41:**245.

Klareskog, L., Rask, L., Fohlman, J., and Peterson, P.A., 1978, Heavy HLA-DR (Ia) antigen chain is controlled by the MHC region, *Nature (London)* **275:**762.

Klein, J., 1975, Central regions of the H-2 complex, in: *Biology of the Mouse Histocompatibility*, pp. 389–489, Springer-Verlag, New York.

Klein, J., Flaherty, L., Vandeberg, J.L., and Shreffler, D.C., 1978, H-2 haplotypes, genes, regions, and antigens: First listing, *Immunogenetics* **6:**489.

Laemmli, U.K., 1970, Cleavage of structural proteins during the assembly of the head of bacteriophage T_4, *Nature (London)* **227:**680.

Lieberman, R., Paul, W.E., Humphrey, W., and Stimpfling, J.W., 1972, H-2-linked immune response (*Ir*) genes: Independent loci for Ir-IgG and Ir-IgA genes, *J. Exp. Med.* **136:**1231.

Maizel, J.V., Jr., 1966, Acrylamide gel electropherograms by mechanical fractionation: Radioactive adenovirus proteins, *Science* **151:**988.

Marrack, P., and Kappler, J.W., 1977, Anti-Ia inhibits the activity of B cells but not a T cell derived helper mediator, *Immunogenetics* **4:**541.

McMillan, M., Cecka, J.M., Murphy, D.B., McDevitt, H.O., and Hood, L., 1978, Partial amino acid sequences of murine Ia antigens of the I-EC^d subregion, *Immunogenetics* **6:**137.

Meo, T., David, C.S., Rijnbeck, A.M., Nabholz, M., Miggiano, V., and Shreffler, D.C., 1975, Inhibition of mouse MLR by anti-Ia sera, *Transplant. Proc.* **7:**127.

Merryman, C.F., and Maurer, P.H., 1974, Characterization of a new Ir-GLT gene and its location in the I region of the H-2 complex, *Immunogenetics* **1**:549.

Munro, A.J., and Taussig, M.J., 1975, Two genes in the major histocompatibility complex control immune response, *Nature (London)* **256**: 103.

Murphy, D.B., 1978, The I-J subregion of the murine H-2 gene complex, *Springer Semin. Immunopathol.* **1**:111.

Murphy, D.B., Herzenberg, L.A., Okumura, K., Herzenberg, L.A., and McDevitt, H.O., 1976, A new I subregion (I-J) marked by a locus (Ia-4) controlling surface determinants on suppressor T lymphocytes, *J. Exp. Med.* **144**:699.

Niederhuber, J.E., and Frelinger, J.A., 1976, Expression of Ia antigens on T and B cells and their relationship to immune-response functions, *Transplant. Rev.* **30**:101.

Niederhuber, J.E., Frelinger, J.A., Dugan, E., Coutinho, A., and Shreffler, D.C., 1975, Effects of anti-Ia serum on mitogenic responses. I. Inhibition of the proliferative response to B cell mitogen, LPS, by specific anti-Ia sera, *J. Immunol.* **115**:1672.

Okuda, K., and David, C., 1978, A new lymphocyte activating determinant locus expressed on T cells and mapping in I-E subregion, *J. Exp. Med.* **147**:1028.

Pierce, C.W., Kapp, J.A., and Benacerraf, B., 1976, Regulation by the H-2 gene complex of macrophage–lymphoid cell interactions in secondary antibody responses *in vitro*, *J. Exp. Med.* **144**:371.

Pierres, M., Germain, R.N., Dorf, M.E., and Benacerraf, B., 1978, *In vivo* effects of anti-Ia alloantisera. I. Elimination of specific suppression by *in vivo* administration of antisera specific for I-J controlled determinants, *J. Exp. Med.* **147**:656.

Press, J.L., Klinman, N.R., and McDevitt, H.O., 1976, Expression of Ia antigens on hapten-specific B cells. I. Delineation of B-cell subpopulations, *J. Exp. Med.* **144**:414.

Rich, S.S., David C.S., and Rich, R.T., 1978. Regulatory mechanisms in cell mediated-immune responses. VII. Presence of I-C subregion determinants on mixed leukocyte reaction suppressor factor, *J. Exp. Med.* **149**:114.

Rosenthal, A.S., 1978, Determinant selection and macrophage function in genetic control of the immune response, *Immunol. Rev.* **40**:136.

Sachs, D.H., and Cone, J.L., 1973, A mouse B-cell alloantigen determined by gene(s) linked to the major histocompatibility complex, *J. Exp. Med.* **138**:1289.

Sachs, D.H., Berzofsky, J.A., Pisetsky, D.S., and Schwartz, R.H., 1978, Genetic control of the immune response to staphylococcal nuclease, *Springer Semin. Immunopathol.* **1**:51.

Schwartz, B.D., and Cullen, S.E., 1978, Chemical characterization of Ia antigens, *Springer Semin. Immunopathol.* **1**:85.

Schwartz, B.D., Kask, A.M., Sharrow, S.O., David, C.S., and Schwartz, R.H., 1977, Partial chemical characterization of Ia antigens derived from murine thymocytes, *Proc. Natl. Acad. Sci. U.S.A.* **74**:1195.

Schwartz, B.D., Vitetta, E.S., and Cullen, S.E., 1978, Labeling characteristics and separation of Ia antigen subunits, *J. Immunol.* **120**:671.

Schwartz, R.H., David, C.S., Sachs, D.H., and Paul, W.E., 1976a, T lymphocyte-enriched murine peritoneal exudate cells. III. Inhibition of antigen-induced T lymphocyte proliferation with anti-Ia antisera, *J. Immunol.* **117**:531.

Schwartz, R.H., Dickler, H.B., Sachs, D.H., and Schwartz, B.D., 1976b, Studies of Ia antigens on murine peritoneal macrophages, *Scand. J. Immunol.* **5**:731.

Schwartz, R.H., Dorf, M.E., Benacerraf, B., and Paul, W.E., 1976c, The requirement for two complementary Ir-GLΦ immune response genes in the T-lymphocyte proliferative response to poly-($Glu^{53}Lys^{36}Phe^{11}$), *J. Exp. Med.* **143**:897.

Schwartz, R.H., David, C.S., Dorf, M.E., Benacerraf, B., and Paul, W.E., 1978a, Inhibition of dual Ir gene-controlled T-lymphocyte proliferative response to poly ($Glu^{56}Lys^{35}Phe^{9}$)n with anti-Ia antisera directed against products of either I-A or I-C subregion, *Proc. Natl. Acad. Sci. U.S.A.* **75**:2387.

Schwartz, R.H., Yano, A., and Paul, W.E., 1978b, Antigen presentation in the T-lymphocyte proliferation assay: Requirement for genetic identity at the MHC, in: *Ir Genes and Ia Antigens* (H.O. McDevitt, ed.), pp. 297–304, Academic Press, New York.

Schwartz, R.H., Yano, A., Stimpfling, J.H., and Paul, W.E., 1978c, Gene complementation in the T lymphocyte proliferative response to poly ($Glu^{55}Lys^{36}Phe^{9}$)n: A demonstration that both immune response gene products must be expressed in the same antigen-presenting cell, *J. Exp. Med.* **149:**40.

Shreffler, D.C., and David, C., 1975, The H-2 major histocompatibility complex and the I immune response region: Genetic variation, function and organization, *Adv. Immunol.* **20:**125.

Shreffler, D., David, C., Götze, D., Klein, J., McDevitt, H.O., and Sachs, D.H., 1974, Genetic nomenclature for new lymphocyte antigens controlled by the *I* region of the H-2 complex, *Immunogenetics* **1:**189.

Shreffler, D.C., David, C.S., Cullen, S.E., Frelinger, J.A., and Niederhuber, J.E., 1976, Serological and functional evidence for further subdivision of the I regions of the H-2 gene complex, *Cold Spring Harbor Symph. Quant. Bio.* **41:**477.

Silver, J., Cecka, J.M., McMillan, M., and Hood, L., 1976, Chemical characterization of products of the H-2 complex, *Cold Spring Harbor Symp. Quant. Biol.* **41:**369.

Silver, J., Walker, L.E., Reisfeld, R.A., Pellegrino, M.A., and Ferrone, S., 1979, Structural studies of murine I-E/C and human DR antigens, *J. Mol. Immunol.* **16:**1.

Springer, T.A., Kaufman, J.F., Terhorst, C., and Strominger, J.L., 1977, Purification and structural characterization of human HLA-linked B-cell antigens, *Nature (London)* **268**(213.

Tada, T., Taniguchi, M., and David, C.S., 1976, Properties of the antigen-specific suppressive T-cell factor in the regulation of antibody response of the mouse. IV. Special subregion assignment of the gene(s) that codes for the suppressive T-cell factor in the H-2 histocompability complex, *J. Exp. Med.* **144:**713.

Tosi, R., Tanigaki, N., Centis, D., Ferrara, G.B., and Pressman, D., 1978, Immunological dissection of human Ia molecules, *J. Exp. Med.* **148:**1592.

Vitetta, E.S., and Cook, R.G., 1979, Surface expression and synthesis of *I-A* and *I-E/C* encoded molecules by B lymphocytes and Ig-secreting cells, *J. Immunol.* **122:**2122.

Vitetta, E.S., Baur, S., and Uhr, J.W., 1971, Cell surface Ig. II. Isolation and characterization of Ig from mouse splenic lymphocytes, *J. Exp. Med.* **134:**242.

Vitetta, E.S., Capra, J.D., Klapper, D.G., Klein, J., and Uhr, J.W., 1976a, The partial amino acid sequence of an H-2K molecule, *Proc. Natl. Acad. Sci. U.S.A.* **73:**905.

Vitetta, E.S., Forman, J., and Kettman, J.R., 1976b, Cell surface Ig. XVIII. Functional differences of B lymphocytes bearing different cell surface immunoglobulin isotypes, *J. Exp. Med.* **143:**1055.

16

Ia Antigens

Molecular Components in Immune Regulation?

Susan E. Cullen, Stephen M. Rose, and
Cathy S. Kindle

1. Identity of Ia Molecules

Ia alloantigens are surface glycoproteins found on lymphocytes and macrophages and probably some other cell types (Shreffler and David, 1975; Hammerling *et al.*, 1975; Cowing *et al.*, 1978). They are antigenically quite variable, and their structure is encoded in genes mapping in the *I* (immune-response) region of the murine major histocompatibility complex (MHC). They are detected with the aid of alloantisera, and each molecule is antigenically complex, bearing several different antigenic determinants (Cullen *et al.*, 1976). There are two groups of Ia molecules that are readily detected on homozygous lymphocytes, and these are currently called I-A and I-E molecules (Cullen *et al.*, 1974, 1979; B.D. Schwartz and Cullen, 1978; Cook *et al.*, 1978). These names are derived from the genetic subregion of origin of these molecules, but as will be seen in Section 4, it is not strictly true that the I-E molecule is derived only from the *I-E* subregion.

It is almost certain that there are cell-surface structures determined by the other *I* subregions, particularly *I-J* and *I-C*. These subregions control immunoregulatory traits, particularly suppressor functions (Tada *et al.*, 1976; Murphy *et al.*, 1976). Antisera raised between mouse strains differing only in these subregions are capable of inhibiting these suppressor functions (Tada *et al.*, 1976; Murphy *et al.*, 1976; Rich and Rich, 1976;

Susan E. Cullen, Stephen M. Rose, and Cathy S. Kindle • Department of Microbiology and Immunology, Washington University School of Medicine, St. Louis, Missouri 63110.

Okumura *et al.*, 1976; Frelinger *et al.*, 1976, Okuda *et al.*, 1977; Okuda and David; 1978), which strongly implies the presence of a surface constituent(s) important to suppressor action. However, no molecules encoded by these subregions have been isolated, and this chapter will deal only with I-A and I-E molecules.

2. Subunit Structure of Ia Molecules

Ia molecules are composed of two glycopeptide chains called α and β. The α chain has a molecular weight of about 33,000–35,000 and the β chain a molecular weight of about 24,000–27,000. Both chains are glycosylated, and contain mannose, galactose, and fucose (Cullen and Nathenson, 1974). The molecular weight of the carbohydrate is approximately 3300 daltons, and it appears to be rather homogeneous (Freed and Nathenson, 1977). The glycopeptide chains are associated by noncovalent interactions both on the cell surface and in nonionic-detergent solution. The interaction of the α and β chains of Ia molecules is sometimes stabilized during solubilization by formation of intrachain disulfide bonds (Cullen *et al.*, 1974). These are not native features of the molecules, since their formation can be prevented by iodoacetamide treatment during solubilization (Cullen *et al.*, 1979; Cook *et al.*, 1978). This type of covalent linkage is seen only between the α and β chains of I-A molecules and not between the α and β chains of I-E molecules, but among I-A molecules, it has been observed in every haplotype examined. Thus, despite its artificial nature, the process of disulfide linkage distinguishes I-A from I-E molecules, and shows that there is some consistent structural feature in I-A molecules that permits formation of the bond.

The α and β chains of I-E molecules are not linked through disulfide bonds, but examination of these molecules under very mild conditions of sodium dodecyl sulfate (SDS) dissociation shows that the α and β chains can be found together in a 58,000-dalton form.

It has been further shown that in detergent and on the cell surface, both I-E α and β chains and I-A α and β chains can be deliberately covalently cross-linked by the bifunctional reagent dimethyl 3′,3′-dithiobispropionimidate (DTBP) (Dancey *et al.*, 1979). The cross-linking produces complexes of about 55,000–60,000 daltons that can be shown to contain an α and a β chain by cleaving the reduction-sensitive cross-link. Higher-order interactions have not been seen, and linkage of I-A and I-E components to one another has not been observed.

Thus, it seems quite clear that the natural form of Ia molecules is a dimer composed of noncovalently associated α and β chains. Another conclusion is that I-A and I-E type molecules have distinctive features that are shared by all the members within the type.

3. Further Evidence That the Two Types of Ia Molecules Have "Type-Specific" Structural Features

Isoelectric focusing (IEF) in a gel system can be used to examine radiolabeled immunoprecipitated Ia molecules or isolated Ia α and β subunits. Antigen preparations were made as we reported earlier (Cullen and Schwartz, 1976; *et al.*, B.D. Schwartz, 1978). For performing IEF analysis, [^{35}S]methionine labeled I-A and I-E molecules were precipitated. For example, precipitates from B10.HTT (I-A^{s}, I-E^{k}) were applied to 10% polyacrylamide gels in SDS, and the α and β chains were separated by electrophoresis. The chains were isolated by eluting gel slices with SDS and pooling appropriate fractions. The samples were then dialyzed exhaustively to remove SDS, lyophilized, and resuspended in a urea Nonidet P-40/ampholine mixture in preparation for IEF. The IEF was performed in a slab gel using the method of O'Farrell (1975), and pH 3.5–10 ampholines (LKB Produkter, AB, Sweden). As can be seen from Fig. 1A, the α chains were of restricted heterogeneity and migrated between pH 5 and 6 as indicated by direct pH measurement. The I-A α chains were somewhat more acidic than the I-E α chains. The β chains from both I-A and I-E molecules showed a more complex pattern and migrated at a pH greater than 6. This finding is consistent for numerous haplotypes, and when immune precipitates are examined directly, the pH of migration and the banding pattern permit identification of α and β chains by inspection. One can compare the I-A- and I-E-type molecules in different haplotypes side by side on the same IEF gel. When such a comparison is made (Fig. 1B), it appears to be generally true that the α chains are more acidic when they come from I-A molecules than when they derive from I-E molecules. This is not to say that the α chains are identical when they come from the same type of molecule, but it indicates closer relatedness among α chains from one type of Ia molecule than exists between α chains from the two types of molecules.

The finding of some structural consistency among related chains by IEF is supported by the results of tryptic peptide analysis of isolated α and β chains. We are performing tryptic peptide analysis by high-pressure liquid chromatography (HPLC) using modifications of methods described by Hancock *et al.* (1978). Immunoprecipitated [^{3}H]leucine-labeled α and β chains isolated from SDS gels were reduced and alkylated in the presence of bovine gamma-globulin (BGG) carrier protein, precipi-

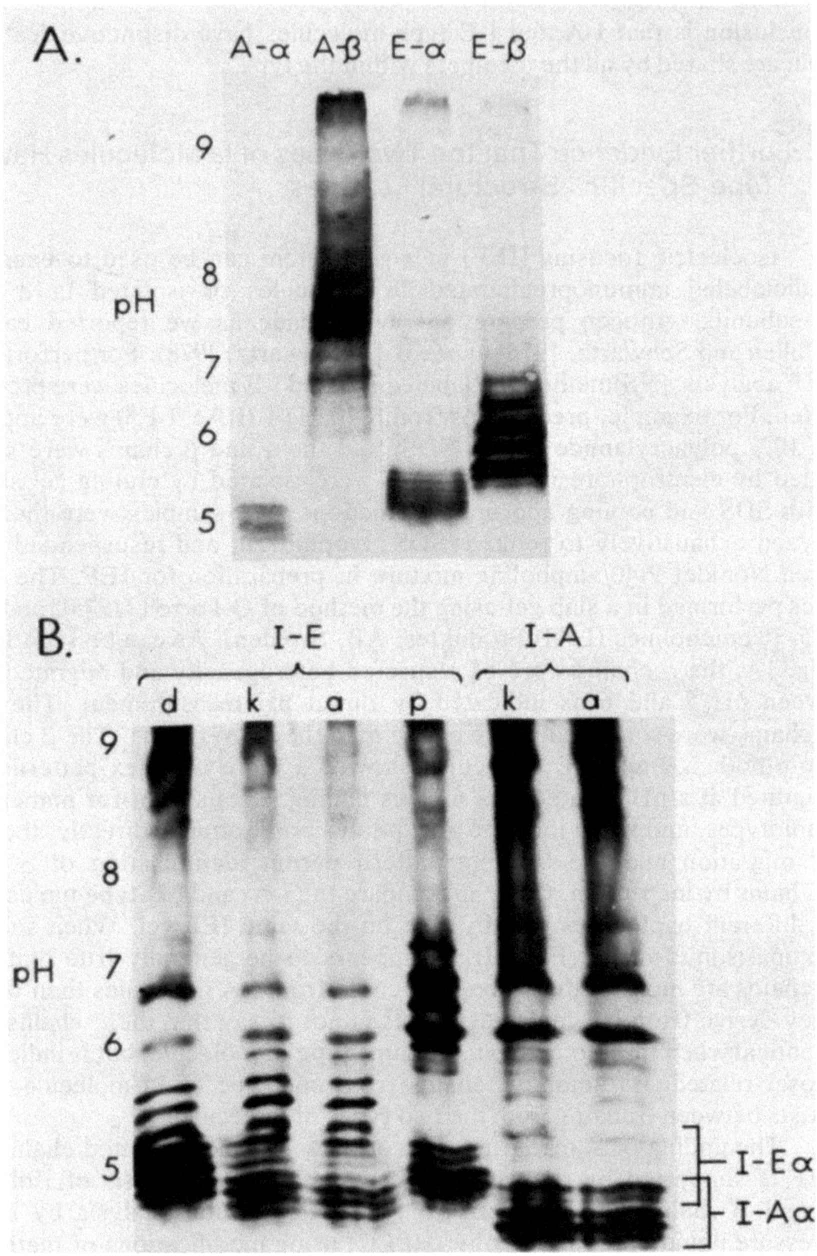

Figure 1. IEF in 10% polyacrylamide slab gels. (A) Isolated α and β chains from I-A and I-E molecules of strain B10.HTT; (B) comparison of immunoprecipitated I-A and I-E molecules from various haplotypes.

tated with trichloroacetic acid, extracted to remove SDS, and digested with trypsin treated with L-(tosylamide-2-phenyl) ethyl chloromethyl ketone, using the conditions employed by Brown *et al.* (1974). The digests were lyophilized, dissolved in 5% acetonitrile in 0.1% phosphoric acid, and injected onto a Waters fatty acid analysis column equilibrated in the same solvent. The instrument used was a Spectra-physics 8000 equipped to monitor optical density at 206 nm. Electronically generated gradients of acetonitrile in 0.1% phosphoric acid were employed for elution of peptides, and the gradients were varied as indicated. Fractions of 0.25 ml were collected at a flow rate of 0.5 ml/min, scintillation fluid was added, and the samples were counted.

Monitoring optical density of the column effluent revealed the peptide profile of the BGG carrier protein, and this profile provided two important internal controls. First, the completeness of the trypsin digestion could be assured by determining that the profile showed the same appearance from one digest to the next. Second, although radiolabeled peptide profiles from separate runs were compared using the acetonitrile gradients as a primary guide, the BGG profiles were also examined to determine that they were correctly in register in order to verify the correct alignment of radiolabeled peptide profiles.

Comparisons of peptides from α chains isolated from I-A and I-E molecules were carried out, and it was noted that for I-A α chains, there were certain recurrent or "typical" peptides that were absent from I-E α chains, but present in the I-A α chains of several strains. For example, Fig. 2 shows a profile from B10.BR I-A^k α chain compared to an α-chain profile from the wild mouse strain B10.WR7 (Fig. 2A) and compared to an I-E^k α chain from B10.BR (Fig. 2B). The "typical" I-A α peptides are indicated by arrows, and the sharing of peptides by the wild-strain α chains indicates their relatedness to I-A^k α chains rather than to I-E^k α chains, which share none of the I-A α peptides. The relationship of B10.WR7 α chains to B10.BR I-A α is affirmed by the fact that the B10.WR7 molecules are cross-reactive with alloantisera detecting I-A but not I-E molecules of B10.BR.

This type of finding argues for some kind of shared structure between allelic products. So far, consistency in structure has been easily observed among the α chains, but the peptide maps and the IEF data also clearly show structural variability among α chains that are the products of alleles. Because of this variability, the α chain may bear antigenic determinants, and there is no way to rule out the presence of serological determinants on either α or β chains on the basis of these data. The group of "typical" peptides observed for I-A α chains could be an indication that the variability in α is restricted to a certain part of the molecule, a hypothesis that is certainly amenable to test.

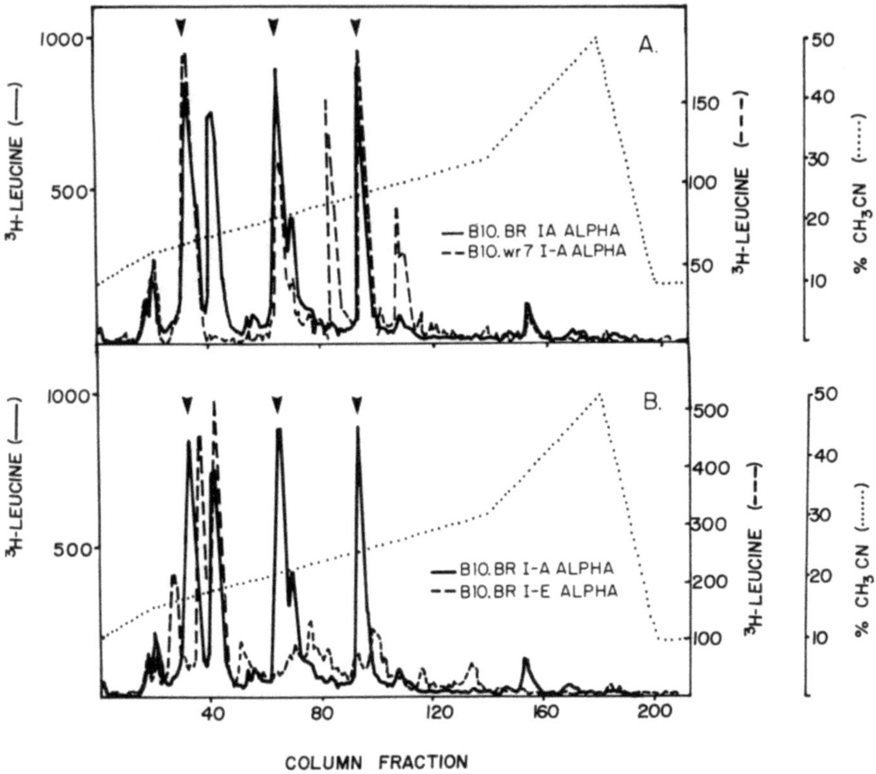

Figure 2. Tryptic peptide analysis of α chains by HPLC. (A) Comparison of isolated α chains from the I-A molecule of strain B10.BR (haplotype *k*) and the presumed I-A molecule of strain B10.WR7 (wild haplotype *wr7*); (B) comparison of isolated α chains from the I-A molecule of strain B10.BR and I-E α chains from the same strain. The arrows mark peaks that appear to be typical of I-A α chains and that are absent from I-E α chains.

4. Evidence for the Presence of the Gene Coding for I-E β Chains outside the *I-E* Subregion

An investigation by Jones *et al.* (1978) had shown that the β chains of I-E molecules showed electrophoretic variability dependent on the *I-A* subregion. To examine this variability further, we used the technique of HPLC peptide mapping to study parental and recombinant strains of mice in which the recombination event is known to be between the *I-A* and *I-E* subregions.

Radiolabeled I-E molecules were precipitated by the same serum [(B10 × HTI) F_1 anti-B10.A (5R)] from strains B10.A (*I-A*^{k}, *I-E*^{k}) and B10.A (5R) (*I-A*^{b}, *I-E*^{k}), and the *α* and β chains were separated, isolated,

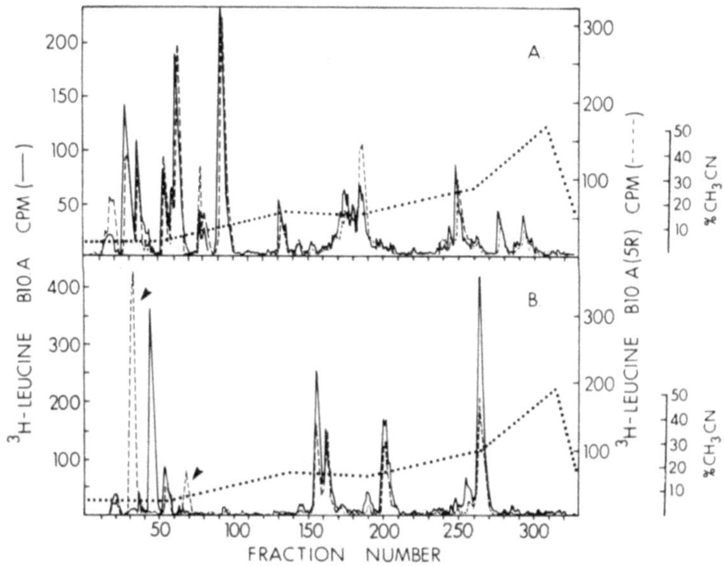

Figure 3. Tryptic peptide analysis of α and β chains from I-E molecules by HPLC. (A) Comparison of β chains from I-E molecules of strain B10.A (*I-A*^{k}, *I-E*^{k}) and recombinant strain B10.A(5R) (*I-A*^{b}, *I-E*^{k}) showing identity of peptide profiles; (B) comparison of β chains from I-E molecules of strain B10.A and B10.A(5R) showing differences in profiles. Peptide peaks present in B10.A(5R) but absent from B10.A are marked by arrows.

and digested with trypsin. The comparisons of α and β chain maps are shown in Fig. 3. The I-E α-chain profiles (Fig. 3A) are identical in both strains. The I-E β-chain profiles, however, show distinct differences that indicate quite clearly that they must be different structures (Fig. 3B). This finding confirms the suggestion made by Jones and co-workers on the basis of electrophoretic data, and provides data complementary to those obtained in ion-exchange peptide mapping systems, in which similar conclusions have been drawn (Cook *et al.*, 1979). Because this strain pair shares all the non-MHC "background" genes, the most likely reason for the difference in the I-E β chains is that the structural gene for this chain

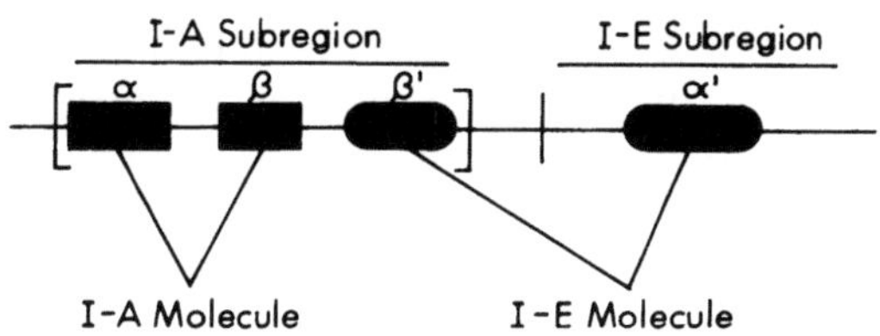

Figure 4. Suggested arrangement of Ia structural genes within the *I* region. No order of genes is implied for the *I-A*-subregion gene cluster.

is in the *I-A* subregion, wherein the two strains differ. This suggestion is diagrammed in Fig. 4. In this diagram, no ordering of the *I-A* subregion genes is implied.

Comparisons of I-A molecules from strain pairs that are of the same haplotype in *I-A* but differ in *I-E* [e.g., B10.A (4R) and B10.A] show total identity of profiles. These data indicate that both I-A α- and β-chain genes are associated with the *I-A* subregion.

According to this model, then, the I-E molecule is composed of two polypeptide chains the determining genes of which lie some distance apart in the MHC, separated by intervening genes. The I-A molecule is composed of α and β chains encoded in the *I-A*-subregion gene cluster, which also includes the I-E β-chain gene.

It is noteworthy that there are a number of haplotypes in which no I-E molecules have been detected by serological analysis or immunochemical testing using alloantisera. Attempts to find I-E molecules in these haplotypes using xenoantisera have also been made (Lafuse *et al.*, 1979), but the molecules with which the xenoantibodies react have not been structurally identified as I-E molecules.

These I-E "nonexpressor" haplotypes (including *b, f, q,* and *s*) apparently do not lack the *I-A*-subregion-encoded I-E β chain, because these β chains can be "rescued" by crossing the I-E nonexpressor haplotype with an expressor haplotype (Jones *et al.*, 1978). The β chains can also be seen in recombinants in which the *I-E* subregion is derived from an expressor haplotype [as in B10.A (5R), in which the I-E β^b chain is expressed in a molecule with I-E α^k chains (see Fig. 3B)] (Cook *et al.*, 1979). It has also been found that certain nonexpressor haplotypes have some electrophoretically identified I-E β chains in the cytoplasm, while others lack the chains totally except in the presence of appropriate I-E α-chain genes (Jones *et al.*, 1978).

5. Implications of the Arrangement of Ia Structural Genes with Regard to Ia Immunogenicity

The finding that I-E molecules derive their β chains from the *I-A* subregion provokes some questions about the way in which I-E molecules are recognized by antiserum. The most logical conclusion to make is that the serological specificities that map to the *I-E* subregion are part of the structure that is encoded in that region, namely, the I-E α chain. I-E molecules from different haplotypes share specificity Ia.7, but also have unique specificities that doubtless reflect structural variability. Peptide mapping shows that structural variability among I-E α chains does exist. Thus, the I-E α chains are a structurally reasonable site for the antigenic specificities recognized by antisera raised between animals differing in their *I-E* subregions. Attempts to examine the serological reactivity of separated α and β chains have not been successful, so that a direct test of this suggestion has not been possible.

Conversely, the β chains of the I-E molecule are not likely to carry the Ia specificities that map to the *I-E* subregion. One could construct a model in which a specificity-bearing β chain from the *I-A* subregion was either not expressed or lacked proper configuration in the absence of I-E α chain. This suggestion cannot explain the consistent serological composition of I-E molecules that come from recombinants differing in *I-A*-subregion source. The I-E molecules from B10.BR ($\alpha^k\beta^k$), B10.HTT (α^k β^s), and B10.A (5R) ($\alpha^k\beta^b$) do not differ in their *I-E*-subregion-associated specificities even though their β chains are all structurally different.

In contrast to the relatively limited serological polymorphism found associated with the *I-E* subregion, the *I-A* subregion is quite antigenically complex. Figure 5 shows the assignment of Ia specificities to the *I* subregions. The specificities assigned to *I-A* are either mapped by recombination or associated with the region by immunochemical analysis of Ia molecules (Cullen *et al.*, 1976; B.D. Schwartz and Cullen, 1978). The specifities in parentheses are excluded from the *I-E* subregion by recombination, and are likely to be associated with the *I-A* subregion, since no Ia molecules from *I-B* or *I-J* have yet been found. The I-A molecules have both α and β chains encoded in the *I-A* subregion, and as in the case of I-E molecules, both chains are structurally variable. A reason for the greater serological complexity of the subregion could be that both α and β chains carry some of the antigenic specificites.

A very obvious question concerns the antibodies potentially elicited by the I-A-encoded β chains of the I-E molecule. They possess structural variability, and there is no obvious reason that they would fail to elicit antibodies. It seemed quite likely to us that they had in fact elicited antibodies, but that these antibodies were systematically excluded from analysis because the usual method for defining specificities of the I-E

I-A	I-B	I-J	I-E	I-C
1,2,3,8,9,11 20 (4,5,10,12, 13,14,16,17, 18,19)			7,21,22,23	6?

Figure 5. Map distribution of Ia serological specificities by *I* subregion. Assignments have been made by serological and immunochemical testing. Specificities in parentheses have been formally excluded from the *I-E* subregion by recombination.

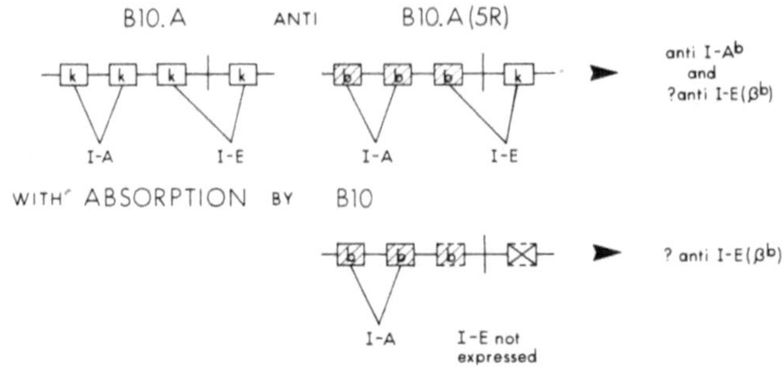

Figure 6. Example of a procedure used to search for antibody activity specific for the β chain of I-E molecules in antisera raised against recombinant haplotypes.

molecule requires the activity to be consistent on a panel of recombinants differing in the *I-A* subregion. We have deliberately searched for such antibodies by taking antirecombinant sera with potential for containing anti-I-E β antibodies, exhaustively absorbing with the I-E nonexpressor parental haplotype to remove antibodies to I-A molecules, and retesting on the recombinant to detect anti-I-E β activity. An example of such a test protocol is shown in Fig. 6. Surprisingly, this method has not revealed anti-I-E β activity in five different sera with potential activity against I-E β^b, β^s, or β^k. It is difficult to judge whether our inability to find antibody stems from a defect in the protocol or from true absence of antibody. For example, it could be that in addition to the intended absorption of antibodies detecting I-A molecules by the apparent I-E nonexpressor strain, antibodies to I-E β are removed as well because of low-level surface or cytoplasmic expression. Further investigation is clearly required to resolve this issue.

Another way in which Ia immunogenicity may manifest itself is in the induction of mixed-lymphocyte response (MLR). The evidence that the *I* region lymphocyte-activating determinants (LADs) are Ia antigens is that anti-Ia antisera are capable of inhibiting MLRs (Meo *et al.*, 1973). If the Ia antigens are themselves the major LADs of the MHC, one might expect to observe MLRs directed against I-E β-chain differences in appropriate combinations.

While no selective study of I-E β as an antigen has been performed in MLR, there have been reports of responses to determinants expressed in F_1 animals, but lacking in either parent (Fathman and Nabholz, 1977; Fathman *et al.*, 1978). These determinants could be on I-E β chains newly expressed in the F_1 because of the simultaneous presence of an I-E α-chain gene of the expressor type in the *trans* position. Not all the features of the MLR described by Fathman and Nabholz (1977) are consistent with this hypothesis, however, since the I-E β chain should also be expressed in appropriate recombinants, and such recombinants failed to induce response in their experiments. The so-called "F_1 determinants" could also result from $\alpha-\beta$ exchange of I-A-molecule chains that might occur in the heterozygous condition. An earlier study of I-A molecules in an F_1 using sequential immunoprecipitation did not demonstrate such exchange (Cullen *et al.*, 1976), but it could have been missed because of quantitative limitations or if the antisera used contained antibodies detecting only one chain.

6. Implications of the Arrangement of Ia Structural Genes for Immune-Response Function

6.1. GLΦ Complementation System

If we suppose that Ia antigens are immune-response (*Ir*)-gene products, the distribution of Ia structural genes establishes a framework for explaining and exploring *Ir*-gene-complementation effects.

The level of response to several antigens (5 of approximately 45 antigens known to be under *Ir*-gene control) has been shown to be affected by two genes, and complementation between genes has been observed. The antigens that are reported to be in this category are GLΦ(GLT, GLIeu) (Dorf *et al.*, 1975, 1976a,b; Merryman *et al.*, 1975), H-2.2 (Stimpfling and Durham, 1972), Thy-1.1 (Zaleski and Milgrom, 1973), cytochrome *c* (R.H. Schwartz *et al.*, 1978a), and LDH_B (Melchers and Rajewsky, 1975). Of these, GLΦ has been studied most systematically, has provided the clearest results, and has been confirmed in two different laboratories. The *Ir-GLΦ* genes are in the *I-A* subregion ("β gene") and the *I-E* subregion ("α gene"). The names for the *Ir* genes are not to be confused with the names for Ia polypeptide chains.

In the GLΦ system, it was observed that crosses of certain nonresponder haplotypes generated responsiveness in the F_1 generation, and that recombination between two nonresponder parental haplotypes could sometimes generate responsiveness. Some results of Dorf and Benacerraf (1975) are summarized in Table 1. The complementation observed was of two types, which were referred to as "α–β complementation" and "β–β complementation."

A clear example of α–β complementation is seen in a recombinant or an F_1 between nonresponder strains A and B10. The defects in A and B10 can be localized to subregions by observing that while the B10.A (4R) recombinant is nonresponsive, the B10.A (5R) recombinant is a good responder. The conclusion from these studies was that strain A is defect-

TABLE 1. Complementation in the Response to GLΦ

			Source of subregion			I-A molecule		I-E molecule	
Strain	Haplotype	GLΦ response[a]	*A*	*E*	Complementation	Chain composition (α/β)	Potential to mediate response	Chain composition[b] (α/β)	Potential to mediate response
B10	*b*	Low	*b*	*b*	—	*bb*	No	None	No
A	*a*	Low	*k*	*k*	—	*kk*	No	*kk*	No
B10.A(4R)	*h4*	Low	*k*	*b*	—	*kk*	No	None	No
B10.A(5R)	*i5*	High	*b*	*k*	α–β	*bb*	No	*kb*	Yes
(B10 × A)F_1	*bxa*	High	*b/k*	*b/k*	α–β	*bb*	No	*kk*	No
						kk	No	*kb*	Yes
						bk	?		
						kb	?		
SJL	*s*	Low	*s*	*s*	—	*ss*	No	None	No
B10.S(8R)	*as1*	Low	*k*	*s*	—	*kk*	No	*kk*	No
B10.HTT	*t3*	High	*s*	*k*	α–β	*ss*	No	*ks*	Yes
(B6 × SJL)F_1	*bxs*	High	*b/s*	*b/s*	β – β	*bb*	No	None	Nc
						ss	No		
						bs	Yes?		
						sb	Yes?		

[a] Data from Dorf and Benacerraf (1975).
[b] "None" signifies that the I-E molecule is not expressed.

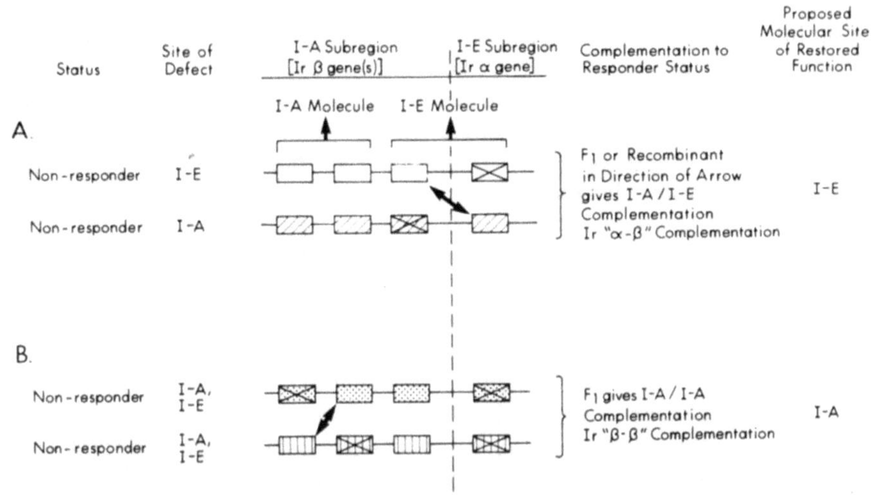

Figure 7. Proposed molecular explanation for *Ir*-gene complementation. (A) α–β complementation, in which function is restored by formation of an I-E molecule different from the molecules present in nonresponder parental types; (B) β–β complementation, in which function is restored by formation of an I-A molecule different from the molecules present in nonresponder parental types.

ive in the *I-A*-subregion gene *Ir-GLΦ-β*^{k}, while B10 is defective in the *I-E*-subregion gene *Ir-GLΦ-α*^{b} (cf. Table 1).

In view of the data now available on Ia gene mapping, it seems possible that GLΦ α–β complementation could result from the formation, either in a recombinant or in an F_1, of functional I-E molecules composed of Ia α and β chains from the two parental haplotypes (see Fig. 7A). The fact that α–β complementation sometimes seems to be more efficient in *cis* than in *trans* would be expected, because recombinant animals are homozygous for the "correct" α- and β-chain genes and would therefore generate a larger proportion of functional molecules than the F_1 heterozygote.

The second (β–β) type of complementation has been less frequently observed but can be explained in terms of Ia molecular structure. So far, it has been found operating only in *trans,* in certain F_1 combinations in which both parental types are known to be defective in the *I-E*-subregion gene *Ir-GLΦ-α*. Thus, in combinations such as (B6 × SJL)F_1, responsiveness is generated, and it was suggested by Benacerraf and Dorf (1976) that complementation may be occurring between the *Ir-GLΦ-β*^{b} and *Ir-GLΦ-β*^{s} genes. Other explanations that they raised included selective complementation by certain β alleles with α alleles that appear defective in most other combinations ("coupled complementation") or complementation between the β genes and an additional heretofore unrecognized *I-E*-subregion locus (second "*Ir-α*" gene).

Since there are several *Ia* genes in the *I-A*-subregion gene cluster, it seems possible that "*Ir* β-β" complementation could be due to mixing of I-A molecule α and β chains from the two haplotypes, generating a "hybrid" I-A molecule that is functional (see Fig. 7B). This complementation would therefore involve two different genes from the *I-A* subregion, one for an α chain and the other for a β chain. In this event, the *Ir*-gene nomenclature ("β-β" complementation) would not indicate complementation by two defective alleles of the same gene—but rather would indicate that two different genes contribute to the molecule required for function. The Ia data thus suggest that the *Ir-GLΦ*-β gene is not a single entity, but may refer to any of the three *I-A*-subregion genes.

The main implication of these suggestions is that *Ir*-gene complementation need not mean that two separate Ia molecules are required for the support of *Ir* function, but could indicate that one appropriately constituted Ia molecule could carry out the function independently. The *Ir*α-β type of complementation would involve I-E molecules and *Ir* α-β complementation would involve I-A molecules. Apparently, GLΦ responsiveness sometimes involves I-A molecules and sometimes involves I-E molecules. Responsiveness that can be mediated through either of two molecules depending on which haplotype is involved could be explained if the GLΦ-antigen molecule, despite its relative chemical simplicity, contained more than one determinant under *Ir*-gene control. The synthetic antigen (T,G)-A--L is known to have multiple determinants (Mozes *et al.*, 1974; Seaver *et al.*, 1976). Thus, in the GLΦ system, we might imagine that I-A molecules promote response to determinant X in some haplotypes, that I-E molecules promote response to determinant Y in other haplotypes, and that in some haplotypes both Ia molecules may be functional, generating both types of responses.

One may ask why two molecules are present if only one is needed to regulate response. This is not easy to answer in concrete terms, since there is no good explanation of how *Ir* systems attain antigen specificity. If the specificity resides in or depends on the Ia-antigen molecules, then broader variability of Ia molecules may permit generation of a wider spectrum of specifically controlled responses, which sould be advantageous to the individual. Duplication is already known in the mouse MHC (Shreffler *et al.*, 1971; Snell *et al.*, 1971). The H-2 transplantation antigens derive from three duplicated genes, and there are probable additional H-2-like duplications among linked genes determining the structurally related Tla (Vitetta *et al.*, 1972; Muramatsu *et al.*, 1973), Qa (Michaelson *et al.*, 1977), and F9 (Vitetta *et al.*, 1975) molecules. In this genetic context, duplication of Ia structural genes is not particularly surprising, and could provide a means of generating a broad spectrum of immune responses.

These remarks represent an attempt to point out ways in which Ia molecules could provide a framework for *Ir* function, and they are intended mainly as an orientation for the design of experiments to confirm or refute the hypothesis that *Ir*-gene function is dependent on one Ia molecule. One must also consider *Ir*-gene-controlled responses to other antigens, to determine whether the hypothesis is generally applicable.

6.2. Other *Ir*-Gene Complementation Systems

When the available data on other two-gene-controlled responses are examined, it is somewhat difficult to determine whether these antigen systems follow the pattern set by GLΦ. The main reason for this is that in the panel of recombinants currently available, responder and nonresponder alleles are informatively recombined for GLΦ and the related antigens GLT and GLleu (45,46), but responder and nonresponder alleles for other antigens are not recombined as frequently. Because GLT and GLleu share an antigenic determinant(s) with GLΦ and the response patterns are so comparable, GLT and GLleu do not provide a good test of the generality of the hypothesis suggested using the GLΦ model.

The other responses reported to be under two-gene control are those against H-2.2, Thy-1.1, cytochrome *c*, and LDH_B. The response to H-2.2 was the earliest-recognized instance of *Ir*-gene complementation (Stimpfling and Durham, 1972), but further study of this response has not been extensive, and is hampered by the fact that the gene encoding the antigen is closely linked to the *Ir* gene(s) regulating response. Some potential responder recombinants cannot be tested because they possess H-2.2, and responsiveness in some strains may be affected by the fact that potential responders have H-2 molecules that share structural features with the molecule bearing the H-2.2 determinant in the immunogen.

The Thy-1.1 system, as currently analyzed, appears to be compatible with an inter-*I-A*-subregion complementation mechanism such as that shown in Fig. 7B. The Thy-1.1 response has been thoroughly examined in two haplotypes and their recombinant derivatives, showing the presence of complementing genes in the *I-A* subregion of haplotypes *b* and *d*. Thus, F_1 animals heterozygous for *b/d* in the *I-A* subregion are better responders than either homozygous parental type (Zaleski and Milgrom, 1973; Zaleski and Klein, 1976). Examination of a broad panel of standard and recombinant haplotypes for responsiveness to Thy-1.1 has not been carried out. The data obtained thus far are therefore compatible with the conclusion that responsiveness to this antigen is mediated through an Ia molecule determined by the *I-A* subregion, but they do not rule out further complexity. The study of MHC-determined *Ir* complementation in this system is also complicated by the presence of an additional *Ir* gene affecting Thy-1.1 response outside the MHC (Zaleski and Klein, 1974).

Response to pigeon cytochrome c has been tested on a fairly broad panel of H-2 haplotypes (R.H. Schwartz *et al.*, 1978a). Response is present only in haplotypes *k* and *a*, which share most of the *I* region. Recombinants derived from *k* that have lost either the $I\text{-}A^k$ subregion [e.g., B10.A(5R)] or the $I\text{-}E^k$ subregion [e.g., B10.A(4R)] are low responders, and an F_1 between the 5R and 4R recombinants has restored responsiveness. These findings are consistent with the conclusion that responsiveness to this antigen is mediated through an Ia molecule of the I-E type, which is composed of β chains encoded in the $I\text{-}A^k$ subregion and α chains encoded in the $I\text{-}E^k$ subregion. This complementation mechanism is the one illustrated in Fig. 7A.

Of all the two-gene systems examined thus far, LDH_B is the most difficult to interpret. Responsiveness in this system was assessed by the quantity of antibody produced. In the first series tested (Melchers *et al.*, 1973), response was classified as low or high, but subsequent analysis of additional haplotypes and of heterozygotes revealed a continuum of response level that was divided somewhat arbitrarily into low, intermediate, high, and superhigh categories (Melchers and Rajewsky, 1975). When the dose of immunogen was varied, both high and low responders increased their antibody production substantially, the low responders increasing to levels that may have overlapped the response level of some but not all "high" responders. These findings are a probable indication of heterogeneity in the system, which could be due to the presence of more than one controlling gene, to the presence of more than one antigenic determinant under *Ir*-gene control on the LDH_B molecule, or to the presence of both types of heterogeneity.

The response levels of various standard haplotypes, recombinants, and heterozygotes, taken from the data of Melchers and Rajewsky (1975) and Melchers *et al.* (1973), are presented in Table 2, along with a description of the types of Ia molecules that could be produced in each case. The low-responder haplotypes are *k* and *a*, which, as stated above, have similar *I* regions. The remaining haplotypes listed are all more responsive than the *k* and *a* haplotypes, and if interpreted according to the hypothesis under consideration, these facts permit several conclusions.

First, it appears that I-A molecules of the composition $\alpha^k\beta^k$ and I-E molecules of the composition $\alpha^k\beta^k$ are both nonfunctional with respect to LDH_B. Second, because they are present in responder haplotypes that are I-E nonexpressors, I-A molecules from haplotypes *b, f, q,* and *s* are probably functional in the response to at least one antigenic determinant

TABLE 2. Potential of Ia Molecules to Mediate Response to LDH_B

Haplotype	LDH_B response[a]	Source of subregion		I-A molecule		I-E molecule	
		A	*E*	Chain composition (αβ)	Potential to mediate response?	Chain composition[b] (αβ)	Potential to mediate response?
k	Low	*k*	*k*	*kk*	No?	*kk*	No
a	Low	*k*	*k*	*kk*	No?	*kk*	No
b	High	*b*	*b*	*bb*	Yes	None[b]	No
f	High	*f*	*f*	*ff*	Yes	None	No
q	High	*q*	*q*	*qq*	Yes	None	No
s	High	*s*	*s*	*ss*	Yes	None	No
h2	Low	*k*	*k*	*kk*	No?	*kk*	No
t3	Intermediate	*s*	*k*	*ss*	Yes	*ks*	?
i5	High	*b*	*k*	*bb*	Yes	*kb*	?
h4	High	*k*	*b*	*kk*	No?	None	No
t3xa	High	*s/k*	*k/k*	*ss*	Yes	*ks*	?
				kk	No?	*kk*	No
				sk	?		
				ks	?		
t3xb	Superhigh	*s/b*	*k/b*	*ss*	Yes	*ks*	?
				bb	Yes	*kb*	?
				sb	?		
				bs	?		

[a] Data from Melchers and Rajewsky (1975) and Melchers *et al.* (1973).
[b] "None" signifies that the I-E molecule is not expressed.

on LDH_B. It is difficult to explain the high response of B10.A(4R), a recombinant that is $I\text{-}A^k$ and $I\text{-}E^b$ and that does not express I-E molecules. Complementation of the $\alpha-\beta$ type could be invoked, but if this type of complementation requires the formation of new I-E molecules (in this case, $\alpha^k\beta^k$), this explanation is not acceptable because the strain is an I-E nonexpressor. An alternative explanation is that I-A molecules of the *k* haplotype ($\alpha^k\beta^k$) are in fact functional with respect to the LDH_B response, but that response in the *k* haplotype is suppressed by a gene(s) to the right of the *I-A* subregion. Thus, in the B10.A(4R) recombinant, absence of this suppressor gene(s) would allow a response mediated by $I\text{-}A^k$ molecules to occur. This explanation would implicate the *I-A* subregion as the main site controlling responsiveness to LDHB, with *b, f, q, s,* and *k* being responder alleles. Suppression of immune response mapping in the *I* region (*Is* genes) has been observed in responses to GAT (Kapp *et al.*, 1974), lysozyme (Kipp *et al.*, 1975), and GT (Benacerraf and Dorf, 1976), and thus it is not unreasonable to propose that this type of regulation may exist in the LDH_B system.

Although one can assume that I-A molecules may control at least part of the response to LDH_B, there is no result from any animal tested by Melchers and co-workers that either demonstrates or rules out involvement of I-E molecules other than those of the *k* and *a* haplotypes in the response to LDH_B.

Table 2 shows that among the haplotypes examined by Melchers and co-workers, many carry molecules that are clearly associated with responsiveness, and, in addition, some carry one or more Ia molecules that have potential for mediating response but that have not been, or cannot be, selectively examined with currently available recombinants. In the light of present information, it would be desirable to reexamine the LDH_B system, using animals chosen to selectively test the potential roles of different Ia molecules in the response, and to search for possible suppression in the system. In view of the quantitative variation in response level, it is also of importance to determine whether more than one antigenic determinant is involved in LDHB responsiveness.

Some of the protein antigens that elicit responses controlled by MHC-linked *Ir* genes, and that were recognized to be under complex control, were subsequently understood to be composed of more than one antigenic determinant. An example of this is staphylococcal nuclease, which has been shown to contain several different antigenic determinants that can be at least partly isolated by selective cleavage of the completely sequenced nuclease molecule (Berzofsky *et al.*, 1977a,b). Two of the different antigenic determinants of nuclease are contained within the fragments spanning amino acids 99–149 and 1–126, and these fragments can be tested by reaction with anti-whole nuclease antibodies raised in different strains of mice.

When immunizations of B10.A and B10 mice (haplotypes *a* and *b*) by intact nuclease are made, an initial low dose of immunogen elicits response to whole nuclease in B10.A but not B10. However, boosting shows that response can eventually be elicited in B10. Thus, in this system, as in the LDH_B system mentioned above, the level of responsiveness is not absolute. It was found that when the individual fragments of nuclease were used to bind anti-whole nuclease antibody, the pattern of responsiveness changed. B10 proved to be a responder to fragment 1–126 and a nonresponder to 99–149, while B10.A was responsive to the very immunogenic 99–149 fragment, as well as to 1–126. This pattern explains the early responsiveness seen when B10.A is immunized with whole protein (response is primarily anti-99–149, with a late-appearing anti-1–126 component) and the more sluggish response of B10 (response is anti-1–126, but only after boosting).

Although the response to five different nuclease fragments has also been tested in a T-cell-proliferation assay using appropriate recombinants, the specific mapping sites for the response genes to individual nuclease determinants could not be definitively localized within the *I* region, although dual-gene control is possible in some instances (R.H. Schwartz *et al.*, 1978b). The uncertainty in mapping is probably due to antigenic heterogeneity of the fragments and to the capacity of some of the responder haplotypes to respond to more than one of the nuclease determinants. In retrospect, it is somewhat amazing that the response to antigens as complex as nuclease could be perceived to be under *Ir*-gene control at all.

In summary, the data on complementation of immune response are consistent with the idea that responsiveness to a single determinant can be mediated by a single Ia molecule. Although there are gaps in the data, one could conclude that I-A molecules can mediate response to an antigenic determinant(s) on GLΦ, Thy-1.1, and LDH_B, and that I-E molecules can mediate response to a determinant on GLΦ, and cytochrome c. When antigens bearing several determinants are examined, it is more difficult to discern the subregions on which *Ir* control is dependent.

7. Future Direction of Structural Analysis

The limited review of MHC-linked immune-response control presented in Section 6 shows that data accumulated by many investigators are compatible with the idea that *Ir*-gene control is dependent—in some way as yet unexplained—on a single Ia-antigen molecule. In many cases, complete information is not available, but there is no case that contradicts this hypothesis. Because this proposal seems viable, it is important to design experiments analyzing *Ir* function with the current view of *Ia* genes and molecules in mind. It is equally important to let our subsequent analysis of Ia structure be attuned to recognition of structural features that could help to explain biological action of the molecule.

In this regard, it is of interest to characterize further the consistent structural differences between I-A and I-E molecules, and to pursue the hint that certain areas of the molecules may be conserved from one haplotype to another. Is part of the Ia molecule relatively invariant, and if it is, what is the extent and type of heterogeneity existing elsewhere in the structure?

If invariant and variable portions of the molecule are found, can they be shown to serve a function? Possible functions could include selection of membrane location and orientation, interaction with other cellular components for triggering of specialized function within the cell, specific antigen binding, coupling of Ia molecules to selected subpopulations of antigen receptors on interacting cells involved in the immune response, and so on. Contributions from structural and functional analyses should allow a better understanding of the mechanism of immune-response control.

ACKNOWLEDGMENTS: The authors are grateful to Dr. B.D. Schwartz for critical comments and to Ms. Lorraine Bourisaw and Ms. Judy Craig for meticulous preparation of the manuscript.

NOTE ADDED IN PROOF: The discussion in Section 5 does not reflect more recent data (Lafuse, W.P., McCormick, J.F., and David, C.S., 1980, Serological and biochemical identification of hybrid Ia antigens, *J. Exp. Med.* **151**:709) which do suggest that serological specificities Ia.22 and 23, which are associated with I-E molecules, are either β-chain-derived or result from β-chain interaction with I-E α. Of these two specificities, Ia.22 had been studied more extensively, and earlier failure to recognize it as an *I-A*-subregion-dependent (β-chain-dependent) specificity resulted from the fact that it is a relatively public determinant. I-E molecule β chains derived from *I-A* subregions of haplotypes *k*, *s*, and *b* all generate Ia.22.

The finding that some I-E-molecule-associated specificities depend on β chains from particular haplotypes raises another issue, however. In all studies using recombinant haplotypes to define *I-A* subregion contributions to I-E molecules, it is important to confirm by independent means that the I-E molecule β chains from the recombinant animal are of the expected *I-A* subregion origin, and have not resulted from inter-*I-A* subregion recombination.

References

Benacerraf, B., and Dorf, M.E., 1976, Genetic control of specific immune responses and immune suppressions by *I*-region genes, *Cold Spring Harbor Symp. Quant. Biol.* **41**:465.

Berzofsky, J., Schechter, A.N., Shearer, G.M., and Sachs, D.H., 1977a, Genetic control of the immune response to Staphylococcal nuclease. III. Time-course and correlation between the response to native nuclease and the response to its polypeptide fragments, *J. Exp. Med.* **145**:111.

Berzofsky, J., Schechter, A.N., Shearer, G.M., and Sachs, D.H., 1977b, Genetic control of the immune response to Staphylococcal nuclease. IV. *H-2* linked control of the relative proportions of antibodies produced to different determinants of native nuclease, *J. Exp. Med.* **145**:123.

Brown, J.L., Kato, K., Silver, J., and Nathenson, S.G., 1974, Notable diversity in peptide composition of murine H-2K and H-2D alloantigens, *Biochemistry* **13**:3174.

Cook, R.G., Uhr, J.W., Capra, J.D., and Vitetta, E.S., 1978, Structural studies on the murine Ia alloantigens. II. Molecular weight characterization of the *I-A* and *I-E/C* subregions, *J. Immunol.* **121**:2205.

Cook, R.G., Vitetta, E.S., Uhr, J.W., and Capra, J.D., 1979, Structural studies on murine Ia alloantigens. V. Evidence that the structural gene for the I-E/C beta polypeptide is encoded within the *I-A* subregion, *J. Exp. Med.* **149**:981.

Cowing, C., Schwartz, B.D., and Dickler, H.B., 1978, Macrophage Ia antigens. I. Macrophage populations differ in their expression of Ia antigens, *J. Immunol.* **120**:378.

Cullen, S.E., and Nathenson, S.G., 1974, Further characterization of Ia (immune response region associated antigen molecules), in: *The Immune System: Genes, Receptors, Signals* (E.E. Sercarz, A.R. Williamson, and C.F. Fox, eds.), p. 191, Academic Press, New York.

Cullen, S.E., and Schwartz, B.D., 1976, An improved method for isolation of H-2 and Ia alloantigens using immune precipitation induced by protein A-bearing *Staphylococci*, *J. Immunol.* **117**:136.

Cullen, S.E., David, C.S., Shreffler, D.C., and Nathenson, S.G., 1974, Membrane molecules determined by the *H-2* associated immune response region: Isolation and some properties, *Proc. Natl. Acad. Sci. U.S.A.* **71**:648.

Cullen, S.E., David, C.S., Cone, J.L., and Sachs, D.H., 1976, Evidence for more than one Ia antigenic specificity on molecules determined by the *I-A* subregion of the mouse major histocompatibility complex, *J. Immunol.* **116**:549.

Cullen, S.E., Kindle, C.S., and Littman, D.R., 1979, Structural comparison of murine Ia antigens determined by the *I-A* and *I-E* subregions, *J. Immunol.* **122**:855.

Dancey, G.F., Cutler, J., and Schwartz, B.D., 1979, Chemical cross-linking of Ia alloantigen α and β chains with dimethyl 3′, 3′-dithiobispropionimidate, *J. Immunol.* **123**:870.

Dorf, M.E., and Benacerraf, B., 1975, Complementation of *H-2* linked *Ir* genes in the mouse, *Proc. Natl. Acad. Sci. U.S.A.* **72**:3671.

Dorf, M.E., Stimpfling, J.H., and Benacerraf, B., 1975, Requirement for two *H-2* complex *Ir* genes for the immune response to the L-glu, L-lys, L-phe terpolymer, *J. Exp. Med.* **141**:1459.

Dorf, M.E., Maurer, P.H., Merryman, C.F., and Benacerraf, B., 1976a, Inclusion group systems and cis-trans effects in response controlled by the two complementing *Ir-GLφ* genes, *J. Exp. Med.* **143**:889.

Dorf, M.E., Twigg, M.B., and Benacerraf, B., 1976b, Genetic control of the immune response to the random linear terpolymer of L-glutamic acid, L-lysine and L-leucine (GLleu) by complementing *Ir* genes, *Eur. J. Immunol.* **6**:552.

Fathman, C.G., and Nabholz, M., 1977, *In vitro* secondary mixed lymphocyte reaction (MLR). II. Interaction MLR determinants expressed by F_1 cells, *Eur. J. Immunol.* **7**:370.

Fathman, C.G., Watanabe, T., and Augustin, A., 1978, *In vitro* secondary MLR. III. Hybrid histocompatibility determinants, *J. Immunol.* **121**:259.

Freed, J.H., and Nathenson, S.G., 1977, Similarity of the carbohydrate structures of H-2 and Ia glycoproteins, *J. Immunol.* **119**:477.

Frelinger, J.A., Niederhuber, J.E., and Shreffler, D.C., 1976. Effects of anti-Ia sera on mitogenic responses. III. Mapping the genes controlling the expression of Ia determinants on Con A reactive cells to the *I-J* subregion of the H-2 complex, *J. Exp. Med.* **144**:1141.

Hammerling, G.J., Mauve, G., Goldberg, E., and McDevitt, H.O., 1975, Tissue distribution of Ia antigens: Ia on spermatozoa, macrophages, and epidermal cells, *Immunogenetics* **1**:428.

Hancock, W.S., Bishop, C.A., Prestidge, R.L., and Hearn, M.T.W., 1978, The use of high pressure liquid chromatography (HPLC) for peptide mapping of proteins, *Anal. Biochem.* **88**:203.

Jones, P.P., Murphy, D.B., and McDevitt, H.O., 1978, Two-gene control of the expression of a murine Ia antigen, *J. Exp. Med.* **148**:925.

Kapp, J.A., Pierce, C.W., Schlossman, S., and Benacerraf, B., 1974, Genetic control of immune responses *in vitro.* V. Stimulation of suppressor T cells in non-responder mice by the terpolymer L-glutamic acid ^{60}-L-alanine^{30}-L-tyrosine^{10} (GAT), *J. Exp. Med.* **140**:648.

Kipp, D.E., Sercarz, E.E., and Miller, A., 1975, Multigenic, *H-2* linked control of the mouse immune response to human lysozyme (HUL), *Fed. Proc. Fed. Am. Soc. Exp. Biol.* **35**:825 (abstract).

Lafuse, W., Neely, B., McKean, D., and David, C., 1979, Biochemical studies of Ia gene products with xenoantisera, Fed. Proc. *Fed. Am. Soc. Exp. Biol.* **38**:1423 (abstract).

Melchers, I., and Rajewsky, K., 1975, Specific control of responsiveness by two complementing *Ir* loci in the *H-2* complex, *Eur. J. Immunol.* **5**:753.

Melchers, I., Rajewsky, K., and Shreffler, D.C., 1973. *Ir-LDHB:* Map position and functional analysis, *Eur. J. Immunol.* **3**:754.

Meo, T., David, C.S., Rijnbeek, A.M., Nabholz, M., Miggiano, V., and Shreffler, D.C., 1973, Inhibition of mouse MLR by anti-Ia antisera, *Transplant. Proc.* **7**:127.

Merryman, C.F., Maurer, P.H., and Stimpfling, J.H., 1975, Unigenic and multigenic *I* region control of the immune responses of mice to the GAT^{10} and GLϕ-GLT terpolymers, *Immunogenetics* **2**:441.

Michaelson, J., Flaherty, L., Vitetta, E., and Poulik, M.D., 1977, Molecular similarities between the Qa-2 alloantigen and other gene products of the 17th chromosome of the mouse, *J. Exp. Med.* **145**:1066.

Mozes, E., Schwartz, M., and Sela, M., 1974, Antibody response of inbred mouse strains to ordered tetrapeptides of tyrosine and glutamic acid attached to multichain polyalanine or polyproline, *J. Exp. Med.* **140**:349.

Muramatsu, T., Nathanson, S.G., Boyse, E.A., and Old, L.J., 1973, Some biochemical properties of thymus leukemia antigens solubilized from cell membranes by papain digestion, *J. Exp. Med.* **137**:1256.

Murphy, D.B., Herzenberg, L.A., Okumura, K., Herzenberg, L.A., and McDevitt, H.O., 1976, A new I subregion (*I-J*) marked by a locus (*Ia-4*) controlling surface determinants on suppressor T lymphocytes, *J. Exp. Med.* **144**:699.

O'Farrell, P.H., 1975, High resolution two-dimensional electrophoresis of proteins, *J. Biol. Chem.* **250**:4007.

Okuda, K., and David, C.S., 1978, A new lymphocyte activating determinant locus expressed on T cells, and mapping in the *I-C* subregion, *J. Exp. Med.* **147:**1028.

Okuda, K., David, C.S., and Shreffler, D.C., 1977, The role of gene products of the *I-J* subregion in mixed lymphocyte reactions, *J. Exp. Med.* **146:**1561.

Okumura, K., Herzenberg, L.A., Murphy, D.B., McDevitt, H.O., and Herzenberg, L.A., 1976, Selective expression of *H-2 (I* region) loci controlling determinants on helper and suppressor T lymphocytes, *J. Exp. Med.* **144:**685.

Rich, S.S., and Rich, R.R., 1976. Regulatory mechanisms in cell mediated immune responses. III. *I* region control of suppressor cell interaction with responder cells in mixed lymphocyte reactions, *J. Exp. Med.* **143:**672.

Schwartz, B.D., and Cullen, S.E., 1978, Chemical characteristics of Ia antigens, *Semin. Immunopathol.* **1:**85.

Schwartz, B.D., Vitetta, E.S., and Cullen, S.E., 1978, Labeling characteristics and separation of Ia antigen subunits, *J. Immunol.* **120:**671.

Schwartz, R.H., Solinger, A.M., Ultee, M., and Margoliash, E., 1978a, Genetic control of the T-lymphocyte proliferative response to cytochrome c, in: Immunobiology of proteins and peptides, I (M.Z. Atassi and A.B. Stavitsky, eds.), *Adv. Exp. Med. Biol.* **98:**371.

Schwartz, R.H., Berzofsky, J.A., Horton, C.L., Schechter, A.N., and Sachs, D.H., 1978b, Genetic control of the T-lymphocyte proliferative response to staphylococcal nuclease: Evidence for multiple MHC-linked *Ir* gene control, *J. Immunol.* **120:**1741.

Seaver, S.S., Brown, A., Hammerling, G., and McDevitt, H.O., 1976, Genetic control of the immune response: Ability of antigens of defined amino acid sequence to be recognized by the *Ir-1* gene system, *Eur. J. Immunol.* **6:**502.

Shreffler, D.C., and David, C.S., 1975, The H-2 major histocompatibility complex and the I immune response region: Genetic variation, function, and organization, *Adv. Immunol.* **20:**125.

Shreffler, D.C., David, C.S., Passmore, H.C., and Klein, J., 1971, Genetic organization and evolution of the mouse *H-2* region: A duplication model, *Transplant. Proc.* **3:**176.

Snell, G.D., Cherry, M., and Demant, P., 1971, Evidence that H-2 private specificities can be arranged in two mutually exclusive systems possibly homologous with two subsystems of HLA, *Transplant. Proc.* **3:**183.

Stimpfling, J.H., and Durham, T., 1972, Genetic control by the *H-2* gene complex of the alloantibody response to to H-2 antigen, *J. Immunol.* **108:**947.

Tada, T., Taniguchi, M., and David, C.S., 1976, Properties of the antigen-specific suppressive T cell factor in the regulation of antibody response of the mouse. IV. Special subregion assignment of the gene(s) that codes for the suppressive T cell factor in the *H-2* histocompatibility complex, *J. Exp. Med.* **144:**713.

Vitetta, E.S., Uhr, J.W., and Boyse, E.A., 1972, Isolation and characterization of H-2 and TL alloantigens from the surface of mouse thymocytes, *Cell. Immunol.* **4:**187.

Vitetta, E.S., Artzt, K., Bennett, D., Boyse, E.A., and Jacob, F., 1975, Structural similarities between a product of the *T/t* locus isolated from sperm and teratoma cells, and H-2 antigens isolated from splenocytes, *Proc. Natl. Acad. Sci. U.S.A.* **73:**3215.

Zaleski, M., and Klein, J., 1974, Immune response of mice to Thy-1.1 antigen: Genetic control by alleles at the *Ir-5* locus loosely linked to the *H-2* complex, *J. Immunol.* **113:**1170.

Zaleski, M.B., and Klein, J., 1976, Immune response of mice to the Thy-1.1 antigen: Intra-*H-2* mapping of the complemeentary *Ir–Thy-1* loci, *J. Immunol.* **117:**814.

Zaleski, M., and Milgrom, F., 1973, Complementary genes controlling immune response to θ-AKR antigen in mice, *J. Immunol.* **110:**1238.

17

Structure of H-2 Major Histocompatibility Complex Products

Recent Studies on the H-2K^b Glycoprotein and on the H-2K^b MHC Mutants

Stanley G. Nathenson, Bruce M. Ewenstein, Hiroshi Uehara, John M. Martinko, John E. Coligan, and Thomas J. Kindt

1. Introduction

The immune response is a reaction to a foreign or nonself substance. Intricately involved in this highly specific and tightly regulated protective-reaction mechanism are the gene products of the major histocompatibility complex (MHC) (Klein, 1975; Snell *et al.*, 1976; Paul and Benacerraf, 1977; Götze, 1977; Snell, 1978). This genetic system was referred to as the *H-2* locus when it was initially recognized as a determinant of transplantation acceptance or rejection nearly 45 years ago by P.A. Gorer (1936). The serological and genetic features were gradually unraveled over the ensuing years. The complexity, both in terms of number of genes and in terms of polymorphism, led to the use of the term *H-2* major histocompatibility complex to refer to this chromosomal region in the mouse. Similar MHC complexes have been found in other species (Götze, 1977).

Stanley G. Nathenson, Bruce M. Ewenstein, Hiroshi Uehara, and John M. Martinko • Department of Microbiology and Immunology and Department of Cell Biology, Albert Einstein College of Medicine, Bronx, New York 10461. John E. Coligan and Thomas J. Kindt • Laboratory of Immunogenetics, National Institutes of Health, Bethesda, Maryland 20205.

In the *H-2* MHC, the present genetic map in its most simplified form consists of the following regions, listed in order of their distance from the centromere: *K, I, S, G, D, L, Qa-1, Qa-2,* and *TL* (Klein, 1975; Snell *et al.*, 1976; Klein, 1978). The glycoprotein products of the *K* and *D* genes have a molecular weight of 44,000 and carry two carbohydrate chains with a molecular weight of 3100, and exist *in vivo* tightly integrated into the matrix of the cell surface (Schwartz *et al.*, 1973; Snell *et al.*, 1976; Nathenson and Cullen, 1974). In the cell membrane, the glycoproteins are noncovalently associated with β_2-microglobulin (β_2m) (Rask *et al.*, 1974; Silver and Hood, 1974; Natori *et al.*, 1975). The serologically detected alloantigenicity of the H-2 glycoproteins resides in their protein structure (Nathenson and Muramatsu, 1971).

2. Studies on the Primary Structure of the H-2K^b Glycoprotein

2.1. General Methodology and Preparation of H-2K^b

The approach developed for the present studies arose from the need to analyze the primary structure of proteins that are normally insoluble or membrane-bound *in situ* and that are available in extremely small amounts. Previously, classic techniques in protein chemistry have required hundreds of milligrams of purified protein to determine the sequence of a polypeptide chain of about 300–350 amino acids in length. Because of the extremely small amounts of the H-2 antigens available for analysis and because of the great difficulty in obtaining these molecules in purified form, several approaches have been tried in various laboratories.

One approach has been the development of bulk cell-culture techniques to isolate kilogram quantities of cells from which milligram quantities of antigens can be isolated (Acton and Lynn, 1977). Sequences have been determined for extensive parts of several HLA molecules isolated from cultured human lymphoblastoid-cell lines (Pleogh *et al.*, 1978). Another type of approach based on improvements of amino acid sequence techniques developed by Wittman-Liebold (1973) was described by Hood and associates (Hunkapiller and Hood, 1978), in which extensive data can be obtained with only a few milligrams of protein.

The technique that we have successfully utilized for the H-2 MHC antigens was a logical extension of our previous analysis of radiolabeled alloantigens for peptide mapping studies (Brown *et al.*, 1974). This method of sequence analysis has also been used previously for partial structure studies on small proteins such as hormones (Jacobs *et al.*, 1974) and viral peptides (McKean *et al.*, 1974). The methodology (schematically described in Fig. 1) involves the use of intrinsically labeled proteins ob-

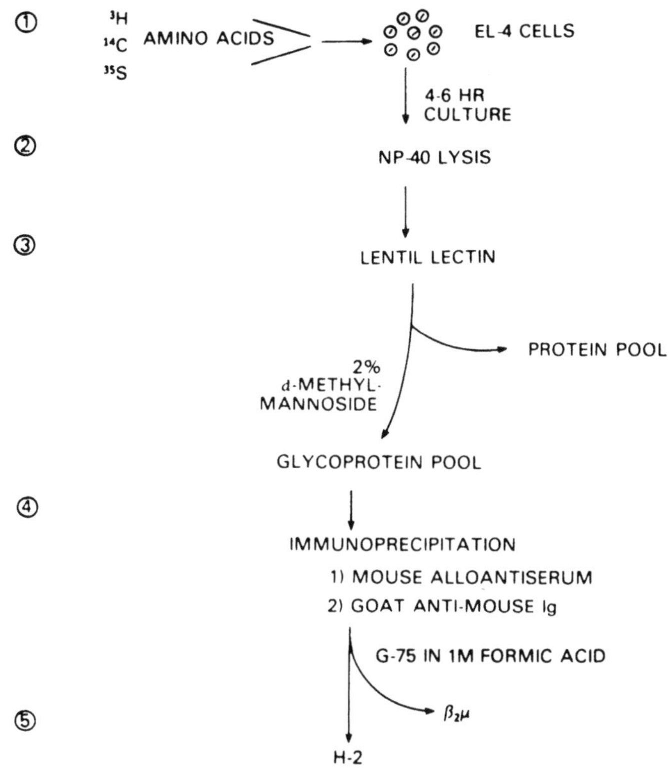

Figure 1. Scheme for isolation of the H-2K^b glycoprotein.

tained from cells cultured in the presence of radioactive amino acids. The cells are then extracted with nonionic detergent to solubilize the membrane-integrated antigen, and a partial purification of about 10-fold is effected by affinity chromatography on a lentil lectin–Sepharose column. This fractionation step enriches for the H-2 glycoproteins, which are then isolated from this mixture by immune complex formation using alloantisera, followed by a second antibody for precipitation. The immune precipitate is dissolved in formic acid and fractionated by G-75 Sephadex chromatography to separate the H-2 molecules from the β_2m (Ewenstein *et al.*, 1978).

This approach is universal in its applicability to any protein that can be metabolically radiolabeled and isolated by a specific affinity agent. The radiolabeled protein obtained can be analyzed using routine procedures for sequence analysis. A limitation of this technique is that the various amino acids are incorporated at different levels.

2.2. Isolation and Biochemical Characterization of the CNBr Fragments of the H-2K^b Glycoprotein

To obtain peptide fragments for amino acid sequence analysis of the K^b glycoprotein, the molecule was treated with cyanogen bromide (Gross, 1967). This treatment results in cleavage at the C-terminal side of most methionine residues in a protein. Nine unique fragments could be isolated by a series of gel filtration and ion-exchange chromatographic separations (Fig. 2). The first step in their isolation was chromatography of the CNBr digests on Sephadex G-100 in the presence of 6 M guanidine

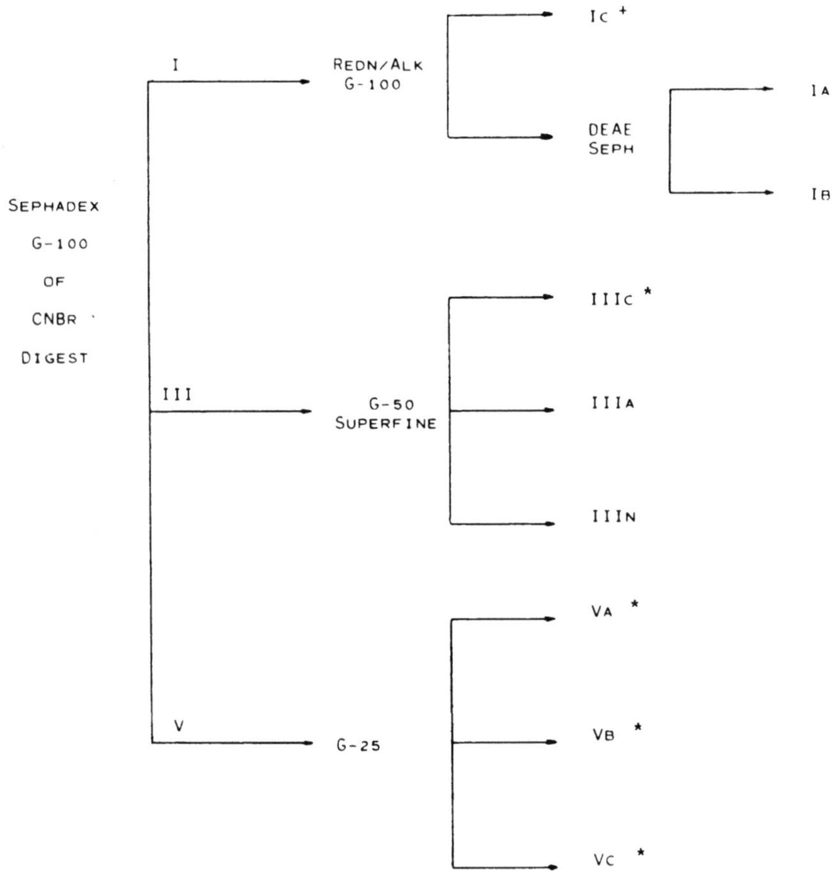

Figure 2. Purification scheme for CNBr fragments from H-2K^b. *Fragments not present in papain-solubilized molecule; $^+$size reduced when isolated from papain-solubilized molecule.

hydrochloride (Fig. 3A). Three major fractions (I, III, V) and a variable amount of uncleaved material (A) were separated. Pool I, eluting with chymotrypsinogen, was subjected to reduction and alkylation to cleave any disulfide bonds among the large peptides in this mixture. Following this treatment, the Pool I peptides were again subjected to chromatography on the same Sephadex G-100 Column (Fig. 3B). This resulted in two fractions, one of which contained a pure peptide designated Ic and the other of which contained two peptides (Iab), plus some partially cleaved material (Ix). It was observed that the molecular weight of peptide Ic changed when the molecule was subjected to digestion with papain prior to isolation. This indicated that the Ic peptide included the C terminus of the molecule, which was lost on papain cleavage. The other pool, Pool Iab, was subjected to chromatography on DEAE Sephadex and yielded two pure glycopeptides (Ia and Ib).

Pool III (Fig.2) from the first G-100 column was subjected to chromatography on Sephadex G-50 (superfine), yielding three peptides designated IIIc, IIIa, and IIIn. The peptide designated IIIc was not present in digests of papain-treated K^b molecules. Amino acid sequence analysis indicated that the IIIn peptide had the sequence of the amino terminus of

Figure 3. Chromatography of fragments labeled with tritiated amino acid (Ser, Ile, Gly, His, Thr, Val, and Trp) from the H-2K^b molecule on a Sephadex G-100 column (135 × 1.5 cm) in 6 M guanadine hydrochloride (Gdn • HCl). (A) Unreduced CNBr fragments; (B) rechromatography of Pool I after reduction and akkylation with iodoacetamide. Molecular-weight markers: (BSA) bovine serum albumin (M_r = 68,000); (CHYM), bovine chymotrypsinogen (M_r = 25,700); (MGB) sperm whale myoglobin (M_r = 17,800); (CYT C) cytochrome *c* (M_r = 14,200); (INS B) bovine pancreas insulin B (M_r = 3,400); (LEU) leucine (M_r = 131). Reprinted by permission of the National Academy of Sciences from Ewenstein *et al.* (1978), which should be consulted for further details.

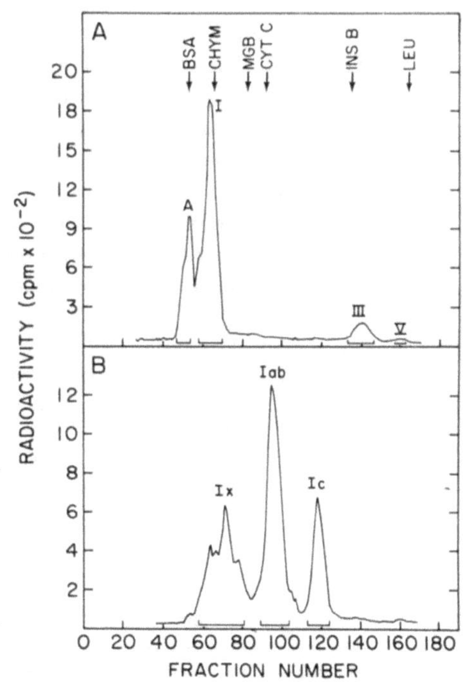

the K^b molecule and that the IIIa peptide had the sequence beginning with position 24 in the intact molecule. Pool V from the original Sephadex G-100 column contained at least three peptides that could be separated by gel-filtration chromatography on Sephadex G-25. These peptides were not present in papain-digested molecules, and probably represent regions C-terminal to the papain-cleavage site. They are presently being studied in greater detail.

The characteristics of the major CNBr fragments of H-2K^b are shown in Table 1. The five fragments listed comprise the entire N-terminal portion of the papain-cleaved molecule. In the carbohydrate-containing fragments, Ia and Ib, similar fucose incorporation levels suggest that equal amounts of carbohydrate are present in each. Since the amount of carbohydrate reported in purified papain-cleaved material isolated from mouse spleens was about 12% (Shimada and Nathenson, 1969), it can be estimated that one carbohydrate unit of 3100 daltons is present in each of these CNBr fragments. This finding of two carbohydrate moieties represents a significant difference from the HLA-A2 and HLA-B7 glycoproteins, for which only one carbohydrate unit has been observed (Parham *et al.*, 1977).

2.3. Alignment of the CNBr Fragments of H-2K^b

CNBr fragments of K^b were aligned as shown in Fig. 4. The alignment of IIIn and IIIa was determined by comparison of the amino acid sequence of these peptides with that of the amino terminal of the intact glycoprotein. For example, by automatic sequence determination, it was possible to assign positions 23 and 52 as methionine, as well as to make definitive assignments for Arg and Tyr in order to confirm this alignment.

To align the remaining CNBr fragments, tryptic peptides labeled in both [^{35}S]-Met and in several tritiated amino acids were isolated and their sequences determined. The unambiguous assignments of overlapping

TABLE 1. Characterization of Major CNBr Fragments of H-2K^b

Fragment	M_r	Spanning positions	NH_2 terminus	Carbohydrate
IIIn	2,500	1–23	Gly Pro His	–
IIIa	3,200	24–52	Glu Val Gly	–
Ib	11,500[a]	53–138	Glu Gln Glu	+
Ia	12,000[a]	139–228	Ala Ala Leu	+
Ic	5,800[a]	229–283	Glu Leu Val	–

[a]Molecular weights were estimated for these fragments.

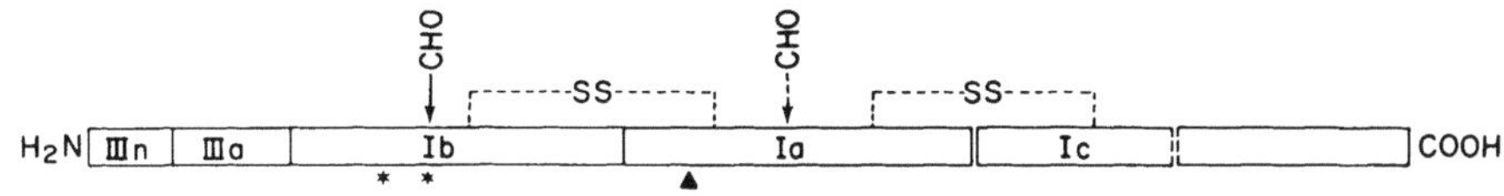

Figure 4. Hypothetical model of the structure of the H-2K^b glycoprotein. The five major CNBr fragments found in the papain solubilized molecule include: IIIn, IIIa, Ib, Ia, and Ic. Fragments IIIb, Va, Vb, and Vc are absent in the papain-solubilized molecule and are contained in the region C-terminal to the Ic fragment. (CHO) Carbohydrate moiety; (SS) cysteine disulfide bridge. *Mutations found in bm 3 mutant; ▲, mutations found in bm 1 mutant.

peptides have to date proved the alignment of all CNBr peptides except for the Ia–Ic junction.

Thus far, it has not been possible to unambiguously align the four CNBr fragments of the K^b glycoprotein that fit in the unmarked region carboxy-terminal to Ic (Fig. 4). However, it was previously demonstrated that the apparent molecular weight of fragment Ic is decreased by approximately 1000 when this fragment is obtained from the papain-treated molecule. Thus, it is possible to place fragment Ic at the carboxy terminal of the 37,000-molecular-weight fragment. Because fragments IIIc, Va, Vb, and Vc are absent from the papain-cleaved molecule, they are placed carboxy-terminal to the site of papain cleavage of the 45,000-molecular-weight glycoprotein.

Although formal studies aimed at the determination of the disulfide bridges have not yet been completed, several lines of reasoning have led to the arrangement shown. It has been demonstrated that in K^b, the CNBr fragments Ia, Ib, and Ic are connected by disulfide bonds. In a mutant molecule, H-2K^{bj} (bm 10) (B. Ewenstein, unpublished observation), a Met–Val interchange at residue 165 results in a new cleavage for CNBr. The characterization of the CNBr peptides from the H-2K^{bj} glycoprotein strongly supports the presence of two linear cysteine bridges, as has been reported for HLA-A2 and HLA-B7 (Ferguson *et al.*, 1979). The positions of the carbohydrate moieties have been determined by isolation and analysis of the tryptic glycopeptides.

2.4. Amino Acid Sequence Studies of the CNBr Fragments of the H-2K^b Glycoprotein

To obtain the complete sequence of the K^b glycoprotein, it was necessary to develop a total strategy based on radioactive sequence techniques. A primary consideration in radioisotope sequence analysis of a protein concerns the choice of radioactive amino acids to be added to a cell culture in order to radiolabel the protein. Tritium-labeled amino acids

TABLE 2. Combinations of Radiolabeled[a] Amino Acids Analyzed for H-2K[b]

Group	I	Phe, Leu, Lys, Cys, Pro,[b] Ala[a]
	II	His, Trp, Thr, Ile, Val, Ser,[b] Gly[b]
	III	Glu, Pro, Arg
	IV	Gly, Ser
	V	Gln, Glu, Pro
	VI	Met, Tyr
	VII	Ala, Cys

[a] All amino acids, except Cys and Met, were radiolabeled with ^3H.
[b] Incorporated at levels too low for reliable sequence analysis.

were chosen in our study because of the high specific activity and the low cost relative to the ^{14}C-labeled amino acids. The question of how many different amino acids are to be added to the cell culture is difficult to answer and requires experimental data for an appropriate solution. The alternative extremes of adding either one amino acid or all 20 amino acids are usually not practical. With a single-amino-acid-labeled protein, all peptides would have to be purified and their sequences determined a minimum of 20 times. This would represent a time-consuming and expensive effort. With 20 amino acids radiolabeled, complete sequence determinations for each peptide could be done after one or two isolations. However, identification of the derivatives of the radioactive amino acids from each sequenator step would require very precise analysis, and any significant inequalities among the specific activities of the radioactive amino acids could lead to errors. Clearly, a compromise must be effected.

In our original studies (Coligan *et al.*, 1978), groups of six or seven amino acids were chosen for incorporation. The relative amount of each radioactive amino acid incorporated into cellular proteins was determined by sequence analysis of the β_2m, which is a by-product of an earlier purification step for the H-2 molecule. Mouse β_2m has a known amino-terminal sequence for approximately 35 residues, and these residues include all but 2 of the 20 amino acids normally found in mammalian proteins (Kimball *et al.*, 1979). Analysis of the radiolabeled β_2m then indicated that certain amino acids (Ala, Gly, Pro) have relatively low incorporation rates. Further, the phenylthiohydantoin derivatives of Gly and Ser are particularly problematic, since normal conversion procedures often destroy Ser and the tritium in radiolabeled Gly appears to be lost with excessive heating, especially during evaporation of the butyl chloride from the thiazolinone. Because of these problems, the amino acids mentioned above were incorporated in individual experiments as shown in Table 2, and the molecules radiolabeled with these residues were analyzed separately.

The sequence analysis of β_2m and subsequently that of the H-2 molecule has shown that with the EL-4 cell line, certain amino acids are biosynthetically converted during growth in culture. The most important of these interconversions are listed in Table 3. Similar interconversions have been seen with other cell lines (Kimball *et al.*, 1979).

It was further observed that certain radiolabeled amino acids were incorporated at higher rates than others. The amino acid with best incorporation was Arg, with as much as 80% of the added radioactivity observed in cell protein. At the bottom of the list would be Asp, which has incorporation of under 1%. This difficulty with Asp has made it the only amino acid for which data are not at present available in the K^b molecule. Asn has only recently been available in high specific activity, but there appears to be no difficulty with its incorporation, and it is anticipated that Asn positions will be assigned shortly.

The results of the amino-terminal sequence analysis of the CNBr fragments are shown in Fig. 5. The X symbols are used for positions that have not been directly identified, but it can be assumed that many of these positions will be occupied by Asp or Asn. The lengths of CNBr fragments Ia and Ic were estimated by reference to HLA sequences and are in substantial agreement with the molecular weights of these fragments obtained by molecular-sieve chromatography in 6 M Gdn • HCl. The position of the carbohydrate unit of peptide Ib has been assigned to position 86 from the amino terminus. There is a second carbohydrate moiety pre-

TABLE 3. Interconversion of ^{3}H Amino Acids In EL-4 Cell Cultures

Added to culture	Radioactive Amino acids in β_2m[a]	Relative activity
Glu	Glu	10
	Pro	0.64
	Arg	0.18
Gln	Gln	1.0
	Glu	0.22
	Pro	0.09
Ser	Ser	1.0
	Gly	0.1
Gly	Gly	1.0
	Ser	0.5

[a]Detected by NH_2-terminal sequence analysis of the β_2m separated from H-2K^b by gel filtration.

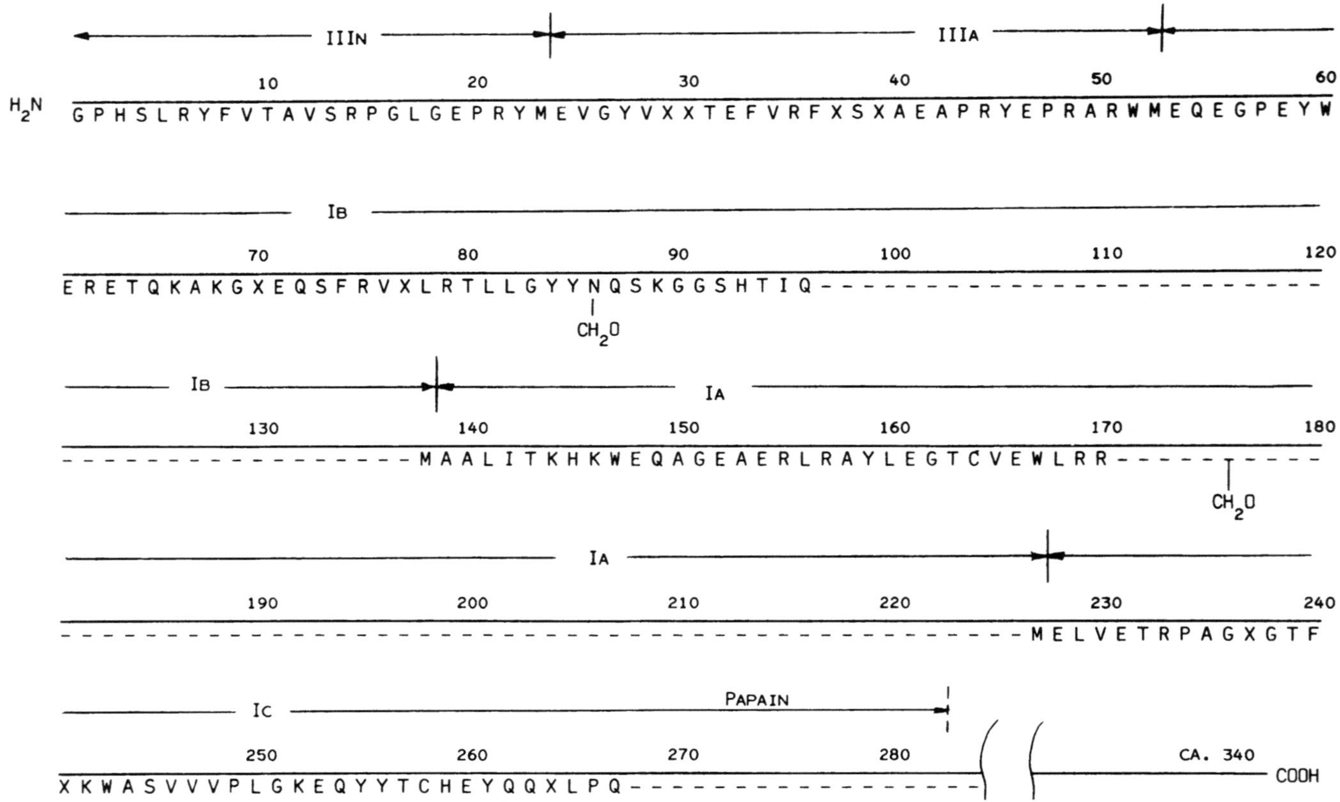

Figure 5. Schematic representation of the H-2K^b molecule depicting the approximate regions of known sequence as described previously. Details were taken from references by Ewenstein *et al.* (1978) and Coligan *et al.* (1978, 1979). Arrows delimit CNBr fragments. The site of papain cleavage is not known, but it is depicted in the region 270–275. Amino acids are designated by the standard one-letter symbols: (A) Ala; (C) Cys; (D) Asp; (E) Glu; (F) Phe; (G) Gly; (H) His; (I) Ile; (K) Lys; (L) Leu; (M) Met; (N) Asn; (Q) Gln; (R) Arg; (S) Ser; (T) Thr; (V) Val; (W) Tyr.

sent in peptide Ia, but this unit has not yet been precisely localized, although our present evidence suggests that it is attached at position 176.

2.5. Comparison of H-2K^b with Other Transplantation Antigens

2.5.1. Comparison with Other H-2 Antigens

A comparison of the NH_2-terminal 27 residues of K^b with those of several other H-2 antigens is shown in Table 4.

Although the data are not yet extensive for any mouse histocompatibility antigen other than K^b, several patterns have already emerged. It is obvious that a striking degree of homology exists among all the molecules thus far examined. In particular, of the 20 positions that can be compared between K^b (EL-4) and K^k or K^q, 17 appear to be identical (85% homology). Similarly, a comparison of K^b with D^d reveals that of the 20 positions that can be evaluated, 18 appear to be identical (90% homology), and for another K to D comparison (K^b vs. D^b), 11 of 13 are identical (85%). Thus, no greater similarities are evident between individual K products than between K and D products, and no particular patterns can be used to define a biochemical difference between D and K products. However, a pattern of possible significance is that the observed amino acid interchanges occur at rather discrete places. Residues 9 and 22 appear to be particularly interesting because of the possibility that the interchanges at these two positions may be coupled to each other (Vitetta and Capra, 1978).

TABLE 4. Comparison of H-2K^b to Other H-2 Molecules in the NH_2-Terminal Region[a]

	1				5					10					15					20						25	
H-2K^b	G	P	H	S	L	R	Y	F	V	T	A	V	S	R	P	G	L	G	E[b]	P	R	Y	M	E	V	G	Y
H-2K^k	[c]	–	–	–	–	–	–	–	H	–	–	–	–	–	–		–			–	–	F	[c]				–
H-2K^q	(–)	–	–	–	–	–	–	–	H	–	–	–	–	–	–		–			–	–	F					–
H-2K^d	M		–		–	–	–			(–)				(–)			–			(–)	–	F					–
H-2D^b		–			M	–	–	–			–	–		–			–			–	–	F					–
H-2D^d	–	S	–	–	–	–	–	–	–	–		–	–	–	,–	F	–			–	–	–				–	

[a]Data taken from Cook *et al.* (1976), Henning *et al.* (1976), Silver and Hood (1976), Vitetta *et al.* (1976), Vitetta and Capra (1978), and Dr. R. Nairn, personal communication (H-2D^d). The standard one-letter symbols are used to designate amino acids (IUPAC-IUB Commission on Biochemical Nomenclature). A dash (—) is used where the amino acid residue is identical to that of H-2K^b. Parentheses indicate tentative assignment.

[b]Position 19 has been reported by Vitetta *et al.* (1976) to be Lys for K^b.

[c]Previously assigned as Met, now unassigned (Vitetta *et al.*, 1976).

2.5.2. Comparison with HLA

The first extensive comparison of amino acid sequences of human and mouse histocompatibility antigens has been made possible by the structural data recently reported by Ploegh *et al.* (1978). Comparison of regions of HLA-A2 or -B7 for which continuous amino acid sequences have been reported are shown in Table 5 compared to the amino acid sequences for corresponding segments of K^b. Comparison of K^b with A2 at positions 1–96 shows that the amino acids at 63 of the comparable 89 positions are identical, for a homology of 70%. Further comparison of the K^b molecule between positions 228 and 267 to homologous regions of the B7 molecule indicates identity of 77%, with 30 of 39 compared positions. In these comparisons, Asx (Asp or Asn) was substituted in all positions in K^b where it was felt that if any other amino acid residue occurred it would have been detected by our sequence analysis. Of the 9 presumptive Asx residues that have been inserted in the K^b sequence, 7 are homologous to those present in the HLA.

It is of interest that where differences exist, most of the interchanges minimally require only single base substitutions at the nucleic acid level. Another striking aspect of the sequence variation observed with the HLA-A2, HLA-B7, and K^b comparisons is the apparent nonrandom distribution of the differences. For example, in the amino terminal, two clusters of differences can be seen encompassing residues 41–45 and 67–75. These residues consist of 13 (15%) of the 89 compared positions, but account for about half the observed differences. The overall impressions to be drawn from this comparison are of course preliminary, since only one H-2 and one HLA sequence have been reported. Nonetheless, the striking clustering of differences suggests possible functional significance.

An amino acid sequence homology of greater than 70% between H-2 and HLA molecules would appear not to be greatly different from the 80–85% homology observed among H-2 molecules from different haplotypes, as determined by NH_2-terminal sequence determination and extrapolation from tryptic peptide comparisons (Brown *et al.*, 1974).

2.6. Division of K^b Into Intramolecular Regions

A convenient way to view the structural organization of the K^b protein is suggested in Fig. 6, in which the molecule has been subdivided into four regions of approximately 90 residues each. The three NH_2-terminal regions, N (amino terminal), C_1 (first cysteine-disulfide-linked), and C_2 (second cysteine-disulfide-linked), are presumed to be exterior to the cell surface and show some features of similarity to each other. The fourth region (TM, or transmembrane) is strikingly different and appears to be

TABLE 5. Comparison between Mouse and Human Histocompatibility Antigens[a]

	10 20 30
H-2K^b	G P H S L R Y F V T A V S R P G L G E P R Y M E V G Y V B B T E F V R
HLA-A2	— S —— M ——— F — S ———— R ——— F I A ————————
	40 50 60 70
K^b	F B S B A E A P R Y E P R A R W M E Q E G P E Y W E R E T Q K A K G B
A2	———— A S Z — M ——— P — I ——— S —— X X — X X X — V — A H
	80 90
K^b	E Q S F R V B L R T L L G Y Y B Q S K G G S H T I Q
A2	A H T V ——— G ————— Z A ——— V —
	230 240 250 260
K^b	E L V E T R P A G B G T F Q K W A S V V V P L G K E X Y Y Y T C H X Y Q
HLA-B7	———— R ———— A [] ——— X — X X X R ———— V O H
	267
K^b	Q G L P
B7	E ——

[a]Data taken from Coligan *et al.* (1979) and Pleogh *et al.* (1978).

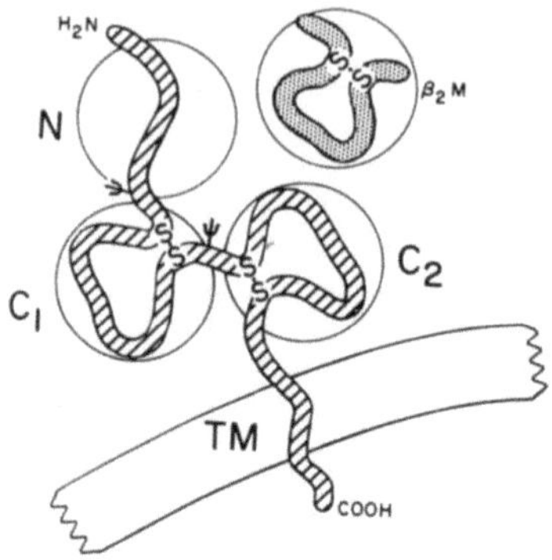

Figure 6. Hypothetical structural organization of the K^b protein. H-$2K^b$ is depicted as containing four regions: (N) N-terminal region; (C_1) first cysteine-disulfide-linked region; (C_2) second cysteine-disulfide-linked region; (TM) transmembrane region. β_2-Microglobulin (β_2m, stippled) is shown in noncovalent association with the H-$2K^b$ glycoprotein heavy chain. (SS) Cysteine-disulfide-linked; (Ψ) carbohydrate moieties.

involved with membrane anchorage and possibly cytoplasmic interactions. The most salient feature of the two central regions, C_1 and C_2,, is that each contains a single disulfide bridge that comprises a loop of approximately 60 amino acid residues. The N region contains no cysteine, but has a single carbohydrate unit at a position homologous to the single carbohydrate unit of the C_1 region.

Physical evidence arising from differential susceptibility to proteolytic cleavage and consistent with the postulated intramolecular organization in K^b has been obtained in a number of experiments. Earlier studies on the release of H-2 molecules from cell membranes by proteolytic digestion with papain revealed that the antigenic activity resided on fragments (designated Class I and Class II) of two distinct molecular weights (Shimada and Nathenson, 1969). The Class I fragments, including that derived from K^b , have an estimated $M_r = 37{,}000$. Papain digests of the isolated membrane-free detergent-solubilized K^b have also yielded the amino-terminal fragment of approximately $M_r = 37{,}000$. Such data suggest that these treatments have resulted in the removal of the fourth region. Papain cleavage between regions C_1 and C_2 does not appear to occur in H-$2K^b$. However, similar treatment of D^b results in a 26,000-molecular-weight NH_2-fragment (Class II fragment) consistent with the model shown (Shimada and Nathenson, 1969; Uehara, unpublished observation). Experiments essentially in agreement with this model have also been reported (Peterson *et al.*, 1975) demonstrating that a variety of proteolytic enzymes, including trypsin, papain, and thermolysin-subfragmented papain yielded solubilized H-2 molecules yielding peptides of approximately 20,000 and 13,000 daltons. The 20,000-dalton fragment was thought to have been derived from the amino-terminal molecule and to contain all the carbohydrate of the intact protein (Peterson *et al.*, 1975). The differential susceptibility to proteolytic cleavage suggests, but does not prove, that there exist limited regions of less tightly folded polypeptide analogous to the hinge or switch region of the immunoglobulin chain (Gally, 1973).

The question of primary-structure homology among these regions remains to be elucidated. Cursory inspection of the amino acid sequences presented in this review indicates that such homology, if present, will not be very high. On the other hand, this low degree of homology at the primary-structural level may be a reflection of an accumulation of amino acid substitutions that do not significantly alter the secondary and tertiary structural features of the molecule. Thus, the ultimate evaluation of this model will probably require the application of X-ray crystallographic techniques.

3. Structural Analysis of H-2K^b Products from H-2K^b Mutants

3.1. Background

While the genetic and functional properties of the *K* and *D* gene products have not yet been fully defined, it is already clear that these products are intimately involved in the specificity of cell–cell interactions in immune recognition and response. For example, *K* and *D* gene products are targets for allograft rejection and graft-vs.-host (GVH) reactivity. Also, evidence strongly suggests that these same products can serve as both stimulators in the mixed-lymphocyte reaction (MLR) and targets in cell-mediated lympholysis (CML). Finally, it is increasingly clear that the K and D antigens are part of the recognition complex in the immune reaction to a variety of non-H-2 antigens, including viral polypeptides, chemically modified antigens, and minor histocompatibility antigens (for reviews, see Klein, 1975; Snell *et al.*, 1976; Paul and Benacerraf, 1977). It seems reasonable that the extreme polymorphism of the MHC system plays a role in the specificity of such interactions, and it is polymorphism that is one of the most striking properties of the H-2K and H-2D glycoproteins.

The amino acid substitutions among the *K* and *D* gene products, as revealed by previous structural studies, are extensively distributed throughout the molecule (Brown *et al.*, 1974). Because of the large number of amino acid differences (as many as 40–50) estimated to exist between the *K* and *D* gene products of standard haplotypes, a straightforward correlation between structure and function has not been possible. In order to examine a genetic situation in which it was hoped that the number of structural alterations might be small, but one in which a specific biological activity could be measured, we began to analyze a series of mouse haplotypes carrying mutations in their *K* and *D* gene products. The most extensive study involves the *H-2K^b* series, in which strong reciprocal histogenic activity can be readily observed. Over 11 such mutants in the gene of the *H-2K^b* allele have been discovered by skin-graft rejection

(Bailey and Kohn, 1965; Egorov, 1967; Melvold and Kohn, 1976, Kohn *et al.*, 1978; reviews by McKenzie *et al.*, 1977; Klein, 1978). These mutant strains show GVH reactivity, positive reactivity in MLR and CML, and in some cases altered H-2 associative recognition.

In the following section, we wish to review some of our recent results on the overall properties and primary structure of the *K* products from two of the mutants of the $H\text{-}2K^b$ series. Previous published structural studies of two K^b mutants, bm 1* (Hzl, B6.C-H-2^{ba}) and bm 3 (M505, B6-H-2^{bd}), demonstrate the presence of limited biochemical alterations in each of the mutant glycoproteins (Brown and Nathenson, 1977). In comparisons of the *K* gene products of each of these mutant lines with that of the *K* product of the standard C57BL/6 strain, it was found that the H-2 glycoproteins exhibited unaltered behavior in a number of purification procedures, including lentil lectin–Sepharose affinity chromatography, immune precipitation, and gel filtration on BioGel A 0.5 M in the presence of sodium dodecyl sulfate. However, ion-exchange chromatography of the tryptic peptides of each of these H-2 molecules on Spherix resin revealed differences among these proteins involving two to three peptides.

The approach undertaken to further biochemically characterize the K^b molecules of the mutant mouse strains involves the use of the same CNBr fragmentation and purification scheme outlined in Section 2. In such studies, spleen cells from parent and mutant animals are labeled in short-term tissue culture with either ^{3}H- or ^{14}C-labeled Arg or Lys. Following purification of the H-2 glycoprotein and CNBr fragmentation, each individual CNBr fragment is subjected to further digestion by trypsin. The resultant tryptic peptides are then compared in a paired-label experiment by co-chromatography using ion-exchange techniques. Because the individual CNBr fragments contain only a few Lys or Arg residues, chromatographic patterns are relatively simple. In addition, on the strength of the extensive sequence studies that have been performed on the purified CNBr fragments and the tryptic peptides of the K^b glycoprotein derived from the EL-4 cell line (Ewenstein *et al.*, 1978; Coligan *et al.*, 1978), these patterns are often readily interpretable in terms of amino acid alterations. Moreover, CNBr fragmentation has allowed some preliminary sequence studies to be carried out on the mutant K^b molecules themselves in an attempt to confirm models of mutational events based on the tryptic mapping technique.

When a protein is labeled in Arg or Lys and digested with trypsin, it is in theory possible to visualize every peptide with one exception, the carboxy-terminal tryptic peptide of that intact molecule. However, on

*Designations conform with H-2 Mutant Workshop Agreements (Kohn *et al.*, 1978).

prior digestion with CNBr, additional unlabeled regions of the proteins are created at the carboxy terminal of each CNBr fragment. This limitation has, in part, been overcome in this work by also performing tryptic maps of the intact mutant and parent K^b glycoprotein labeled in [^{35}S]- or [^{3}H]methionine.

Finally, it should also be mentioned that the tryptic peptide analyses performed thus far have principally involved the five CNBr fragments that constitute the papain-derived fragment of K^b (regions N, C_1, and C_2). These fragments collectively represent that portion of the H-2 molecule thought to be exposed on the outside of the cell and account for approximately 280 of the estimated 350 residues of the intact molecule. In addition, they span what is believed to be the entire serologically defined antigenic portion of the molecule.

3.2. Structural Studies of the K Products from the bm 1 and bm 3 Mutants

In studies on bm 1, following purification of CNBr fragments from $K^{bm\,1}$ and K^b differentially radioactively labeled at either Arg or Lys residues, the fragments were subjected to tryptic digestion and the resultant peptides compared. The peptide differences between parent- and mutant-derived molecules were localized to CNBr fragment Ia (Fig. 7). Two peptides (Loss) containing labeled Arg were seen to be lacking in the peptide map of mutant-derived material that were present in the profile obtained from the parent strain. On the other hand, a new Arg-labeled peptide (Gain) was present in the tryptic map of CNBr fragment Ia derived from $K^{bm\,1}$ that is absent from the K^b molecule (Nisizawa *et al.*, 1980).

The amino acid sequence of the peptides missing in the mutant molecule but present in the parent have been determined in the course of a sequence analysis of the K^b glycoprotein of EL-4. These peptides are thought to encompass residues 147–155 and 156–157. The loss of two adjacent tryptic peptides and the concomitant gain of a single new peptide is most simply explained by a mutation of the Arg at position 155 of the parent molecule to an amino acid that is not susceptible to tryptic cleavage. Such an event would produce a single peptide in the mutant spanning residues 147–157, which could still contain the carboxy-terminal Arg residue. To test this hypothesis, the N-terminal sequence of CNBr fragment Ia labeled in [^{3}H]-Arg from the mutant H-2$K^{bm\,1}$ was determined. [^{14}C]-Arg-labeled CNBr Ia from K^b was included as an internal control. The results confirmed the suspected loss of Arg in position 17 of the Ia fragment corresponding to residue 155 of the K^b molecule. Tryptic peptide profiles of the other CNBr fragments and of Met-containing peptides

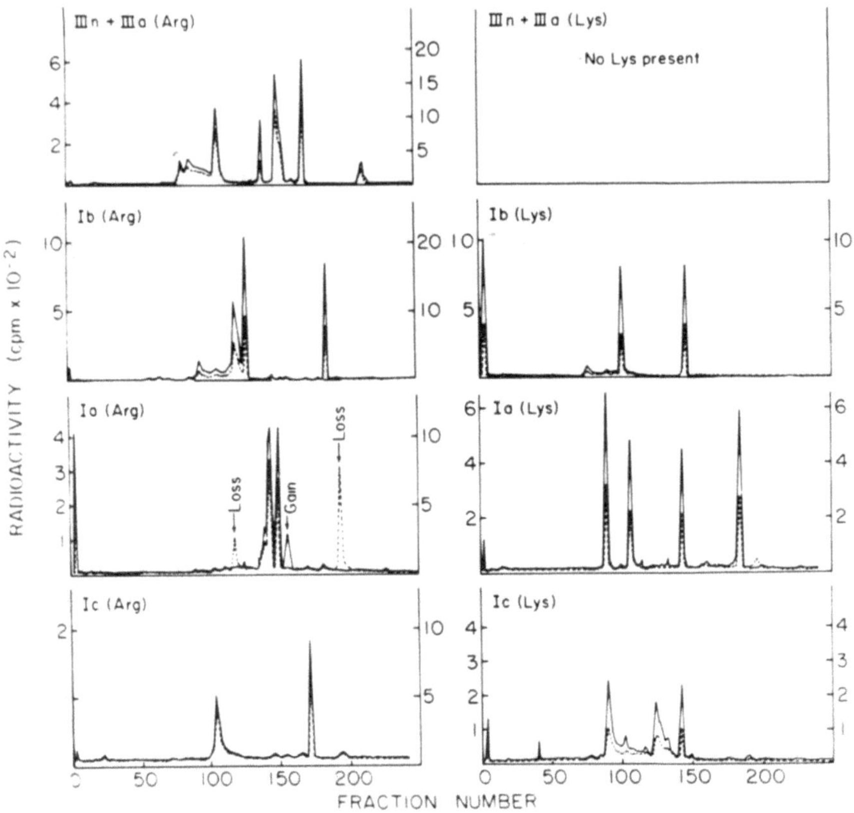

Figure 7. Comparative tryptic peptide profile of the five NH_2-terminal CNBr fragments of H-2K^b and H-2K$^{bm\ 1}$. CNBr fragments were purified from [^{3}H]-Arg H-2K$^{bm\ 1}$ [^{14}C]-Arg H-2K^b and from [^{3}H]-Lys H-2K$^{bm\ 1}$/[^{14}C]-Lys H-2K^b, subjected to digestion with [L-(tosylamido-2-phenyl) ethyl chloromethyl ketone treated] (TPCK–trypsin, and analyzed by ion-exchange chromatography on Spherix XX-80-60-00 resin. Further details are provided in Nisizawa *et al.* (1981), from which this figure is taken.

from intact molecules showed no differences. Thus, on the basis of these studies, it is suggested that all the biological alterations noted in the K$^{bm\ 1}$ mutant molecule can be explained by a change at residue 155 in which an Arg was mutated to a Tyr and at residue 156 in which an Leu was changed to a Tyr.

When the CNBr fragments of K$^{bm\ 3}$ from the bm 3 mutant were prepared and analyzed in the same fashion as described for bm 1, peptide differences were again noted in only one fragment. However, in contrast to the results obtained for the K$^{bm\ 1}$ molecule, tryptic peptide differences in K$^{bm\ 3}$ were localized to the Ib CNBr fragment. Two Arg-labeled peptides present in the parent were lacking in the mutant. However, two peptides were seen in fragment Ib derived from $K^{bm\ 3}$ that were not found in the K^b of the parent. Examination of Lys-labeled tryptic fragments revealed the absence in the mutant of a single Ib-derived peptide present in the parent molecule (Ewenstein *et al.*, 1980).

Amino acid sequence studies suggest that one amino acid alteration of the $K^{bm\ 3}$ glycoprotein affects the tryptic peptides spanning positions 80–89 and 90–108 of the parent K^b molecule. The presumptive alteration is thus a substitution of the Lys residue at position 89, generating a new peptide in the mutant that spans positions 80–108 and contains the carbohydrate moiety.

The second altered amino acid in the $K^{bm\ 3}$ mutant was localized to the peptide from 76 to 79. The amino acid sequence analysis of this peptide labeled with Val, Leu, and Arg from the mutant was identical with that of the parent at positions 76, 78, and 79. Thus, the altered amino acid is at position 77. Although the precise nature of the mutation cannot as yet be ascertained, it is tempting to speculate, on the basis of the comparatively retarded elution of the derived peptide from the ion-exchange column, that it involves a substitution of a less acidic for a more acidic amino acid.

3.3. Discussion and Conclusion

The *H-2* MHC mutations are relevant to our understanding of the nature, generation, and maintenance of the polymorphism in the *H-2K* and *H-2D* gene product system, provide a tool to enhance the resolution power of *H-2* fine-structure analysis, and provide a unique probe for function–structure relationships. Our structural studies on the bm 1 and bm 3 mutants clearly document that the *K* gene product of each of these mutant lines, when isolated by a standard antiserum directed against the major private specificity of the parental K^b gene products, reveals specific and unique alterations. In the case of bm 1, amino acid exchanges are present at position 155 and 156, and in the case of bm 3, two amino acid changes are noted, one at position 89 and the other at position 77. As diagrammed in Fig. 4, the mutation sites are present in the amino terminal one half of the K^b molecule. The two mutation sites in bm 3 are rather close to one another and located near the first carbohydrate moiety. The mutation site for bm 1 is distinct and separate from the mutational sites for bm 3.

Insofar as we can tell, except for the amino acid changes discussed above, these two K^b glycoproteins are identical to the K^b molecule in amino acid sequence and in every other respect studied. Thus, while we cannot rule out the possibility that changes undetected by our present methodology may be present, the most likely conclusion of these studies is that one or at most two point mutations have occurred.

It is of considerable interest that the structural differences that we see are distinct and unique; that is, the bm 1 K glycoprotein has at positions 155 and 156 amino acids different from the parent and from the bm 3 K glycoproteins. Similarly, positions 77 and 89 in the bm 3 glycoprotein differ from the parent and from the bm 1 mutant. This unique primary structure thus correlates with the specific pattern of histogenic reactivity between the mutants themselves and the parent cells. Such observations would be expected, and correlate with the notion that they represent the structural basis by which immunological specificity and recognition occur between cells of these haplotypes. The findings thus reveal the potential of such apparently small and discrete primary structural alterations to effect a major change in the specificity in the H-2 interaction situation.

These data also bear on the question of polymorphism of the *H-2* genes. The finding of point mutations suggests that the polymorphism is generated by an accumulation of such discrete alterations that seem to occur in restricted regions of the molecule. It is of interest in this regard that the position of one mutation site in the bm 3 mutant glycoprotein occurs close to a cluster of differences noted between the HLA-A2 molecule and a K^b molecule (see Table 5). At present, we do not have an explanation for the finding of two amino acid exchanges in the bm 3 mutant. It seems likely that these two mutations occurred independently and then became fixed together in the germ line.

Currently, 14 mutants of the $H\text{-}2^b$ haplotype have been reported, 11 of which are in the *K* gene. It is clear that this series provides an intriguing model system for probing structure–function relationships of the cell surface. Studies are in progress to determine the precise location and nature of the structural alterations in the products of these MHC mutants.

ACKNOWLEDGMENTS. The investigations discussed in this chapter were partly supported by NIH grants AI-07289 and AI-10702 to S.G.N. B.M.E. is a medical scientist trainee supported by grant 5T5-GM-1674. The expert technical assistance of Mss. Diane McGovern and Selma Schumacher and the skilled clerical assistance of Ms. Catherine Whelan are gratefully acknowledged. We also wish to thank Drs. Roderick Nairn and Karen Yamaga for their enlightening discussions and for their review of the manuscript.

NOTE ADDED IN PROOF. To update the information in this chapter, see Nairn, R., Yamaga, K., and Nathenson, S.G., 1980, *Ann. Rev. Genet.* **14**:241, and Vehara, H., Ewenstein, B.M., Kindt, T.J., and Coligan, J.E., 1981, *Ann. Rev. Biochem.* (in press).

References

Acton, R.T., and Lynn, J.D. (eds.), 1977, *Cell Culture and Its Application*, Academic Press, New York.

Bailey, D.W., and Kohn, H.I., 1965, Inherited histocompatibility changes in progeny of irradiated and unirradiated inbred mice, *Genet. Res.* **6:**330.

Brown, J.L., and Nathenson, S.G., 1977, Structural differences between parent and mutant H-2K glycoproteins from two H-2K gene mutants: B6.C-H-2^{ba} (Hzl) and B6-H-2^{bd} (M505), *J. Immunol.* **118:**98.

Brown, J.L., Kato, K., Silver, J., and Nathenson, S.G., 1974, Notable diversity in peptide composition of murine H-2K and H-2D alloantigens, *Biochemistry* **13:**3174.

Coligan, J.E., Kindt, T.J., Ewenstein, B.M., Uehara, H., Nisizawa, T., and Nathenson, S.G., 1978, Primary structure of murine major histocompatibility complex alloantigen: Amino acid sequence studies of the cyanogen bromide fragments of the H-$2K^b$ glycoprotein, *Proc. Natl. Acad. Sci. U.S.A.* **75:**3390.

Coligan, J.E., Kindt, T.J., Ewenstein, B.M., Uehara, H., Martinko, J.M., and Nathenson, S.G., 1979, Further structural analysis of the murine H-$2K^b$ glycoprotein using radiochemical methodology, *Mol. Immunol.* **16:**3.

Cook, R.G., Vitetta, E.S., Uhr, J.W., Klein, J., Wilde, C.E., III, and Capra, J.D., 1978, Structural studies on protein products of murine chromosome 17. III. Partial amino sequence of an H-$2K^q$ molecule, *J. Immunol.* **121:**1015.

Egorov, I.K., 1967, A mutation of the histocompatibility-2 locus in the mouse, *Genetika* **9:**136.

Ewenstein, B.M., Nisizawa, T., Uehara, H., Nathenson, S.G., Coligan, J.E., and Kindt, T.J., 1978, Primary structure of murine major histocompatibility complex alloantigens: Isolation, biochemical characterization and preliminary alignment of CNBr fragments from the H-$2K^b$ glycoprotein, *Proc. Natl. Acad. Sci. U.S.A.* **75:**2909.

Ewenstein, B.M., Uehara, H., Nisizawa, T., Nathenson, S.G., Melvold, R.W., and Kohn, H.I., 1980, Biochemical studies on the H-2K antigens of the MHC mutants bm 3 and bm 11, *Immunogenetics* **11:**383.

Ferguson, W.S., Terhorst, C.T., Robb, R.J., and Strominger, J.L., 1979, Localization of the disulfide bridges of human histocompatibility antigens, *Mol. Immunol.* **16:**23.

Gally, J.A., 1973, Structure of immunoglobulins, in: *The Antigens*, Vol. I (M. Sela, ed.), pp. 161–298, Academic Press, New York.

Gorer, P.A., 1936, The detection of antigenic differences in mouse erythrocytes by the employment of immune sera, *Brt. J. Exp. Pathol.* **17:**42.

Götze, D. (ed.), 1977, *The Major Histocompatibility System in Man and Animals*, Springer-Verlag, Berlin and New York.

Gross, E., 1967, The cyanogen bromide reaction, in: *Methods in Enzymology* (C.H.W. Hirs, ed.), pp. 238–255, Academic Press, New York.

Henning, R., Milner, R.J., Reske, K., Cunningham, B.A., and Edelman, G.M., 1976, Subunit structure, cell surface orientation and partial amino acid sequences of murine histocompatibility antigens, *Proc. Natl. Acad. Sci. U.S.A.* **73:**118.

Hunkapiller, M.W., and Hood, L.E., 1978, Direct micro sequence analysis of polypeptides using an improved sequenator, a nonprotein carrier (Polybrene) and high pressure liquid chromatography, *Biochemistry* **17:**2122.

Jacobs, J.W., Kemper, B., Niall, H.D., Habener, J.F., and Potts, J.J., Jr., 1974, Structural analysis of human proparathyroid hormone by a new micro sequencing approach, *Nature (London)* **249:**155.

Kimball, E.S., Coligan, J.E., and Kindt, T.J., 1979, Structural characterization of antigens encoded by rabbit RLA-11 histocompatibility genes, *Immunogenetics* **8:**201.

Klein, J., 1975, *Biology of the Mouse H-2 Complex*, Springer-Verlag, New York.

Klein, J., 1978, H-2 mutations: Their genetics and effect on immune functions, *Adv. Immunol.* **26:**55.

Kohn, H.I., Klein, J., Melvold, R.W., Nathenson, S.G., Pious, D., and Shreffler, D.C., 1978, The First H-2 Mutant Workshop, *Immunogenetics* **7:**279.

McKean, D.J., Peters, E.H., Waldby, J.I., and Smithies, O., 1974, Amino acid sequence determination with radioactive proteins, *Biochemistry* **13:**3048.

McKenzie, I.F.C., Pang, T., and Blanden, R.V., 1977, The use of H-2 mutants as models for the study of T cell activation, *Immunol. Rev.* **35:**181.

Melvold, R.W., and Kohn, H.I., 1976, Eight new mutations associated with the H-2 complex, *Immunogenetics* **3:**185.

Nathenson, S.G., and Cullen, S.E., 1974, Biochemical properties and immunochemical–genetic relationships of mouse H-2 alloantigens, *Biochim. Biophys. Acta* **344:**1.

Nathenson, S.G., and Muramatsu, T., 1971, Properties of the carbohydrate portion of mouse H-2 alloantigen glycoproteins, in: *Glycoproteins of Blood Cells and Plasma* (G.A. Jamieson and T.J. Greenwalt, eds.), pp. 245–262, J.B. Lippincott, Philadelphia.

Natori, T., Tanagaki, N., Appella, E., and Pressman, D., 1975, Amino acid composition and physicochemical properties of mouse β_2-microglobulin, *Biochem. Biophys. Res. Commun.* **65:**611.

Nisizawa, T., Ewenstein, B.M., Uehara, H., and Nathenson, S.G., 1981, Biochemical studies on the H-2K antigen of the MHC bm 1, *Immunogenetics* **12:**33.

Parham, P., Alpert, B.N., Orr, H.T., and Strominger, J.L., 1977, Carbohydrate moiety of HLA antigens: Antigenic properties and amino acid sequences around the site of glycoprotein, *J. Biol. Chem.* **252:**7555.

Paul, W.E., and Benacerraf, B., 1977, Functional specificity of thymus-dependent lymphocytes, *Science* **195:**1293.

Peterson, P.A., Rask, L., Sege, K., Klareskog, L., Anundi, H., and Ostberg, L., 1975, Evolutionary relationship between immunoglobulins and transplantation antigens, *Proc. Natl. Acad. Sci. U.S.A.* **72:**1612.

Pleogh, H.L., Orr, H.R., Robb, R., and Strominger, J.L., 1978, Structure of HLA antigens, in: *Biological Markers of Neoplasia* (H. Ruddon, ed.), pp. 201–211, North Holland, New York.

Rask, L., Lindstrom, J.B., and Peterson, P.A., 1974, Subunit structure of H-2 alloantigens, *Nature (London)* **249:**833.

Schwartz, B.D., Kato, K., Cullen, S.E., and Nathenson, S.G., 1973, H-2 histocompatibility alloantigens: Some biochemical properties of the molecules solubilized by NP-40 detergent, *Biochemistry* **12:**2157.

Shimada, A., and Nathenson, S.G., 1969, Murine histocompatibility-2 (H-2) alloantigens: Purification and some chemical properties of soluble products from H-2^b and H-2^d genotypes released by papain digestion of membrane fractions, *Biochemistry* **8:**4048.

Silver, J., and Hood, L., 1974, Detergent-solubilized H-2 alloantigen is associated with a small molecular weight polypeptide, *Nature (London)* **249:**764.

Silver, J., and Hood, L.E., 1976, Structure and evolution of transplantation antigens: Partial amino acid sequences of H-2K and H-2D alloantigens, *Proc. Natl. Acad. Sci. U.S.A.* **73:**599.

Snell, G.D., 1978, T-cells, T-cell recognition structures and the major histocompatibility complex, *Immunol. Rev.* **38:**3.

Snell, G.D., Dausset, J., and Nathenson, S.G., 1976, *Histocompatibility*, Academic Press, New York.

Wittman-Liebold, B., 1973, Amino acid sequence studies on 10 ribosomal proteins of *E. coli* with an improved sequenator equipped with an automatic conversion device, *Hoppe-Seyler's Z. Physiol. Chem.* **354:**1415.

Vitetta, E., and Capra, J.D., 1978, The protein products of the murine 17th chromosome: Genetics and structure, *Adv. Immunol.* **26:**147.

Vitetta, E.S., Capra, J.D., Klapper, D.G., Klein, J., and Uhr, J.W., 1976, The partial amino acid sequence of an H-2K molecule, *Proc. Natl. Acad. Sci. U.S.A.* **73:**905.

18

Are the Classic Transplantation Antigens Primitive Cell-Surface Antibodies?

Per A. Peterson and Olle Kämpe

1. Introduction

The existence of a well-developed immune system is restricted to the vertebrates. Foreign substances are recognized by antibodies that exhibit an almost endless variety of antigen-combining sites. Although some of the antibody variability may be due to somatic mutations, the vertebrate genome contains substantial numbers of genes coding for immunoglobulin variable regions (see Seidman *et al.*, 1978). It appears possible that these sets of genes evolved under environmental selection by a gradual expansion of duplicated and mutated genes. At some time during the course of this development, the gene products may have occurred as a family of proteins displaying a restricted genetic polymorphism. These ancestral proteins may have participated in recognitive processes such as the discrimination between self and nonself wherein genetic polymorphism should have provided a selective advantage. Assuming that the evolution of the variable regions included organisms lacking a circulatory system, it can be envisaged that the predecessors of the immunoglobulins were cell-surface proteins.

The major histocompatibility complex (MHC) controls the expression of an array of genetically polymorphic cell-membrane glycoproteins that participate in several immunobiological events (see Shreffler and

Per A. Peterson and Olle Kämpe • Department of Cell Research, The Wallenberg Laboratory, University of Uppsala, S-751-22 Uppsala, Sweden.

David, 1975; Peterson *et al.*, 1977). Some of these proteins appear to be involved in the immunological recognition of foreign antigens by T lymphocytes. Although T cells, particularly T helper and T killer cells, display antibodylike receptors for foreign antigens (Binz and Wigzell, 1977), they do not seem to be able to react with the antigens directly. Available information suggests that T helper cells can recognize foreign material only if the foreign substances are presented to the T helper cells together with MHC-coded molecules located on the surface of macrophages (see Rosenthal, 1978). Moreover, T killer cells cannot become activated unless foreign antigens are presented jointly with the MHC-controlled, classic transplantation antigens (Doherty *et al.*, 1976; Shearer *et al.*, 1975).

The central role of the MHC in the immune system together with its extensive genetic polymorphism raises the important question whether this genetic region, which may have counterparts in invertebrate species (Hildemann *et al.*, 1977), is the ancestor of the highly sophisticated antigen-recognition system of vertebrates. In this chapter, data are summarized that demonstrate that the classic transplantation antigens (called HLA-A, -B, and -C antigens in man) are structurally similar to antibodies and that they may interact directly with foreign substances such as bacteria and virus proteins. These data argue for an interrelated evolution for immunoglobulins and transplantation antigens and suggest that the transplantation antigens may function as primitive cell-surface antibodies.

2. Immunoglobulinlike Structure of HLA-A, -B, and -C Antigens

2.1. HLA-A, -B, and -C Antigens Are Composed of Immunoglobulinlike Domains

The HLA-A, -B, and -C antigens consist of one heavy and one light chain (Nakamuro *et al.*, 1973; Grey *et al.*, 1973; Peterson *et al.*, 1974). The light chain, β_2-microglobulin, is the common subunit of all HLA-A, -B, and -C antigens (Rask *et al.*, 1976; Snary *et al.*, 1977). It has been called a "free immunoglobulin domain" (Peterson *et al.*, 1972), since its primary structure is homologous to those of constant domains of IgG (Smithies and Poulik, 1972; Peterson *et al.*, 1972; Cunningham *et al.*, 1973).

Papain-solubilized HLA-A, -B, and -C antigens, which account for about 80% of the intact molecule (see Springer and Strominger, 1976), were isolated from about 4000 g of peripheral-blood lymphocytes (Trägårdh *et al.*, 1979b). The heavy chains were separated from β_2-microglobulin and subjected to acid cleavage (Terhorst *et al.*, 1977). This treatment resulted in the almost quantitative cleavage of the heavy chains. Two dominating fragments with apparent molecular weights of 22,000 and 11,000 could be isolated by gel chromatography under denaturing conditions (Trägårdh *et al.*, 1979a). Amino acid analyses demonstrated that each fragment contained two half-cystines, but only the 22,000-dalton fragment contained hexoseamine. All the methionines of the papain-solubilized heavy chain were confined to the larger, carbohydrate-containing fragment. Since acid preferentially cleaves aspartyl–prolyl bonds (Hill, 1965), these data strongly suggest that most if not all heavy-chain allotypes display an invariant aspartyl–prolyl sequence. This confirms and extends the observations fo Terhorst *et al.* (1977), who obtained similar fragments after acid cleavage of a few defined HLA-A and -B antigen heavy chains.

Since the 22,000-dalton acid-cleavage fragment contained methionyl residues, it was further subjected to CNBr cleavage in 70% formic acid (Gross and Witkopf, 1962). After gel chromatography under denaturing conditions, two partially resolved protein peaks were obtained. Rechromatography of each of the peaks provided two CNBr fragments that were obtained in highly purified form. One fragment, with an apparent molecular weight of 14,000, contained hexoseamine but no half-cystines as determined by amino acid analysis. The other CNBr fragment, with an apparent molecular weight of 9000, contained two half-cystines but was devoid of carbohydrate.

2.2. Disulfide-Bond Distribution in the HLA-A, -B, and -C Antigens

Previous data have suggested that HLA-A and -B antigen heavy chains of a few defined specificities display immunoglobulin-like disulfide loops (Peterson *et al.*, 1975; Springer and Strominger, 1976; Terhorst *et al.*, 1977). To verify that the disulfide bonds of the genetically polymorphic heavy chains are an invariant feature of most if not all allotypes, we have examined their distribution in pooled HLA-A, -B, and -C antigens derived from thousands of individuals (Trägårdh *et al.*, 1979a; Wiman *et al.*, 1979).

To analyze the distribution of disulfide bridges in the HLA-A, -B, and -C antigens, the papain-solubilized antigen subunits and the acid and CNBr fragments of the heavy chains were labeled with ^{125}I under denaturing conditions to maximize incorporation of radioactivity. The subunits and the fragments were separately cleaved with 2-nitro-5-thiocyanobenzoic acid (NTCB), which selectively cleaves peptide bonds at cysteinyl residues (Jacobson *et al.*, 1973), and were then subjected to gel chromatography. The papain-solubilized HLA-A, -B, and -C antigen heavy-chain mixture gave rise, after cleavage at cysteinyl residues, to four well-resolved radioctive peaks with apparent molecular weights of 14,000, 6500, 4500, and 1700, respectively (Fig. 1A). β_2-Microglobulin was cleaved to yield two easily discernible peptides with apparent molecular weights of 6500 and 2500 (not shown). The latter result demonstrated that the cleavage was quantitative and specific, since the two half-cystines of β_2-microglobulin occur in positions 25 and 81 (Cunningham *et al.*, 1973), which theoretically should yield peptides with molecular weights of about 6600, 2800, and 2400. Obviously, the two smaller fragments were not resolved on gel chromatography, since ion-exchange chromatography on DEAE–Sephadex A-25 demonstrated that both peptides had incorporated radioactivity. NTCB did not affect the molecular weight of the 14,000-dalton CNBr fragment (not shown), but the 9000-dalton CNBr peptide was cleaved to yield radioactive peaks with apparent molecular weights of 6500 and 2200 (Fig. 1B). The 11,000-dalton acid-cleavage fragment gave rise to three radioactive peptides with molecular weights of 6500, 2200, and 1700 (Fig. 1C). The 22,000-dalton acid-cleavage fragment was broken down by NTCB into peptides with molecular weights of 14,000, 6500, and 2500 (not shown).

The results of the fragmentation of the papain-solubilized HLA-A, -B, and -C antigen heavy chains are summarized in Fig. 2. The ordering of the fragments was accomplished by the peptide patterns obtained and by the amino acid sequence determinations (see below). The amino acid sequence data clearly demonstrated that the 22,000-dalton acid-cleavage fragment is the NH_2-terminal fragment. Since the combined molecular weight of the two acid-cleavage fragments is identical to that of the pa-

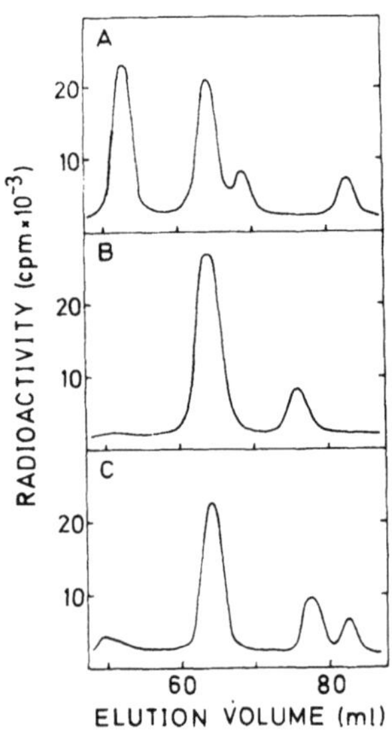

Figure 1. Gel chromatography of NTCB-cleaved papain-solubilized HLA-A, -B, and -C antigen heavy chains (A), the 9,000-dalton CNBr fragment (B), and the 11,-000-dalton acid-cleavage fragment (C) on a 110 × 1.1 cm column of Sephadex G-100. The column was equilibrated with 0.05 M sodium acetate buffer (pH 5.0) containing 6 M guanidine hydrochloride. The fragments were isolated as described in the text and were labeled with ^{125}I under denaturing conditions to maximize incorporation of radioactivity.

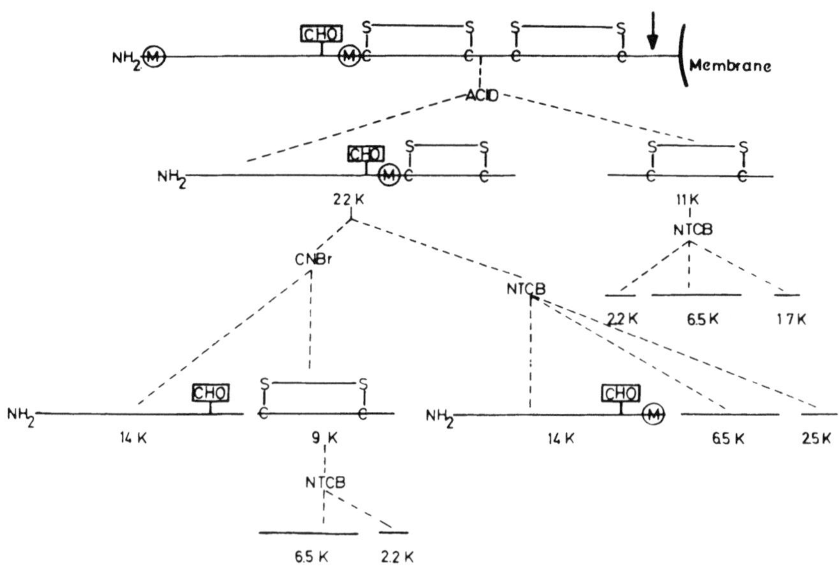

Figure 2. Schematic picture of the papain-solubilized HLA-A, -B, and -C antigen heavy chains. (↓) Position of papain cleavage. The various fragments obtained to construct the model are indicated. For further details, see the text. (22K, 11K, etc.) Apparent molecular weights of the fragments.

pain-solubilized heavy chain and since proline is the NH_2-terminal residue of the 11,000-dalton fragment, it is reasonable to conclude that the acid-cleavage fragments account for the whole of the papain-solubilized heavy chain. Amino acid sequence determinations demonstrated that the most NH_2-terminal half-cystine occurs in position 20 of the 11,000-dalton acid-cleavage fragment, which is in keeping with the notion that the half-cystines are separated by some 55–60 amino acid residues. Consequently, COOH-terminal to the last half-cystine in the 11,000-dalton fragment, some 15 amino acid residues should occur.

The 22,000-dalton acid-cleavage fragment yielded CNBr peptides with molecular weights of 14,000 and 9000 (see above). The 14,000-dalton CNBr fragment is preceded by a five-membered peptide that is the NH_2-terminal one as revealed by the amino acid sequence analyses. The 14,000-dalton fragment contained all the carbohydrate but no half-cystines. The COOH-terminal homoserine of this fragment resided in the only carbohydrate-containing tryptic peptide that could be isolated (see below), and the most NH_2-terminal half-cystine in the 9000-dalton CNBr fragment occurred in position 3. These data are consistent only with the interpretation that the 14,000-dalton peptide generated on NTCB cleavage of the 22,000-dalton acid-cleavage fragments represents most of the NH_2-terminal portion of the molecule and demonstrate that one of the methionyl residues is separated by only two amino acids from the first half-cystinyl residue. That the 6500-dalton NTCB peptide of the 22,000-dalton acid-cleavage fragment and of the 9000-dalton CNBr fragment is NH_2-terminal to the 2200-dalton fragment was supported by amino acid sequence analyses.

The outline of the HLA-A, -B, and -C antigen heavy chains, as shown in Fig. 3, is fully concordant with previous models based on less extensive information (Peterson *et al.*, 1975; Terhorst *et al.*, 1977). It is apparent that the chain contains two immunoglobulinlike disulfide bridges, each encompassing some 55–60 amino acid residues. The NH_2-terminal portion of the molecule lacks the repetitive disulfide bridge, and amino acid sequence analyses do not support the idea that this portion of the heavy chain is similar to immunoglobulin chains in structure (see below). However, it is likely that the two immunoglobulinlike regions of the heavy chain are independently folded into compact domains like the immunoglobulin homology regions (Poljak, 1975), since the HLA-A, -B, and -C antigen heavy chains can be cleaved by limited proteolysis at a position between the disulfide bridges (Peterson *et al.*, 1975; Wiman *et al.*, 1979). Obviously, acid also cleaves the HLA-A, -B, and -C antigen heavy chains at about the same position (Terhorst *et al.*, 1977). Interestingly,

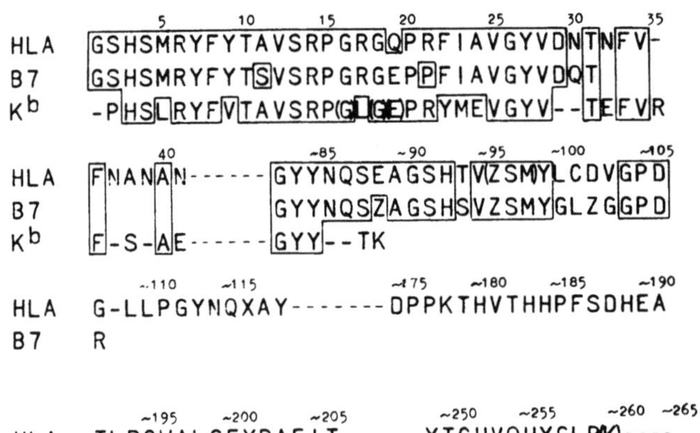

Figure 3. Amino acid sequence of the polymorphic HLA-A, -B, and -C antigen heavy-chain mixture (HLA). For comparison, corresponding sequences reported for the HLA-B7 antigen (Terhorst *et. al.*, 1977; Parham *et al.*, 1977) and the murine H-2K^b antigen (Coligan *et al.*, 1978) are shown, and identical residues are boxed. After residue 41, the numbering is tentative. Letters in parentheses denote residues inferred from the amino acid composition. The sequence information is given in the one-letter code (see Dayhoff *et al.*, 1976).

rabbit immunoglobulin light chains are cleaved similarly by acid (Poulsen *et al.*, 1972). β_2-Microglobulin is associated with one of the two disulfide-containing regions of the heavy chain, although ambiguity still remains as to its precise location.

2.3. Amino Acid Sequence Homology between the HLA-A, -B, and -C Antigen Subunits and Immunoglobulin G Constant Domains

The results of the amino acid sequence determinations are summarized in Fig. 3. A total of 121 positions were investigated representing about half the sequence of the papain-solubilized heavy chain. Since the analyzed material comprised a mixture of allotypes derived from the *HLA-A, -B,* and *-C* loci, multiple amino acid residues were expected. Approximately 25% of the positions in the NH_2-terminus of the intact chain (residues 1–41) and of the 9000-dalton CNBr fragment (residues 98–117) displayed variations (see Trägårdh *et al.*, 1978, 1979a). Only one of the 31 positions examined in the 11,000-dalton fragment (residues 174–205) gave multiple residues. However, apart from positions 35 and 107, one quantitatively dominating residue could always be easily identified.

The main sequence obtained is in excellent agreement with that for the HLA-B7 antigen (Terhorst *et al.*, 1977; Parham *et al.*, 1977). Only 9 of 56 positions available for comparison were not identical. The most NH_2-terminal half-cystine of the heavy chain was observed in position 100 from the NH_2 terminus. The corresponding position in the HLA-B7 antigen is occupied by leucine (Parham *et al.*, 1977). This discrepancy is surprising inasmuch as the NTCB cleavage results suggested that most if not all heavy chains display half-cystine residues in invariant positions (see above). However, the HLA-B7 antigen may be an exception to this. The homology with the murine H-$2K^b$ antigen (Coligan *et al.*, 1978) is approximately 70% for the 40 positions compared (Fig. 3).

The amino acid sequence homology between the heavy chain and the constant IgG domains was examined. The NH_2-terminal third of the heavy chain is devoid of the typical immunoglobulinlike disulfide bridge, and no homology was observed in this region. The 9000-dalton CNBr fragment exhibits the disulfide bridge, but no convincing homology with constant and variable immunoglobulin domains was found. However, the amino acid sequence of the 11,000-dalton acid-cleavage fragment was as similar to those of β_2-microglobulin and the $C\kappa$, $C\lambda$, C_H1, C_H2, and C_H3 domains as the latter are to one another (Table 1). When aligned as in Fig. 4, the 11,000-dalton fragment displays between 23 and 42% identical residues with the corresponding regions of the immunoglobulin domains and β_2-microglobulin. It is particularly noteworthy that 8 positions are com-

TABLE 1. Number of Identical Residues among the Sequences of the HLA Antigen Heavy-Chain 11,000-Dalton Acid-Cleavage Fragment, β_2-Microglobulin, and the Constant-Homology Regions of IgG[a]

	HLA	β_2m	Cκ	Cλ	C_H	C_H	C_H3
HLA	—						
β_2m	18 (42)	—					
Cκ	17 (39)	14 (29)	—				
Cλ	17 (39)	16 (33)	25 (49)	—			
C_H1	14 (32)	14 (29)	20 (39)	18 (35)	—		
C_H2	10 (23)	12 (25)	13 (25)	17 (33)	17 (33)	—	
C_H3	17 (39)	21 (44)	21 (41)	19 (36)	16 (31)	14 (26)	—

[a]The sequences were aligned as shown in Fig. 4, and the alignment was kept constant for all comparisons. Values in parentheses are the number of residues expressed as percentages of the number of residues compared. For further details, see the Fig. 4 caption.

pletely invariant in the immunoglobulin structures shown, and both β_2-microglobulin and the 11,000-dalton heavychain fragment exhibit the invariant residues in the corresponding positions.

These data argue for the idea that the HLA-A, -B, and -C antigen heavy chains and β_2-microglobulin are immunoglobulinlike in structure. The amino acid sequence analyses lend support to the view that the HLA-A, -B, and -C antigen subunits and the immunoglobulin chains have evolved from the same ancestral gene (Gally and Edelman, 1972; Bodmer, 1972; Peterson *et al.*, 1975). Available information does not formally allow the conclusion that the HLA-A, -B, and -C antigen heavy chains have arisen by a gene-duplication event, but the conspicuous distribution of the disulfide bridges makes this idea attractive. However, further amino acid sequence determinations of the 9000-dalton CNBr fragment are required to establish its possible homology with the 11,000-dalton fragment. Further structural analyses will also reveal whether the genetic polymorphism is restricted in distribution rather than disseminated throughout the molecule.

3. Interaction between the Classic Transplantation Antigens and Foreign Substances

Despite several lines of indirect evidence for a physical interaction between transplantation antigens and foreign substances—such as cocapping experiments (Schrader *et al.*, 1975; Henning *et al.*, 1976; Zarling *et al.*, 1978), antiserum-induced inhibition of T-cell-dependent cytolysis (Koszinowski and Ertl, 1975a, b; Germain *et al.*, 1975; Schrader and

Edelman, 1976; Hale *et al.*, 1978), and selective incorporation of transplantation antigens into enveloped viruses (Hecht and Summers, 1976; Bubbers *et al.*, 1978)—convincing data at the molecular level have been lacking.

3.1. Binding of HLA-A, -B, and -C Antigens to Bacteria

In view of the structural similarity between HLA-A, -B, and -C antigens and immunoglobulins, it seems of importance to investigate whether there exists a functional similarity as well. Since HLA-A, -B, and -C antigens normally occur anchored in the lipid bilayer of the membrane, highly purified HLA antigens were inserted into liposomes (Klareskog *et*

				~175					~180
HLA 11K acid cleavage fragment			ASP	PRO	PRO	LYS	THR	HIS	VAL
β_2-microglobulin	ILE	GLN	ARG	THR	PRO	LYS	ILE	GLN	VAL
C_λ constant region	PRO	LYS	ALA	ALA	PRO			SER	VAL
C_κ constant region	THR	VAL	ALA	ALA	PRO			SER	VAL
C_H1 homology region	SER	THR	LYS	GLY	PRO			SER	VAL
C_H2 homology region	LEU	LEU	GLY	GLY	PRO			SER	VAL
C_H3 homology region	GLN	PRO	ARG	GLU	PRO			GLN	VAL

												~185					~190
HLA		THR	HIS	HIS	PRO							PHE	SER	ASP	HIS	GLU	ALA
β_2m	TYR	SER	ARG	HIS	PRO	ALA		GLU					ASN	GLY	LYS	SER	ASN
C_λ	THR	LEU	PHE	PRO	PRO	SER	SER	GLU	GLU			LEU	GLN	ALA	ASN	LYS	ALA
C_κ	PHE	ILE	PHE	PRO	PRO	SER	ASP	GLU	GLN			LEU	LYS	SER	GLY	THR	ALA
C_H1	PHE	PRO	LEU	ALA	PRO	SER	SER	LYS	SER			THR	SER	GLY	GLY	THR	ALA
C_H2	PHE	LEU	PHE	PRO	PRO	LYS	PRO	LYS	ASP	THR	LEU	MET	ILE	SER	ARG	THR	PRO
C_H3	TYR	THR	LEU	PRO	PRO	SER	ARG	GLU	GLU			MET	THR	LYS	ASN	GLN	VAL

					~195					~200					~205	
HLA	THR	LEU	ARG	CYS	TRP	ALA	LEU	GLY	PHE	TYR	PRO	ALA	GLU	ILE	THR	-----
β_2m	PHE	LEU	ASN	CYS	TYR	VAL	SER	GLY	PHE	HIS	PRO	SER	ASP	ILE	GLU	-----
C_λ	THR	LEU	VAL	CYS	LEU	ILE	SER	ASP	PHE	TYR	PRO	GLY	ALA	VAL	THR	-----
C_κ	SER	VAL	VAL	CYS	LEU	LEU	ASN	ASN	PHE	TYR	PRO	ARG	GLU	ALA	LYS	-- --
C_H1	ALA	LEU	GLY	CYS	LEU	VAL	LYS	ASP	TYR	PHE	PRO	GLU	PRO	VAL	THR	-----
C_H2	GLU	VAL	THR	CYS	VAL	VAL	VAL	ASP	VAL	SER	HIS	GLU	ASP	PRO	GLN	-----
C_H3	SER	LEU	THR	CYS	LEU	VAL	LYS	GLY	PHE	TYR	PRO	SER	ASP	ILE	ALA	-----

			~250					~255									
HLA	TYR	THR	CYS	HIS	VAL	GLN	HIS	TYR	GLY	LEU			PRO				(LYS)
β_2m	TYR	ALA	CYS	ARG	VAL	ASN	HIS	VAL	THR	LEU	SER	GLN	PRO				LYS
C_λ	TYR	SER	CYS	GLN	VAL	THR	HIS	GLU	GLY	SER	THR	VAL	GLU				LYS
C_κ	TYR	ALA	CYS	GLU	VAL	THR	HIS	GLN	GLY	LEU	SER	SER	PRO	VAL	THR		LYS
C_H1	TYR	ILE	CYS	ASN	VAL	ASN	HIS	LYS	PRO	SER	ASN	THR	LYS	VAL		ASP	LYS
C_H2	TYR	LYS	CYS	LYS	VAL	SER	ASN	LYS	ALA	LEU	PRO	ALA	PRO	ILE		GLU	LYS
C_H3	TYR	SER	CYS	SER	VAL	MET	HIS	GLU	ALA	LEU	HIS	ASN	HIS	TYR	THR	GLN	LYS

Figure 4. Comparison of the primary structure of the HLA-A, -B, and -C antigen heavy-chain 11,000 dalton acid-cleavage fragment with the structures of β_2-microglobulin, C_κ, C_λ, C_H1, C_H2, and C_H3. The alignments of the sequences were made to maximize the homologies. The β_2-microglobulin and the C_κ sequences are from Cunningham *et al.* (1973) and Wikler *et al.* (1967); the other four sequences are from the γG-immunoglobulin Eu (Edelman, 1970).

al., 1978) to ascertain conditions as physiological as possible. The liposomes were mixed with various strains of bacteria, which in this case were used as foreign material, and the binding of the liposomes to the bacteria was recorded (Klareskog *et al.*, 1978). Figure 5 shows that two strains of *Neisseria catharralis* and one strain of *Haemophilus influenzae* bound the HLA-antigen-containing liposomes to a significant extent, whereas two strains of *E. coli* bound only small amounts of liposomes, if any. To demonstrate that the binding of the liposomes was due to their content of HLA-A, -B, and -C antigens, the HLA antigens were reacted with various concentrations of antigen-binding fragment (Fab) specific for the two subunits. Figure 6 shows that with increasing concentration of Fab directed against the HLA-A, -B, and -C antigen heavy chains, the interaction between the liposomes and the bacteria was progressively impeded. In contrast, Fab directed against β_2-microglobulin, although of higher avidity, had no or only very weak impeding activity (Fig. 6). These and related observations (see Klareskog *et al.*, 1978) suggest that the HLA-A, -B, and -C antigens may interact with foreign material such as bacterial surface components. It seems likely that this interaction is preferentially brought about by the HLA antigen heavy chains, since antibody fragments against β_2-microglobulin had little effect on the binding process.

It is doubtful whether the observed interaction between HLA antigens and some strains of bacteria is of pathophysiological importance, since several strains of bacteria display tissue-specific binding. However,

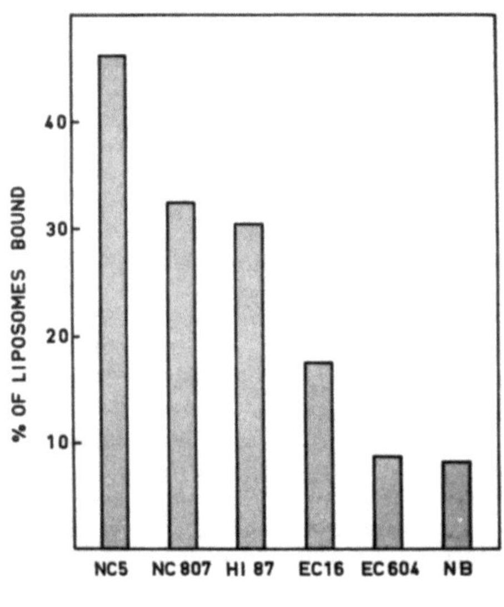

Figure 5. Binding of HLA-A, -B, and -C-antigen-containing liposomes to some strains of bacteria (adapted from Klareskog *et al.*, 1978). The liposomes, containing ^{125}I-labeled HLA antigens, were incubated with the bacteria. Liposomes remaining bound to the bacteria after centrifugation and three washings were measured. (NC) *Neisseria catharralis* strains 5 and 807; (HI) *Haemophilus influenzae* strain 87; (EC) *E. coli* strains 16 and 604; (NB) no bacteria.

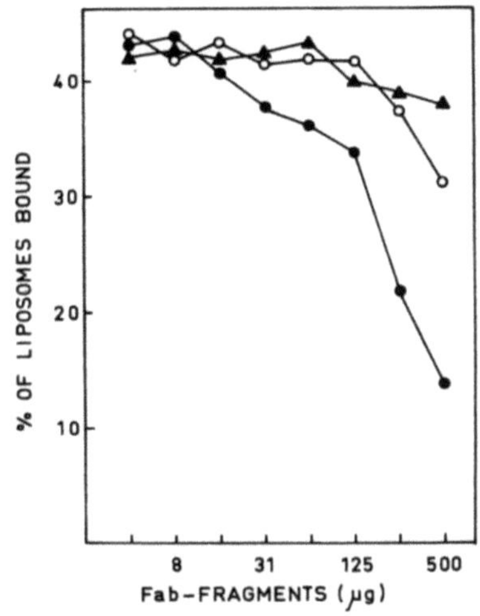

Figure 6. Inhibition of binding of HLA-A, -B, and -C-antigen-containing liposomes to bacteria of the *Neisseria catharralis* 5 strain. The liposomes, containing ^{125}I-labeled antigens, were preincubated for 30 min with Fab against β_2-microglobulin (○), the HLA-A, -B, and -C antigen heavy chains (●), and Fab (▲) from normal rabbit IgG prior to the addition of the bacteria.

the demonstrated interaction between bacteria and HLA antigens may reflect a general property of the HLA antigens to interact with any type of foreign material. Thus, with use of HLA-A- and -B-antigen-containing liposomes similar to those described here, Helenius *et al.* (1978) demonstrated that Semliki Forest virus proteins interacted with the HLA antigens. It seems likely that a great number of materials containing multiple foreign determinants will display similar types of interactions with the HLA antigens (see Section 4).

3.2. Association between an Early Adenovirus-2 Protein and Transplantation Antigens

T killer cells react with cell surface substances (Doherty *et al.*, 1976; Shearer *et al.*, 1975). It has been argued that the T killer cells may interact with molecular complexes consisting of self and nonself structures. To directly examine this possibility, we have investigated some adenovirus-transformed rat cell lines with regard to syngeneic T-cell cytolysis and cell-surface antigen expression.

Properly immunized T killer cells specific for the transformed cell line A2T2C4 could be obtained from syngeneic rats (Kvist *et al.*, 1978b). These cells were cytotoxic for the transformed cells, but not for syngeneic rat fibroblasts. The cytolytic activity of the T cells was abrogated by antisera directed against the Ag-B antigens (the rat equivalents of the HLA-A, -B, and -C antigens), as shown in Fig. 7. A rabbit antiserum against the two Ag-B antigen subunits was very efficient in blocking the lysis of the adenovirus-transformed target cells. Antibodies against β_2-

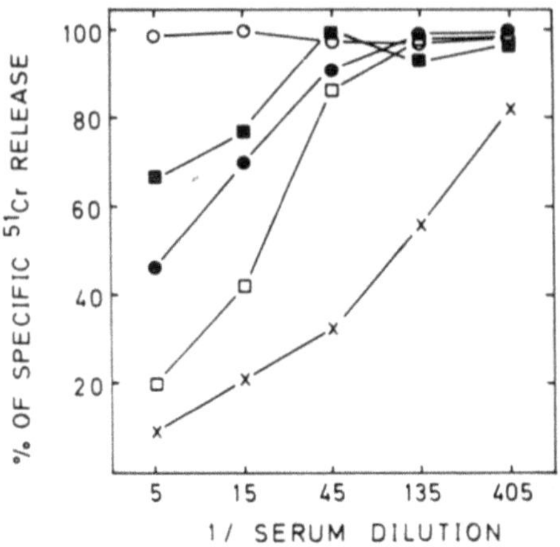

Figure 7. Inhibition of T-cell-dependent cytolysis of the adenovirus-2-transformed fibroblast cell line A2T2C4 by various dilutions of normal rabbit serum (○), rabbit anti-rat β_2-microglobulin (■), Lewis anti-August spleen cell serum (●), syngeneic antiserum against A2T2C4 cells (□), and rabbit anti-AgB antigen serum (×). All antisera have been characterized earlier (see Kvist *et al.*, 1978a). Male Hooded-Lister rats were immunized intraperitoneally with 5×10^6 untreated A2T2C4 cells. The rats were used as spleen-cell donors after 6 weeks, when T lymphocytes were prepared and 3×10^7 cells were cultured together with 3×10^6 A2T2C4 cells previously irradiated with 5000 rads. The cytolytic activity was measured by incubating 1×10^4 educated T lymphocytes with 1×10^3 ^{51}Cr-labeled A2T2C4 cells, which had been preincubated for 30 min with the dialyzed antisera. The incubations proceeded for 5 hr at 37°C, and the ^{51}Cr released was measured after centrifugation. A release of 100% represents the amount of radioactivity recovered in the supernatant after incubation of the T lymphocytes in the absence of added serum. This release amounted to 76% of that obtained after Triton X-100 treatment of the target cells. The background release (15% of the maximum) was subtracted from all values. The experimental points are the averages of analyses performed in quadruplicate. The standard error of the mean never exceeded 12%.

microglobulin were relatively poor inhibitors, whereas alloantibodies against the Ag-B antigen heavy chain expressed on the target cells were more efficient in impeding the cytolytic activity (Fig. 7). The antigen-binding capacity of the anti-β_2-microglobulin serum was about 10-fold greater than that of the rabbit anti-Ag-B antigen serum. The latter serum displayed a titer that was about 5-fold greater than that of the alloantiserum. By taking this information into consideration, it may be suggested that antibodies that bind to the Ag-B antigen heavy chain are more efficient in interfering with the action of the cytolytic T lymphocytes than are antibodies directed against β_2-microglobulin.

Figure 7 also shows that a syngeneic antiserum raised against the transformed cells impeded the cytolysis. This antiserum did not react with normal cells, as evidenced by indirect immunoprecipitation analyses of radioactively labeled membrane glycoproteins (Fig. 8C), but precipitated three types of molecules from the transformed cells (Fig. 8D). Thus, components with molecular weights of 12,000, 19,000, and 45,000 were visualized after sodium dodecyl sulfate–polyacrylamide gel electrophoresis (SDS-PAGE). Interestingly, an alloantiserum against the Ag-B antigen allotype of the transformed cell line precipitated the same type of molecules when tested against glycoproteins of the transformed cells (Fig. 8B), but reacted only with the expected components—i.e., the 12,000- and 45,000-molecular-weight Ag-B antigen subunits—when tested against normal fibroblast glycoproteins (Fig. 8A).

Further data have demonstrated that the two types of antisera do indeed precipitate the same molecules from the transformed cell line. Thus, fingerprint analyses unambiguously showed that the 45,000-dalton chain is the Ag-B antigen heavy chain and that the 12,000-dalton chain is β_2-microglobulin. The 19,000-dalton glycoprotein is coded for by the adenovirus-2 genome (H. Persson and L. Philipson, personal communication) and belongs to the early adenovirus proteins (Walter and Maizel, 1974). These data demonstrate at the molecular level that transplantation antigens may display the general property to interact physically with foreign substances, and lend credence to the view that T killer cells recognize molecular complexes, partly comprised of self structures (Doherty *et al.*, 1976). Recently, Callahan *et al.* (1979) have shown that another virus protein can also be isolated in a physical complex with H-2 antigens, and it is to be anticipated that this will be a finding of some generality also with regard to other virus proteins.

4. Conclusions

The amino acid sequence homology between the HLA-A, -B, and -C antigens and the immunoglobulin constant domains is, with available information, not extended to the immunoglobulin variable regions. However, it is generally agreed that the immunoglobulin variable- and constant-region genes have evolved from the same ancestor (Hill *et al.*, 1966; Singer and Doolittle, 1966), so it seems reasonable to assume that immu-

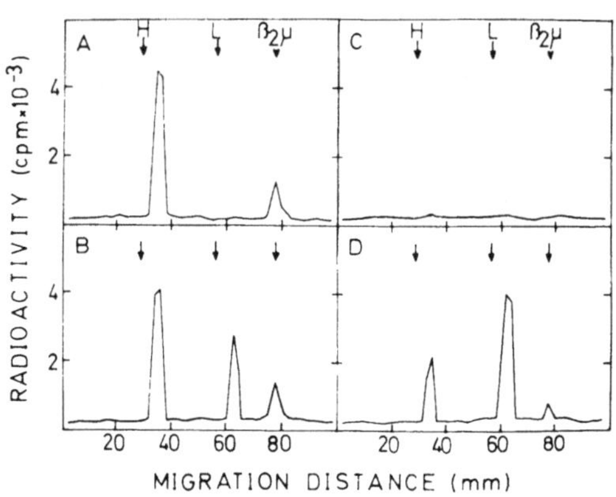

Figure 8. SDS–PAGE of cell-surface proteins reactive with a Lewis anti-August spleen cell antiserum reactive with AgB antigens (A,B) and a syngeneic antiserum against A2T2C4 cells (C,D). Glycoproteins, internally labeled with [^{3}H]tyrosine, were derived from primary Hooded-Lister rat fibroblasts (A,C) and from A2T2C4 cells (B,D). Normal rat serum did not bind measurable amounts of radioactive proteins (not shown).

noglobulin variable-region genes are as related to the HLA-A, -B, and -C antigen genes as they are to immunoglobulin constant-region genes. Indeed, the genetic polymorphism of the HLA-A, -B, and -C antigens may reflect one stage in the evolution of the immunoglobulin variability, and a substantial part of the variability would thus be endowed in the germ line.

The genetic polymorphism of the HLA-A, -B, and -C antigens poses certain structural constraints on the molecules: (1) Variable amino acids will most probably not occur in positions containing residues in contact with β_2-microglobulin. (2) Amino acid variations may to a large extent occur on the surface of the molecule, since they are recognized by alloantibodies. (3) The allotypic amino acid substitutions must preferentially occur in portions of the heavy chain that are of little importance for the overall three-dimensional structure, since sensitive probes of the tertiary structure such as xenoantibodies raised against one allotype react about equally well with other allotypes (Rask *et al.*, 1976; Kvist *et al.*, 1978a). An immunoglobulinlike structure of the HLA-A, -B, and -C antigens would easily encompass these features provided the amino acid variations were distributed like the hypervariable regions in immunoglobulins (Edelman and Gall, 1969). In such a case, allotypic amino acids would be confined to relatively restricted regions of the molecule that would not influence the general structure of the allotypically different HLA-A, -B, and -C antigens.

The immunoglobulinlike structure of the HLA-A, -B, and -C antigens, which is apparent at the level of both primary and tertiary structure, as evidenced by amino acid sequence analyses (Trägårdh *et al.*, 1978) and chiroptical examinations (Trägårdh *et al.*, 1979b), may explain the association of virus proteins and other foreign substances, such as bacteria, with transplantation antigens. It is obvious that these types of interactions cannot be as specific as those between antibodies and antigens. Whereas an individual heterozygous at each *HLA* locus may express perhaps some ten HLA-A, -B, and -C and similar antigens, it is likely that he will be able to manufacture as many as one million different antibodies. However, it is possible that each individual antibody may bind many different antigens with varying strength and that an antiserum always displays greater specificity than a single antibody. The heterogeneity of an antibody population raised against a given antigen would thus reduce the concentration of each individual species so that chance reactions with unrelated antigens will occur below the level of detection. These ideas, first proposed by Talmage (1959), have been examined theoretically (Inman, 1974) and have received some experimental support (Richards *et al.*, 1975). According to this concept, the HLA-A, -B, and -C antigens would be "primitive antibodies" with broad although limited specificity. The genetic polymorphism and the resulting heterozygosity would allow an extension of the specificity range and would accordingly confer a selective advantage over the homozygous state (Bodmer, 1972). The strength of the binding between an antibody and an unrelated antigen is generally low (Richards *et al.*, 1974), and it is likely that HLA-A, -B, and -C antigens also bind foreign substances with weak forces. However, viruses and bacteria have multiple copies of antigens on their surface, and HLA-A, -B, and -C antigens, like most cell-surface proteins, are mobile in the plane of the membrane (Neauport-Sautes *et al.*, 1973). Multipoint binding involving many individually weak interactions may therefore cause strong associations. This may serve as a focusing device for some foreign antigens so that endocytosis is induced. That T killer cells may require physical association between HLA-A, -B, and -C antigens and foreign substances for activation was discussed above.

It is obvious that the suggestion that the HLA-A, -B, and -C antigens act as primitive cell-surface antibodies, if extended to the HLA-DR (Ia) antigens (see Klareskog *et al.*, 1978), easily explains a number of observations such as the association between the MHC and certain diseases, the requirements for stimulation of T lymphocytes, the high proportion of T lymphocytes responsive against foreign MHC antigens, and so on. However, extensive structural analyses of HLA-A, -B, and -C as well as -DR antigens are required to test these ideas.

NOTE ADDED IN PROOF. The complete amino acid sequence of pooled papain-solubilized HLA-A, -B, and -C antigens (Trägårdh *et al.*, 1979c, 1980) and the HLA-B7 antigen (Orr *et al.*, 1979a,b,c; López de Castro *et al.*, 1979) were recently published. The data are in accord with the preliminary sequence information presented here.

ACKNOWLEDGMENTS. We are greatly indebted to our collaborators who have provided most of the information in this article. Work cited from the authors' laboratory was supported by grants from the Swedish Cancer Society. This chapter is dedicated to the late Dr. Ingemar Berggård, whose discovery of β_2-microglobulin has greatly influenced studies on the structure of the HLA-A, -B, and -C antigens.

References

Binz, H., and Wigzell H., 1977, Idiotypic, alloantigen-reactive T lymphocyte receptors and their use to induce specific transplantation tolerance, *Prog. Allergy* **23:**154–198.

Bodmer, W.F., 1972, Evolutionary significance of the HLA system, *Nature (London)* **237:**139–145.

Bubbers, J.E., Chen, S., and Lilly, F., 1978, Nonrandom inclusion of the H-2K and H-2D antigens in Friend virus particles from mice of various strains, *J. Exp. Med.* **147**:340–351.

Callahan, G.N., Allison, J.P., Pellegrino, M.A., and Reisfeld, R.A., 1979, Physical association of histocompatibility antigens and tumor-associated antigens on the surface of murine lymphoma cells, *J. Immunol.* **122**:80–81.

Coligan, J.E., Kindt, T.J., Ewenstein, B.M., Uehara, H., Nisizawa, T., and Nathenson, S.G., 1978, Primary structure of murine major histocompatibility complex alloantigens: Amino acid sequence studies of the cyanogen bromide fragments of the H-2 K^b glycoprotein, *Proc. Natl. Acad. Sci. U.S.A.* **75**:3390–3394.

Cunningham, B.A., Wang, J.L., Berggård, I., and Peterson, P.A., 1973, The complete amino acid sequence of β_2-microglobulin, *Biochemistry* **12**:4811–4822.

Dayhoff, M.O., Hunt, L.T., Barker, W.C., and Orcutt, B.C., 1976, *Atlas of Protein Sequence and Structure*, Vol. 5 (M.O. Dayhoff, ed.), Suppl. 1 and 2, National Biomedical Research Foundation, Washington, D.C.

Doherty, P.A., Blanden, R.V., and Zinkernagel, R.M., 1976, Specificity of virus-immune effector T-cells for H-2K or H-2D compatible interactions: Implications for H-antigen diversity, *Transplant. Rev.* **29**:89–124.

Edelman, G.M., 1970, The covalent structure of a human IgG-immunoglobulin. XI. Functional implications, *Biochemistry* **9**:3197–3205.

Edelman, G.M., and Gall, W.E., 1969, The antibody problem, *Annu. Rev. Biochem.* **38**:415–466.

Gally, J.A., and Edelman, G.M., 1972, The genetic control of immunoglobulin synthesis, *Annu. Rev. Genet.* **6**:1–46.

Germain, R.N., Dorf, M.E., and Benacerraf, B., 1975, Inhibition of T-lymphocyte mediated tumor-specific lysis by alloantisera directed against the H-2 serological specificities of the tumor, *J. Exp. Med.* **142**:1023–1028.

Grey, H.M., Kubo, R.T., Colon, S.M., Poulik, M.D., Cresswell, P., Springer, T., Turner, M., and Strominger, J.L., 1973, The small subunit of HL-A antigens is β_2-microglobulin, *J. Exp. Med.* **138**:1608–1612.

Gross, E., and Witkopf, B., 1962, Nonenzymatic cleavage of peptide bonds: The methionine residues in bovine pancreatic ribonuclease, *J. Biol. Chem.* **237**:1856–1860.

Hale, A.H., Whitte, O.W., Baltimore, D., and Eisen, H.N., 1978, Vesicular stomatitis virus glycoprotein is necessary for H-2-restricted lysis of infected cells by cytotoxic T-lymphocytes, *Proc. Natl. Acad. Sci. U.S.A.* **75**:970–974.

Hecht, T.T., and Summers, D.F., 1976, Interactions of vesicular stomatitis virus with murine cell surface antigens, *J. Virol.* **19**:833–845.

Helenius, A., Morein, B., Fries, E., Simons, K., Robinson, P., Schirrmacher, V., Terhorst, C., and Strominger, J.L., 1978, Human (HLA-A and HLA-B) and murine (H-2K and H-2D) histocompatibility antigens are cell surface receptors for Semliki Forest virus, *Proc. Natl. Acad. Sci. U.S.A.* **75**:3846–3850.

Henning, R., Schrader, J.E., and Edelman, G.M., 1976, Antiviral antibodies inhibit the lysis of tumor cells by anti-H-2 sera, *Nature (London)* **263**:689–691.

Hildemann, W.H., Raison, R.L., Cheong, G., Hull, C.J., Akaka, L., and Okamoto, J., 1977, Immunological specificity and memory in a scleractinian coral, *Nature (London)* **270**:219–223.

Hill, R.L., 1965, Hydrolysis of proteins, *Adv. Protein Chem.* **20**:37–107.

Hill, R.L., Delaney, R., Fellows, R.E., Jr., and Lebovitz, M.E., 1966, The evolutionary origins of the immunoglobulins, *Proc. Natl. Acad. Sci. U.S.A.* **56**:1762–1769.

Inman, J.K., 1974, Multispecificity of the antibody combining region and antibody diversity, in: *The Immune System* (E.E. Sercarz, A.R. Williamson, and C.F. Fox, eds.), pp. 37–52, Academic Press, New York.

Jacobson, G.R., Schaffer, M.H., Stark, G.R., and Vanaman, T.C., 1973, Specific chemical cleavage in high yield at the amino peptide bonds of cysteine and cystine residues, *J. Biol. Chem.* **248**:6583–6591.

Klareskog, L., Banck, G., Forsgren, A., and Peterson, P.A., 1978, Binding of HLA antigen-containing liposomes to bacteria, *Proc. Natl. Acad. Sci. U.S.A.* **75**:6197–6201.

Koszinowski, U., and Ertl, H., 1975a, Lysis mediated by T cells and restricted by H-2 antigen of target cells infected with vaccinia virus, *Nature (London)* **255**:552–554.

Koszinowski, U., and Ertl, H., 1975b, Target cell-dependent T cell-mediated lysis of vaccinia virus-infected cells, *Eur. J. Immunol.* **5**:245–251.

Kvist, S., Östberg, L., and Peterson, P.A., 1978a, Reactions and crossreactions of a rabbit anti-H2 antigen serum, *Scand. J. Immunol.* **7**:265–276.

Kvist, S., Östberg, L., Person, H., Philipson, L., and Peterson, P.A., 1978b, Molecular association between transplantation antigens and a cell surface antigen in an adenovirus-transformed cell line, *Proc. Natl. Acad. Sci. U.S.A.* **75**:5674–5678.

López de Castro, J.A., Orr, H.T., Robb, R.J., Kostyk, T.G., Mann, D.L., and Strominger, J.L., 1979, Complete amino acid sequence of papain-solubilized human histocompatibility antigen, HLA-B7. 1. Isolation and amino acid composition of fragments and of tryptic and chymotryptic peptides, *Biochemistry* **18**:5704–5711.

Nakamuro, K., Tanigaki, N., and Pressman, D., 1973, Multiple common properties of human β_2-microglobulin and the common portion fragment derived from HL-A antigen molecules, *Proc. Natl. Acad. Sci. U.S.A.* **70**:2863–2865.

Neauport-Sautes, C., Lilly, F., Silvestre, D., and Kourilsky, F.M., 1973, Independence of H-2K and H-2D antigenic determinants on the surface of mouse lymphocytes, *J. Exp. Med.* **137**:511–526.

Orr, H.T., Lancet, D., Robb, R.J., López de Castro, J.A., and Strominger, J.L., 1979, The heavy chain of human histocompatibility antigen, HLA-B7, contains an immunoglobin-like region, *Nature* **282**:266–270.

Orr, H.T., López de Castro, J.A., Parham, P., Pleogh, H.L., and Strominger, J.L., 1979a Comparison of amino acid sequences of two human histocompatibility antigens, HLA-A2 and HLA-B7: Location of putative alloantigenic sites, *Proc. Natl. Acad. Sci. U.S.A.* **76**:4395–4399.

Orr, H.T., López de Castro, J.A., Lancet, D., and Strominger, J.L., 1979b, Complete amino acid sequence of a papain-solubilized histocompatibility antigen, HLA-B7. 2. Sequence determination and search for homologies, *Biochemistry* **18**:5711–5720.

Parham, P., Alpert, B.W., Orr, H.T., and Strominger, J.L., 1977, Carbohydrate moiety of HLA-antigens, *J. Biol. Chem.* **252**:7555–7567.

Peterson, P.A., Cunningham, B.A., Berggård, I., and Edelman, G.M., 1972, β_2-Microglobulin—a free immunoglobulin domain, *Proc. Natl. Acad. Sci. U.S.A.* **69**:1697–1701.

Peterson, P.A., Rask, L., and Lindblom, J.B., 1974, Highly purified papain-solubilized HLA-antigens contain β_2-microglobulin, *Proc. Natl. Acad. Sci. U.S.A.* **71**:35–39.

Peterson, P.A., Rask, L., Sege, K., Klareskog, L., Anundi, H., and Ostberg, L., 1975, Evolutionary relationship between immunoglobulins and transplantation antigens, *Proc. Natl. Acad. Sci. U.S.A.* **72**:1612–1616.

Peterson, P.A., Östberg, L., and Rask, L., 1977, β_2-Microglobulin and the major histocompatibility complex, *Adv. Cancer Res.* **24**:115–163.

Poljak, R.J., 1975, Three-dimensional structure, function and genetic control of immunoglobulins, *Nature (London)* **256**:373–376.

Poulsen, K., Fraser, K.J., and Haber, E., 1972, An active derivative of rabbit antibody light chain composed of the constant and the variable domains held together only by a native disulfide bond, *Proc. Natl. Acad. Sci. U.S.A.* **69**:2495–2499.

Rask, L., Lindblom, J.B., and Peterson, P.A., 1976, Structural and immunological similarities between HLA antigens for three loci, *Eur. J. Immunol.* **6**:93–100.

Richards, F.F., Anzel, L.M., Konigsberg, W.H., Manjula, B.N., Poljak, R.J., Rosenstein, R.W., Saul, F., and Varga, J.M., 1974, Polyfunctional antibody combining regions, in: *The Immune System* (E.E. Sercarz, A.R. Williamson, and C.F. Fox, eds.), pp. 53–68, Academic Press, New York.

Richards, F.F., Konigsberg, W.H., Rosenstein, R.W., and Varga, J.M., 1975, On the specificity of antibodies, *Science* **187:**130–137.

Rosenthal, A., 1978, Determinant selection and macrophage function in genetic control of the immune response, *Immunol. Rev.* **40:**136–152.

Schrader, J.W., and Edelman, G.M., 1976, Participation of the H-2 antigens of tumor cells in their lysis by syngeneic T cells, *J. Exp. Med.* **143:**601–604.

Schrader, J.W., Cunningham, B.A., and Edelman, G.M., 1975, Functional interactions of viral and histocompatibility antigens at tumor cell surfaces, *Proc. Natl. Acad. Sci. U.S.A.* **72:**5066–5070.

Seidman, J.G., Leder, A., Nav, M., Norman, B., and Leder, P., 1978, Antibody diversity, *Science* **202:**11–17.

Shearer, G.M., Rehn, T.G., and Garbarino, C.A., 1975, Cell-mediated lympholysis of trinitrophenyl-modified antologous lymphocytes, *J. Exp. Med.* **141:**1348–1364.

Shreffler, D., and David, C.S., 1975, The H-2 major histocompatibility complex and the I immune response region: Genetic variation, function and organization, *Adv. Immunol.* **20:**125–196.

Singer, S.J., and Doolittle, R.F.,1966, Antibody active sites and immunoglobulin molecules, *Science* **153:**13–25.

Smithies, O., and Poulik, M.D., 1972, Initiation of protein synthesis at an unusual position in an immunoglobulin gene?, *Science* **175:**187–189.

Snary, D., Barnstable, C.J., Bodmer, W.F., and Crumpton, M.J., 1977, Molecular structure of human histocompatibility antigens: The HLA-C-series, *Eur. J. Immunol.* **8:**580–585.

Springer, T.A., and Strominger, J.L., 1976, Detergent-soluble HLA-antigens contain a hydrophilic region at the COOH-terminus and a penultimate hydrophobic region, *Proc. Natl. Acad. Sci. U.S.A.* **73:**2481–2485.

Talmage, D.E., 1959, Immunological specificity, *Science* **129:**1643–1648.

Terhorst, C., Robb, R., Jones, C., and Strominger, J.L., 1977, Further structural studies of the heavy chain of HLA-antigens and its similarity to immunoglobulins, *Proc. Natl. Acad. Sci. U.S.A.* **74:**4002–4006.

Trägårdh, L., Klareskog, L., Curman, B., Rask, L., and Peterson, P.A., 1978, Isolation and properties of detergent-solubilized HLA antigens obtained from platelets, *Scand. J. Immunol.* **8:**563–568.

Trägårdh, L., Wiman, K., Rask, L., and Peterson, P.A., 1979a, Fragmentation of human transplantation antigen heavy chains by limited proteolysis, acid cleavage and cyanogen bromide treatment, *Biochemistry* **18:**1322–1328.

Trägårdh, L., Curman, B., Wiman, K., Rask, L., and Peterson, P.A., 1979b, Chemical, physical–chemical, and immunological properties of papain-solubilized human transplantation antigens, *Biochemistry* **18:**2218–2226.

Trägårdh, L., Rask, L., Wiman, K., Fohlman, J., and Peterson, P.A., 1979c, Amino acid sequence of an immunoglobulin-like HLA antigen heavy chain domain, *Proc. Natl. Acad. Sci. U.S.A.* **76:**5839–5842.

Trägårdh, L., Rask, L., Wiman, K., and Peterson, P.A., 1979d, Primary structure of pooled, papain-solubilized HLA-A, -B, and -C antigens, *Scand. J. Immunol.* **10:**597–600.

Trägårdh, L., Rask, L., Wiman, K., Fohlman, J., and Peterson, P.A., 1980, Complete amino acid sequence of pooled papain-solubilized HLA-A, -B, and -C antigens: Relatedness to immunoglobulins and internal homologies, *Proc. Natl. Acad. Sci. U.S.A.* **77:**1129–1133.

Walter, G., Maizel, J.V., Jr., 1974, The polypeptides of adenovirus, *Virology* **57**:402–408.

Wikler, M., Titani, K., Shinoda, T., and Putnam, F.W., 1967, The complete amino acid sequence of a λtype Bence-Jones protein, *J. Biol. Chem.* **242**:1668–1670.

Wiman, K., Trägårdh, L., Rask, L., and Peterson, P.A., 1979, Similarities between immunoglobulins and transplantation antigens in amino acid sequence and disulfide bond distribution, *Eur. J. Biochem.* **95**:265–273.

Zarling, D.A., Keshet, I., Watson, A., and Bach, F.H., 1978, Association of mouse major histocompatibility and Rauscher murine leukemia virus envelope glycoprotein antigens on leukemia cells and their recognition by syngenic virus-immune cytotoxic T-lymphocytes, *Scand. J. Immunol.* **8**:497–508.

19

Functional Implications of the Structural Diversity of Murine Ia and Human DR Antigens

Jack Silver

1. Introduction

The survival of an organism depends on the ability of its cells to recognize each other and their immediate environment. The immune responses found in most vertebrates are prime instances of vitally important interactions among subpopulations of cells. In the sophisticated immune system of mammals, the generation of immune responses requires interactions among T cells, B cells, and macrophages. The *I* and *HLA-D* regions of the murine and human major histocompatibility complexes (MHC) contain genes that regulate these cell interactions. This role for these genes was recognized with the observation that subpopulations of immune cells from individuals possessing different forms (haplotypes) of the MHC failed to interact. The cellular interactions genetically regulated by the MHC are apparently mediated by cell-surface glycoproteins known as Ia antigens in mice and HLA-DR antigens in humans. These molecules display a high degree of serological and structural polymorphism, a consequence of the high degree of polymorphism of the MHC. The genetic restrictions placed on cellular interactions by the MHC presumably reflect the requirement for recognition of haplotype-specific Ia or HLA-DR antigens. Consequently, molecular analysis of the structural diversity of Ia and HLA-DR antigens provides a basis for understanding how cells

---

Jack Silver • Department of Cellular and Developmental Immunology, Scripps Clinic and Research Foundation, La Jolla, California 92037.

recognize and communicate with each other. This chapter summarizes current knowledge concerning the molecular diversity of murine Ia and human HLA-DR antigens and some of the interesting implications involved.

2. The Murine MHC Codes for Two Groups of Structurally Different Ia Molecules

By genetic analysis, the murine *I* region may be subdivided into a number of subregions: *I-A*, *I-B*, *I-J*, *I-E*, and *I-C* (Shreffler and David, 1975). Immunoprecipitation with antiserum prepared by cross-immunizing *I*-region-disparate strains of mice has until now permitted identification of only two groups of cell-surface Ia molecules, one determined by the *I-A* subregion and the other by the *I-E* subregion (Cullen *et al.*, 1976; Silver *et al.*, 1976, 1977; McMillan *et al.*, 1977). Both consist of two noncovalently associated polypeptide chains, the larger and smaller subunits of each being designated α and β, respectively (Fig. 1). Despite this similarity in subunit structure, the I-A- and I-E-subregion molecules are biochemically separate and distinct. Under nonreducing conditions, a large proportion of the two polypeptides, A_α and A_β, that comprose I-A-subregion molecules exist as a disulfide-linked αβ dimer with a molecular

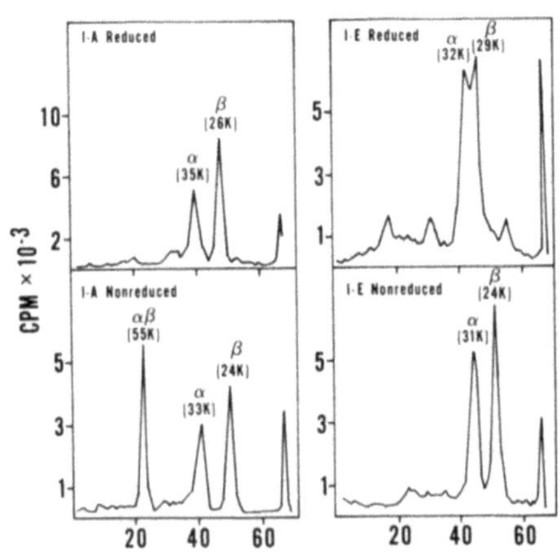

Figure 1. SDS-PAGE profiles of immunoprecipitated I-A and I-E molecules.

weight of 55,000. In contrast, no such dimer is observed for the I-E-subregion molecules. However, under nonreducing conditions, the migration rate on sodium dodecyl sulfate–polyacrylamide gel electrophoresis (SDS-PAGE) of the smaller subunit, designated E_β, changes dramatically, although the migration rate of the larger chain, designated E_α, changes only minimally. Neither the A_α nor the A_β subunit undergoes such a change. The more rapid migration rate of the E_β chain under nonreducing conditions presumably reflects the presence of an intrachain disulfide bond that keeps the molecule in a compact form.

Even more striking are the differences that these two groups of molecules display by amino acid sequence and peptide map analysis. Partial N-terminal sequence analysis fails to reveal any significant degree of similarity between I-A and I-E molecules (Fig. 2). Concordant with this is the lack of any striking similarity by peptide mapping (Cullen *et al.*, 1976; Freed *et al.*, 1978) (Fig. 3). Thus, the murine *I* region codes for two groups of Ia molecules that are biochemically quite different.

3. Human HLA-DR Antigens Are the Homologues of Murine I-E-Subregion Molecules

Membrane antigens determined by a gene closely linked to the *HLA-D* region of the MHC have been identified by serological analysis of human lymphocytes and designated HLA-DR. The cell-surface molecules displaying these antigens may be isolated by conventional purification procedures or immunoprecipitation with anti-DR serum (Cresswell and Geier, 1975; Humphreys *et al.*, 1976; Geier and Cresswell, 1977; Springer *et al.*, 1977a,b; Snary *et al.*, 1977; Klareskog *et al.*, 1977; Nilsson *et al.*, 1977; Allison *et al.*, 1978). The HLA-DR molecules consist of two polypeptides, DR_α and DR_β, with molecular weights similar to those of murine I-E-subregion molecules (Fig. 4). In addition, the nonreduced DR_β chain migrates more rapidly on SDS-PAGE than the reduced chain. This anomalous behavior of the DR_β subunit, which is also displayed by the murine E_β subunit, suggests that the two are homologous products of different species. Partial N-terminal sequence analysis of human DR- and murine I-E-subregion molecules confirms this proposal (Allison *et al.*, 1978; Silver *et al.*, 1979). The E_α and DR_α polypeptides display a high degree of sequence homology, as do the E_β and DR_β polypeptides, providing an amino acid is deleted from the N terminus of the DR_β subunit (Fig. 5).

STEP NUMBER

	1	2	3	4	5	6	7	8	9	10	11	12	13	14	15	16	17	18	19	20	21	22	23	24	25	26	27
I-A_α	-			ile		ala	-	-	val	-		tyr	-	-	-	val	tyr									tyr	
I-E_α	ile			-	his	-	ile	ile	-	ala		phe	tyr	leu	leu	pro	-					phe	met	phe		phe	
I-A_β	-				arg			val	tyr		-	-				tyr			-							tyr	
I-E_β	val					pro		phe	leu		tyr	val						phe	tyr						val		

Figure 2. Comparisons of the partial amino-terminal sequences of I-A and I-E molecules. (—) Denotes the absence of a residue found in the other molecule.

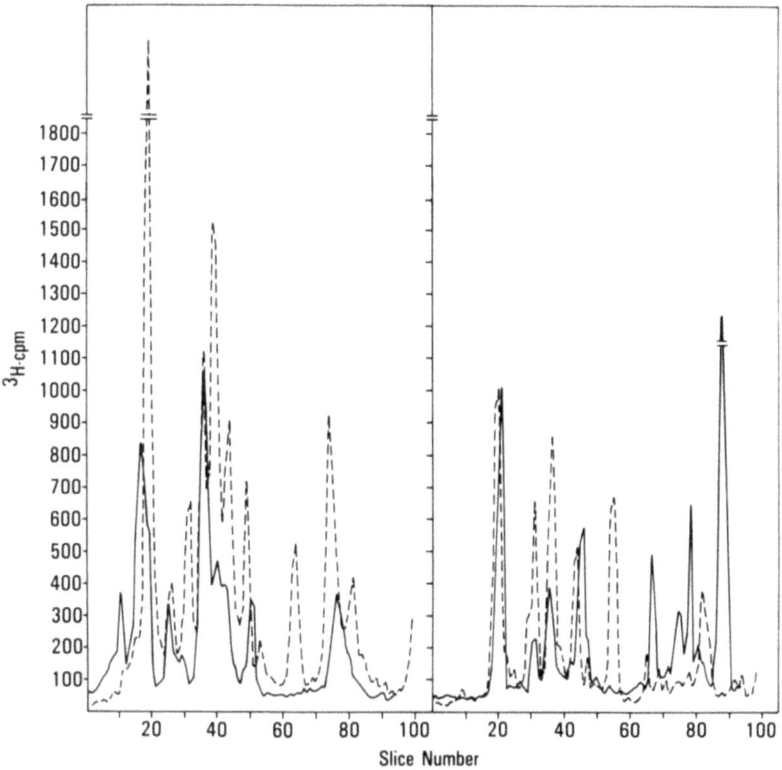

Figure 3. Comparisons of tryptic peptide profiles of α (*left*) and β (*right*) polypeptides derived from I-A (—) and I-E (----) molecules.

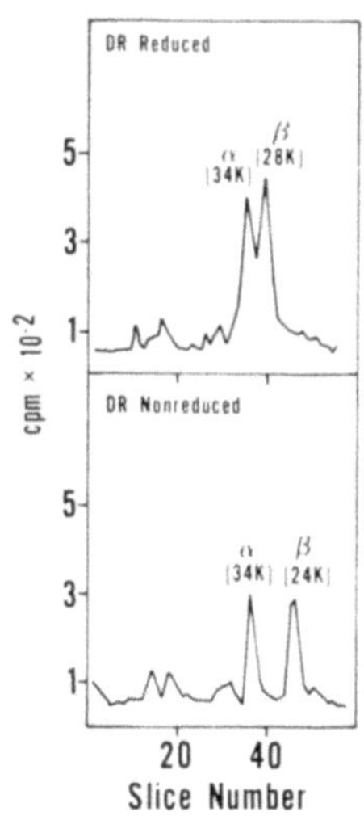

Figure 4. SDS-PAGE profiles of human HLA-DR antigens.

STEP NUMBER

	1	2	3	4	5	6	7	8	9	10	11	12	13	14	15	16	17	18	19	20	21	22	23	24	25	26	27	28	29	30	31	32
$E_{\alpha}^{d,k}$	ile				* his	-	ile	ile		ala		* phe	* tyr	* leu	leu	* pro						* phe	* met	* phe		* phe						
DR_{α}					his	val						phe	tyr	leu		pro						phe	met	phe		phe						
E_{β}^{k}	val					* pro		* phe	* leu	-	* tyr	* -						* phe	* tyr						* val		* -	* leu			* tyr	* phe
DR_{β}	[ ]					pro		phe	leu	tyr	tyr	val						phe	tyr						val		(phe)	leu			tyr	(phe)
E_{β}^{d}	val					pro		phe	leu	-	tyr	val						phe	tyr						val		phe	leu			phe	-

Figure 5. Comparisons of the partial amino-terminal sequences of human HLA-DR and murine I-E molecules. (*) Denotes sequence identity of murine and human antigens.

4. The Structural Diversity of Murine I-E-Subregion Molecules Is Restricted to the Small (β) Subunit

Comparisons of the structures of allotypic I-E-subregion molecules isolated from murine strains that differ at the *I* region but are otherwise genetically identical leads to a very intriguing observation: the E_α polypeptides are apparently invariant in structure, but the E_β polypeptides display a high degree of variability. Partial N-terminal sequence analysis reveals several amino acid sequence differences between E^k and E^d polypeptides and no apparent differences between the E_α polypeptides (Fig. 6). Peptide map analysis of allotypic I-E-subregion molecules confirms the dichotomy in the degree of structural variation; the peptide maps of E^k and E^d polypeptides are virtually identical, yet the E^k and E^d polypeptides display several salient differences (Fig. 7). Similar observations have been made by others (McMillan *et al.*, 1978; Cook *et al.*, 1979a,b). The structural constancy of the E_α polypeptide is presumably a reflection of some common function that requires an invarient structure. However, since the location of the gene encoding the E_α chain is unknown and may in fact be outside the MHC, the structural identity may merely reflect the fact that the allotypic I-E-subregion molecules were isolated from mice that are MHC congenic (genetically identical outside the MHC).

5. Most of the Structural Diversity Displayed by Human DR Antigens Is Found in the Small (β) Subunit

As observed with the murine I-E-subregion molecules, allotypic DR molecules differ primarily in the structure of their β subunits. Peptide maps of DR molecules, isolated by immunoprecipitation with anti-DR serum, from three human lymphoblastoid cell lines that express differing DR antigens, are shown in Fig. 8. Peptide maps of the three DR_β polypeptides are strikingly different; in contrast, the DR_α peptide maps are very similar, with only minor differences apparent. These data are consistent with data obtained from partial N-terminal sequence analysis (Springer *et al.*, 1977a; Silver *et al.*, 1979). The DR_β chains isolated from Victor and RPMI 4265 lymphoblastoid cell lines differ in four of seven positions that can be compared, but the DR_α chains display only a single tentative difference among the five residues that can be compared (Fig. 9). The limited variation in structure of DR_α subunits cannot be explained on the basis of genetic identity created by genetic manipulation, as may be proposed for the murine E_α subunits, since the three human cell lines presumably differ genetically outside the MHC. Thus, functional or evo-

STEP NUMBER

	1	2	3	4	5	6	7	8	9	10	11	12	13	14	15	16	17,	18	19	20	21	22	23	24	25	26	27	28	29	30	31	32
E^k_α										Ala		Phe	Tyr	Leu	(Leu)	Pro						Phe		Phe		Phe						
E^d_α										Ala		Phe	Tyr	Leu	(Leu)	Pro						Phe		Phe		Phe						
E^k_β	Val					Pro		Phe	Leu		Tyr	-						Phe	Tyr						Val		-	Leu			Tyr	Phe
E^d_β	Val					Pro		Phe	Leu		Tyr	Val						Phe	Tyr						Val		Phe	Leu			Phe	-

Figure 6. Comparisons of the partial amino-terminal sequences of two allotypic I-E molecules. (—) Denotes the absence of a residue found in the other allele. Boxed residues denote sequence differences between alleles.

lutionary pressures, or both, have apparently created and maintained the dichotomy in the degree of structural variation displayed by the DR_{α} (E_{α}) and DR_{β}(E_{β}) subunits.

6. Allotypic I-A-Subregion Molecules of the Mouse Display Structural Diversity in Both Subunits

Partial N-terminal sequence analysis of allotypic I-A-subregion molecules isolated from B10.A(4R) and B10.A(5R) mice by immunoprecipitation fails to reveal any differences between the A_{α} chains and documents

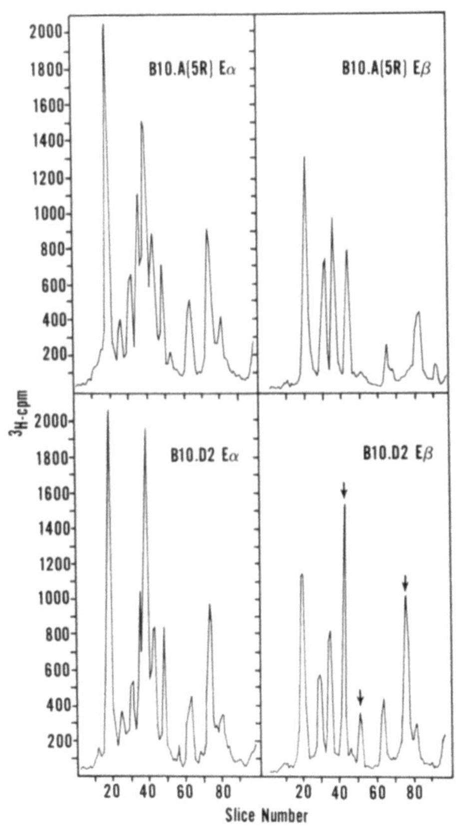

Figure 7. Comparisons of the tryptic peptide profiles of allotypic I-E molecules isolated from B10.D2 and B10.A(5R) mice. Arrows denote conspicuous differences.

only two differences between the A_β chains (Fig. 10). The absence of any sequence differences between the A_α chains is probably due to the fact that only a small number of sequence data are available, since peptide map analyses reveal that both A_α and A_β subunits display a significant degree of structural diversity (Figs. 11 and 12).

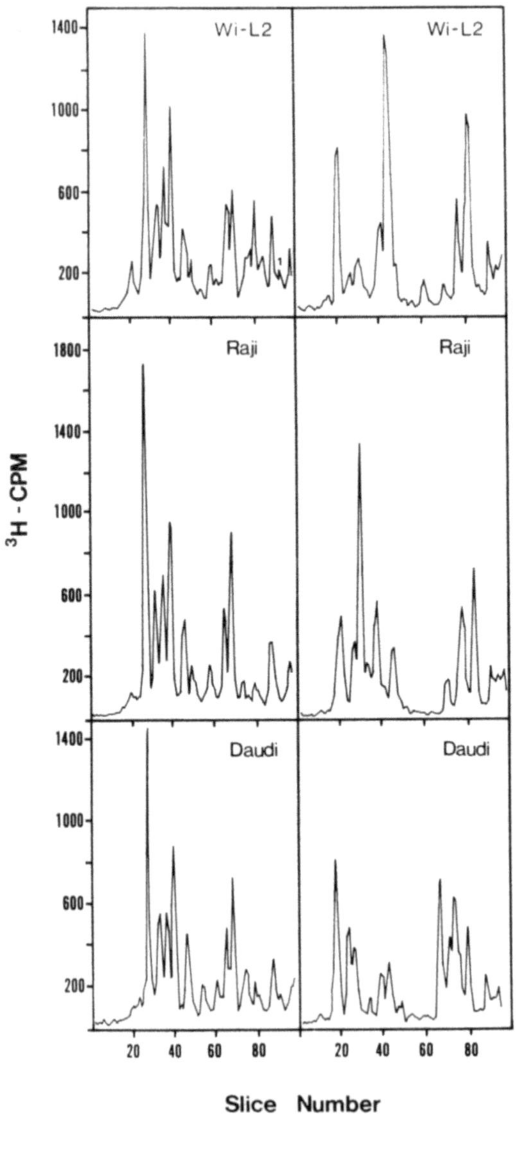

Figure 8. Comparisons of tryptic peptide profiles of DR_α *(left)* and DR_β *(right)* polypeptides isolated from lymphoblastoid cell lines with different HLA-DR phenotypes.

STEP NUMBER

	1	2	3	4	5	6	7	8	9	10	11	12	13	14	15
DR_α					His	Val						Phe	Tyr	Leu	
p34	Ile	Lys	Glu	Glu	(Arg)	Val	Ile		Gln	Ala	Glu	Phe	Tyr	Leu	Asn
DR_β	[]			-	-	Pro		Phe	Leu	Tyr	Tyr	Val			
p29	[]	Gly	Asp	Val	Pro	-		Phe	Leu	Glu	Glu	Val			

Figure 9. Comparisons of the partial amino-terminal sequences of DR antigens isolated from Victor and RPMI 4265 lymphoblastoid cell lines. (—) Denotes the absence of a residue found in the other allele. Boxed residues denote sequence differences between alleles.

7. The Small Subunit of an I-A-Subregion Molecule Determines the Allospecificity Recognizable by a Monoclonal Antibody

Each allotypic I-A-subregion molecule may be serologically distinguished by a group of antigenic specificities. Some of these are common to other allotypic I-A-subregion molecules and are denoted "public" specificities; some are unique to that particular I-A-subregion molecule and are denoted "private" specificities (Shreffler *et al.*, 1976). On the basis of sequential immunoprecipitation experiments, "public" and "private" specificities reside on the same molecular complex (Cullen *et al.*, 1976; Shreffler *et al.*, 1976). The series of experiments described below demonstrate that the "public" specificity Ia.17 detectable by a monoclonal antibody, 10-2.16, on I-A-subregion molecules isolated from B10.A(4R) mice is determined by the small (β) subunit.

7.1. Allotypic I-A-Subregion Molecules May Be Immunoprecipitated from B10.A(4R) and B10.A(5R) Mice

I-A-subregion molecules from B10.A(4R) mice express the "public" specificity Ia.17 and are immunoprecipitable with the relevant monoclonal antibody, 10-2.16 (Fig. 13a). However, the I-A-subregion molecules from B10.A(5R) mice do not express Ia.17 and are not immunoprecipitated with monoclonal antibody 10-2.16; consequently, it is necessary to use for this purpose an alloantiserum, (B10.A × A)F_1 anti B10.A(5R), that recognizes multiple antigenic specifities (Fig. 13).

STEP NUMBER

	1	2	3	4	5	6	7	8	9	10	11	12	13	14	15	16	17	18	19	20	21	22	23	24	25	26	27
$I\text{-}A^b_\alpha$				ile		ala			val			tyr				val	tyr									tyr	
$I\text{-}A^k_\alpha$				ile		ala			val			tyr				val	tyr									tyr	
$I\text{-}A^b_\beta$					arg			val	tyr							tyr										tyr	
$I\text{-}A^k_\beta$					arg			val	-							tyr										-	

Figure 10. Comparisons of the partial amino-terminal sequences of two allotypic I-A molecules. (—) Denotes the absence of a residue found in the other allele. Boxed residues denote sequence differences between alleles.

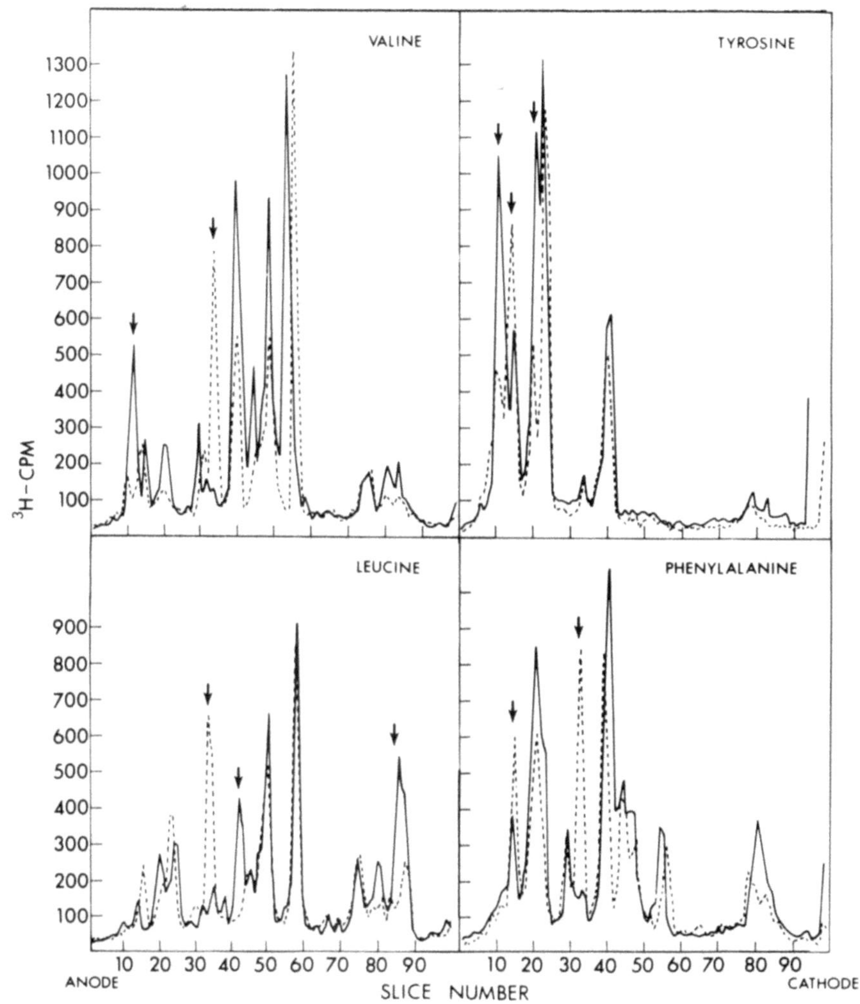

Figure 11. Comparisons of tryptic peptide profiles of allotypic A_α polypeptides radiolabeled with different tritiated amino acids and isolated from 4R (——) and 5R (----) mice. Arrows denotes conspicuous differences.

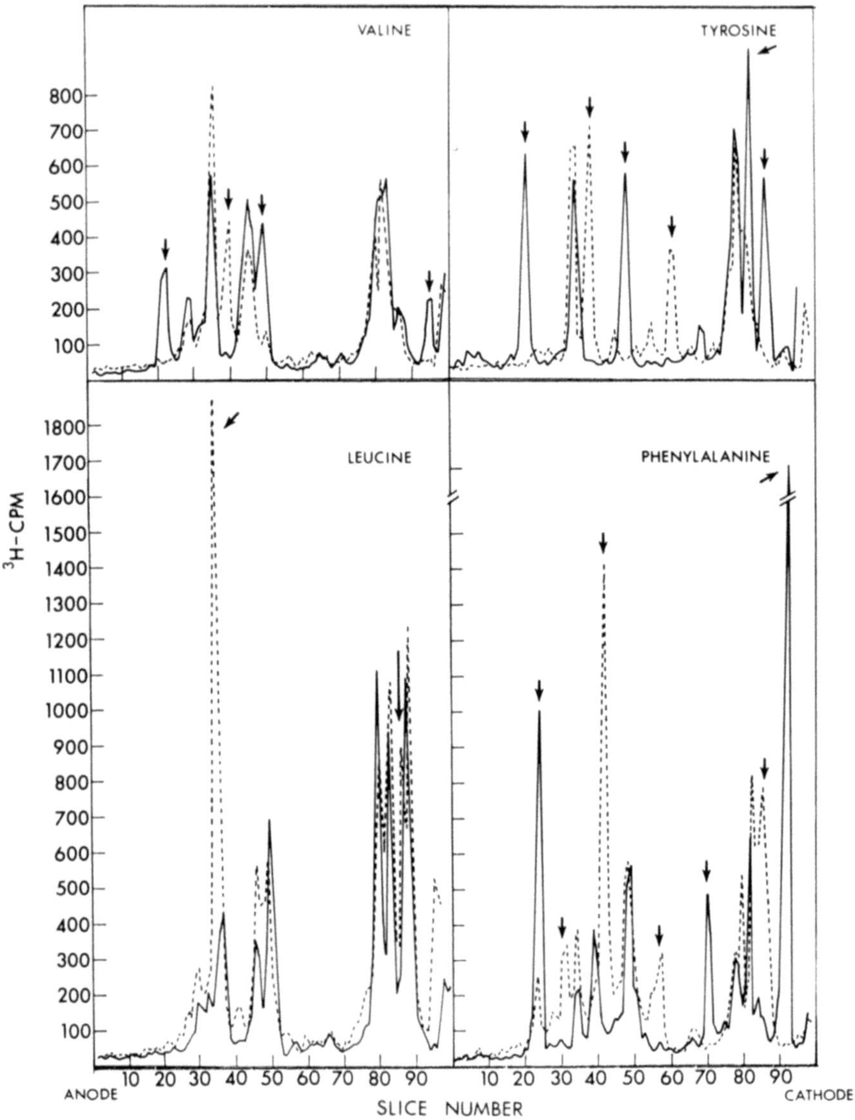

Figure 12. Comparisons of tryptic peptide profiles of allotypic A_{β} polypeptides radiolabeled with different tritiated amino acids and isolated from 4R (——) and 5R (------) mice. Arrows denote conspicuous differences.

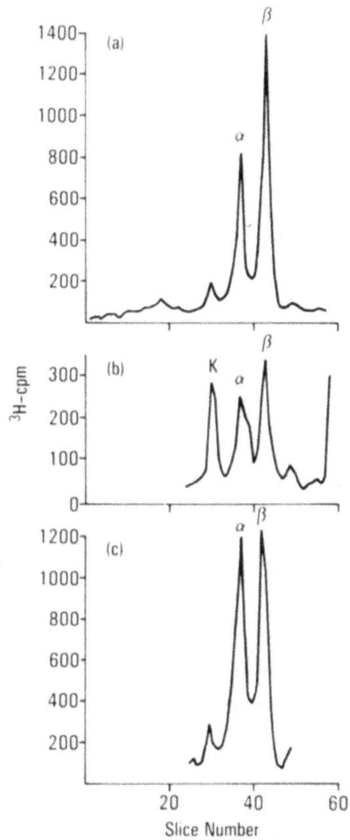

Figure 13. SDS-PAGE profiles of I-A molecules immunoprecipitated from 4R (a), 5R (b), and F_1 (c) mice.

7.2. Allotypes of A_α and A_β Chains Isolated from 4R and 5R Mice Are Distinguishable According to Their Peptide Maps

The A_α chain isolated from B10.A(5R) mice (designated A_α^b) displays a peptide peak (I) that is absent from the A_α chain isolated from B10.A(4R) mice (designated A_α^k) (Fig. 14A). Similarly, A_β chains from these two strains may be distinguished by their peptide maps (Fig. 15A). The A_β chain isolated from B10.A(5R) mice (designated A_β^b) displays several unique peptides (III and IV); the A_β chain isolated from B10.A(4R) mice (designated A_β^k) also has one unique peptide (II).

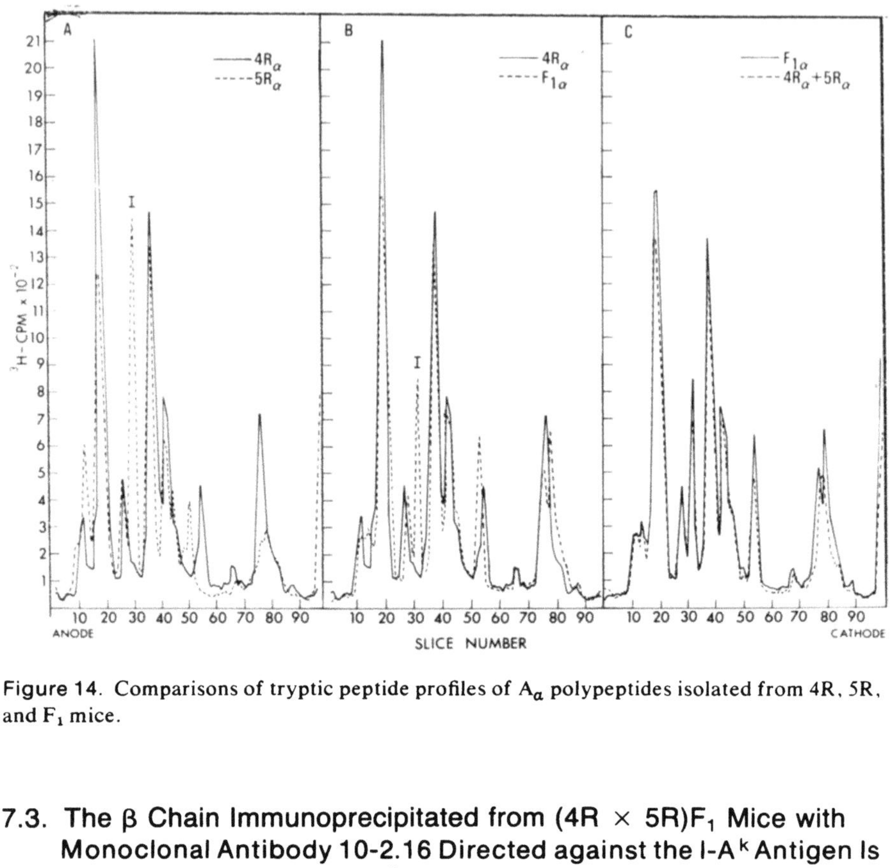

Figure 14. Comparisons of tryptic peptide profiles of A_α polypeptides isolated from 4R, 5R, and F_1 mice.

7.3. The β Chain Immunoprecipitated from (4R × 5R)F_1 Mice with Monoclonal Antibody 10-2.16 Directed against the I-A^k Antigen Is Comprised Solely of the A^k_β Chain

This is demonstrated by the fact that the peptide maps of A_β chains isolated from (4R × 5R)F_1 and B10.A(4R) mice are virtually identical (Fig. 15B). Clearly, the A_β chain isolated from (4R × 5R)F_1 mice does not comprise a mixture of A^b_β and A^k_β chains, since its peptide map is different from that derived from the mixed A^b_β and A^k_β chains (Fig. 15C).

7.4. The α Chain Immunoprecipitated from (4R × 5R)F_1 Mice with Monoclonal Antibody 10-2.16 Consists of Both the A^k_α and A^b_α Chains

The peptide map of the A_α chain isolated from (4R × 5R)F_1 mice displays peak I, which is unique to the A^b_β chain (Fig. 14B). Furthermore, this peptide map is virtually identical to that derived from a mixture of the A^b_α and A^k_α chains (Fig. 15C).

These results indicate that I-A-subregion antigens precipitated from $(4R \times 5R)F_1$ mice with antiserum directed against the I-A-subregion antigen of the 4R parent are composed of the β chain derived from the 4R parent and a mixture of the α chains derived from both parents. The absence of an A^b_β chain in the immunoprecipitate is not due to the inability of these F_1 mice to express the A^b_β chain; to the contrary, antiserum directed against I-A^b antigens precipitates the A^b_β chain of F_1 mice (unpublished observations).

These observations indicate that the allospecificity, Ia.17, recognized by monoclonal antibody 10-2.16 is conferred on the molecular complex by the β chain, since the antibody displays specificity for the A^k_β chain, but none for α chains. Coprecipitation of both α chains cannot be due to recognition of both by monoclonal antibody 10-2.16, because if this were the case, one would expect antibody 10-2.16 to immunoprecipitate I-A-subregion molecules from B10.(5R) mice, which it does not. However, we cannot entirely rule out the possibility that the antigenic determinant recognized by monoclonal antibody 10-2.16 actually resides on the α chain and is generated by association with the specific A^k_β chain.

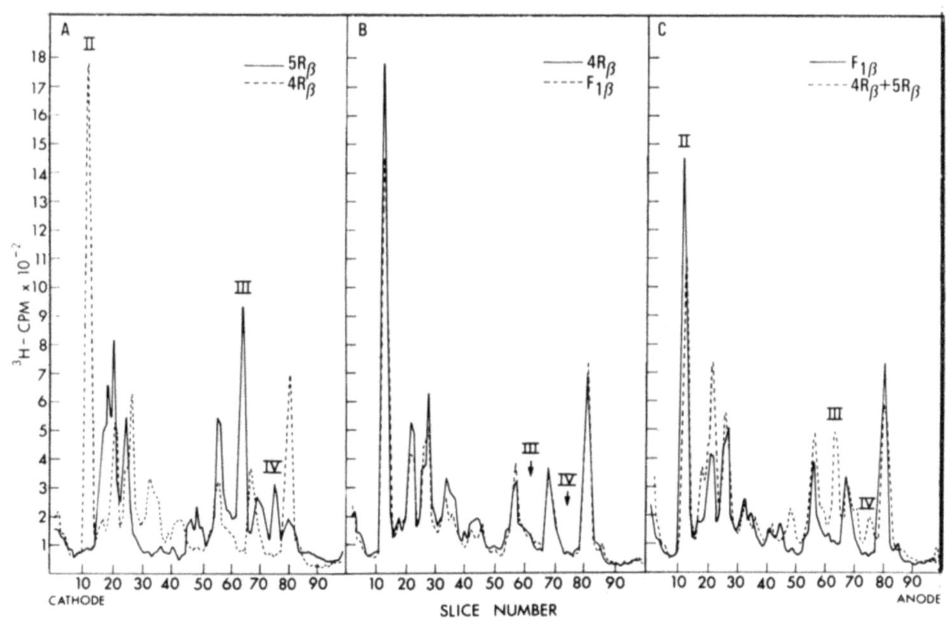

Figure 15. Comparisons of tryptic peptide profiles of A_β polypeptides isolated from 4R, 5R, and F_1 mice. (B) Arrows denote positions where one would expect to find peaks III and IV derived from the 5R β chain.

8. Functional Implications

In the past ten years, functional analysis of the genetic region known as the MHC has led to a number of fascinating discoveries. It is now well established that the MHC contains a number of genetic loci that regulate cell–cell interactions. Interactions between cytotoxic T cells and target cells are regulated by the *K* and *D* loci of the murine MHC (Bevan, 1975; Gordon *et al.*, 1975; Zinkernagel *et al.*, 1976), and T–B cell (Katz *et al.*, 1975) and T cell–macrophage (Erb and Feldmann, 1975; Bergholtz and Thorsby, 1978) interactions are regulated by the *I* and *HLA-D* regions of the murine and human MHC, respectively. These discoveries were virtually made possible by the observation that the interactions are genetically restricted by the MHC; that is, potentially interacting cells must be genetically identical at the appropriate MHC region to develop the appropriate response.

Molecular analyses of the cell-surface components that mediate these interactions have yielded equally fascinating discoveries. All these cell-interaction components are composed of two noncovalently associated polypeptide chains. In addition, the murine K,D and I-E molecules and the human analogues, the HLA-A,B and HLA-DR molecules, display another feature in common. Their structural diversity is restricted to one subunit; one subunit manifests a high degree of structural differences when comparisons are made among allotypic molecules, but the other subunit is relatively constant in structure. Thus, the genetic restrictions imposed on these interactions is paralleled by a restriction of structural diversity to one subunit, leading to the logical conclusion that only one of the two subunits is recognized in a haplotype-specific fashion when two cells interact.

The similarity in structural organization of the K,D and I-E molecules (and of their human analogues) suggests that they have a common mechanism of action in cellular interactions. The facts that only one of the two juxtaposed polypeptide subunits displays extensive diversity and that this dichotomy has withstood evolution imply that diversity is important to the function of these molecules. In addition, this dichotomy in degree of structural diversity suggests that a dichotomy in fuction also exists. The structural dichotomy of immunoglobulins (i.e., variable and constant regions) is paralleled by a functional dichotomy in which variable components mediate antigen-specific recognition while a constant portion mediates a common effector function (e.g., complement fixation). The only substantial difference is that in immunoglobulins, variable and constant portions are covalently linked, but in K,D and I-E molecules (and in their human analogues), the two components are noncovalently associated. Thus, it is tempting to propose that one component of K,D and I-E molecules is involved in the specificity of recognition while the other component is involved in mediating some common effector function.

The murine I-A-subregion molecules have properties different from those of the other MHC membrane products in that both subunits display a significant degree of structural diversity. However, the experiments on antigen–antibody recognition demonstrating that only one subunit (A_β) determines the antigenic specificity Ia.17 recognizable by a monoclonal antibody suggests that the structural diversity of the A_β subunit alone may be important for conferring uniqueness on I-A molecules recognized in cell interactions. This proposal is based on the premise that recognition of I-A molecules by antibody is analogous to recognition of I-A molecules by a putative receptor. Obviously, additional studies with monoclonal antibodies directed against other determinants are necessary to determine the validity of this hypothesis. However, confirmation of this proposal would imply that all the MHC membrane components involved in cell interactions display the common property of having only one of two subunits determining the specificity of haplotype recognition. The other subunit may exert some common effect that results either in triggering the differentiation of T and B cells or in the lysis of virus-infected syngeneic cells.

It is interesting to note that a number of other regulatory molecules (i.e., polypeptide hormones) and plant and bacterial toxins display very similar structural properties. The pituitary gonadotropins, follicle-stimulating hormone and luteinizing hormone; the pituitary thyrotropin, thyroid-stimulating hormone; and the placental gonadotropin, human chorionic gonadotropin, all consist of two polypeptides, α and β, one of which (β) determines target-cell specificity and binds to specific receptors on the target cell and the other of which (α) regulates adenyl cyclase activity (Stewart and Stewart, 1977). The α polypeptides, the structures of which are essentially constant, are generally interchangeable with the various β polypeptides, the structures of which are different, without eliminating biological activity. The bacterial and plant toxins (i.e., abrin, ricin, diphtheria and cholera toxin) also either consist of two polypeptides or may be enzymatically cleaved into two units, one of which binds to specific receptors on the cell surface, while the other exerts its toxic effect either by inhibiting protein synthesis or by modifying adenyl cyclase activity (Olsnes *et al.*, 1974; van Heyningen, 1976; Pappenheimer, 1978).

Thus, it is tempting to speculate that the structural organization of MHC products involved in cell interactions may turn out to be a general property of other molecules that mediate heterotypic cell interactions in eukaryotic organisms. Additional studies will determine whether this generalization is true and should improve understanding of the molecular basis of cell–cell interaction. At present, one important and intriguing question that remains is what functional necessity provides the impetus for these molecules to develop such a high degree of structural polymorphism.

ACKNOWLEDGMENTS. This work was supported by ACS grant IM-132, AHA grand-in-aid 76-1036, and NIH grant CA 23030. Jack Silver is a recipient of an American Heart Association Established Investigatorship Award. This is publication number 140 from the Department of Cellular and Developmental Immunology and publication number 1967 from the Immunology Departments, Scripps Clinic and Research Foundation, La Jolla, California 92037.

References

Allison, J.P., Walker, L.E., Russell, W.A., Pellegrino, M.A., Ferrone, S., Reisfeld, R.A., Frelinger, J.A., and Silver, J., 1978, Murine Ia and human DR antigens: Homology of amino-terminal sequences, *Proc. Natl. Acad. Sci. U.S.A.* **75**:3953.

Bergholtz, B.O., and Thorsby, E., 1978, HLA-D restriction of the macrophage-dependent response of immune human T lymphocytes to PPD *in vitro*: Inhibition by anti-HLA-DR antisera, *Scand. J. Immunol.* **8**:63.

Bevan, M.J., 1975, The major histocompatibility complex determines susceptibility to cytotoxic T cells directed against minor histocompatibility antigens, *J. Exp. Med.* **142**:1349.

Cook, R.G., Siegelman, M.H., Capra, J.D., Uhr, J.W., and Vitetta, E.S., 1979a, Structural studies on the murine Ia alloantigens. IV. NH_2-terminal sequence analysis of allelic products of the I-A and I-E/C subregions, *J. Immunol.* **122**(6):2232.

Cook, R.G., Vitetta, E.S., Uhr, J.W., and Capra, J.D., 1979b, Structural studies on the murine Ia alloantigens. III. Tryptic peptide comparisons of allelic products of the I-E/C subregion, *Mol. Immunol.* **16**:29.

Cresswell, P., and Geier, S.S., 1975, Antisera to human B-lymphocyte membrane glycoproteins block stimulation in mixed lymphocyte culture, *Nature (London)* **257**:147.

Cullen, S.E., Freed, J.H., and Nathenson, S.C., 1976, Structural and serological properties of murine Ia alloantigens, *Transplant. Rev.* **30**:236.

Erb, P., and Feldmann, M., 1975, The role of macrophages in the generation of T-helper cells, *J. Exp. Med.* **142**:460.

Freed, J.H., David, C.S., Shreffler, D.C., and Nathenson, S.G., 1978, Structural studies of the protein portion of the H-2-linked Ia glycoprotein antigens of the mouse: Tryptic peptide comparison of products from the *I-A* and *I-C* subregions of B10.HTT, *J. Immunol.* **121**(1):91.

Geier, S.S., and Cresswell, P., 1977, Rabbit antisera to human B cell alloantigens: Effects on the mixed lymphocyte response, *Cell. Immunol.* **28**:341.

Gordon, R.D., Simpson, E., and Samelson, L.E., 1975, *In vitro* cell-mediated immune responses to the male specific (H-Y) antigen in mice, *J. Exp. Med.* **142**:1108.

Humphreys, R.E., McCune, J.M., Chess, L., Herrman, H.C., Malenka, D.J., Mann, D.L., Parham, P., Schlossman, S.F., and Strominger, J.L., 1976, Isolation and immunologic characterization of a human B-lymphocyte specific, cell surface antigen, *J. Exp. Med.* **144**:98.

Katz, D.H., Graves, M., Dorf, M.E., Dimuzio, H., and Benacerraf, B., 1975, Cell interactions between histocompatible T and B lymphocytes, *J. Exp. Med.* **141:**263.

Klareskog, L., Sandberg-Trägårdh, L., Rask, L., Lindblom, J.B., Curman, B., and Peterson, P.A., 1977, Chemical properties of human Ia antigens, *Nature (London)* **265:**248.

McMillan, M., Cecka, J.M., Murphy, D.B., McDevitt, H.O., and Hood, L., 1977, Structure of murine Ia antigens: Partial NH_2-terminal amino acid sequences of products of the *I-E* or *I-C* subregion, *Proc. Natl. Acad. Sci. U.S.A.* **74**(11):5135.

McMillan, M., Cecka, J.M., Murphy, D.B., McDevitt, H.O., and Hood, L., 1978, Partial amino acid sequences of murine Ia antigens of the I-EC subregion, *Immunogenetics* **6:**137.

Nilsson, S., Schwartz, B.D., Waxdal, M., Green, I., Cullen, S.E., and Mann, D.L., 1977, A human alloantiserum precipitates Ia-like molecules from chronic lymphocytic leukemia cells, *J. Immunol.* **118**(4):1271.

Olsnes, S., Refsnes, K., and Pihl, A., 1974, Mechanism of action of the toxic lectins abrin and ricin, *Nature (London)* **249:**627.

Pappenheimer, A.M., Jr., 1978, Diphtheria: Molecular biology of an infectious process, *Trends Biochem. Sci.* **1978:**N 220.

Shreffler, D.C., and David, C.S., 1975, The H-2 major histocompatibility complex and the *I* immune response: Genetic variation, function and organization, *Adv. Immunol.* **20:**125.

Shreffler, D.C., David, C.S., Cullen, S.E., Frelinger, J.A., and Niederhuber, J.E., 1976, Serological and functional evidence for further subdivision of the *I* region of the *H-2* gene complex, *Cold Spring Harbor Symp. Quant. Biol.* **41:**477.

Silver, J., Cecka, J.M., McMillan, M., and Hood, L.E., 1976, Chemical characterization of products of the H-2 complex, *Cold Spring Harbor Symp. Quant. Biol.* **41:**369.

Silver, J., Russell, W.A., Reis, B.L., and Frelinger, J.A., 1977, Chemical characterization of murine Ia alloantigens determined by the I-E/C subregions of the H-2 complex, *Proc. Natl. Acad. Sci. U.S.A.* **74:**5131.

Silver, J., Walker, L.E., Reisfeld, R.A., Pellegrino, M.A., and Ferrone, S., 1979, Structural studies of murine I-E and human DR antigens, *Mol. Immunol.* **16:**37.

Snary, D., Barnstable, C.J., Bodmer, W.F., Goodfellow, P.N., and Crumpton, M.J., 1977, Cellular distribution, purification and molecular nature of human Ia antigens, *Scand. J. Immunol.* **6:**439.

Springer, T.A., Kaufman, J.F., Terhorst, C., and Strominger, J.L., 1977a, Purification and structural characterization of human *HLA*-linked B-cell antigens, *Nature (London)* **268:**213.

Springer, T.A., Kaufman, J.F., Siddoway, L.A., Mann, D.L., and Strominger, J.L., 1977b, Purification of *HLA*-linked B lymphocyte alloantigens in immunologically active form by preparative sodium dodecyl sulfate-gel electrophoresis and studies on their subunit association, *J. Biol. Chem.* **252**(17):6201.

Stewart, M., and Stewart, F., 1977, Constant and variable regions in glycoprotein hormone beta subunit sequences: Implications for receptor binding specificity, *J. Mol. Biol.* **116:**175.

van Heyningen, S., 1976, The structure of bacterial toxins, *Trends Biochem. Sci.* **1976:**114.

Zinkernagel, R.M., Dunlop, M.B.C., Blanden, R.B., Doherty, P.C., and Shreffler, D.C., 1976, *H-2* compatibility requirements for virus-specific T-cell-mediated cytolysis, *J. Exp. Med.* **144:**519.

20

Complete Primary Structure of Human Histocompatibility Antigen HLA-B7

Its Evolutionary and Functional Implications

Jack L. Strominger, Victor H. Engelhard, Braydon C. Guild, Thomas G. Kostyk, Doron Lancet, José A. Lopez de Castro, Harry T. Orr, Peter Parham, Hidde L. Ploegh, and Jordan S. Pober

1. Introduction

Tissue grafts cannot be exchanged successfully in the absence of immuno-suppression, except between syngeneic strains or identical twins. From a biochemical standpoint, each individual of a species carries on the surface of its cells substances now known to be glycoproteins that are recognized by every other individual of that species as foreign. These glycoproteins are the products of a highly polymorphic genetic system, first discovered through mouse-breeding studies. Largely through the efforts of Peter Gorer in England and George Snell in Bar Harbor, a region was identified, called the *H-2* region, differences at which are the two major histocompatibility antigens, called H-2K and H-2D, were products of two genetic loci in the *H-2* region on the 17th mouse chromosome.

Jack L. Strominger, Victor H. Engelhard, Braydon C. Guild, Thomas G. Kostyk, Doron Lancet, José A. Lopez de Castro, Harry T. Orr, Peter Parham, Hidde L. Ploegh, and Jordan S. Pober • Biological Laboratories, Harvard University, Cambridge, Massachusetts 02138.

Subsequently, a variety of other loci have been identified that are in some manner involved in graft rejection or acceptance. This region is organized similarly in all species that have been examined and is now called the major histocompatibility complex (MHC).

In man, the MHC is on the 6th chromosome. The genes that have been identified in this region include the *HLA-A* and *HLA-B* genes, the human analogues of the mouse *H-2K* and *H-2D* genes. A third closely linked locus coding for similar products has been identified both in man (*HLA-C*) and in the mouse (*H-2L*). A variety of other genes have been identified in this region in man, as well as in the corresponding region in the mouse; it is striking that many of these genes have something to do with immune functions or with cell-surface proteins. In man, the structural genes for a number of complement components are located in this region, as are those for Chido and Rogers (rare red-cell antigens now thought to be determinants on the C4 component of complement), the complement receptors, and the HLA-D antigens (the analogues of the murine Ia antigens).

The most striking feature of the *HLA-A* and *-B* genes is their extreme polymorphism. Over 20 alleles have now been identified at each of the *HLA-A* and *-B* loci. The *HLA-C* locus and the *HLA-D* locus have been studied more recently, and the number of alleles now known at these loci is in the range of 10 and is increasing slowly. As far as is known, the products of *HLA-A*, *-B*, and *-C* genes are expressed codominantly on most cells in the organism. Since any individual may therefore have a selection for among 10–30 alleles at each locus, giving rise to 6 surface glycoproteins on all cells, the potential for biological variability in outbred populations is extreme. The frequency of these alleles in different populations is very different. Some alleles have a close association with human disease. The most striking of these is the very close association of ankylosing spondylitis and a number of other autoimmune diseases with the occurence of the *HLA-B27* allele. The most interesting question about the system is: what is the natural function of these molecules and what was the evolutionary pressure that gave rise to the polymorphism? Clearly, it was not the exchange of surgical grafts that led to the discovery of the system in mice and has promoted the most interest in it in man. It must be related to some phenomenon or phenomena of enormous importance to the species (for a review, see Bodmer, 1978).

It should be noted that only a limited number of references, mainly from the authors' laboratory, have been provided in this chapter. However, complete documentation and a full reference list can be found in an extensive review (Strominger *et al.*, 1980).

2. Purification of HLA-A and -B Antigens after Papain Solubilization

Efforts to isolate these molecules and elucidate their structure were initiated in our laboratory in the belief that from a knowledge of their structure, some information about their function might be obtained. It was initially discovered that the murine H-2 antigens can be solubilized by papain. Correspondingly, the first step in solubilzing the HLA-A, -B, and -C antigens from cell membranes is treatment of membranes with papain. After solubilization with papain, the purification of HLA-A and -B antigens is a relatively straightforward biochemical procedure, requiring only three additional steps to obtain pure antigens from the membranes of cultured human B-lymphoblastoid cell lines (Turner *et al.*, 1975; Parham *et al.*, 1977). This procedure requires only about 100-fold purification of the HLA-A and -B antigens; i.e., these antigens represent about 1% of the total membrane protein. Their density on the cultured cells is about 20 times that on normal peripheral-blood (or spleen) lymphocytes. About 30 mg of each of the HLA-A and -B specificities can be obtained from 1 kg of cultured cells. The use of a doubly homozygous cell line (*HLA-A2,2; -B7,7*) established from an individual, J.Y., from the highly inbred Indiana Amish community, has greatly simplified the problem of separation of specificities.

The first interesting discovery was that the purified material contains two polypeptide chains (Cresswell *et al.*, 1973). One of these chains is a glycoprotein with a molecular weight of about 34,000 and the other is a small protein with a molecular weight of 12,000. The small subunit was identical to a small urinary protein called β_2-microglobulin, first isolated from nephrotic human urine. It was subsequently sequenced in several laboratories and was found to have sequence homology to immunoglobulin domains, particularly to the C_3H domain of immunoglobulins (Moller, 1974). Therefore, early in these studies, there were discovered several striking similarities of the cell-bound histocompatibility antigens to the circulating immunoglobulins. They include the limited proteolysis by papain, the two-chain structure, and the sequence homology of the small chain to immunoglobulin sequences. An additional similarity is the content of disulfide bridges. The heavy chain, which is about three times the size of an immunoglobulin domain, contains 4 cysteine residues in two intrachain disulfide bridges (Strominger *et al.*, 1974). Later, it was shown that these two intrachain disulfide linkages are linearly arranged as they are in immunoglobulins and have about the same size as immunoglobulin loops (Terhorst *et al.*, 1977; Ferguson *et al.*, 1979).

3. Dissection of the Papain-Solubilized Heavy Chain into Three Regions by Chemical Cleavages

For further structural work on the large extracellular portion of the molecule released by papain, the heavy chains (p34) of papain-solubilized HLA-A and -B antigens were cleaved further. Most of these antigens (including HLA-B7, but not HLA-A2) have a single acid-cleavable linkage, fortuitously located between the two disulfide bridges (Terhorst *et al.*, 1977). After cleavage with acid, two large fragments (ac-1 and ac-2) were separated from HLA-B7. They each contained an intrachain disulfide. Therefore, the disulfide bridges in histocompatibility antigens are linearly arranged. HLA-B7 also has two methionine residues that can be cleaved with CNBr (Terhorst *et al.*, 1977). This cleavage results in formation of two equal-sized fragments from ac-1, together with the unimportant loss of the N-terminal pentapeptide. The N-terminal region carries the single asparagine-linked glycan of the whole molecule and contains no cysteine residues (Parham *et al.*, 1977; Terhorst *et al.*, 1977). The acid and CNBr cleavages together dissect the molecule into three fragments of approximately equal size, containing the N-terminal glycosylated region, the first disulfide-loop region, and the second disulfide-loop region. With the reagent 2-nitro-5-thiocyanobenzoic acid (NTCB), which cleaves at Cys residues, it was further established that the size of the two disulfide loops is similar to the size of disulfide loops in immunoglobulins (Ferguson *et al.*, 1979). Further tryptic and chymotyptic cleavages of the three fragments gave all the peptides required for sequencing (Lopez de Castro *et al.*, 1979; Orr *et al.*, 1979b).

4. Complete Primary Sequence of,HLA-B7

The complete primary sequence of a human histocompatibility antigen, HLA-B7, is shown in Fig. 1 (Orr *et al.*, 1979a,b). About 70% of the HLA-A2 sequence has also been obtained (Orr *et al.*, 1979). Although these two antigens are encoded by genes that are about 1 centimorgan apart on the 6th human chromosome, their sequence homology is 85%. One of the most interesting questions about the structure is the location of the alloantigenic site. In the HLA-A and -B antigens, the alloantigenic determinants are encoded in the polypeptide, and not in the carbohydrate (as they are in the red-cell ABO system) (Parham *et al.*, 1977). A clustering of differences between HLA-A2 and -B7 occurs in the region of residues 65–80 (9 of 15 residues different). A second cluster difference is found between residues 102 and 114 (8 of 13 residues different). There-

```
                 10        20        30        40        50        60        70        80        90
HLA-B7  NH2-GSHSMRYFYTSVSRPGRGEPRFISVGYVDDTQFVRFDSDAASPREEPRAPWIEQEGPEYWDRNTQIYKAQAQTDRESLRNLRGYYNQSEA
HLA-A2  NH2-——————F——————————A————————————————Z-M————— ——————————     KV—H-H-V-VD-GT———————————
H2-Kb   NH2--P—L———V-A————L————YME——————E——————————EN—Y————R-M——————————E-E—KA-GNE-SF-VD—T-L————————KG

                100       110       120       130       140       150       160       170       180
HLA-B7      GSHTLQSMYGCDVGPDGRLLRGHDQYAYDGKDYIALNEDLRSWTAADTAAQITQRKWEAAREAEQRRAYLEGECVEWLRRYLENGKDKLE
HLA-A2      ——————R——— —S-W-F——YH——————————K——————————M——————KH——————V————————T———
H-2Kb       ———I—                                        M—L—KH——Q-G—RL—————T——————— -K

                190       200       210       220       230       240       250       260       270
HLA-B7      RADPPKTHVTHHPISDHEATLRCWALGFYPAEITLTWQRDGEDQTQDTELVETRPAGDRTFEKWAAVVVPSGEEQRYTCHVQHEGLPKPLT

H-2Kb                                                    M———————————G— —S —L-K- Y-
```

Figure 1. Complete amino acid sequence of HLA-B7 pap and partial sequences of HLA-A2 pap and H-2K^b pap.

fore, in comparing HLA-B7 and HLA-A2, a pattern of highly conserved regions separating two clusters of variability is seen. How these clusters relate to a given alloantigenic specificity awaits additional evidence.

The structure of H-2K^b antigen is also being elucidated (Coligan *et al.*, 1979; Vehara *et al.*, 1980). There is 72 or 74% homology between human HLA-A2 or -B7 antigens and the sequences at present available for H-2K^b. Clearly, the structure of these histocompatibility antigens has been greatly conserved during the evolution of species. A clustering of differences between HLA-A2 or -B7 and H-2K^b also occurs at residues 60–80 (10 or 11 of 20 residues different). Thus, between HLA-A2 or -B7 and H-2K, the same region stands out as a region that is highly variable in the comparison of the human and mouse antigen.

5. Sequence Homology to Immunoglobulin Sequences

A structural relationship between histocompatibility antigens and immunoglobulins has been postulated for some time. Only recently have enough sequence data for HLA been obtained so that meaningful comparisons can be made. The ac-2 fragment containing the last 88 residues of the papain-solubilized molecule was the first sequence available of sufficient size to compare to immunoglobulin sequences in a critical way (Orr *et al.*, 1979c; Strominger *et al.*, 1980b). This region also appears to be highly conserved between human and mouse; there is about 80% homology with sequences at present available for the corresponding H-2K^b region (Coligan *et al.*, 1979). Without question, the ac-2 fragment (α_3), a region that is the size of an immunoglobulin domain and that contains the second disulfide loop of HLA-B7, is highly homologous in sequence to immunoglobulin constant domain. Using the PROPHET computer system, alignments based only on identities were obtained. A maximum of 35% sequence homology with a number of immunoglobulin domain sequences was found (Strominger *et al.*, 1980b). These alignments also included the important features of matches at the rare amino acids, 2 Cys, 1 His, and 1 Trp. [For a discussion of the critical importance both of matches at rare amino acids and of statistical evaluation of homology data, see Strominger *et al.* (1980)].

Identities are not the only way to compare sequences. Beale and Feinstein (1976), in their analysis of the structure of immunoglobulins based on crystallographic data, identified a number of residues that are very important in chain-folding of immunoglobulin domains and that were conserved in the sense that substitutions were permitted only within a closely related group of hydrophobic amino acids, Phe, Pro, Met, Val, Leu, Ile, and to some extent Ala and Gly. A second series of alignments were obtained by computer in which the number of gaps and residues in gaps were minimized and in which consideration was given to conservative substitutions (Orr *et al.*, 1979c). In this alignment (Fig. 2), 6 of the 7 highly conserved immunoglobulin residues are conserved in the ac-2 sequence. These 7 residues appear in 80% of all known immunoglobulin sequences. Of the 19 residues in immunoglobulin domains pointed out by Beale and Feinstein (1976) as being conserved within a hydrophobic group of amino acids, 15 are also conserved in the ac-2 fragment. The clustering and location of these residues also point to the fact that most probably the ac-2 region of HLA-B7 folds in the β-pleated sheet structure, as do immunoglobulin domains (Fig. 3). Circular dichroism spectra had already been carried out and revealed the high content of β-pleated sheet structure in HLA-A2 and -B7 (Lancet and Strominger, 1979; Lancet *et al.*, 1979).

Z scores were calculated by the method of Barker and Dayhoff (1972), comparing immunoglobulin domain sequences with sequences of the various regions of HLA-B7 (Table 1). To a first approximation, the Z score is a measure of the probability that the homology observed is sta-

Figure 2. Alignment of the ac-2 fragment of HLA-B7 with the human-derived sequences of the superfamily of immunoglobulin constant domains and related proteins. Conserved residues in the Ig and β_2-m sequences indicated in (a) by (–) occur in $^{6}/_{12}$–$^{7}/_{12}$; (=) occur in $^{8}/_{12}$–$^{9}/_{12}$; (= occur in $^{10}/_{12}$–$^{11}/_{12}$ and (=), occur in 12 12 sequences; (b) (▲) indicates positions of hydrophobic residues (Phe, Ala, Tyr, Pro, Met, Val, Leu, Ile, or Cys) whose side chains are found to fill the internal space in folded Ig domain (see references in Orr *et al.*, 1979c); (*) indicates that an identical (a) or homologous (b) residue occurs in ac-2. Residues are indicated using the single-letter code.

Human Ig C domains																														
Light chains										10										20										30
1 kappa	—	T	V	A	A	P	S	**V**	F	I	F	**P**	P	S	—	D	E	Q	L	K	—	S	G	T	**A**	S	V	V	**C**	L
2 lambda	Q	P	K	A	A	P	S	**V**	**T**	L	F	**P**	P	S	—	S	E	E	L	Q	—	A	N	K	**A**	**T**	**L**	V	**C**	L
Heavy chains																														
3 $C_\gamma 1$	A	S	T	K	G	P	S	**V**	F	P	L	**A**	P	S	—	S	**K**	S	T	**S**	—	G	G	T	**A**	A	**L**	G	**C**	L
4 $C_\mu 1$	G	S	A	S	A	P	T	L	F	P	L	V	S	C	—	E	B	S	B	P	—	S	S	T	V	A	V	G	**C**	L
5 $C_\mu 2$	Z	L	**P**	**P**	**K**	V	S	**V**	F	V	—	**P**	P	R	—	B	G	F	F	G	B	P	R	K	S	**K**	**L**	I	**C**	Q
6 $C_\gamma 3$	E	L	L	G	G	P	S	**V**	F	L	F	**P**	P	K	P	K	D	T	L	M	I	S	R	T	P	E	V	T	**C**	V
7 $C_\mu 3$	D	Z	B	T	A	I	R	**V**	F	A	I	**P**	P	S	—	F	A	S	**I**	F	L	T	K	S	T	**K**	**L**	T	**C**	L
8 $C_\epsilon 3$	S	**D**	**P**	R	G	V	S	A	Y	L	S	R	P	S	P	F	D	—	L	F	I	R	K	S	P	**T**	I	T	**C**	L
9 $C_\gamma 4$	Q	P	R	—	E	P	Q	**V**	Y	T	L	**P**	P	S	—	R	E	E	M	T	—	K	N	Q	V	S	**L**	T	**C**	L
10 $C_\mu 4$	V	A	L	H	R	P	D	**V**	Y	L	L	**P**	P	A	—	R	E	Q	L	N	L	R	E	S	**A**	**T**	I	T	**C**	L
11 $C_\epsilon 4$	—	P	R	A	A	P	E	**V**	Y	A	F	A	T	P	—	E	W	P	G	**S**	—	R	D	K	R	**T**	L	A	**C**	L
HLA chains																														
12 β_2m	I	Q	R	—	T	P	K	I	Q	V	Y	S	R	H	—	P	A	E	N	G	—	K	S	N	F	—	L	N	**C**	Y
13 B7, ac-2	/	**D**	**P**	**P**	**K**	**T**	**H**	V	**T**	**H**	**H**	**P**	—	—	—	—	—	—	**I**	**S**	—	**D**	**H**	**E**	**A**	**T**	**L**	**R**	**C**	**W**
(a)						=	—	•=	—			•—	=	—													•—	—	•≡≡	—
(b)						▲		•▲		▲															•▲		•▲		•▲	

Human Ig C domains																														
Light chains										40										50									60	
1 kappa	L	N	N	**F**	**Y**	**P**	R	**E**	—	—	A	K	V	Q	**W**	K	V	—	—	**D**	N	A	L	**Q**	S	G	N	S	Q	—
2 lambda	I	S	D	**F**	**Y**	**P**	G	A	—	—	V	**T**	V	A	**W**	K	A	—	—	**D**	S	S	P	V	K	A	G	V	—	—
Heavy chains																														
3 $C_\gamma 1$	V	K	D	Y	F	**P**	E	P	—	—	V	**T**	V	S	**W**	—	—	—	—	N	S	G	A	L	**T**	S	G	V	—	—
4 $C_\mu 1$	**A**	Q	D	**F**	L	**P**	D	S	—	—	**I**	**T**	F	S	**W**	K	Y	K	B	N	S	D	I	—	—	S	S	T	—	—
5 $C_\mu 2$	**A**	T	**G**	**F**	S	**P**	R	Q	—	—	**I**	Q	V	S	**W**	L	**R**	—	—	E	**G**	K	Q	V	G	S	G	V	T	**T**
6 $C_\gamma 3$	V	V	D	V	S	H	E	D	P	Q	V	K	F	N	**W**	Y	V	—	—	**D**	**G**	V	Q	V	H	N	—	—	—	A
7 $C_\mu 3$	V	T	D	L	T	—	Y	D	—	S	V	**T**	I	S	**W**	T	**R**	—	—	Q	D	G	E	A	V	K	—	—	—	**T**
8 $C_\epsilon 3$	V	V	B	L	A	**P**	S	K	G	T	V	B	**L**	**T**	**W**	S	**R**	—	—	A	S	G	K	P	V	B	—	—	—	H
9 $C_\gamma 4$	V	K	**G**	**F**	**Y**	**P**	S	D	—	—	**I**	A	V	E	**W**	E	S	—	—	N	D	G	E	P	E	N	—	—	—	Y
10 $C_\mu 4$	V	T	**G**	**F**	S	**P**	**A**	D	—	—	V	F	V	Q	**W**	**Q**	M	—	—	Q	R	G	Q	P	L	S	P	E	K	Y
11 $C_\epsilon 4$	I	Q	N	**F**	M	**P**	E	D	—	—	**I**	S	V	Q	**W**	L	H	—	—	N	E	V	Q	L	P	D	—	A	R	H
HLA chains																														
12 β_2m	V	S	**G**	**F**	H	**P**	S	D	—	—	**I**	E	V	D	L	L	K	—	—	**D**	**G**	**E**	R	I	E	K	—	—	—	V
13 B7, ac-2	**A**	**L**	**G**	**F**	**Y**	**P**	**A**	**E**	—	—	**I**	**T**	**L**	**T**	**W**	**Q**	**R**	—	—	**D**	**G**	**E**	**D**	**Q**	**T**	**Q**	**D**	—	—	**T**
(a)	—			•=		•≡		—			—		=		•≡															
(b)	•▲			•▲							•▲		•▲		•▲															▲

Human Ig C domains																														
Light chains										70										80										90
1 kappa	**E**	S	**V**	T	E	Q	D	S	K	**D**	—	—	S	**T**	Y	S	L	S	S	T	L	T	L	S	K	A	D	Y	E	—
2 lambda	**E**	T	T	T	P	S	K	Q	S	N	—	—	N	K	Y	A	A	S	S	Y	L	S	L	T	P	E	Q	W	K	—
Heavy chains																														
3 $C_\gamma 1$	H	T	F	P	A	V	L	Q	S	S	—	—	G	L	Y	S	L	S	S	V	**V**	T	**V**	**P**	**S**	S	S	L	—	—
4 $C_\mu 1$	R	G	F	P	S	V	L	R	**G**	—	—	—	G	K	Y	A	A	T	S	Q	**V**	L	L	**P**	**S**	K	D	V	M	Q
5 $C_\mu 2$	N	E	**V**	Z	A	Z	A	K	E	S	G	P	T	**T**	Y	K	V	T	S	T	L	T	I	K	E	S	B	W	L	—
6 $C_\gamma 3$	K	T	K	P	R	E	Q	Q	Y	**B**	—	—	S	**T**	Y	R	V	V	S	V	L	T	**V**	L	H	Q	N	W	L	—
7 $C_\mu 3$	H	T	B	I	S	Z	S	H	P	**B**	—	—	A	**T**	**F**	S	A	V	G	E	A	S	I	C	E	B	B	W	N	—
8 $C_\epsilon 3$	S	T	R	K	E	E	K	Q	R	**B**	—	—	G	**T**	L	T	V	T	S	T	L	P	**V**	G	T	R	B	W	I	—
9 $C_\gamma 4$	K	T	T	P	P	V	L	D	S	**D**	—	—	G	S	**F**	F	L	Y	S	K	L	T	**V**	D	K	S	R	W	Q	—
10 $C_\mu 4$	V	T	S	A	P	M	**P**	E	P	Q	A	P	G	R	Y	F	A	H	S	I	L	T	**V**	S	E	E	E	W	N	—
11 $C_\epsilon 4$	S	T	T	Q	P	**R**	K	T	K	G	—	—	S	G	**F**	F	V	F	S	R	L	E	**V**	T	R	A	E	W	Q	—
HLA chains																														
12 β_2m	**E**	H	S	D	L	S	F	S	K	**D**	—	—	W	S	**F**	Y	L	L	Y	S	Y	T	E	F	T	P	T	—	—	—
13 B7, ac-2	**E**	**L**	**V**	**E**	**T**	**R**	**P**	**A**	**G**	**D**	—	—	**R**	**T**	**F**	**E**	**K**	**W**	**A**	**A**	**V**	**V**	**V**	**P**	**S**	**G**	—	—	—	—
(a)		=								•—					—				≡		=	—	•—					=		
(b)															•▲		▲				•▲		•▲							

Human Ig C domains																																
Light chains										100										110										120		
1 kappa	—	K	H	K	V	**Y**	A	**C**	E	**V**	T	**H**	Q	**G**	**L**	S	S	**P**	—	—	V	T	K	S	F	N	R	G	E	C	—	22
2 lambda	—	S	H	R	S	**Y**	S	**C**	Q	**V**	T	**H**	**E**	**G**	—	—	S	T	—	—	V	E	K	T	V	A	P	T	E	C	S	20
Heavy chains																																
3 $C_\gamma 1$	G	T	Q	—	T	**Y**	I	**C**	N	**V**	N	**H**	K	P	S	N	T	K	—	—	V	D	K	R	V	E	P	K	S	C	/	17
4 $C_\mu 1$	G	T	N	E	H	V	V	**C**	K	**V**	Z	**H**	P	B	G	B	—	K	—	—	—	E	K	D	V	—	P	L	P	V	I	14
5 $C_\mu 2$	—	S	Q	S	M	E	**T**	**C**	R	**V**	D	**H**	R	**G**	**L**	T	F	Q	Q	—	—	B	A	S	S	M	C	V	P	—	—	24
6 $C_\gamma 3$	-	D	G	K	E	**Y**	K	**C**	K	**V**	S	N	**K**	A	**L**	**P**	A	**P**	—	—	I	E	K	T	I	S	K	A	**K**	G	—	15
7 $C_\mu 3$	—	S	G	E	**R**	F	**T**	**C**	T	**V**	T	**H**	T	D	**L**	**P**	S	**P**	—	—	L	K	Q	T	I	S	R	P	**K**	G	—	20
8 $C_\epsilon 3$	—	**E**	G	E	T	**Y**	Z	**C**	R	**V**	T	**H**	P	H	**L**	**P**	R	A	—	—	L	M	R	S	T	T	K	T	S	G	—	19
9 $C_\gamma 4$	—	Q	G	N	V	F	S	**C**	S	**V**	M	**H**	**E**	A	**L**	H	N	H	Y	**T**	—	Q	K	S	L	S	L	S	P	G	—	19
10 $C_\mu 4$	—	T	G	E	T	**Y**	**T**	**C**	V	**V**	A	**H**	**E**	A	**L**	**P**	N	R	V	**T**	—	E	R	T	V	D	K	S	T	G	K	22
11 $C_\epsilon 4$	--	**E**	K	D	E	F	I	**C**	R	A	V	**H**	**E**	A	A	S	P	S	Q	**T**	V	Q	R	A	V	S	V	N	P	G	K	17
HLA chains																																
12 β_2m	—	**E**	K	D	E	**Y**	A	**C**	R	**V**	N	**H**	V	T	**L**	S	Q	**P**	K	—	I	V	K	—	W	D	R	D	M	—	—	19
13 B7, ac-2	—	**E**	**E**	**Q**	**R**	**Y**	**T**	**C**	**H**	**V**	**Q**	**H**	**E**	**G**	**L**	**P**	**K**	**P**	**L**	**T**	/											
(a)						•—		•≡≡		•≡		•≡			•=																	
(b)						•▲		•▲		•▲																						

tistically significant. A Z score of 3 or higher is considered as indicative of significant homology. The α_3 or ac-2 fragment sequence was compared with different immunoglobulin-domain sequences and with the β_2-microglobulin (β_2m) sequence. When compared with the sequences of immunoglobulin constant (C)-region domains, Z scores as high as 11 were obtained (Orr *et al.*, 1979c). Similarly, a comparison of the α_3 region with β_2-microglobulin gave a Z score of 8.4. These values and the other features of the homology leave no doubt that the α_3 region of HLA-B7, β_2-microglobulin, and C-region domains of immunoglobulins belong to the same superfamily of polypeptides. No homology of α_3 to immunoglobulin variable (V) regions occurs (Z score 0.8).

Interestingly, the α_1 region (the N-terminal fragment) has no sequence homology to immunoglobulin V- or C-region sequences and homology of borderline significance to the α_3 fragment (Z score 2.7). The α_2 fragment (containing the first disulfide loop) also has no sequence homology to immunoglobulin C- or V-region domain sequences, even though the size of its disulfide loop, 63 residues, is in the range of V-region loop sizes. The α_2 fragment has no sequence homology to α_3 but α_1 and α_2 have a statistically significant homology to each other (Z score

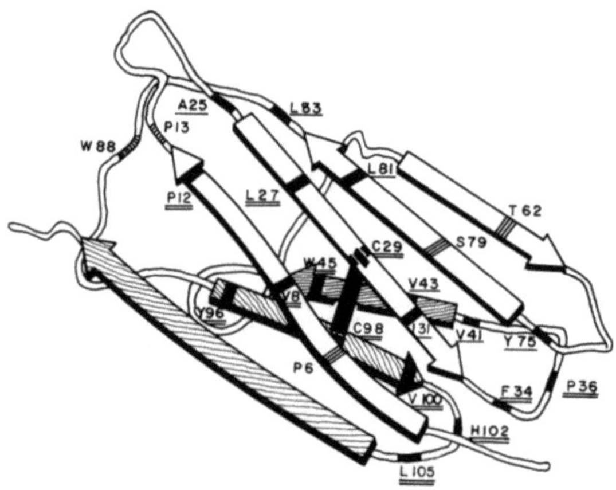

Figure 3. Folding scheme of a constant immunoglobulin domain, as obtained by X-ray crystallographic studies of the Mcg λ human light-chain dimer. Arrows denote the location and direction of strands in the β-pleated sheet structure (open arrows, the four-stranded sheet; hatched arrows, the three-stranded sheet). The solid bar between positions 29 and 98 represents the intradomain disulfide bond. Numbering is according to Fig. 2. Solid bars denote residues that are invariable in all or most immunoglobulin constant domains and appear in the second disulfide region of HLA-B7 (double-scored) or are restricted to a group of hydrophobic residues in all the above (single-scored). Hatched bars denote residues that are highly conserved in immunoglobulin constant domains, but different in the second disulfide region.

TABLE 1. Z Scores for HLA Regions and Immunoglobulin Domains[a]

	$\alpha 1$	$\alpha 2$	$\alpha 3$	β_2m	C	V
α_1	—	**5.2**	*2.7*	1.1	1.5	0.0
α_2	**5.2**	—	0.1	0.9	1.1	0.6
α_3	*2.7*	0.1	—	**8.4**	**8.7**	0.8
β_2m	1.1	0.9	**8.4**	—	**5.5**	1.0
C	1.5	1.1	**8.7**	**5.5**	**11.8**	1.6
V	0.0	0.6	0.8	1.0	1.6	**10.5**

[a]The values for V and C regions of Ig are averages of several different domain comparisons, and obviously C vs. C and V vs. V are comparisons of different V and C region domains.

2.9 or 5.2, the higher score being obtained by placing a single gap in α_2). These data are highly suggestive of internal homology of α_1 and α_2 and perhaps of α_1 and α_3.

Thus, HLA-A and -B antigens appear to be made up of regions that either are derived from different genes or in which α_1 and α_2 have undergone considerably more evolution than α_3. The data lead to the speculation that like the immunoglobulins, the heavy chains of HLA antigens may be synthesized from a spliced gene product.

One other very interesting and speculative point relates to the role of β_2-microglobulin. It may function to hold the HLA heavy chain in its alloantigenic conformation. When β_2-microglobulin is released from the molecule by denaturation, the heavy chain irreversibly unfolds (Lancet *et al.*, 1979). The circular dichroism spectrum is only partially restored in efforts to renature the molecule, and it has so far been impossible to reassociate the two chains and restore alloantigenic reactivity.

6. Purification of HLA-A and -B Antigens after Detergent Solubilization

A second way of solubilizing membrane proteins make use of detergent rather than proteolysis. Two different methods for purification after detergent solubilization were developed (Springer *et al.*, 1974; Robb *et al.*, 1976). One employed ordinary chromatographic methods (Springer *et al.*, 1974), and the other used immunoaffinity chromatography on an anti-β_2-microglobulin column (Robb *et al.*, 1976). The separation of allelic specificities with detergent-soluble antigen is especially difficult (but see below). Again, two chains were obtained in the purified HLA antigen preparation, one of molecular weight about 44,000 and the other of molecular weight 12,000. The light chain was identical to that obtained after papain solubilization. The heavy chain was 10,000 daltons larger than the heavy chain obtained after papain solubilization. Most important, the occurrence of a two-chain structure for HLA-A and -B antigens after detergent solubilization showed that this structure was not an artifact of papain proteolysis.

Recently, more elegant methods for separating the detergent-soluble antigens from the J.Y. cell line have been developed (Parham, 1979). Monoclonal antibodies, specifically recognizing HLA-A2 and HLA-B7 (Parker and Bodmer, 1978; Broasky *et al.*, 1979), were obtained using the technique described by Kohler and Milstein (1975). When mice were hyperimmunized with the papain-solubilized purified HLA-A and -B antigens obtained as described above before the cell fusion was carried out, the identification of the appropriate clones synthesizing monoclonal HLA-A2 and HLA-B7 antibodies was greatly facilitated. For the purification, cells are lysed in detergent and the extract applied to a monoclonal anti-HLA-A2 immuno-affinity column. Pure HLA-A2 was eluted by raising the pH of the column. The effluent was applied to an immunoaffinity column to which the monoclonal anti-HLA-B7 was bound and that effluent then applied to a column containing the W6/32 monoclonal antibody (Barnstable *et al.*, 1978), which recognizes all HLA-A, -B, and -C specificities. The small amount of eluate from the last column could be an *HLA-C*-locus antigen.

The heavy chain of the detergent-soluble isolated histocompatibility antigens is cleaved by papain to the 34,000-molecular-weight species; an intermediate of 39,000 molecular weight is formed in the process (Springer *et al.*, 1974). The native molecule (p44), the intermediate (p39), and the final product (p34) were isolated. From their amino acid compositions, it was deduced that the peptide removed by the first papain cleavage was a highly hydrophilic peptide, containing a large number of Asp, Glu, Ser, Lys, and Arg residues and virtually no hydrophobic amino acids. The second peptide removed, by contrast, had a very large amount of hydrophobic residues and virtually no charged residues. In fact, the molecule spans the membrane. The N-terminal extracellular portion is very large (p34). The penultimate hydrophobic peptide lies within the membrane, and the C-terminal hydrophilic peptide is inside the cell (Fig. 4).

7. Structure of the Penultimate Hydrophobic and C-Terminal Hydrophilic Peptides

A tentative sequence of the hydrophobic region is available (Robb, 1977). It is 25 residues long and contains only hydrophobic residues, essentially Val, Ile, Leu, and Ala. The sequence of the hydrophilic region, the internal piece, has a number of interesting structural features (Robb *et al.*, 1978). One is the clustering of positively charged amino acids near the membrane interface, similar to that found in the red-cell-membrane protein glycophorin, which also spans the membrane. Another extremely interesting structural feature of the internal piece is its unusually high content of serine residues. The occurrence of these residues led to the discovery that one of these serine residues is phosphorylated *in vivo* (Pober *et al.*, 1978). Similarly, membranes of the J.Y. cell line contain an enzyme that phosphorylates the C-terminal region in the endogenous histocompatibility antigens using γ-[^{32}P]-ATP as the phosphate donor. Microphosphate analyses of isolated HLA-B7 antigen (kindly carried out by Dr. O.H. Lowry) revealed that there was 0.68 nmol organic phosphate/nmol HLA-B7 in the steady state. The location of this phosphate residue may point to some function of these molecules. They are oriented in the membrane so that they have the potential for signaling from outside the cell to inside. Such signaling could be reflected by turnover of the phosphate residue at the inside of the cell. It has been suggested that H-2K and H-2D antigens are associated with intracellular actin (Koch and Smith, 1978). The capping of HLA-A and -B antigens is associated with coincident rearrangement of actin, myosin, and tubulin (Guild and Strominger, 1981: manuscript submitted). This laboratory has recently developed an *in vitro* biophysical assay to demonstrate an association of cytoskeletal ele-

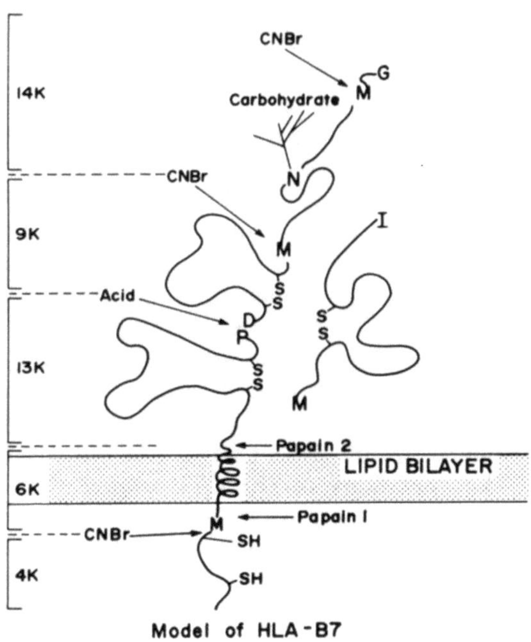

Figure 4. A model of HLA-B7. Cyanogen bromide (CNBr) and acid (+H) cleavage points are indicated. Also shown are the positions of the carbohydrate moiety and the arrangement of the disulfide loops.

ments with detergent-purified HLA-A and -B molecules labeled with a fluorescent reporter group in the intracellular domain (Pober *et al.*, 1981: manuscript submitted). The phosphorylation of HLA-A and -B antigens may play an important role in these cytoskeletal reactions.

8. Use of HLA-A and -B Antigens Reconstituted in Liposomes to Study Function

If purified HLA-A and -B antigens are isolated in or exchanged into a dialyzable detergent, such as octyl glucoside or deoxycholate, removal of detergent by dialysis in the presence of phospholipid results in the formation of phospholipid vesicles containing HLA-A and -B antigens (Englehard *et al.*, 1978a). In these liposomes, the protein molecules appear to orient with the hydrophobic region in the lipid bilayer and the bulk of the molecule outside the liposome, just as they are oriented in the cell membrane.

These liposomes can be used to generate secondary cytotoxic T lymphocytes (CTL) *in vitro* after appropriate primary immunization of mice (Englehard *et al.*, 1978b). These secondary CTL, when assayed on different target cells carrying a number of HLA allospecificities, are highly specific for the alloantigens that were inserted in the liposomes during the stimulation. The ability to generate CTL by HLA-containing liposomes is nearly equivalent to the ability to generate them using membranes that have been solubilized and then reconstituted. Similarly, *HLA-D*-locus antigens can be inserted in liposomes and are able to generate secondary CTL *in vitro* (Burakoff *et al.*, 1980).

When membranes or cells are used for stimulation, CTL are generated that recognize both the HLA-A and -B antigens and the structurally different HLA-D antigens (Burakoff *et al.*, 1980). The CTL generated by the HLA-A2 and -B7 antigens in liposomes are directed against HLA-A and -B determinants on the target cells, since cytotoxicity is blocked by antiserum to these molecules (the monoclonal W6/32 antibody), but not by antisera against HLA-D (anti-p29,34 serum). In contrast, the second class of CTL that are generated, those that are stimulated by HLA-D liposomes, are blocked by anti-p29,34 serum (the anti-HLA-D serum) and not by W6/32. The specificity of the CTL argues that they are being stimulated directly by the antigen-containing liposome, rather than by nonspecific helper factors, as has been suggested. Since the CTL are capable of distinguishing among different -A, -B, and -D alloantigens, they should be useful tools for probing the location of the alloantigenic site(s) on these molecules. Correspondingly, the purified antigens are very useful tools with which to carry out functional studies.

HLA-A and -B antigens in vesicles have also been used as a tool to examine the interaction of Semliki Forest virus (SFV) glycoprotein with its cell-surface receptor (Helenius *et al.*, 1978). Because antisera against HLA and H-2 inhibited the binding of the isolated glycoprotein to cells, it was thought that histocompatibility antigens might be the receptors on the cell surface for the virus. Direct interaction between HLA and the SFV glycoprotein can be shown in a number of ways, and this interaction is particularly strong if one or both proteins have been reconstituted into phospholipid vesicles. This suggests that the interaction between the virus and HLA or the cell surface involves multiple attachments to a single viral particle. These results are very intriguing and suggest that HLA may in fact be the surface receptor for SFV. However, it has yet to be demonstrated that blocking the HLA on the cell surface will block viral infection, showing that this interaction is physiologically significant.

9. Conclusion

The histocompatibility antigens and the immunoglobulins are both probably descendents of some common ancestral gene that may have originally coded for a cell-bound defense molecule. The development of animals with circulatory systems and duplication of that gene resulted later in evolution in the secretion of the products of one of these genes, i.e., the immunoglobulins, into the circulation. The product of the other gene remained membrane-bound and probably went on to evolve to become the histocompatibility antigens. Presumably, like their cousins the immunoglobulins, the histocompatibility antigens also serve a defense function for the organism. In this case, the cell-bound defense mechanism may serve to protect the organism from invasion by closely related cells, perhaps serving in primitive organisms to maintain colonial identity on the sea floor. There is increasing evidence that in higher evolutionary forms, a major function of this system is to participate in the control of proliferation of modified syngeneic cells, in particular virus-infected and/or tumor cells. Still later in evolution, the Placentalie emerged as a subspecies of Mammalia. With this development came another need for rejecting foreign haploidentical cells, i.e., the need to prevent the invasion of the maternal organism by foreign tissue containing paternal antigens derived from the highly invasive trophoblast. Thus, a variety of situations in which the organism needs to protect itself from closely related invading foreign cells occurs. It seems likely that the substances called histocompatibility antigens have evolved to serve that need.

References

Barker, W.C., and Dayhoff, M.O., 1972, Detecting distant relationships: Computer methods and results, in: *Atlas of Protein Sequence and Structure*, Vol. 5 (M.O. Dayhoff, ed.), pp. 101–110, National Biomedical Research Foundation, Washington, D.C.

Barnstable, C.J., Bodmer, W.F., Brown, G., Galfe, G., Milstein, C., Williams, A.F., and Ziegler, A., 1978, Production of monoclonal antibodies to group A erythrocytes, HLA and other human cell surface antigens—new tools for genetic analysis, *Cell* **14**:9.

Beale, D., and Feinstein, A., 1976, Structure and function of the constant regions of immunoglobulins, *Q. Rev. Biophys.* **9**:135.

Bodmer, W.F. (ed.), 1978, The HLA system, *Br. Med. Bull.* **34**:213–309.

Brodsky, F.M., Parham, P., Barnstable, C.J., Crumpton, M.J., and Bodmer, W.F., 1979, Monoclonal antibodies for analysis of the HLA system, *Immunol. Rev.* **47**:3–61.

Burakoff, S.J., Engelhard, V.H., Kaufman, J., and Strominger, J.L., 1980, Induction of secondary cytotoxic T lymphocytes by liposomes containing HLA-DR antigens, *Nature (London)* **283**:495–497.

Coligan, J.E., Kindt, T.J., Ewenstein, B.M., Uehara, H., Martinko, J.M., and Nathenson, S.G., 1979, Further structural analysis of the murine H-2K^b glycoprotein using radiochemical methodology, *Mol. Immunol.* **16**:3.

Cresswell, P., Turner, M.J., and Strominger, J.L., 1973, Papain-solubilized HL-A antigens from cultured human lymphocytes contain two peptide fragments, *Proc. Natl. Acad. Sci. U.S.A.* **70**:1603.

Engelhard, V.H., Guild, B.C., Helenius, A., Terhorst, C., and Strominger, J.L., 1978a, Reconstitution of purified detergent soluble HLA-A and -B antigens into phospholipid vesicles, *Proc. Natl. Acad. Sci. U.S.A.* **75**:3230.

Engelhard, V.H., Strominger, J.L., Mescher, M., and Burakoff, S., 1978b, Induction of secondary cytotoxic T lymphocytes using purified HLA-A and HLA-B antigens reconstituted into phospholipid vesicles, *Proc. Natl. Acad. Sci. U.S.A.* **75**:5688.

Ferguson, W.S., Terhorst, C.T., Robb, R.J., and Strominger, J.L., 1979, Localization of the disulfide bridges of human histocompatiblity antigens, *Mol. Immunol.* **16**:23.

Helenius, A., Morein, B., Fries, E., Simons, K., Robinson, P., Schirr-macher, V., Terhorst, C., and Strominger, J., 1978, Human (HLA-A and -B) and murine (H-2K and -D) histocompatibility antigens are cell surface receptors for Semliki Forest virus, *Proc. Natl. Acad. Sci. U.S.A.* **75**:3846.

Koch, G.L.E., and Smith, M.J., 1978, An association between actin and the major histocompatibility antigen H-2, *Nature (London)* **273**:274.

Lancet, D., and Strominger, J.L., 1979, Conformation and chain interaction of human histocompatibility antigens, in: *Molecular Mechanisms of Biological Recognition* (M. Balaban, ed.), pp. 289–298, Elsevier/North-Holland, Berlin.

Lancet, D., Parham, P., and Strominger, J.L., 1979, The heavy chain of HLA-A and HLA-B antigens is conformationally labile: A possible role for β_2-microglobulin, *Proc. Natl. Acad. Sci. U.S.A.* **76**:3844.

Lopez de Castro, J.A., Orr, H.T., Robb, R.J., Kostyk, T.G., Mann, D.L., and Strominger, J.L., 1979, Complete amino acid sequence of a papain-solubilized human histocompatibility antigen, HLA-B7. I. Isolation and amino acid composition of fragments, and of tryptic and chymotryptic peptides, *Biochemistry* **18**:5704–5711.

Moller, G. (ed.), 1974, β_2-Microglobulin and HL-A antigen, *Transplant. Rev.* **21**.

Orr, H.T., Lopez de Castro, J.A., Parham, P., Ploegh, H.L., and Strominger, J.L., 1979a, Comparison of amino acid sequences of two human histocompatibility antigens, HLA-A2 and HLA-B7: The location of putative alloantigenic sites, *Proc. Natl. Acad. Sci. U.S.A.* **76**:4395.

Orr, H.T., Lopez de Castro, J.A., Lancet, D., and Strominger, J.L., 1979b, Complete amino acid sequence of a papain-solubilized human histocompatibility antigen, HLA-B7. II. Sequence determination and search for homologies, *Biochemistry* **18**:5711–5720.

Orr, H.T., Lancet, D., Robb, R.J., Lopez de Castro, J.A., and Strominger, J.L., 1979c, The heavy chain of a human histocompatibility antigen (HLA-B7) contains an immunoglobulin-like region, *Nature (London)* **282**:266–270.

Parham, P., 1980, Isolation of immunologically active HLA-A and B antigens by a series of monoclonal antibody columns, *J. Biol. Chem.* **254:**8709–8712.

Parham, P., and Bodmer, W.F., 1978, Monoclonal antibody to a human histocompatibility antigen, HLA-A2, *Nature (London)* **276:**397.

Parham, P., Alpert, B.N., Orr, H.T., and Strominger, J.L., 1977, The carbohydrate moiety of HLA antigens: Antigenic properties and amino acid sequences around the site of glycosylation, *J. Biol. Chem.* **252:**7555.

Pober, J.S., Guild, B.C., and Strominger, J.L., 1978, Phosphorylation *in vivo* and *in vitro* of human histocompatibility antigens (HLA-A and HLA-B) in the carboxy-terminal intracellular domain, *Proc. Natl. Acad. Sci. U.S.A.* **75:**6002.

Robb, R.J., 1977, Structural studies on the HLA-A and HLA-B human histocompatibility antigens, Ph.D. thesis, Harvard University.

Robb, R.J., Strominger, J.L., and Mann, D.L., 1976, Rapid purification of detergent-solubilized HLA antigen by affinity chromatography employing anti-β_2-microglobulin serum, *J. Biol. Chem.* **251:**5427.

Robb, R.J., Terhorst, C., and Strominger, J.L., 1978, Sequence of the COOH-terminal hydrophilic region of histocompatibility antigens HLA-A2 and HLA-B7, *J. Biol. Chem.* **253:**5319.

Springer, T.A., Strominger, J.L., and Mann, D., 1974, Partial purification of detergent soluble HL-A antigen and its cleavage by papain, *Proc. Natl. Acad. Sci. U.S.A.* **71:**1539.

Strominger, J.L., Cresswell, P., Grey, H., Humphreys, R.E., Mann, D., McCune, J., Parham, P., Robb, R., Sanderson, A.R., Springer, T.A., Terhorst, C., and Turner, M.J., 1974, The immunoglobulin-like structure of human histocompatibility antigens, *Transplant. Rev.* **21:**126.

Strominger, J.L., Engelhard, V.H., Fuks, A., Guild, B.C., Hyafil, F., Kaufman, J.F., Korman, A.J., Kostyk, T.G., Krangel, M.S., Lancet, D., Lopez de Castro, J.A., Mann, D.L., Orr, H.T., Parham, P., Parker, K.C., Ploegh, H.L., Pober, J.S., Robb, R.J., and Shackelford, D.A., 1980, The biochemical analysis of products of the major histocompatibility complex, in: *The Role of the Major Histocompatibility Complex in Immunobiology* (B. Benacerraf and M.E. Dorf, eds.), pp. 115–171, Garland Press, New York.

Strominger, J.L., Orr, H.T., Robb, R.J., Parham, P., Ploegh, H.L., Mann, D.L., Bilofsky, M., Saroff, H.A., Wu, T.T., and Kabat, E.A., 1980b, Homology of amino acids in human histocompatibility antigens (HLA-A and HLA-B) with those in immunoglobulins, *Scan. J. Immunol.* **11:**573–592.

Terhorst, C., Robb, R., Jones, C., and Strominger, J.L., 1977, Further structural studies of the heavy chain of HLA antigens and its similarity to immunoglobulins, *Proc. Natl. Acad. Sci. U.S.A.* **74:**4002.

Turner, M.J., Cresswell, P., Parham, P., Strominger, J.L., Mann, D.L., and Sanderson, A.R., 1975, Purification of papain-solubilized histocompatibility from a cultured human lymphoblastoid line, RPMI 4265, *J. Biol. Chem.* **250:**4512.

Vehara, H., Ewenstein, B.M. Martinko, S.M. Nathenson, S.G., Coligan, J.E., and Kindt, T.S., 1980, Primary structure of murine major histocompatibility complex alloantigens: Amino acid sequence of the amino-terminal one hundred and seventy-three residues of the H-2K^b glycoprotein, *Biochemistry* **19:**306.

21

Antigenic Structures of HLA(A,B,C) Antigens

Chymotryptic Glycopeptides Carrying HLA(A,B,C) Determinants

Nobuyuki Tanigaki, Nobuhiko Tada, and David Pressman

1. Introduction

HLA(A,B,C) antigens,* i.e., the human classic histocompatibility antigens, form a unique group of human cell-surface antigens that are controlled by allelic genes of three loci, *HLA-A, HLA-B,* and *HLA-C,* located in the human major histocompatibility complex. It is a highly polymorphic alloantigen system, and a total of 50 allospecificities have been defined. The alloantigens in this system are composed of two noncovalently bound component peptides, one of 43,000 daltons and another of 11,000 daltons (Rask *et al.*, 1974; Strominger *et al.*, 1974; Tanigaki and Pressman, 1974). The 11,000-dalton component is a simple protein and is known to be identical to human β_2-microglobulin (Grey *et al.*, 1973; Naka-

*We refer to *HLA-A*, *-B*, and *-C* gene products bound to β_2-microglobulin as "HLA(A,B,C) antigens"—briefly, "HLA antigens." The gene products themselves will be termed "HLA(A,B,C) alloantigenic components"—briefly, "HLA(A,B,C) components," these portions of the HLA(A,B,C) antigen molecules are also named HLA large subunits or HLA heavy polypeptide chains by others.

Nobuyuki Tanigaki, Nobuhiko Tada, and David Pressman • Department of Immunology Research, Roswell Park Memorial Institute, Buffalo, New York 14263. Dr. Tada's present address is: Memorial Sloan-Kettering Institute for Cancer Research, New York, New York 10021.

muro *et al.*, 1973; Tanigaki *et al.*, 1973; Peterson *et al.*, 1974). No allospecificity has been found in this portion of any HLA antigens. The 43,000-dalton component is a glycoprotein and carries a determinant(s) that is responsible for the HLA(A,B,C) allospecificity and is indeed the HLA gene product (Nakamuro *et al.*, 1975a). This alloantigenic component of the HLA(A,B,C) alloantigens is referred to as the "HLA(A,B,C) component" in this chapter.

Previously, we isolated the HLA(A,B,C) components from papain-solubilized HLA preparations carrying different HLA allospecificity by a specific procedure that utilized dissociation of HLA antigens induced in the reaction with rabbit antibodies directed to the β_2-microglobulin portion of HLA antigens (Nakamuro *et al.*, 1975a,b). The process is mild and appears to be the result of a competitive binding of anti-β_2-microglobulin antibodies and the HLA(A,B,C) components to the β_2-microglobulin portion of HLA antigens.

The HLA components isolated in such a way retain to a large extent the HLA allospecificity carried by the parental HLA antigens (Nakamuro *et al.*, 1975a). Moreover, the HLA components obtained in this way retain a unique specificity that is detected with xenoantiserum raised against HLA antigens (Nakamuro *et al.*, 1975b). The xenospecificity is native to the HLA alloantigenic component portion of intact HLA antigens and is expressed in common on the HLA(A,B,C) components regardless of their polymorphic HLA allospecificity. We refer to the determinant(s) responsible for this particular HLA specificity as the "HLA common determinant."

Other procedures such as exposure to acid pH or treatment with denaturants—for example, sodium iodide, sodium thiocyanate, sodium dodecyl sulfate (SDS), guanidine-HCl, or urea—also induce dissociation of HLA antigens. However, the HLA components obtained by these methods are apparently denatured and do not carry either the HLA allospecificity or the HLA xenospecificity characteristic of intact HLA antigens in a level comparable to that carried by the HLA components obtained by the "antibody dissociation" method. Instead, the HLA components obtained by chemical dissociation acquire xenospecificity that is detected with rabbit antiserum raised against acid-exposed HLA components and is characteristic of denatured HLA antigens (Tanigaki *et al.*, 1974). The determinant(s) responsible for this type of HLA xenospecificity has been termed the "HLA cryptic determinant."

The present work was undertaken to reveal more detailed antigenic structures of HLA antigens. The specific aim was to determine the location of the HLA alloantigenic determinant, the HLA common determinant, and the HLA cryptic determinant on HLA(A,B,C) components. To this end, HLA(A,B,C) components were isolated from papain-solubilized

HLA preparations by the antibody dissociation method and fragmented by enzymatic digestion with chymotrypsin. The digests were found to contain two glycopeptide fragments, one of 24,000 daltons and another of 34,000 daltons that retained HLA allospecificity and HLA xenospecificity. The 34,000-dalton fragments were apparently the original HLA(A,B,C) components that had not been digested under the conditions used. On the other hand, the 24,000-dalton fragments were split by cyanogen bromide treatment but not by formic acid treatment, indicating their close resemblance to the similar-size glycopeptide fragments obtained from formic-acid-treated HLA large subunits and labeled as fragment B by Terhorst *et al.* (1977). Because fragment B has been shown to be the NH_2-terminal fragment of the HLA large subunit, our results indicate that the determinant responsible for HLA allospecificity and a part, if not all, of the determinants responsible for HLA xenospecificity are located at the distal portion of the HLA(A,B,C) component and also in proximity to the point at which the carbohydrate chain is attached to the HLA(A,B,C) polypeptide chain.

2. Preparation of HLA(A,B,C) Components

HLA(A,B,C) antigens were solubilized by papain digestion from crude membrane materials of cells of a human B-cell type cell line, RPMI 1788 (HLA phenotype: A2, B7, B14), and purified by a sequence of procedures involving hypotonic dialysis, ion-exchange chromatography, gel filtration, and column electrophoresis (Miyakawa *et al.*, 1971). They were further purified by affinity chromatography on *Lens culinaris* hemagglutinin (LcH)-coupled Sepharose as described first by Hayman and Crumpton (1972). Two preparations were obtained by following HLA-A2 specificity and HLA-B7 specificity. The preparations were labeled with radioactive iodine ^{125}I by the chloramine-T method (Greenwood *et al.*, 1963) and subjected to LcH affinity chromatography. The labeled HLA antigens were completely retarded on the chromatography. They were eluted with a 5% α-methyl-D-mannoside solution. The level of specific radioactivity was about 20 mCi/mg antigen, and the level of iodine labeling showed an average of 5.5 atoms of iodine per molecule of antigen.

HLA(A,B,C) components were isolated from the radiolabeled HLA preparations, following reaction with rabbit anti-human β_2-microglobulin antibodies to remove the β_2-microglobulin portion of HLA antigens and release the HLA(A,B,C) components. The isolation was carried out as follows: 600 μl of an ^{125}I-labeled HLA preparation (a total of 6 μg antigen containing radioactivity of about 120 μCi) was incubated with an excess (360 μl in this case) of rabbit anti-human β_2-microglobulin antiserum for

48 hr at 4°C. The precipitates that appeared during incubation were removed by centrifugation. The supernatant was gel-filtered on a column (12 × 550 mm) of Bio-Gel A1.5 M (Bio-Rad, Richmond, California) prewashed with Tris-HC1 buffer (Tris 0.075 M, pH 7.8) containing 0.02% bovine serum albumin (BSA). The HLA(A,B,C) components were eluted as a single peak of radioactivity. The molecular size estimated by SDS-polyacrylamide gel electrophoresis (SDS-PAGE) was 34,000 daltons. These "antibody-dissociated" HLA(A,B,C) component preparations were apparently intact in antigenic conformation with respect to the HLA allospecificity and HLA xenospecificity native to the intact HLA antigens. This is shown in Table 1 for a HLA-B7 component preparation that was analyzed in detail in the subsequent experiments.

TABLE 1. Binding Properties[a] of HLA(A,B,C) Components and Their Chymotryptic Fragments

	Binding by indicated antiserum (%)		
Substance assayed	Human alloantiserum Betz	Rabbit anti-HLA(A,B,C) 6095	Rabbit anti-denatured HLA(A,B,C) 5996
HLA(A,B,C) component[b]	39.7	75.5	38.9
Whole chymotrypsin digest of the HLA componant	9.3	13.2	3.9
LcH-bound fraction	41.5	60.1	7.5
Fragment I	59.0	78.2	11.1
Fragment II	46.3	55.0	17.9
Fragment III	0.2	0.6	9.4
LcH-unbound fraction	0.2	0.6	0.5
Fragment IV	0.2	0.8	0.2
Fragment V	0.0	0.1	0.2
Fragment VI	0.4	0.1	0.1

[a]Binding properties were determined by the direct binding reaction as follows: A 20-μl sample of a given ^{125}I-labeled specimen of about 4000 cpm was incubated overnight at 4°C with 10 μl alloantiserum or 4 μl rabbit antiserum (diluted twice with normal rabbit serum). The immune complex was precipitated by an excess of goat anti-human IgG or goat anti-rabbit IgG antiserum. The radioactivity in the precipitate was determined and expressed as the percentage of the added radioactivity. A control with the same amount of normal human serum or of normal rabbit serum was included. The values are the percentages of binding from which the control value of each ^{125}I-labeled specimen, −0.1 to 1.1% for normal human serum and −0.1 to 0.7% for normal rabbit serum, has been subtracted.

[b]This HLA(A,B,C) component was isolated from a radioiodinated preparation of papain-solubilized HLA-B7 antigen molecule, following reaction with rabbit anti-human β_2-microglobulin antibodies to remove the β_2-microglobulin portion of the HLA molecule and release the HLA(A,B,C) component.

3. Chymotrypsin Digestion of HLA(A,B,C) Components and Subsequent Separation of the Chymotryptic Fragments

HLA(A,B,C) component preparations were digested with α-chymotrypsin. The digests were subjected to LcH affinity chromatography followed by gel filtration. Six fragments of different molecular size were separated. Three were glycopeptides and the others were simple peptides.

^{125}I-labeled HLA component preparations contained about 1.2 A_{280} units protein/ml. The protein present was largely the BSA used as a carrier protein and rabbit serum proteins derived from rabbit anti-human β_2-microglobulin antiserum that was used for dissociation of HLA antigens (see above). These proteins were taken to compose the substrates for the subsequent chymotrypsin digestion, because the amount of HLA(A,B,C) components present was negligibly small. Two different enzyme/substrate (E/S) ratios, 1:10 and 1:40, were used. The digestion was carried out at pH 9.0 in the presence of 0.1 M $CaCl_2$. After 1 hr digestion at 37°C, the reaction was terminated by use of Kunitz-type bovine pancreatic trypsin inhibitor.

The digests (a total volume of about 3 ml containing radioactivity of about 36 μCi) were subjected to affinity chromatography on an LcH-coupled Sepharose column (7 × 110 mm). The patterns for an HLA-B7 component preparation are shown in Fig. 1. In the case of the 1:10 digest (Fig. 1a), the LcH-unbound fraction and the LcH-bound fraction accounted for, respectively, 70 and 30% of the radioactivity recovered. The values obtained for the 1:40 digest (Fig. 1b) were 63 and 36%, respectively.

The major portion (2.4–3.0 ml) of each of the LcH-unbound and LcH-bound fractions, as indicated by the hatching in Fig. 1, was concentrated to about 0.6 ml by ultrafiltration with a UM-2 membrane filter (Amicon Corp., Lexington, Massachusetts) and then fractionated by gel filtration on a Sephadex G-75 superfine column (12 × 600 mm). As shown in Fig. 2 for the 1:10 digest of HLA-B7 component preparation, the LcH-bound fraction gave three peaks of radioactivity, one of 34,000 daltons, one of 24,000 daltons, and one of 8400 daltons, as estimated on the gel column by use of papain-solubilized HLA antigens of 45,000 daltons and human β_2-microglobulin of 11,800 daltons (Fig. 2a). The LcH-unbound fraction also showed three discernible peaks of radioactivity, but all were less than 5500 daltons (Fig. 2b). Almost identical patterns were obtained for the 1:40 digest (patterns not shown). The major fractions of each peak were pooled as indicated by the hatching in Fig. 2. The fragments in each pool were designated in the order of elution, Fragments I, II, and III for those from the LcH-bound fraction, and Fragments IV, V, and VI for those from the LcH-unbound fraction.

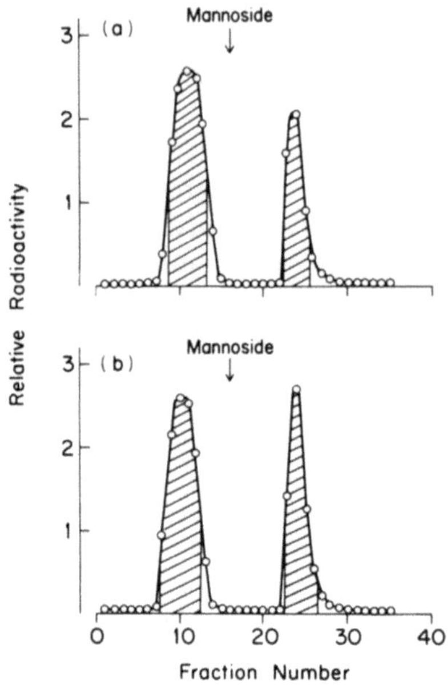

Figure 1. Affinity chromatography of chymotrypsin-digested HLA(A,B,C) components on LcH-coupled Sepharose. (a) Digests at an E/S ratio of 1:10; (b) digests at an E/S ratio of 1:40. An ^{125}I-labeled HLA-B7(A,B,C) component preparation was digested with α-chymotrypsin at an E/S ratio of 1:10 or 1:40 (see the text for details). The digests (a total volume of about 3 ml containing radioactivity of about 36 μCi) were subjected to affinity chromatography on a column (7 × 110 mm) of LcH-coupled Sepharose (4 mg LcH/ml gel) prewashed with Tris-HCl buffer (Tris 0.075 M, pH 7.8) containing 0.5 M NaCl. The LcH-unbound fragments were washed away with the same buffer containing 0.02% BSA. A 5% solution of α methyl-D-mannoside in the same BSA-containing buffer was applied as indicated by the arrow to elute the LcH-bound fragments. The curves are plots of ^{125}I-radioactivity (relative radioactivity) against fraction number (fraction size 0.6 ml).

4. Binding Properties of HLA(A,B,C) Components and Their Chymotryptic Fragments

The HLA(A,B,C) fragments that were obtained by chymotrypsin digestion of HLA-B7 component preparation were examined by the direct binding assay to determine whether they carry HLA allospecificity or HLA xenospecificity or both. Of the six fragments, two fragments that were apparently glycopeptides in view of their affinity to LcH carried both HLA allospecificity and HLA xenospecificity.

HLA allospecificity was assayed by use of a human alloantiserum Betz that is polyspecific but has been found to have a high level of binding with HLA-B7 preparations. HLA xenospecificity was assayed by use of a rabbit antiserum raised against papain-solubilized HLA antigens [rabbit anti-HLA(A,B,C) antiserum] and a rabbit antiserum raised against HLA(A,B,C) components isolated from papain-solubilized HLA antigens by acid dissociation [rabbit anti-denatured HLA(A,B,C) antiserum]. The former antiserum has been used to detect HLA common determinant(s), i.e., a determinant(s) responsible for HLA xenospecificity that is native and common to HLA antigens regardless of the HLA allospecificity carried (Nakamuro *et al.*, 1975b); the latter antiserum has been used to detect an HLA cryptic determinant(s) that is characteristic of denatured HLA(A,B,C) components of HLA antigens (Tanigaki *et al.*, 1974). In addition to the assay of the chymotryptic fragments, the original HLA-B7 component preparation, the whole chymotrypsin digests, and the LcH-unbound and LcH-bound fractions were also assayed at the same time.

The direct binding assay was carried out as follows: 20 μl of each assay specimen of about 5000 cpm was incubated with 10 μl alloantiserum in a total volume of 70 μl. After incubation overnight at 4°C, an excess (70 μl in this case) of goat anti-human IgG antiserum was added. After further incubation for 1 hr at room temperature, the immune precipitate was washed and the radioactivity was determined. A control with the same amount of normal human serum was included. The test with rabbit antiserum was the same, except that 4 μl rabbit antiserum (diluted twice with

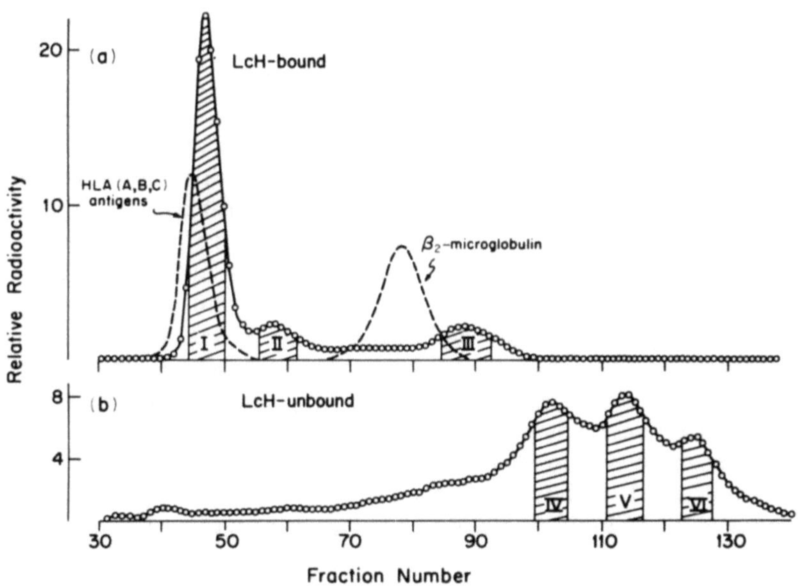

Figure 2. Gel filtration of chymotrypsin-digested HLA(A,B,C) components on Sephadex G-75. (a) LcH-bound fraction; (b) LcH-unbound fraction. The major portion (2.4–3.0 ml) of each of the LcH-unbound and LcH-bound fractions of chymotrypsin-digested ^{125}I-labeled HLA-B7 components (see Fig. 1) was concentrated to about 0.6 ml and fractionated by gel filtration on a Sephadex G-75 superfine column (12 × 600 mm). The patterns are shown by the solid line for the digests at an E/S ratio of 1:10, and are plots of ^{125}I radioactivity (relative radioactivity) against fraction number (fraction size 0.48 ml). The same column was calibrated by use of papain-solubilized HLA antigens of 45,000 daltons and human β_2-microglobulin of 11,800 daltons. The pattern is shown by the dashed line in plot (a). Note that the LcH-bound fraction gives three radioactive peaks of 34,000, 24,000, and 8400 daltons and that the LcH-unbound fraction also shows three discernible peaks, but all are less than 5500 daltons.

normal rabbit serum) was used and 40 μl of goat anti-rabbit IgG antiserum was added to precipitate the immune complex. The results are shown in Table 1 for the 1:10 digest as the percentage of the added radioactivity carried down in the precipitate.

In the reaction with alloantiserum Betz, the original HLA-B7 component preparation gave a substantial level of binding, 39.7%. When the preparation was digested with chymotrypsin and assayed, the value reduced to 9.3%. The active fragments in the digest that are responsible for this 9.3% binding were entirely recovered in the fraction that has an affinity for LcH. The binding level of the LcH-bound fraction was 41.5%. Of the three fragments separated by gel filtration of the LcH-bound fraction, Fragment I of 34,000 daltons and Fragment II of 24,000 daltons accounted for all the binding activity. The percentage binding was 59.0% for Fragment I and 46.3% for Fragment II. No significant binding activity was found with Fragment III of 8400 daltons. As expected from 0.2% binding of the LcH-unbound fraction, Fragments IV, V, and VI obtained from the LcH-unbound fraction were totally lacking in binding activity.

The binding properties of these preparations with rabbit anti-HLA(A,B,C) antiserum were very similar, except that the values of percentage binding were higher than those obtained with alloantiserum Betz. The binding level of the original component preparation was 75.5%. The values obtained for Fragments I and II were 78.2 and 55.0%, respectively.

In the reaction with rabbit anti-denatured HLA(A,B,C) antiserum, the original HLA-B7 component preparation showed a value of 38.9%. This value was unexpectedly high, because usual HLA(A,B,C) component preparations prepared in a similar manner give a value less than 15%, mostly less than 10%. However, when the present preparation was digested with chymotrypsin, the value decreased to 3.9%. This binding activity was recovered in the LcH-bound fraction of the digest. Here again, Fragments I and II isolated from the LcH-bound fraction possessed binding activity. The binding level was 11.1% for Fragment I and 17.9% for Fragment II. When these two fragments were exposed to pH 2.3 and assayed, the binding levels were raised to 31.8 and 31.9%, respectively (data not included in Table 1). These results indicate that both Fragment I and Fragment II have a potential HLA cryptic determinant and that Fragment II already expresses it partially.

Almost identical results were obtained for the 1:40 digests. Thus, of the six chymotryptic fragments, two glycopeptide fragments of 34,000 daltons and 24,000 daltons carried HLA allospecificity and HLA xenospecificities, both HLA common and HLA cryptic. No fragments were found that carried only one HLA specificity, either allospecificity or xenospecificity.

5. Characterization of HLA(A,B,C) Chymotryptic Glycopeptide Fragments

The two glycopeptide fragments carrying both HLA allospecificity and HLA xenospecificity, Fragment I of 34,000 daltons and Fragment II of 24,000 daltons, were examined for susceptibility to treatment with formic acid and with cyanogen bromide. Fragment I was split by both treatments, whereas Fragment II was split only by the cyanogen bromide treatment. These results indicate that Fragment I of 34,000 daltons is apparently the original HLA(A,B,C) component that was not digested under the conditions used and that Fragment II of 24,000 daltons is indeed a chymotrypsin-split fragment that is similar to a 23,000-dalton fragment isolated from formic-acid-treated HLA large subunits, i.e., HLA(A,B,C) components, of several HLA allospecificities and labeled as fragment B by Terhorst *et al.* (1977).

The treatments were carried out as follows: Two equal portions of each glycopeptide preparation, about 22,000 cpm for the Fragment I preparation and about 8000 cpm for the Fragment II preparation, were lyophilized. To one specimen, 50 μl of 70% formic acid was added, and to the other specimen the same amount of 70% formic acid and a small amount of solid cyanogen bromide were added. The former mixture was incubated at 37°C for 35 hr and the latter mixture at 25°C for 24 hr. As the control, another equal portion of each glycopeptide preparation was incubated with 50 μl of 70% formic acid at 25°C for 24 hr. After incubation, the reaction mixtures were diluted 10 times with distilled water and lyophilized. Each specimen was treated with 50 μl of a 3% SDS solution containing 2-mercaptoethanol at 37°C for 1 hr and subjected to electrophoresis on a 14% polyacrylamide gel containing 0.1% SDS (Laemmli, 1970). Before treatment with SDS, a small amount of an ^{131}I-labeled preparation of papain-solubilized HLA antigens, about 20,000 cpm, was added to each specimen as an internal size marker. In the presence of SDS, the ^{131}I-label dissociates and gives the two component peptides, the HLA(A,B,C) component of 34,000 daltons and the β_2-microglobulin of 11,800 daltons. The patterns obtained are depicted in Figs. 3 and 4 along with those of the untreated Fragment I and Fragment II preparations.

On SDS-PAGE, the untreated Fragment I preparation gave a single radioactive peak of 34,000 daltons (Fig. 3a). No other peaks were seen. When treated with formic acid at 37°C, the preparation split and yielded two radioactive peaks, one of 20,000 daltons and another of 12,000 daltons (Fig. 3b). These two major peaks were each followed by a minor shoulderlike peak and preceded by a small peak of 34,000 daltons apparently due to the unsplit residual fragments. Cyanogen bromide treatment also split the preparation. In this case, at least three radioactive peaks of about 18,000, 13,000, and 9000 daltons were discernible (Fig. 3c). They were also preceded by a peak of 34,000 daltons. These splittings were not produced by treatment with formic acid at 25°C.

The untreated Fragment II preparation showed a major radioactive peak of 23,000 daltons and an additional minor peak of 16,000 daltons (Fig. 4a). With this preparation, formic acid treatment at 37°C as well as at 25°C had no effect. The patterns, as shown for the preparation treated at 37°C (Fig. 4b), were essentially the same as that of the untreated Fragment II preparation. However, on treatment with cyanogen bromide, the preparation split and gave three radioactive peaks of about 16,000, 11,000, and 9000 daltons (Fig. 4c).

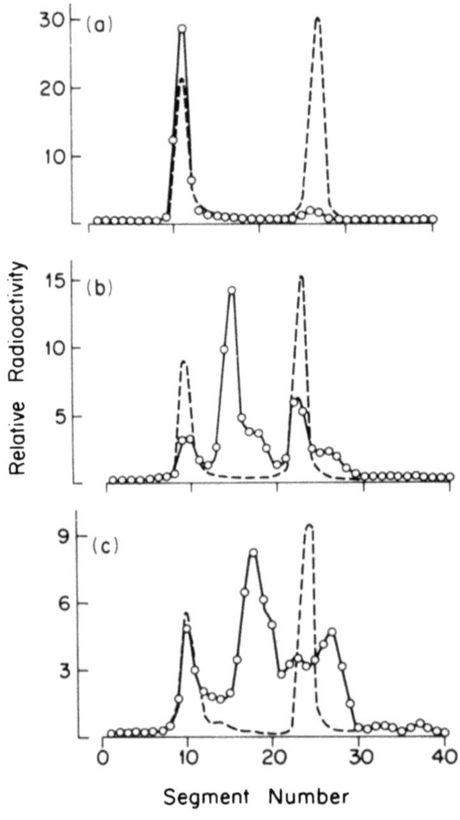

Figure 3. SDS-PAGE of HLA(A,B,C) chymotryptic glycopeptide fragments of 34,000 daltons. (a) Untreated; (b) treated with formic acid; (c) treated with cyanogen bromide. A small amount of a glycopeptide preparation of 34,000 daltons isolated by LcH affinity chromatography and gel filtration from chymotrypsin digests of an ^{125}I-labeled HLA-B7 component preparation was treated with formic acid or with cyanogen bromide (see the text for details) and subjected to electrophoresis on a 14% polyacrylamide gel (6 × 85 mm) containing 0.1% SDS. The untreated preparation was examined in a parallel run. The gel was sliced into 40 segments from the cathode end by an automatic gel divider. (—) Plots of ^{125}I-radioactivity (relative radioactivity) against segment number; (----) positions of two components, the HLA(A,B,C) component (34,000 daltons) and human β_2-microglobulin (11,800 daltons), of ^{131}I-labeled papain-solubilized HLA(A,B,C) antigens added as internal size markers. Note that this glycopeptide preparation is susceptible to both treatments and splits to give smaller fragments.

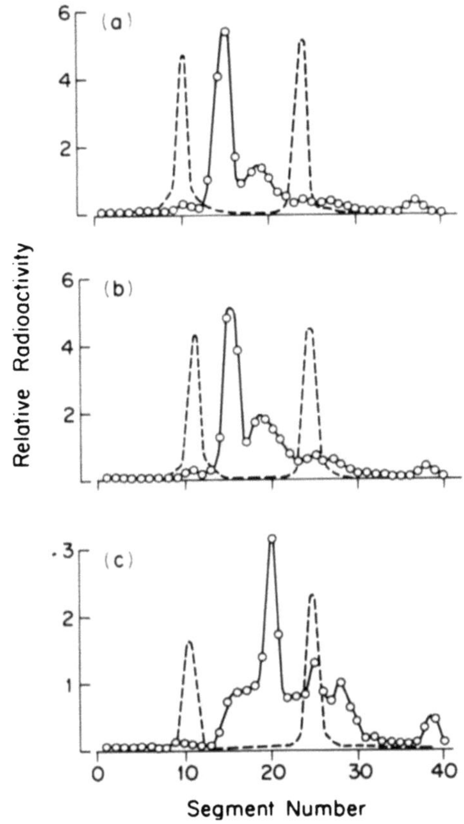

Figure 4. SDS-PAGE of HLA(A,B,C) chymotryptic glycopeptide fragment of 24,000 daltons. (a) Untreated; (b) treated with formic acid; (c) treated with cyanogen bromide. Another glycopeptide preparation of 24,000 daltons isolated from chymotrypsin digests of an ^{125}I-labeled HLA-B7 component preparation was treated and analyzed in the same manner as described for the 34,000-dalton preparation in Fig. 3. Note that this preparation is resistant to formic acid treatment but susceptible to cyanogen bromide treatment.

6. Discussion

The results presented herein from antigenic analysis of the fragments obtained by enzymatic digestion of HLA(A,B,C) alloantigenic components, when combined with those from excellent chemical analysis by Terhorst *et al.* (1977) of the fragments obtained by chemical cleavage of HLA large subunits, indicate that the determinant responsible for HLA allospecificity and a part, if not all, of the determinants responsible for HLA xenospecificity are located on the distal half (in relation to the cell membrane matrix) of HLA(A,B,C) component and also in proximity to the carbohydrate chain bound to the HLA polypeptide chain. This conclusion is deduced from the following facts: (1) a fragment of 23,000 daltons isolated from chymotrypsin digests of HLA(A,B,C) component carries HLA allospecificity and also HLA xenospecificity and (2) the fragment is very similar to a fragment obtained by mild acid treatment of HLA(A,B,C) component and shown to be the NH_2-terminal fragment. The similarities are as follows: (1) both fragments have a molecular size of about 23,000 daltons; (2) both fragments have an affinity for lentil lectin and thus contain carbohydrates; (3) both fragments do not contain acid-labile peptide bonds, even though the chymotryptic fragment may have such peptide bonds in the very peripheral portion of the fragment; and (4) both fragments are susceptible to treatment with cyanogen bromide. These similarities are quite enough to establish the near-identity of the two fragments.

In addition to the experiments described herein, we also carried out an experiment in which whole molecules of papain-solubilized HLA(A,B,C) antigens were digested with chymotrypsin. The major purpose was to obtain smaller HLA(A,B,C) antigen molecules that contain β_2-microglobulin. We could not find such moieties in the digests, although the digests contained a 23,000-dalton fragment carrying HLA specificities that was similar to that obtained by chymotrypsin digestion of HLA(A,B,C) components.

In studies on Ag-B antigen, i.e., the rat classic histocompatibility antigens, we found that limited papain digestion of cell membranes of a rat strain produces two molecules, one of 25,000 daltons and another of 35,000 daltons, both carrying the Ag-B allospecificity, besides the 59,000-dalton Ag-B antigen molecules that correspond to papain-solubilized HLA antigens of 48,000 daltons (Katagiri *et al.*, 1975). The 25,000-dalton molecule did not contain rat β_2-microglobulin. It was apparently a fragment of Ag-B alloantigenic component. This fragment may be a kind of rat homologue of the 23,000-dalton HLA(A,B,C) fragment obtained by chymotrypsin digestion in the present work. On the other hand, the 35,000-dalton molecule dissociated on short-term exposure to acid and gave two component fragments of 20,000 and 11,000 daltons. The 20,000-dalton fragment was a fragment of Ag-B alloantigenic component, because it carried the Ag-B allospecificity. The 11,000-dalton fragment was rat β_2-microglobulin. These results allow us to draw a conclusion that in rat Ag-B antigens, the β_2-microglobulin binds to the Ag-B component, situated in proximity to a segment carrying the alloantigenic determinant on the Ag-B component. A very similar positioning would be possible for HLA(A,B,C) antigens, because the structural homology of the classic histocompatibility antigens in mammalian species seems to be very high. Such a possibility has been indicated by Peterson *et al.* (1975). They found that treatment of papain-solubilized heavy HL-A polypeptide chain with trypsin, pepsin, chymotrypsin, or thermolysin invariably yielded two distinct fragments. One fragment had a molecular weight similar to that of β_2-microglobulin, whereas the other fragment displayed a molecular weight of approximately 20,000. This latter fragment could be the same as our 23,000-dalton chymotryptic HLA(A,B,C) fragment. Very interestingly, they reported that the 20,000-dalton fragment formed a complex with β_2-microglobulin.

Besides the 23,000-dalton glycopeptide fragment carrying HLA specificities, we found another glycopeptide fragment of about 8400 daltons in the present experiments. This smaller fragment did not carry HLA allospecificity or HLA xenospecificity at levels detectable by the direct binding assay. Earlier, Sanderson *et al.* (1971) reported that a similar-sized glycopeptide can be produced by enzymatic digestion of HLA(A,B,C) antigens. Their glycopeptide did show HLA alloantigenic activity. In the pioneer study on enzymatic fragmentation of HLA(A,B,C) antigen, they digested papain-solubilized HLA glycoproteins (antigens) with insoluble pronase and fractionated the digests by gel filtration on a Sephadex G-50 column. They found that gel fractions in an early, barely included peak of a probable molecular weight of 8000–10,000 daltons carries HLA alloantigenic activity that accounted for 8–20% of the activity of the original glycoprotein preparations. These fractions contained a major portion of the carbohydrates but less than 10% of the amino acids of the original glycoprotein preparations. Since HLA(A,B,C) component contains only one carbohydrate chain of about 4000 daltons (Henriksen *et al.*, 1976; Terhorst *et al.*, 1977), the glycopeptide they found should be a part of our 23,000-dalton chymotryptic fragment carrying HLA specificities, and moreover it may be the same as our 8400-dalton chymotryptic glycopeptide fragment. The lack of HLA activity in this latter fragment may not be contradictory because the direct binding assay used here by us for assay of HLA activity is obviously less suitable for detection of a minor residual activity than the inhibition assay of cytotoxicity used by Sanderson *et al.* (1971) in their work. Extensive analyses of this type of HLA glycopeptides are needed for further classification of antigenic structure of HLA antigens.

7. Summary

HLA alloantigenic components were isolated from papain-solubilized HLA preparations carrying different HLA allospecificities by a specific procedure that utilized dissociation of HLA antigens by reaction with rabbit antibodies directed to the β_2-microglobulin portion of HLA antigens. The HLA components isolated in such a way retain to a large extent the HLA allospecificity and HLA xenospecificity of the parental HLA antigens.

The HLA components were digested with α-chymotrypsin and subjected to lentil lectin affinity chromatography followed by gel filtration. Of the six chymotryptic fragments isolated, two glycopeptide fragments, one of 34,000 daltons and another of 24,000 daltons, carried both HLA allospecificity and HLA xenospecificity. No fragments were found that carried only HLA allospecificity or only HLA xenospecificity. Treatment with either formic acid or cyanogen bromide split the 34,000-dalton fragment. The 24,000-dalton fragment was split only by the cyanogen bromide treatment. These results indicate that the 34,000-dalton fragment is apparently the original HLA component that was not digested under the conditions used and that the 24,000-dalton fragment is indeed a chymotrypsin-split fragment. This latter fragment appears to be very similar to a 23,-000-dalton fragment that was isolated from formic-acid-treated HLA subunits, i.e., HLA components, and was shown to be the NH_2-terminal fragment of the HLA large subunits by Terhorst *et al.* (1977).

ACKNOWLEDGMENTS. This investigation was supported by USPHS Grants CA 17276, CA 17609, and AI08899, awarded by the National Cancer Institute and the National Institute of Allergy and Infectious Diseases, Department of Health, Education and Welfare. A part of this chapter was presented at the 60th Annual Meeting of the American Association of Immunologists, Anaheim, California, 1976.

References

Greenwood, F.C., Hunter, W.M., and Glover, J.S., 1963, The preparation of ^{131}I-labeled human growth hormone of high specific radioactivity, *Biochem. J.* **89:**114.

Grey, H.M., Kubo, R.T., Colon, S.M., Poulik, M.D., Cresswell, P., Springer, T., Turner, M., and Strominger, J.L., 1973, The small subunit of HL-A antigens is β_2-microglobulin, *J. Exp. Med.* **138:**1608.

Hayman, M.J., and Crumpton, M.J., 1972, Isolation of glycoproteins from pig lymphocyte plasma membrane using *Lens culinaris* phytohemagglutinin, *Biochem. Biophys. Res. Commun.* **47:**923.

Henriksen, O., Appella, E.A., Smith, D.F., Tanigaki, N., and Pressman, D., 1976, Comparative chemical analyses of the alloantigenic fragments of HL-A antigens, *J. Biol. Chem.* **251:**4214.

Katagiri, M., Tanigaki, N., and Pressman, D., 1975, Papain-solubilized Ag-B antigens. II. Characterization of small sized Ag-B molecules, *Transplantation* **20:**135.

Laemmli, V.K., 1970, Cleavage of structural proteins during the assembly of the head of bacteriophage T4, *Nature (London)* **227:**680.

Miyakawa, Y., Tanigaki, N., Yagi, Y., and Pressman, D., 1971, An efficient method for isolation of HL-A antigens from hematopoietic cells lines, *J. Immunol.* **107:**394.

Nakamuro, K., Tanigaki, N., and Pressman, D., 1973, Multiple common properties of human β_2-microglobulin and the common portion fragment derived from HL-A antigen molecules, *Proc. Natl. Acad. Sci. U.S.A.* **70:**2863.

Nakamuro, K., Tanigaki, N., and Pressman, D., 1975a, Isolation of HL-A 33,000-dalton fragments carrying high HL-A alloantigenic activity, *Transplantation* **19:**431.

Nakamuro, K., Tanigaki, N., and Pressman, D., 1975b, Common antigenic structures of HL-A antigens. VI. Common antigenic determinants located on the 33,000-dalton alloantigenic fragment portion of papain-solubilized HL-A molecules, *Immunology* **29:**1119.

Peterson, P.A., Rask, L., and Lindblom, J.B., 1974, Highly purified papain-solubilized HL-A antigens contain β_2-microglobulin, *Proc. Natl. Acad. Sci. U.S.A.* **71:**35.

Peterson, P.A., Rask, L., Sege, K., Klareskog, L., Anundi, H., and Ostberg, L., 1975, Evolutionary relationship between immunoglobulins and transplantation antigens, *Proc. Natl. Acad. Sci. U.S.A.* **72:**1612.

Rask, L., Ostberg, L., Lindblom, B., Fernstedt, Y., and Peterson, P.A., 1974, The subunit structure of transplantation antigens, *Transplant. Rev.* **21:**85.

Sanderson, A.R., Cresswell, P., and Welsh, K.I., 1971, Involvement of carbohydrate in the immunochemical determinant area of HL-A substances, *Nature (London) New Bio.* **230:**8.

Strominger, J.L., Cresswell, P., Grey, H., Humphreys, R.H., Mann, D., McCune, J., Parham, P., Robb, R., Sanderson, A.R., Springer, T.A., Terhorst, C., and Turner, M.J., 1974, The immunoglobulin-like structure of human histocompatibility antigens, *Transplant. Rev.* **21:**126.

Tanigaki, N., and Pressman, D., 1974, The basic structure and the antigenic characteristics of HL-A antigens, *Transplant. Rev.* **21:**15.

Tanigaki, N., Nakamuro, K., Appella, E., Poulik, M.D., and Pressman, D., 1973, Identity of the HL-A common portion fragment and human β_2-microglobulin, *Biochem. Biophys. Res. Commun.* **55:**1234.

Tanigaki, N., Nakamuro, K., Natori, T., Kreiter, V.P., and Pressman, D., 1974, Common antigenic structures of HL-A antigens. V. An antigenic determinant characteristic of a 33,000-dalton fragment of HL-A molecules, *Transplantation* **18:**74.

Terhorst, C., Robb, R., Jones, C., and Strominger, J.L., 1977, Further structural studies of the heavy chain of HLA antigens and its similarity to immunoglobulins, *Proc. Natl. Acad. Sci. U.S.A.* **74:**4002.

22

Structural Analyses of HLA-DR Antigens

Leslie E. Walker, Soldano Ferrone, Michele A. Pellegrino, and Ralph A. Reisfeld

1. Introduction

There has been considerable progress in the characterization of HLA-DR antigens even though these human counterparts of murine and guinea pig *Ir* gene products were identified only a few years ago. The information available at present concerning the biological, chemical, and structural properties of HLA-DR antigens can be summarized as follows (for a review, see Ferrone *et al.*, 1978).

1. Several allospecificities have been identified by extensive serotyping, a task that was greatly facilitated by the organization of several histocompatibility testing workshops at both the national and international levels.

2. Family studies (Mann *et al.*, 1975, 1976; van Rood *et al.*, 1975, 1977) have shown that the serologically detectable HLA-DR allospecificities are controlled by genes linked to the major histocompatibility complex (MHC) located on the short arm of human chromosome 6 (Breuning *et al.*, 1977; Franche and Pellegrino, 1977).

3. Analogous to HLA-A,B antigens and their murine counterparts, HLA-DR antigens are present in body fluids in an immunologically functional form, since they can specifically bind antibodies *in vitro* and can

Leslie E. Walker, Soldano Ferrone, Michele A. Pellegrino, and Ralph A. Reisfeld • Department of Molecular Immunology, Scripps Clinic and Research Foundation, La Jolla, California 92037 elicit antibodies in xenogeneic combinations (Billing *et al.*, 1976a,b; Ferrone *et al.*, 1977a).

4. HLA-DR antigens are mainly expressed on cells associated with immune functions (Albrechtsen, 1977; Chess *et al.*, 1976; Koide *et al.*, 1977); however, the antigens have also been detected on myeloid cells at certain stages of maturation (Billing *et al.*, 1977; Winchester *et al.*, 1977) and on cells of nonlymphoid origin undergoing malignant transformation (Wilson *et al.*, 1979; Winchester *et al.*, 1978). These findings raise the intriguing possibility that HLA-DR antigens may play a role in the regulation of cell proliferation and in the interaction between the host's immune system and neoplastic cells.

5. HLA-DR antigens are involved in interactions required to generate immune reactions as suggested by the ability of anti-HLA-DR antibodies to inhibit the mixed-leukocyte reaction (MLR) and by the restrictions imposed by HLA-DR antigens on interactions among immune cells (for a review, see Ferrone *et al.*, 1978a). This activity of HLA-DR antigens may be reflected in their association with susceptibility to diseases as well as in the significant functional influence that HLA-DR antigens exert on the fate of kidney grafts (Ting and Morris, 1978; Bodmer, 1978). Thus, an association has been reported between certain HLA-DR specificities and susceptibility to diseases with a known or suspected hereditary element, malignant disorders, and diseases with a possible immunological basis (for a review, see Bodmer, 1978). Furthermore, in renal transplantation, HLA-DR matching results in good allograft survival irrespective of matching for HLA-A and B antigens (Ting and Morris, 1978; Bodmer, 1978).

6. Structural analysis of HLA-DR antigens isolated from lymphoid cells either by conventional biochemical procedures or by indirect immunoprecipitation with specific antisera has shown that HLA-DR antigens are composed of two glycoprotein subunits held by noncovalent bonds: the large chain referred to as the α chain has a molecular weight of approximately 34,000 daltons, while the smaller β chain has an approximate molecular weight of 29,000 daltons when analyzed by sodium dodecyl sulfate–polyacrylamide gel electrophoresis (SDS-PAGE) under reducing conditions (Springer *et al.*, 1977a). Under nonreducing conditions, the small subunit has a faster migration rate and an apparent molecular weight of 24,000 daltons; this change in migration rate may be caused by an intradisulfide bond in the β chain that in unreduced form gives the molecule a more spherical conformation than when this bond is reduced (Allison *et al.*, 1978a).

7. Partial N-terminal amino acid sequence analysis of HLA-DR α and β chains isolated either by immunochemical techniques or by conventional biochemical procedures revealed no homology with the primary

structure of HLA-A,B antigens analyzed thus far (Bridgen *et al.*, 1976; Allison *et al.*, 1978a,b) (see also Chapter 20). In addition, there is no homology between HLA-DR α and β at those positions that can be compared (Allison *et al.*, 1978a). However, the N-terminal amino acid sequence of HLA-DR β chains isolated from cell lines with different phenotypes had several differences, whereas the corresponding α chains were strikingly similar (Allison *et al.*, 1978a; Springer *et al.*, 1977b).

8. The tissue distribution, the involvement in immune function, the subunit structure, and the primary amino acid sequence of HLA-DR are very similar to those of murine *I-E*-subregion antigens (Ferrone *et al.*, 1978a; Allison *et al.*, 1978a; van Rood *et al.*, 1976; Ting *et al.*, 1976; E.A. Jones *et al.*, 1975; Silver *et al.*, 1979). These data, especially the structural properties, suggest that these two sets of histocompatibility antigens have evolved from a common ancestral gene (Allison *et al.*, 1978a; Silver *et al.*, 1979).

We will first present serological and immunochemical data describing the specificity of the xenoantiserum used in our purification procedure; then we will describe the method of isolation of the α and β chains of HLA-DR antigens; finally, we will present data of the tryptic peptide map profiles of α and β polypeptide chains of phenotypically distinct HLA-DR antigens and discuss the implications of our findings.

2. Xenoantisera to Human HLA-DR Antigens

2.1. Production and Serological Characteristics of Xenoantiserum 3634

Antiserum 3634 was produced by immunizing rabbit No. 3634 with antigens solubilized from cultured human B-lymphoid cells WI-L2 with 3 M KCl and partially purified by ultracentrifugal flotation in potassium bromide (KBr) (density 1.21). Since histocompatibility antigens are high-density liproproteins, the top of the KBr gradient contained the majority of the HLA-A,B and -DR antigens, which in this form have been found to be highly immunogenic in xenogeneic combinations (Ferrone *et al.*, 1977b; Allison *et al.*, 1978c). The kinetics of antibody formation during the course of immunization of rabbit No. 3634 are depicted in Fig. 1. An antibody population with low titer reacted with peripheral lymphocytes, whereas a population with high titer reacted with cultured B-lymphoid cells. Following absorption with human red blood cells and cultured human T-lymphoid cells, both of which do not express HLA-DR antigens, the reactivity of the antiserum with peripheral lymphocytes was significantly reduced, while that with B-lymphoid cells did not change significantly. These patterns of reactions suggested that the serum contains a heterogeneous population of antibodies with low titer to surface structures expressed on human T- and B-lymphoid cells and a population of antibodies with high titer to structures expressed on B-lymphoid cells. The following series of serological experiments indicate that the latter type of antibodies react with common determinants expressed on HLA-DR antigens: (1) The absorbed serum was specifically cytotoxic to eight cultured human B-lymphoid cell lines and to enriched preparations of peripheral B lymphocytes from ten unrelated donors. (2) Fab_2 fragments obtained from xenoantiserum 3634 specifically inhibited the cytolytic activity of HLA-DR alloantisera to cultured human B-lymphoid cells (Fig. 2). (3) Antibodies purified from xenoantiserum 3634 by absorption–elution with cultured human B-lymphoid cells Daudi, which express HLA-DR antigens but lack HLA-A, -B, and -C antigens, were cytotoxic to human B-lymphoid cells, but not to human T-lymphoid cells and B-lymphoid cells coated with Fab_2 fragments from a xenoantiserum to common determinants of HLA-DR antigens. (4) Xenoantiserum 3634 reacted with radiochemically pure HLA-DR antigens in a radioimmunoassay; this reactivity was not affected by extensive absorption of the xenoantiserum with human cells lacking HLA-DR antigens, but was significantly reduced following absorption with cultured human B-lymphoid cells.

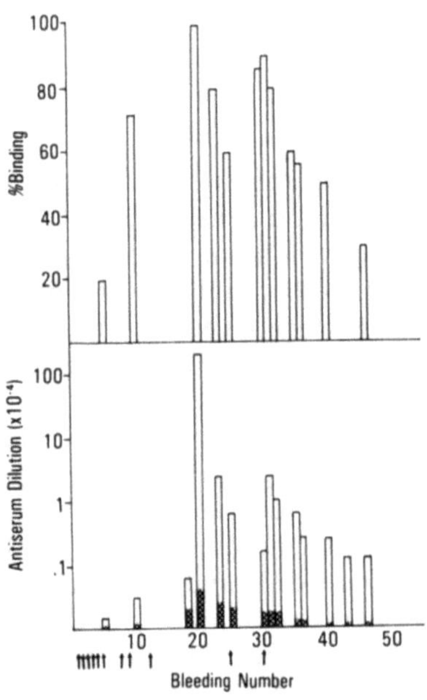

Figure 1. Kinetics of formation of antibodies to HLA-DR antigens. The cytotoxic titer of several bleedings tested in a cytotoxicity test against the cultured human lymphoid cell lines, Wil-Z (□), and against total peripheral lymphocytes, GN (■), is shown in the bottom panel. The percentage of binding of several bleedings tested against radiochemically purified HLA-DR isolated for the cultured human lymphoid-cell line Victor is shown in the top panel. (↑) Time of immunization.

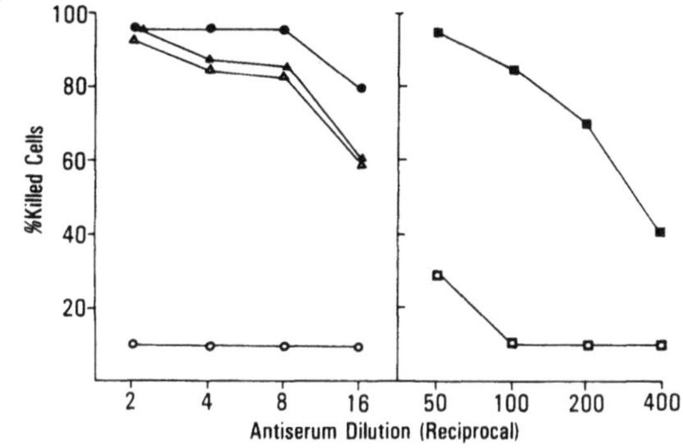

Figure 2. Complement-dependent cytoxicity of alloantiserum PS 512 (anti-HLA-DRw6), alloanti serum Millunzi (anti-HLA-A9), and rabbit antiserum 8812-R2 (anti-common HLA-DR antigens) against cultured human B-lymphoid cells, Victor, coated with Fab_2 fragments from normal rabbit serum (●, ▲, ■) and with Fab_2 fragments from rabbit antiserum 3634 absorbed with the human T-lymphoid cells, Molt 4 (○, △, □).

2.2. Immunochemical Characterization of Xenoantiserum 3634

The xenoantiserum was characterized immunochemically by its reaction in indirect immunoprecipitation with radiolabeled glycoprotein isolated from B-lymphoid cells. Three methods were used to label the cells: (1) intrinsic labeling with [^{35}S]methionine (Callahan *et al.*, 1979); (2) labeling with ^{125}I utilizing the Bolton–Hunter reagent (Bolton and Hunter, 1973); and (3) ^{125}I labeling with the chloramide 1,3,4,6-tetrachloro-3a,6a,-diphenylglycoluril (Fraker and Speds, 1978). The SDS-PAGE profile of the immune complexes formed between xenoantiserum 3634 and glycoproteins purified from cultured human B-lymphoid cell line Victor and labeled by each of the three aforenamed methods is shown in Fig. 3. When glycoproteins labeled with [^{35}S]methionine were used, three peaks with apparent molecular weights of 45,000, 34,000, and 29,000 were observed, corresponding to HLA-A,B heavy chain, the α chain of HLA-DR antigen, and the β chain of HLA-DR antigen, respectively. Indirect immunoprecipitation of glycoproteins labeled with ^{125}I-labeled Bolton–Hunter reagent resulted in the precipitation of only one radioactive peak with an apparent molecular weight of 34,000, i.e., HLA-DR α chain. When the xenoantiserum was reacted with glycoproteins labeled with ^{125}I by the chloramide, three peaks corresponding to the heavy chain of HLA-A,B antigen and the α and β chains of HLA-DR antigen were observed, with the β chain of HLA-DR and the heavy chain of HLA-A,B antigens containing the highest amount of label.

The polypeptides recognized by the xenoantiserum were indeed the α and β chains of HLA-DR antigens, since: (1) The smaller polypeptide reacting with xenoantiserum 3634 migrated faster when SDS-PAGE was performed under nonreducing conditions, as has been reported to occur with the β chain of HLA-DR antigens (Allison *et al.*, 1978a). (2) In sequential immunodepletion experiments, the xenoantiserum removed from glycoproteins purified from B-lymphoid cells those components that react with HLA-DR alloantibodies; the latter were isolated from HLA-DR alloantisera by absorption–elution with cultured human B-lymphoid cells Daudi, since the HLA-DR alloantisera we have tested failed to precipitate sufficient counts in direct immunoprecipitation experiments. (3) Reaction of the radiolabeled glycoprotein with anti-β_2-microglobulin followed by binding of resultant immune complexes by *Staphylococcus aureus* Cowan I strain (SACI) bacteria removed only the 45,000-molecular-weight component, i.e., the heavy chain of HLA-A,B antigens. However, this procedure did not deplete the 34,000- and 29,000-molecular-weight components that reacted specifically with the anti-HLA-DR xenoantiserum. (4) The antigens purified by indirect immuno precipitation using xenoantiserum 3634 show a high degree of homology in their primary amino acid sequence with HLA-DR antigens isolated from B-lymphoid cells by conventional biochemical procedures and with the murine *I-E*-region-coded antigens (Allison *et al.*, 1978a).

3. Isolation and Characterization of HLA-DR Antigens

3.1. Source of HLA-DR Antigens

The cultured human B-lymphoid cell lines RPMI 1788 (Drw4,7) and RPMI 4098 (DRw2,6) used in this study as sources of HLA-DR antigens were selected on the basis of their clearly different phenotypes established by serotyping with DR alloantisera prepared in our laboratory and with those antisera submitted for serological analysis to the 7th International Histocompatibility Workshop and to the 3rd American B-cell Workshop.

3.2. Intrinsic Radiolabeling with [^{3}H]Phenylalanine or [^{3}H]Glucosamine

Both cell lines were radiolabeled intrinsically with [^{3}H]phenylalanine by culturing 2 × 10^8 cells with 2 mCi [^{3}H]phenylalanine (New England Nuclear) in 25 ml phenylalanine-free RPMI 1640 medium supplemented with 10% fetal calf serum (FCS) and buffered to pH 7.2 with 10 mM HEPES. After 16 hr, the cells were washed three times with physiological saline and solubilized with 4 ml 0.5% Nonidet P-40 (NP-40) in 10 mM Tris, 150 mM NaCl, 1mM $CaCl_2$, 1 mM $MgCl_2$, 0.02% sodium azide, 0.02% phenylmethyl sulfonyl fluoride. After 30 min. at 0°C, the extract was centrifuged at 10,000*g* for 20 min, and the supernatant used immediately or frozen at −20°C. Between 20 and 40% of the initial counts were detected in the supernatant.

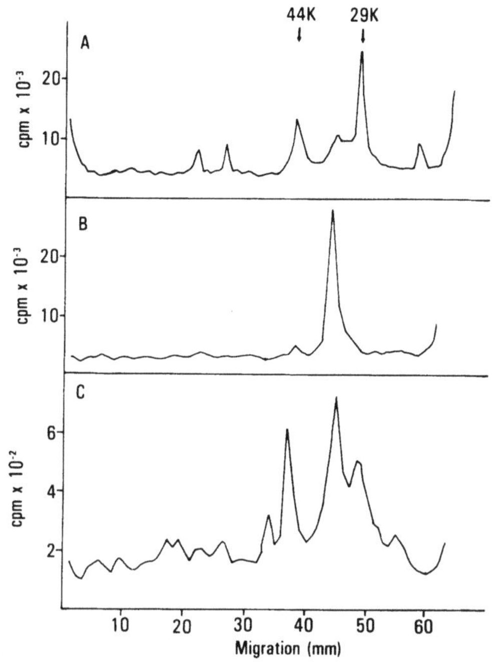

Figure 3. Indirect immunoprecipitation patterns using antiserum 3634 and glycoprotein isolated from the cell line Victor labeled with ^{125}I using a chloramide (A), ^{125}I-labeled Bolton–Hunter reagent (B), and [^{35}S]methionine (C). Antiserum 3634 was loaded onto heat-killed formalin-fixed *Staphylococcus aureus* Cowan I strain bacteria and reacted with the labeled glycoproteins as previously described (Allison *et al.*, 1978b). Bound radioactivity was analyzed on 10% SDS–polyacramide gels as described (Laemmli, 1970).

Intrinsic labeling with [^3H]glucosamine was accomplished by culturing lymphoid-cell line RPMI 4098 with 2 mCi [^3H]glucosamine (Amersham) in RPMI 1640 media with a reduced glucose concentration (50 mg/liter) and supplemented with 10 mM sodium pyruvate and 10% FCS. After being incubated for 16 hr at 37°C, the cells were solubilized as described above. The supernatant contained between 10 and 20% of the original radioactivity.

3.3. Purification of Radiolabeled Glycoprotein by Lectin Affinity

Lens culinaris lectin was coupled to cyanogen-bromide-activated Sepharose-4B at a concentration of 10 mg/ml (Cuatrecasas, 1970). The radiolabeled NP-40 extract of the cultured B-lymphoid cells was chromatographed on a 1 × 5 cm lectin column equilibrated with 0.01 M Tris, 0.15 M NaCl, 1 mM $CaCl_2$, 1 mM $MgCl_2$, pH 8.0, containing 0.25% NP-40. Bound glycoproteins were eluted by equilibration with the above buffer containing 2% α-methyl-D-mannoside.

3.4. Purification of HLA-DR Antigen by Indirect Immunoprecipitation

Antibody-coated heat-killed formalin-fixed SACI bacteria were prepared by incubating 250 μl xenoantiserum 3634 with 2.5 ml of a 10%

suspension of SACI for 1 hr at 4°C followed by three washings with buffer (50 mM Tris, pH 7.4, containing 150 mM NaCl, 0.5 mM EDTA, 1 mg/ml ovalbumin, and 0.25% NP-40). The antibody-coated packed SACI (250 μl) were mixed with either [³H]phenylalanine (10^7 cpm)- or [³H]glucosamine (10^7 cpm)-labeled glycoprotein and allowed to incubate for 2 hr at 4°C with shaking.

After the SACI containing the antigen–antibody complex were washed three times with the above buffer, HLA-DR antigens were eluted by incubating the immuno-adsorbent for 5 min at 100°C with 2.5 ml SDS-PAGE sample buffer (0.0625 M Tris, pH 6.8, containing 2% SDS, 0.02% bromophenol blue, and 10% glycerol). The SACI were removed by centrifugation and the supernatant containing radiolabeled HLA-DR antigens subjected to SDS-PAGE as described by Laemmli (1970) on 5.5 × 80 mm polyacrylamide gels (10%) under nonreducing conditions. After completion of electrophoresis, the gels were sliced into 1-mm sections and each section eluted by incubation with H_2O at 4°C with shaking. The α-chain (mol. wt. 34,000) and β-chain (mol. wt. 24,000) peaks were located by counting aliquots from each tube. Eluates containing the HLA-DR α chains and HLA-DR β chains were each pooled and lyophilized.

Approximately 4×10^5 cpm of each [³H]phenylalanine-labeled α and β chain and 3×10^5 cpm of each [³H]glucosamine-labeled α and β chain were recovered (Table 1).

TABLE 1. Purification of Radiolabeled HLA-DR Antigens

Step	Total cpm	% Total
[³H]phenylalanine-labeled HLA-DR antigen		
NP-40 solubilization	2.5×10^9	100
Lens culinaris lectin–Sepharose	1×10^7	4
SDS-PAGE		
HLA-DR α chain	4×10^5	8×10^{-3}
HLA-DR β chain	4×10^5	8×10^{-3}
[³H]glucosamine-labeled HLA-DR antigen		
NP-40 solubilization	1.1×10^9	100
Lens culinaris lectin–Sepharose	$1. \times 10^7$	9
SDS-PAGE		
HLA-DR α chain	3×10^5	3×10^{-2}
HLA-DR β chain	3×10^5	3×10^{-2}

3.5. Tryptic Digestion of HLA-DR α Chains and HLA-DR β Chains and Peptide Mapping

The purified HLA-DR *α* and HLA-DR β chains were each digested with trypsin essentially as previously described (Silver *et al.*, 1979). Breifly, after lypholization, the samples were dissolved in 1 ml water containing 0.5 mg human gamma-globulin. Solid dithiothreitol was added to each sample to a final concentration of 25 mM. After being incubated at 100°C for 5 min, the samples were purged with nitrogen and incubated at 37°C for 2 hrs. The HLA *α* and β chains were then carboxyamidoethylated by addition of solid iodoacetamide to a final concentration of 50 mM. After 2 hr at 37°C, 0.15 ml of 100% trichloracetic acid was added to each sample to precipitate the HLA-DR chains along with the carrier protein. The pellet formed after centrifugation was washed once with 20% trichloroacetic acid and twice with acetone. After the protein precipitates were dried under a stream of air, 200 μl 0.1 M ammonium bicarbonate buffer, pH 8.0, and 10 μl of 10 mg/ml TPCK-treated trypsin (Worthington) was added to each tube. Following incubation for 12 hr at 37°C, a second 10-μl aliquot of trypsin was added and incubation continued for 4 additional hours. Following this digestion, the samples were lypholized and redissolved in 200 μl 0.5 M sodium phosphate buffer, pH 2.0, and acetone (2:1). Insoluble material, which contained no radioactivity, was removed by centrifugation. The tryptic peptides were separated by high-pressure liquid chromatography (HPLC) essentially as described by McMillan *et al.* (1979) using a Waters Associates instrument. Briefly, the tryptic peptides (15,000 cpm) were chromatographed on a 4.6 mm × 25 cm Zorbax-CN column at room temperature at 1 ml/min. The peptides were eluted with a nonlinear gradient ($y = x^3$) of 0.1 M sodium phosphate buffer, pH 2.1, and 95% acetone (Burdick and Jackson) over a period of 90 min. Fractions were collected at 1-min intervals, dried, and counted in 5 ml Biofluor (New England Nuclear).

4. Structural Analysis of HLA-DR Antigens

4.1. Comparison of Tryptic Peptides of HLA-DR α Chains and HLA-DR β Chains

Comparative analyses of tryptic peptide maps of HLA-DR *α* chains isolated from cultured B-lymphoid cell line RPMI 4098 (DRw2,6) and from RPMI 1788 (DRw4,7) revealed nearly identical profiles (Fig. 4). Both maps show seven major phenylalanine-containing peptides that differ only slightly if at all in retention times on the HPLC column. The only

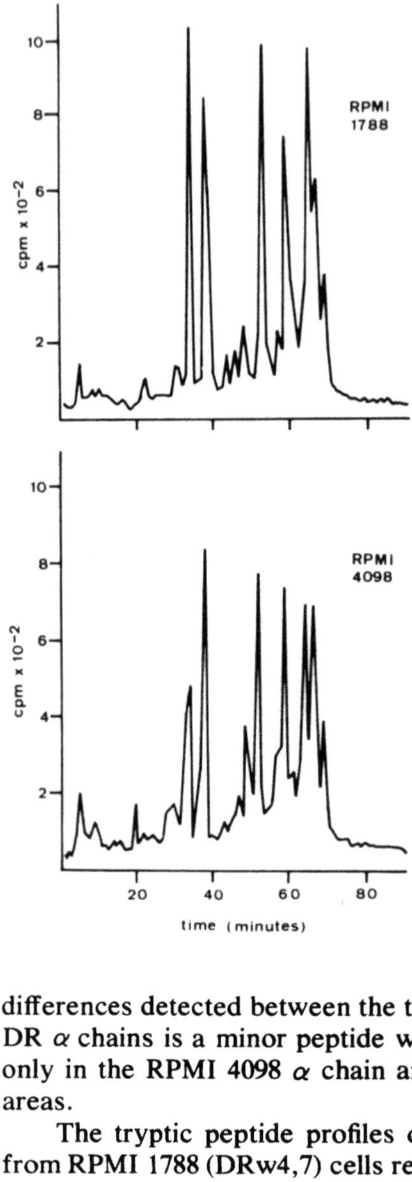

Figure 4. Tryptic peptide maps of HLA-DR α chains labeled with [^{3}H]phenylalanine from the human lymphoid-cell lines RPMI 4098 (DRw2,6) and RPMI 1788 (DRw4,7). The β chains were isolated, digested, and analyzed as described in the text.

differences detected between the tryptic peptide profile of the two HLA-DR α chains is a minor peptide with a retention time of 49 min present only in the RPMI 4098 α chain and a few minor dissimilarities in peak areas.

The tryptic peptide profiles of the two HLA-DR β chains isolated from RPMI 1788 (DRw4,7) cells revealed 9 major [^{3}H]phenylalanine-containing peptides, whereas the HLA-DR β chain isolated from RPMI 4098 (DRw2,6) cells showed 11 peptides (Fig. 5). It is readily apparent that in marked contrast to the peptide profiles of the HLA-DR α chains, the tryptic maps of the HLA-DR β chains show a marked degree of dissimilarity. Even though some peptides have similar retention times, for example, at 47 min, the peak sizes of these peptides vary considerably, indicating that these peptides are probably not homologous. Each typtic peptide map was confirmed by at least one duplicate HPLC analysis and showed excellent reproducibility; retention times varied no more than 1%, and 98–100% of counts applied to the column were recovered.

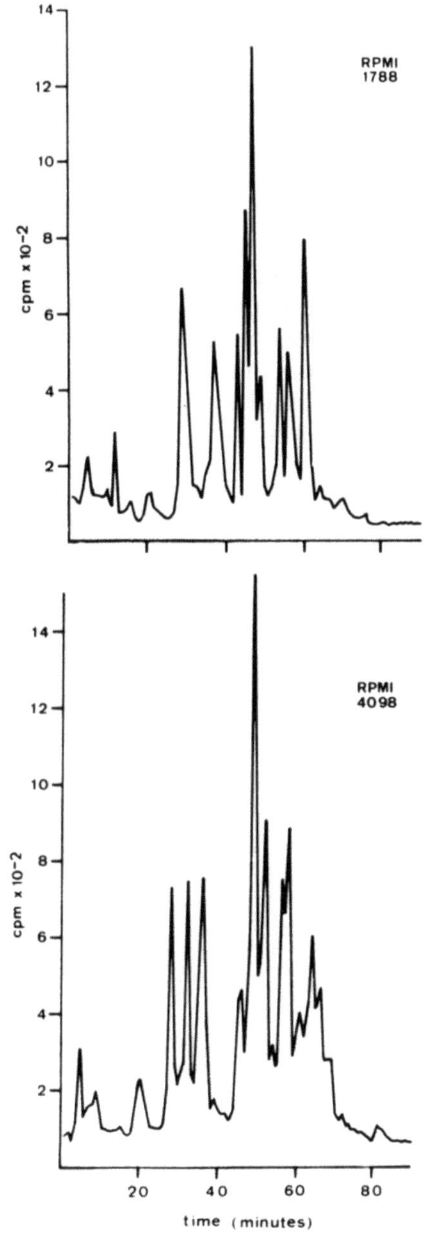

Figure 5. Tryptic peptide maps of HLA-DR β chains labeled with [^{3}H]phenylalanine isolated from the human lymphoid-cell lines RPMI 4098 (DRw2,6) and RPMI 1788 (DRw4,7). The β chains were isolated, digested, and analyzed as described in the text.

4.2. Carbohydrate Structures of HLA-DR α Chains and HLA-DR β Chains

It has been known for some time that both subunits of HLA-DR antigens are glycoproteins, since they were found to contain sialic acid (Springer *et al.*, 1977b). However, the actual number of carbohydrate chains per subunit has not been established. We have attempted to answer this question by determining the number of tryptic peptides of HLA-DR antigens isolated from RPMI 4098 cells that contain [^{3}H]glucosamine and by separating these peptides by HPLC.

One glucosamine-labeled tryptic peptide was detected in the HLA-DR α chain with a retention time of 42 min (Fig. 6). This peptide does not coincide with any of the [^{3}H]phenylalanine-labeled peptides of this same HLA-DR α chain, indicating that it lacks phenylalanine. In marked contrast, the accompanying HLA-DR β chain was found to contain two glucosamine-containing tryptic peptides with retention times of 32 and 46 min, respectively, both of which coincided with [^{3}H]phenylalanine-containing peptides (Fig. 7). This indicates that the HLA-DR β chain has two carbohydrate moieties, both of which contain phenylalanine.

5. Discussion and Conclusion

To assess the structural polymorphism of the two polypeptide subunits of HLA-DR antigens, we have compared tryptic peptide profiles of the α and β chains isolated from cultured B-lymphoid cells with different

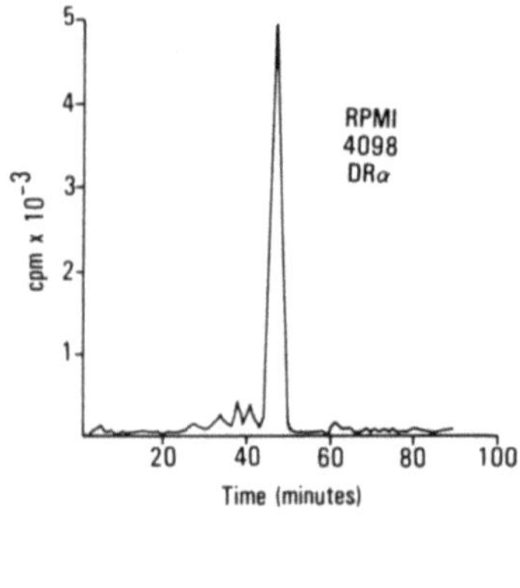

Figure 6. Tryptic peptide maps of HLA-DR α chains labeled with [^{3}H]glucosamine isolated from the human lymphoid-cell line RPMI 4098 (DRw4,6). The α chain was analyzed as described in the text.

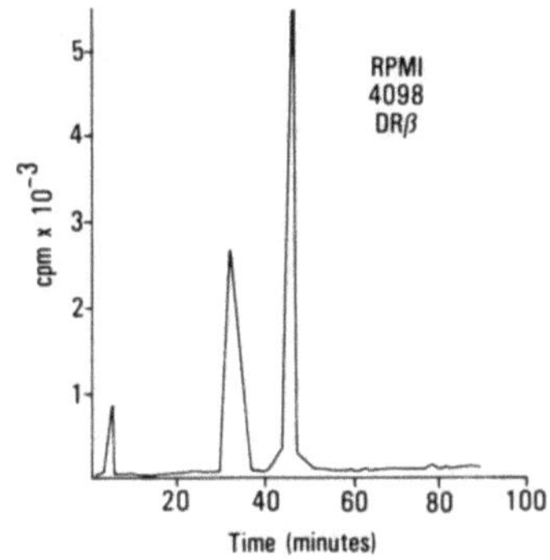

Figure 7. Tryptic peptide maps of HLA-DR β chains labeled with [^{3}H]glucosamine isolated from the human lymphoid-cell line RPMI 4098 (DRw2,6). The β chain was analyzed as described in the text.

phenotypes. This approach provides useful information to determine structural polymorphism of HLA-DR subunits, although the definitive answer will have to come from primary amino acid sequence analysis.

The HLA-DR antigens were isolated by an immunochemical approach utilizing a specific anti-HLA-DR xenoantiserum, since this particular approach has been used successfully by us to probe the N-terminal amino acid sequence of HLA-DR α and β chains (Allison *et al.*, 1978a). This same anti-HLA-DR xenoantiserum was used for the studies described here, since alloantisera proved ineffective for the immunochemical purification of HLA-DR antigens and since the xenoantiserum used by us had been shown to react serologically with the same antigenic structures as DR alloantisera (Ferrone *et al.*, 1977b, 1978b).

The efficiency of this approach will be further improved by the use of monoclonal DR antibodies that have been developed in our laboratory and have already been proven useful to dissect the molecular heterogeneity of HLA-DR antigens.

Among the methods available to establish tryptic peptide profiles, we selected high-pressure liquid chromatography (HPLC), which in our hands proved very sensitive and highly reproducible. HPLC, similar to ion-exchange chromatography, tends to exaggerate differences and minimize homologies between peptides (Vitetta and Capra, 1978). However, it has the advantage over isoelectric focusing in polyacrylamide gels in that it separates peptides not only on the basis of ionic charge difference but also by differences in hydrophobicity and side-chain polarities.

Our analysis of tryptic peptide maps of HLA-DR antigens that bear different allospecificities clearly indicates that the α chains have a highly homologous structure while the β chains are polymorphic. This conclusion is in agreement with results of concurrent studies (Silver and Ferrone, 1979) that utilize an additional four lymphoid cell lines with different HLA-DR phenotypes, a similar methodology, and the same xenoantiserum used in this study. However, these data are in contrast to a report by Klareskog *et al.* (1978), who used HPLC to determine the tryptic peptide profiles of [^{3}H]tyrosine-labeled HLA-DR α and β chains isolated from cultured B-lymphoid cells by indirect immunoprecipitation with a xenoantiserum. The conflicting results cannot be attributed to the source of antigens, since the two cell lines used by Klareskog *et al.* (1978) (Daudi and Raji) were also used in a study that indicated that the major structural polymorphism is restricted to the HLA-DR β chain (Silver and Ferrone, 1979). Additional methodological differences, i.e., method of antigen solubilizing and radioactive amino acids used for labeling of HLA-DR antigens, are not likely to account for these conflicting results. Whether the differing results can be attributed to the use of different xenoantisera for the isolation of HLA-DR antigens can be ascertained only by an exchange of reagents.

Three lines of evidence support our contention that the major structural polymorphism of HLA-DR antigens is exhibited in the β subunit: (1) Comparison of the partial N-terminal amino acid sequence of HLA-DR antigens isolated from two cultured B-lymphoid cell lines revealed several distinct differences between the β chains, whereas the corresponding α chains showed striking similarity (Allison *et al.*, 1978a). (2) Sequence analysis data of the HLA-DR α and β chains isolated from the Victor cell line suggested a single unique amino acid sequence for the α chain and a mixed sequence for the β chain (Walker *et al.*, 1979). (3) Structural studies of *I-E*-subregion antigens, the murine analogue of HLA-DR antigens, have reached a conclusion similar to ours. Specifically, amino acid sequence and peptide mapping analyses of *I-E*-subregion antigens isolated from different strains of mice indicate that the structural polymorphism of I-E antigens is restricted to the β chain (Silver *et al.*, 1979).

Since it has been reported that the serologically detectable HLA-DR alloantigenic specificities are mainly mediated by polypeptide structures, our data offered some insight into the molecular basis for the serological polymorphism and genetic organization of HLA-DR antigens. Our data, revealing the structural polymorphism of the HLA-DR β chain, suggest that this subunit bears the allotypic determinants. This conclusion is in agreement with that of Tosi *et al.* (1978), who analyzed the serological reactivity of isolated HLA-DR α and β chains with alloantisera in a radioimmunassay and found reactivity only with the β chain. However, since the level of antibody-binding in these experiments is low (5–20%), one cannot exclude that (1) the α chain contributes to the alloantigenic expression by maintaining the appropriate configuration of HLA-DR antigens or (2) it carries alloantigenic determinants that were denatured by the stringent procedures used to separate the two HLA-DR subunits.

Since family studies have shown that the HLA-DR allotypic specificities are controlled by genes in the MHC, the apparent structural polymorphism of the β chain implies that the gene coding for this polypeptide is located in the MHC. This contention is supported by data in the murine system assigning the β chain of I-E/C antigens to the MHC region but is in contrast to the data by Barnstable *et al.* (1976) in the human system. These authors prepared somatic-cell hybrids between cultured human lymphoid cells Daudi and murine fibroblasts A9 and analyzed the resulting hybrids for ther content of human chromosomes and their reactivity with alloantisera to HLA-DR specificities and with a xenoantiserum that reacts exclusively with the β chain. Hybrids were found that reacted with HLA-DR alloantisera and contained chromosome 6, but no hybrid reacted with the HLA-DR xenoantiserum. Therefore, the authors concluded that the HLA-DR α subunit carries the allotypic determinants and is encoded by a gene within the MHC. Another important point to be derived from the study by Barnstable *et al.* (1976) is that the polymorphic chain of DR antigens can be expressed independently of the nonpolymorphic chain. If so, then HLA-DR antigens differ from HLA-A, -B, and -C antigens, which can express the alloantigen-bearing subunit only in association with β_2-microgloublin. The results of our structural analysis of HLA-DR α and β subunits do not allow any speculation about which chromosome contains the gene coding for the HLA-DR α chain. Also, parallel studies in our laboratory using somatic-cell-hybridization experiments have failed to answer this question, since hybrids between HLA-DR-bearing cells (i.e., B-lymphoid cells and melanoma cells) and murine fibroblasts do not express HLA-DR antigens as determined by their lack of reactivity with HLA-DR polyclonal and monoclonal xenoantibodies and by their inability to elicit HLA-DR antibodies in xenogeneic combinations.

In mice, structural studies of I-E antigens isolated from appropriate *I*-region recombinant strains have mapped the gene controlling the α chain within the MHC (PP. Jones *et al.*, 1978). If this model also applies to the human DR antigen system, then one has to postulate that the α chain as well as the β chain are encoded by genes within the MHC. If so, then the genetic organization of HLA-DR antigens is different from that of HLA-A, -B, and -C antigens, in which the allotype-bearing chain is coded by the MHC region on chromosome 6 while the common chain is coded by chromosome 15.

Our data indicate that the HLA-DR α chain (34K) isolated from the B-lymphoid cell line RPMI 4098 (DRw2,6) has one carbohydrate subunit. This is a finding similar to that described for the heavy chain of HLA-A,B antigens—which has one carbohydrate moiety—and to both chains of murine I-A and I-E subregion antigens—which, following pronase digestion, were each found to contain one carbohydrate subunit with a molecular weight of 3250—but differs from the H-2K^b heavy chain, which has two carbohydrate subunits (Freed *et al.*, 1977). The HLA-DR β chain (29K) has, however, two carbohydrate-containing tryptic peptides. Two interpretations may be offered for this finding: either (1) each HLA-DR β chain has two carbohydrate subunits or (2) since the β chains are polymorphic, as far as protein structure is concerned, and the B-lymphoid cell line used in our study is heterozygous, it is possible that each β chain has only one carbohydrate subunit either near or within the variable amino acid region that determines each allotypic specificity. This would be analogous to the HLA-A,B heavy chain, in which the single carbohydrate subunit is within one tryptic peptide that encompasses a part of one of the two variable regions (see Chapter 20).

It is clear that the information accumulated on the molecular structures of HLA-DR antigens has provided clues as to their genetic organization, molecular basis of serological polymorphism, and evolution. Further characterization of the physical and chemical properties of HLA-DR antigens will provide significant insight into the molecular mechanisms governing the role of HLA-DR antigens in immune phenomena and may clarify whether the two-chain structure, with one conserved subunit and the other polymorphic, is required for the functional activity of HLA-DR antigens. This information may suggest new studies to manipulate the immune system that may be applied in clinical medicine.

ACKNOWLEDGMENTS. This work was supported by grants from the National Institutes of Health, an American Heart Association Established Investigatorship Award (S.F.), and a Research Career Development Award (M.A.P.). The authors wish to acknowledge the secretarial assistance of Mr. D. Trinko and the editorial assistance of Mrs. P. Minick. This is publication number 2016 from Scripps Clinic and Research Foundation.

References

Albrechtsen, D., 1977, HLA-D-associated "Ia-like" antigens on human macrophages, *Scand. J. Immunol.* **6**:907–912.

Allison, J.P., Walker, L.E., Russell, W.A., Pellegrino, M.A., Ferrone, S., Reisfeld, R.A., Frelinger, J.A., and Silver, J., 1978a, Murine Ia and human DR antigens: Homology of amino terminal sequences, *Proc. Natl. Acad. Sci. U.S.A.* **75**:3953–3956.

Allison, J.P., Ferrone, S., Walker, L.E., Pellegrino, M.A., Silver, J., and Reisfeld, R.A., 1978b, The partial amino acid sequence of HLA-A9 antigen purified with a specific xenoantiserum, *Transplantation* **26**:451–454.

Allison, J.P., Belvedere, M., Reisfeld, R.A., Pellegrino, M.A., and Ferrone, S., 1978c, Serological and immunochemical characterization of HLA-A9 xenoantisera, *J. Immunol.* **121**:579–585.

Barnstable, C.J., Jones, E.A., Bodmer, W.F., Bodmer, J.G., Arce-Gomez, B., Snary, P., and Crumpton, M.S., 1976, Genetics and serology of HLA-linked human Ia antigens, *Cold Spring Harbor Symp. Quant. Biol.* **41**:443–455.

Billing, R.J., Honig, R., Peterson, P., Safani, M., and Terasaki, P.I., 1976a, Blocking of HLA and B lymphocyte alloantigens with $F(ab)_2$ fragments of rabbit antibodies, *J. Immunol.* **117**:2040–2042.

Billing, R., Radezadeh, B., Drew, I., Hartman, G., Gole, R., and Terasaki, P.I., 1976b, Human B-lymphocyte antigens expressed by lymphocytic and myelocytic leukemia cells. I. Detection by rabbit antisera, *J. Exp. Med.* **114**:167–178.

Billing, R., Ting, A., and Terasaki, P.I., 1977, Human B-lymphocyte antigens expressed by lymphocytic and myelocytic leukemia cells. II. Detection by human anti-B-cell alloantisera, *J. Natl. Cancer Inst.* **58**:199–203.

Bodmer, W.F. (ed.), 1978, The HLA system, *Brit. Med. Bull.* **34**:1–316.

Bolton, A.E., and Hunter, W.M., 1973, The labeling of proteins to high specific radioactivities by conjugation to a ^{125}I-containing acylating agent, *Biochem. J.* **133**:529–539.

Breuning, M.H., van den Berg-Loonem, E.M., Bernini, L.F., Bijlsma, J.B., van Loghen, E., Meera Khan, P., and Nyenhuis, L.F., 1977, Localization of HLA on the short arm of chromosome 6, *Hum. Genet.* **37**:131–136.

Bridgen, J., Snary, D., Crumpton, M.J., Barnstable, C., Goodfellow, P., and Bodmer, W.F., 1976, Isolation and N-terminal amino acid sequence of membrane-bound human HLA-A and HLA-B antigens, *Nature (London)* **261**:199–205.

Callahan, G.N., Allison, J.P., and Pellegrino, M.A., 1979, Physical association of histocompatibility antigens and tumor-associated antigens on the surface of murine lymphoma cells, *J. Immunol.* **122**:70–74.

Chess, L., Evans, R., Humphreys, R.E., Strominger, J.L., and Schlosman, S.F., 1976, Inhibition of antibody-dependent cellular cytotoxicity and immunoglobulin synthesis by an antiserum prepared against a human B-cell Ia-like molecule, *J. Exp. Med.* **144**:113–122.

Cuatrecasas, P., 1970, Protein purification by affinity chromatography: Derivatization of agarose and polyacrylamide beads, *Biol. Chem.* **245**:3059–3065.

Ferrone, S., Mittal, K.K., Pellegrino, M.A., Allison, J.P., and Reisfeld, R.A., 1977a, Immunogenicity of HLA antigens purified from serum, *Transplantation* **23**:7–15.

Ferrone, S., Pellegrino, M.A., and Reisfeld, R.A., 1977b, Immunogenicity of human B cell antigens solubilized from cultured-human lymphoid cells, *J. Immunol.* **118**:1036–1041.

Ferrone, S., Allison, J.P., and Pellegrino, M.A., 1978a, Human DR (Ia-like) antigens: Biological and molecular profile, *Contemp. Top. Mol. Immunol.* **7**:239–281.

Ferrone, S., Pellegrino, M.A., Belvedere, M., Reisfeld, R.A., Curry, R., and Allison, J.P., 1978b, Human B cell antigens: Biologic and immunogenic properties, in: *Protides of the Biological Fluids: 25th Colloquium 1977, Proteins and Related Subjects*, Vol. 25 (H. Peters, ed.), p. 645, Pergamon Press, New York.

Fraker, P.J., and Speds, J.C., 1978, Protein and cell membrane iodinations with a sparingly soluble chloramide 1,3,4,6-tetrachloro-3a,6a-diphenyl-glycoluril, *Biochem. Biophys. Res. Commun.* **80**:849–851.

Franche, U., and Pellegrino, M.A., 1977, Assignment of the major histocompatibility complex to a region of the short arm of human chromosome 6, *Proc. Natl. Acad. Sci. U.S.A.* **74**:1147–1151.

Freed, J.H., and Nathenson, S.G., 1977, Similarity of the carbohydrate structures of H-2 and Ia glycoproteins, *J. Immunol.* **119**:477–492.

Jones, E.A., Goodfellow, P.N., Bodmer, J.G., and Bodmer, W.F., 1975, Serological identification of HLA-linked human "Ia-type" antigens, *Nature (London)* **256**:650–652.

Jones, P.P., Murphy, D.S., and McDevitt, H.O., 1978, Two-gene control of the expression of a murine Ia antigen, *J. Exp. Med.* **148**:925–939.

Klareskog, L., Rash, L., Fohlman, J., and Peterson, P.A., 1978, Heavy HLA-DR (Ia) antigen chain is controlled by the MHC region, *Nature (London)* **275**:762–764.

Koide, Y., Takasugi, M., and Billing, R., 1977, B cell antigens on effectors for natural cell-mediated cytotoxicity, *Eur. J. Immunol.* **7**:731–736.

Laemmli, U.K., 1970, Cleavage of structural protein during the assembly of the head of bacteriophage T4, *Nature (London)* **227**:680–682.

Mann, D.L., Abelson, L., Henkart, P., Harris, S., and Amos, D.B., 1975, Serologic detection of B lymphocyte antigens, in: *Histocompatibility Testing, 1975* (F. Kissmeyer-Nielson, ed.), p. 705, Munksgaard Copenhagen.

Mann, D.L., Abelson, L., Harris, S., and Amos, D.B., 1976, Second genetic locus in the HLA region for human B-cell alloantigens, *Nature (London)* **259**:145–147.

McMillan, M., Cecka, J.M., Murphy, D.B., McDevitt, H.O., and Hood, L., 1979, Peptide map analyses of murine Ia antigens of the I-E subregion using high pressure liquid chromatography, *Nature (London)* **277**:663:668.

Silver, J., and Ferrone, S., 1979, Structural polymorphism of human DR antigens, *Nature (London)* **279**:436–439.

Silver, J., Walker, L.E., Reisfeld, R.A., Pellegrino, M.A., and Ferrone, S., 1979, Structural studies of murine I-C and human DR antigens, *Mol. Immunol.* **16**:37–49.

Springer, T.A., Kaufman, J.F., Siddoway, L.A., Gilphart, M., Mann, D.L., Terhorst, C., and Strominger, J.L., 1977a, Chemical and immunological characterization of HL-A-linked B lymphocyte alloantigens, *Cold Spring Harbor Symp. Quant. Biol.* **41**:387–395.

Springer, T.A., Kaufman, J.F., Terhorst, C., and Strominger, J.L., 1977b, Purification and structural characterization of human HLA-linked B-cell antigens, *Nature (London)* **268**:213–218.

Ting, A., and Morris, P.J., 1978, Reactivity of autolymphocytotoxic antibodies from dialysis patients with lymphocytes from chronic lymphocytic leukemia (CLL) patients, *Lancet* **1**:575–577.

Ting, A., Mickey, M.R., and Terasaki, P.I., 1976, B-lymphocyte alloantigens in Caucasiaons, *J. Exp. Med.* **143**:981–986.

Tosi, R., Tanigaki, N., Centis, D., Ferrara, G.B., and Pressman, D., 1978, Immunological dissection of human Ia molecules, *J. Exp. Med.* **148**:1592–1611.

van Rood, J.J., van Leeuwen, A., Parlevliet, J., Termiyelen, A., and Kluning, J.J., 1975, LD typing by serology. IV. Description of a new locus with three alleles, in: *Histocompatibility Testing, 1975* (F. Kissmeyer-Nielson, ed.), p. 629, Munksgaard, Copenhagen.

van Rood, J.J., van Leeuwen, A., and Ploeem, J.S., 1976, Simultaneous detection of two cell populations by two-color fluorescence and application to the recognition of B-cell determinants, *Nature (London)* **262**:795–796.

van Rood, J.J., van Leewven, Kluning, J.J., and Termyelen, A., 1977, Evidence for two series of B-cell antigens in man and their comparison with HLA-D, *Scand. J. Immunol.* **6**:373–384.

Vitetta, E.S., and Capra, J.D., 1978, The protein products of the murine 17th chromosome: Genetics and structure, *Adv. Immunol.* **26**:147–193.

Walker, L.E., Allison, J.P., Silver, J., Pellegrino, J.A., Reisfeld, R.A., and Ferrone, S., 1979, Is serological polymorphism of human DR antigens determined by structural differences in the smaller (β) chain?, in: *Cell Biology and Immunology of Leukocyte Function* (M.R. Quastel, ed.), pp. 271–276, Academic Press, New York.

Wilson, B.S., Indiveri, F., Pellegrino, M.A., and Ferrone, S., 1979, DR (Ia-like) antigens on human melanoma cells: Serological detection and immunological characterization, *J. Exp. Med.* **149**:658–668.

Winchester, R.J., Ross, G.D., Jasowski, C.I., Want, C.Y., Halper, J., and Broxmayer, H.E., 1977, Expression of Ia-like antigen molecules on human granulocytes during early phases of differentiation, *Proc. Natl. Acad. Sci. U.S.A.* **74**:4012–4016.

Winchester, R.J., Wang, C.Y., Gibofsky, A., Kunkel, H.G., Lloyd, D.K., and Old, L.J., 1978, Expression of Ia-like antigens on cultured human malignant melanoma cell lines, *Proc. Natl. Acad. Sci. U.S.A.* **75**:6235–6239.

Index

MIX
Papier aus verantwortungsvollen Quellen
Paper from responsible sources
FSC® C105338

If you have any concerns about our products,
you can contact us on
ProductSafety@springernature.com

In case Publisher is established outside the EU,
the EU authorized representative is:
Springer Nature Customer Service Center GmbH
Europaplatz 3, 69115 Heidelberg, Germany

Printed by Libri Plureos GmbH
in Hamburg, Germany